# Functional MRI

Scott H. Faro, MD
*Professor and Vice-Chairman of Radiology, Director of Functional Brain Imaging Center, Director of Radiology Research and Academics, and Clinical MRI, Temple University School of Medicine, Philadelphia, Pennsylvania*

Feroze B. Mohamed, PhD
*Associate Professor of Radiology, Associate Director of Functional Brain Imaging Center, Temple University School of Medicine, Philadelphia, Pennsylvania*

Editors

# Functional MRI

## Basic Principles and Clinical Applications

With 143 Illustrations in 177 Parts, 134 in Full Color

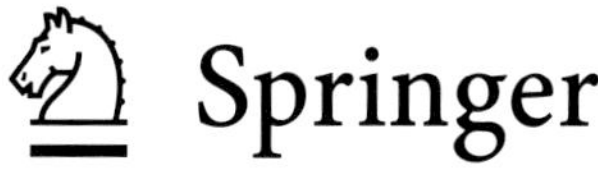
Springer

Scott H. Faro, MD
Professor and Vice-Chairman of Radiology
Director of Functional Brain Imaging Center
Director of Radiology Research and Academics, and Clinical MRI
Temple University School of Medicine
Philadelphia, PA 19140
USA

Feroze B. Mohamed, PhD
Associate Professor of Radiology
Associate Director of Functional Brain Imaging Center
Temple University School of Medicine
Philadelphia, PA 19140
USA

Guest Editor:
Victor Haughton, MD
Professor of Radiology
University of Wisconsin
Madison, WI 53792
USA

Library of Congress Control Number: 2005926700

ISBN 10: 0-387-23046-7
ISBN 13: 978-0387-23046-7

Printed on acid-free paper.



Printed in China. (BS/EVB)

9 8 7 6 5 4 3 2 1

springeronline.com

# Preface

Functional magnetic resonance imaging (fMRI) represents one of the most advanced and enlightening functional imaging techniques that has ever been developed. The past ten years (1990–2000) of scientific research has been designated the decade of the brain and has led to numerous technological developments and the establishment of fundamental clinical protocols to understand brain functions. The next decade, the beginning of the 21$^{st}$ century, will continue the great momentum of brain research. This is currently one of the most exciting and progressive times of scientific advancement in the field of brain function and the development and application of fMRI are the driving forces.

The field of fMRI has two major areas of research interest and applications. The first is within the field of Cognitive Neuroscience, which focuses on understanding all aspects of the mental processes involved in awareness, reasoning, and acquisition of knowledge and behavior. The second is the use of Functional MRI in the Medical Sciences to localize eloquent regions in the brain for a large variety of clinical applications. This book has focused primarily on describing the basic principles of Blood Oxygen Level Dependant (BOLD) imaging and the new and developing clinical applications of fMRI.

This book contains twenty chapters and is separated into three main sections. The first section is an introduction to the physics principles of BOLD imaging as well as a review of fMRI scanning methodologies, data analysis, experimental design, and clinical challenges. The second section is a pictorial Neuroanatomical atlas of the basic motor, sensory, and cognitive activation sites within the brain. This section will give a new clinical scientist a familiarity with some of the more clinically relevant brain activation sites that are discussed in subsequent chapters. The third and final section reviews all the current and future clinical applications of functional MRI. These chapters include the clinical fields of Language, Memory, fMRI WADA, Visual Pathway, Auditory Pathways, Epilepsy, Pain, and Psychiatric Disorders. The cutting edge field of Pharmacological applications of fMRI, including new drug development and drug therapy, is also discussed.

The current clinical fMRI applications include all aspects of pediatric and adult brain imaging. There has never previously been a noninvasive technique with high spatial and temporal resolution to define brain activation. One of the current primary indications for clinical fMRI is evaluation of eloquent areas of the brain such as the cortical spinal tract in relation to a focal parenchymal brain lesion (for example, a neoplasm or arterial venous malformation). Additionally, use of fMRI to localize language centers in the frontal lobe and temporal lobes is becoming a commonplace procedure for presurgical evaluation in temporal lobe epilepsy and regional masses. The concept of a fMRI WADA test is reviewed in detail. Please note that most of the fMRI images are presented in radiologic coordinates (the left side of the image represents the right side of the subject). Images presented in neurologic coordinates (the left side of the image represents the left side of the subject) will be indicated.

The field of fMRI is in its infancy and although the field is relatively young, there has been a discovery of a tremendous body of knowledge. Functional MRI has grown to be a vital tool for clinical and cognitive neuroscience research. It is our hope that this book will give a thorough introduction to this exciting new field and will be a reference, to all physicians and cognitive neuroscientists, for the emerging clinical applications of fMRI.

*Scott H. Faro, MD*
*Feroze B. Mohamed, PhD*

# Acknowledgments

I am grateful to my dear wife Paula for her remarkable patience and continued support of all of my projects.

I would like to thank my dear friend and first scientific mentor, Dr. Anita Pruzan-Hotchkiss who taught me that any question or scientific inquiry, no matter how far fetched it may seem, has merit. I would also like to thank my mentors from my molecular biology graduate program, diagnostic radiology residency, and adult and pediatric neuroradiology fellowship training programs for their encouragement of my academic pursuits. These individuals lead by example and fostered my great interest in teaching and research. I still pass on some of their sayings to my students, such as "Houston we have a problem, little things mean a lot, symmetry is your friend, and quote the literature first and then your experience".

I would also like to thank all of the contributors of this book, for their participation is truly a labor of love, and a special thanks to Feroze Mohamed, my long time friend and colleague who has supported me and our work during the many years of trials and tribulations.

Lastly, I would like to thank all our friends at Springer, especially Rob Albano, who share our goal to produce this timely book on an important and fascinating topic of the principles and clinical applications of fMRI.

*Scott H. Faro, MD*

I am extremely grateful to Shaila for playing the roles of wife, friend, and counselor over the years. She was a great sounding board during the years it took to compile this book. Another person I owe my deepest gratitude is Professor Simon Vinitski, who not only generously guided me in the research project for my doctoral work, but also inspired me to pursue academia with undeterred zeal. I also cannot but mention my parents, Mohamed and Subaidha Ali, without whose encouragement I would not be here writing, and compiling work for, this book.

More specifically, I would like to thank the authors of the various chapters of this book. They should know that this book is essentially a reflection of their work, which, in many instances, is the result of years of research.

I would be remiss if I did not mention Scott Faro, whose friendship and assistance have influenced a good deal of my academic work.

Finally, I wish to express my appreciation to Rob Albano of Springer for his coordination of the efforts of the various people that made this book possible, and to Barbara Chernow for her meticulous editorial work.

*Feroze B. Mohamed, PhD*

# Contents

# Contributors

*Geoffrey K. Aguirre, MD, PhD*
Department of Neurology, Hospital of the University of Pennsylvania, Philadelphia, PA 19104, USA

*Nolan R. Altman, MD*
Department of Radiology, Miami Children's Hospital, Miami, FL 33155, USA

*Bassam A. Assaf, MD*
Department of Neurology, University of Illinois College of Medicine at Peoria, Peoria, IL 61637, USA

*Peter A. Bandettini, PhD*
Unit on Functional Imaging Methods, Functional MRI Facility, National Institute of Mental Health, Bethesda, MD 20892, USA

*Byron Bernal, MD*
Department of Radiology, Miami Children's Hospital, Miami, FL 33155, USA

*Jeffrey R. Binder, MD*
Department of Neurology, Medical College of Wisconsin, Milwaukee, WI 53226, USA

*Susan Y. Bookheimer, PhD*
Department of Psychiatry and Biobehavioral Sciences, Neuropsychiatric Institute, UCLA School of Medicine, Los Angeles, CA 90095, USA

*R. Todd Constable, PhD*
Department of Diagnostic Radiology, Biomedical Engineering Neurosurgery, Yale University School of Medicine, New Haven, CT 06520, USA

*Dietmar Cordes, PhD*
Department of Radiology, University of Washington, Seattle, WA 98195, USA

# Part I

## BOLD Functional MRI

# 1

# Principles of Functional MRI

Seong-Gi Kim and Peter A. Bandettini

## Introduction

The idea that regional cerebral blood flow (CBF) could reflect neuronal activity began with experiments of Roy and Sherrington in 1890.[1] This concept is the basis for all hemodynamic-based brain imaging techniques being used today. The focal increase in CBF can be considered to relate directly to neuronal activity because the glucose metabolism and CBF changes are coupled closely.[2] Thus, the measurement of CBF change induced by stimulation has been used for mapping brain functions. Because cerebral metabolic rate of glucose ($CMR_{glu}$) and CBF changes are coupled, it is assumed that cerebral metabolic rate of oxygen ($CMRO_2$) and CBF changes also are coupled. However, based on positron emission tomographic measurements of CBF and $CMRO_2$ in humans during somatosensory and visual stimulation, Fox and colleagues reported that an increase in CBF surpassed an increase in $CMRO_2$.[3,4] Consequently, a mismatch between CBF and $CMRO_2$ changes results in an *increase* in the capillary and venous oxygenation level, opening a new physiological parameter (in addition to CBF change) for brain mapping. In 1990, based on rat brain studies during global stimulation at 7 Tesla (T), Ogawa and colleagues at AT&T Bell Laboratories reported that functional brain mapping is possible by using the venous blood oxygenation level-dependent (BOLD) magnetic resonance imaging (MRI) contrast.[5–7] The BOLD contrast relies on changes in deoxyhemoglobin (dHb), which acts as an endogenous paramagnetic contrast agent.[5,8] Therefore, changes in the local dHb concentration in the brain lead to alterations in the signal intensity of magnetic resonance images.[5–7,9]

Application of the BOLD contrast to human functional brain mapping followed shortly thereafter.[10–12] Since then, functional magnetic resonance imaging (fMRI) has been the tool of choice for visualizing neural activity in the human brain. The fMRI has been used extensively for investigating various brain functions, including vision, motor, language, and cognition. The BOLD imaging technique is used widely because of its high sensitivity and easy implementation.

Because the BOLD signal is dependent on various anatomical, physiological, and imaging parameters,[13] its interpretation with respect to physiological parameters is qualitative or semi-quantitative. Thus, it is difficult to compare the BOLD signal changes in different brain regions, from the different imaging laboratories, and/or from different magnetic fields. Alternatively, change in CBF can be measured using MRI. Because these fMRI signals are related to a single physiological parameter, its quantitative interpretation is more straightforward.

Functional MRI is a very powerful method to map brain functions with relatively high spatial and temporal resolution. In order to utilize fMRI techniques efficiently and interpret fMRI data accurately, it is important to examine underlying physiology and physics. In this introductory chapter, we will discuss the source of the BOLD signal and improvement of BOLD fMRI techniques.

## Physiological Changes

Because fMRI measures the vascular hemodynamic response induced by increased neural activity, it is important to understand a chain of events from task to fMRI (see Figure 1.1). Task and/or stimulation induce synaptic and electric activities at localized regions, which will trigger an increase in CBF, cerebral blood volume (CBV), $CMRO_2$, and $CMR_{glu}$. Although the exact relationship between neural activity and vascular physiology change is not known, it is well-accepted

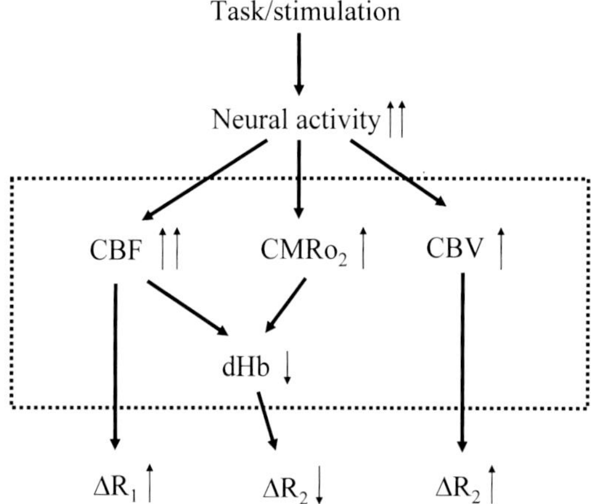


**Figure 1.1.** A schematic of fMRI signal changes induced by stimulation. Task/stimulation increases neural activity and increases metabolic (cerebral metabolic rate of oxygen) and vascular responses (cerebral blood flow and volume). Increase in CBF enhances venous oxygenation level, whereas increase in $CMRO_2$ decreases venous oxygenation level. Because an increase in CBF exceeds an increase in $CMRO_2$, venous oxygenation level increases. These vascular parameter changes will modulate biophysical parameters. Increases in CBF and CBV increase $R_1$ (= $1/T_1$) and $R_2$ (= $1/T_2$), respectively, whereas decrease in dHb contents reduces $R_2$. Changes in biophysical parameters affect MRI signal changes.

that the change in $CMR_{glu}$ is a good indicator of neural activity. Since the $CMR_{glu}$ change is correlated linearly with the CBF change, a change in CBF is a good alternative secondary indicator of neural activity.

Cerebral blood flow and CBV changes are correlated because change in CBF is a multiple of CBV and velocity changes. The relationship between CBF and CBV obtained in monkeys during $CO_2$ modulation can be described as

$$\Delta CBV/CBV = (\Delta CBF/CBF + 1)^{0.38} - 1, \tag{1.1}$$

where $\Delta CBV/CBV$ and $\Delta CBF/CBF$ are relative total CBV and CBF changes.[14] The similar relationship was observed in rat brain during hypercapnia (see Figure 1.2A).[15] Recently, Ito and colleagues measured relative CBF and CBV changes in human visual cortex during visual stimulation and found that the above relationship is reasonally applicable to human stimulation studies.[16] Thus, change in total blood volume can be a good index of the CBF change. Change in total blood volume can be measured by using contrast agents because contrast agents distribute in all vascular system. Because venous blood volume constitutes of 75% of the total blood volume,[15] it is conceivable that the venous blood volume change is dominant. However, based on separate measurements of arterial and venous blood volume changes during hypercapnia by a novel $^{19}F$ NMR technique and video-microscopy, a relative change in venous blood volume is approximately half of the relative total CBV change (see Figure 1.2B).[15]

In the context of BOLD contrast, only venous blood can contribute to activation-induced susceptibility changes because venous blood contains deoxyhemoglobin. The venous oxygenation level is dependent on a mismatch between oxygen supply by CBF and oxygen utilization in tissue. Assuming an arterial oxygen saturation of 1.0, the relative change of venous oxygenation level ($Y$) can be determined from the relative changes of both CBF and $CMRO_2$ in the following manner[17]:

$$\frac{\Delta Y}{1-Y} = 1 - \frac{(\Delta CMR_{O_2}/CMR_{O_2} + 1)}{(\Delta CBF/CBF + 1)}. \tag{1.2}$$

From Equation (1.2), a relative change in $CMRO_2$ can be obtained from information of relative CBF and $Y$ changes. It also is important to recognize that relationship between oxygenation change and blood flow change is linear at low CBF changes,[18,19] but nonlinear at very high CBF changes.[20,21]

## Functional Imaging Contrasts

Magnetic resonance imaging signal in a given voxel can be described as a vector sum of signals from different compartments weighted by functions of $T_1^*$ and $T_2^*$. Thus, MRI signal intensity is

$$S = \sum_i So_i fn(T_{1i}^*) fn(T_{2i}^*), \tag{1.3}$$

($\Delta S_{cont}$) and stimulation periods ($\Delta S_{st}$). Relative CBF changes during task periods can be described as $CBF_{st}/CBF_{cont} = \Delta S_{st}/\Delta S_{cont}$, where $CBF_{st}$ and $CBF_{cont}$ are CBF values during task and control periods, respectively. Functional brain mapping has been obtained successfully during motor, vision, and cognitive tasks (see Figure 1.4 for finger movements). Relative CBF changes measured by FAIR agree extremely with those measured by $H_2{}^{15}O$ positron emission tomography (PET) in the same region and subject during the identical stimulation task.[29] Thus, the perfusion-weighted MRI technique is an excellent approach to detect relative CBF changes induced by neural activity or other external perturbations. Furthermore because small arterioles and capillaries are very close to neuronally active tissue, it is expected that a tissue-specific CBF signal improves a spatial specificity of functional images. Figure 1.5 demonstrates the signal specificity of the perfusion-weighted fMRI technique in an anesthetized cat during single-orientation stimuli. Based on previous 2-DG glucose studies,[30] $CMR_{glu}$ showed patchy, irregular columnar structures with an average inter-column distance of 1.1 to 1.4 millimeters. Cerebral blood flow-based fMRI maps showed similar activation patterns and intercluster distance, suggesting that the CBF response is specific to areas with metabolic increase.[31] It should be noted that the sagittal sinus running between two hemispheres does not show signal changes in CBF-based studies, contrary to conventional BOLD measurements, which has showed the largest signal change in the draining sagittal sinus.[32,33]

Although perfusion-based approaches can be utilized for fMRI studies, there are many shortcomings. First, large vascular contribution

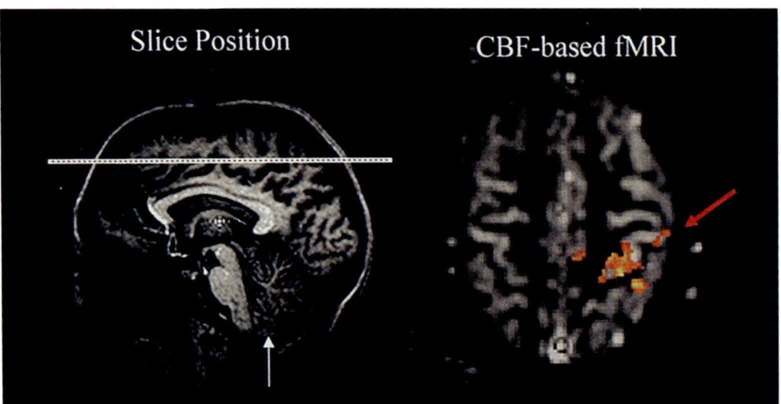


**Figure 1.4.** Cerebral blood flow-weighted functional image during left finger movements.[70] To obtain the perfusion contrast, flow direction (indicated by an up-arrow) has to be considered. Thus, 5-mm–thick transverse planes were selected for CBF-based fMRI studies. The background image was perfusion-weighted; higher signal areas have higher inflow rates. Functional activity areas are located at gray matter in the contralateral primary motor cortex, indicated by a red arrow. Interestingly, no large signal changes were observed at the edge of the brain, which often was seen in conventional BOLD functional maps. Adapted from Kim S-G, Tsekos NV, Ashe J. Multi-slice perfusion-based functional MRI using the FAIR technique: Comparison of CBF and BOLD effects. *NMR in Biomed*. 1997;10:191–196.

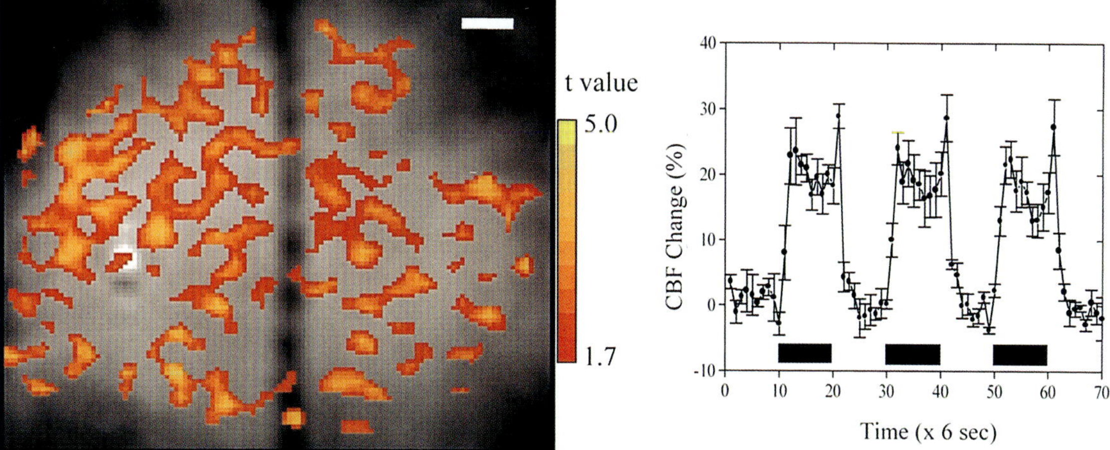


**Figure 1.5.** Application of the CBF-based (FAIR) fMRI technique to isoflurane-anesthetized cat's orientation column mapping.[31] Moving gratings with black and white rectangular single-orientation bars were used for visual stimulation. Unlike the conventional BOLD technique, CBF-weighted fMRI is specific to tissue, not draining vessels. More importantly, active clusters are irregular and column-like based on the size of clusters and the interval between clusters. In addition, single-condition functional regions activated by two orthogonal orientation stimuli are complementary. Scale bar = 1 mm; color vertical bar = *t* value. Time course of activation area is shown. Boxes underneath the time course indicate one-minute–long stimulation periods. Typical CBF change induced by visual stimulation ranges between 15 and 50%. Reprinted with permission from Duong TQ, Kim DS, Ugurbil K, Kim SG. Localized cerebral blood flow response at submillimeter columnar resolution. *Proc Natl Acad Sci USA* 98:10904–10909. Copyright © 2001, National Academy of Sciences, U.S.A.

exists because labeled blood fill up arterial vasculature before it travels into capillaries (see also Figure 1.6).[34] This arterial vascular contribution can be reduced by using spin-echo data collection (see Figure 1.6) or eliminated using bipolar gradients, but this reduces SNR of perfusion-weighted images. Because the dilation of *large* arterial vessels is small,[15] no activation at large vessel areas was found.[35] Thus, for mapping purpose, it may not be necessary to remove large vessel contributions (see Figure 1.5). Second, the proper perfusion contrast is achieved only when enough time is allowed for the labeled arterial spins to travel into the region of interest and exchange with tissue spins. This makes it difficult to detect changes in CBF with a temporal resolution greater than $T_1$ of arterial blood, resulting in ineffective signal averaging. Third, in multi-slice application, transit times to different slices are different, which may cause errors in quantification of relative CBF changes.[28,36] Relative CBF changes measured by multi-slice FAIR agree extremely with those measured by $H_2^{15}O$ PET, suggesting that the change in transit time is not a significant confound.[29]

## $T_2^*$ and $T_2$ Based fMRI

It is well known that, with typical fMRI acquisition parameters, the BOLD response is particularly sensitive in and around large draining veins because the BOLD effect is sensitive to baseline venous blood volume and vessel size.[17,37] To understand the spatial resolution of

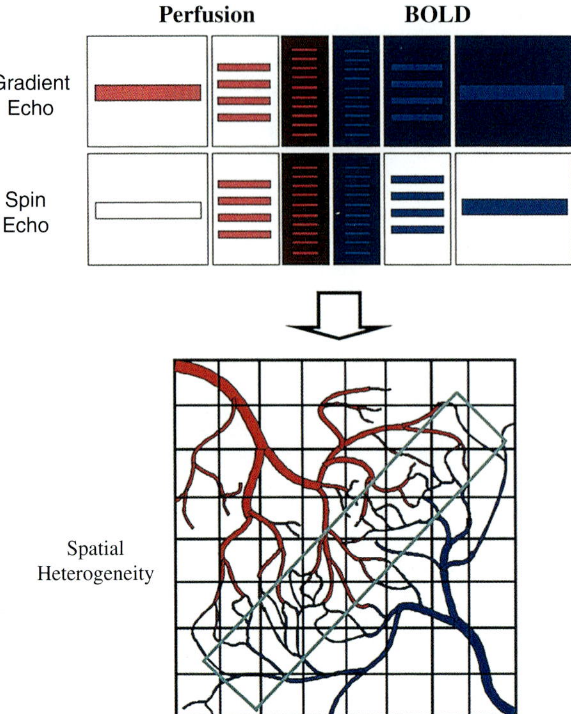


**Figure 1.6.** Intravascular and extravascular signal contributions to perfusion and BOLD signals.[71] In perfusion-weighted images, the IV component of all arterial vessels (red color) and EV component (pink) of capillaries will constitute. When spin-echo data collection is used, spins in large vessels will not be refocused, removing very large artery contribution. Further removal can be achieved by using bipolar flow-crushing gradients. In BOLD images, IV (blue color) and EV (black) components of all size venous vessels will contribute when gradient-echo data collection is used. When spin-echo data collection is utilized, EV effect of large vessels can be minimized. Spatial heterogeneity of vascular distributions exists; in some pixels, large vessels are dominant, whereas some pixels contain mostly capillaries. When neural activity occurs at tissue level, demarked by a green rectangle, only capillary-level signal change will locate the actual neural activity area. Containing large vessels will misleadingly deviate activation to non-specific vessel area. Adapted with permission from Bandettini PA. The temporal resolution of Functional MRI. In: Moonen CTW, Bandettini PA, eds. Functional MRI. New York: Springer 1999: 204–220.

BOLD-based fMRI, it is important to examine the anatomical source of the BOLD signal. The BOLD contrast induced by dHb arises from both intravascular (IV) and extravascular (EV) components. Because the exchange of water between these two compartments (typical lifetime of the water in capillaries greater than 500 milliseconds) is relatively slower compared with the imaging time (echo time less than 100 milliseconds), MRI signals from these are treated as separate pools.

## Intravascular Component

During fMRI measurements, water rapidly exchanges between red blood cells (RBC) with paramagnetic dHb and plasma (average water residence time in RBCs equals approximately five milliseconds) and move along space with different fields by diffusion (e.g., diffusion distance [i.e., (6 × diffusion constant × diffusion time)$^{1/2}$] during ~50 milliseconds measurement time = ~17 micrometers (μm) with diffusion constant of ~1 μm$^2$ per millisecond). Thus, dynamic (time irreversible) averaging occurs over the many different fields induced by dHb. All water molecules inside the vessel will experience the similar dynamic averaging, resulting in reduction of $T_2$ of blood water in the venous pool. A transverse relaxation rate of blood water is affected by exchange of water and diffusion. In both cases, blood $T_2$ can be written as

$$1/T_2 = A_o + K(1-Y)^2, \tag{1.4}$$

where $A_o$ is a field-independent constant term and $K$ would scale quadratically with the magnetic field and depend also on the echo time used in a spin-echo measurement.[38] $T_2$ of blood water at 1.5T is ~127 ms for $Y$ = 0.6[38], whereas $T_2$ is ~12–15 ms at 7T[39,40] and 5 ms at 9.4T.[41] These experimental values are consistent with predictions based on Equation (1.4). $T_2$ values of gray matter water at 1.5T, 7T, and 9.4T are 90 ms,[42] 55 ms,[40] and 40 ms,[41] respectively. When spin-echo time is set to $T_2$ of gray matter, it is evident that the blood contribution to MRI signal decreases dramatically when the magnetic field increases.

In addition to the $T_2$ change induced by deoxyhemoglobin, frequency shift is observed. When a blood vessel is considered as an infinite cylinder, frequency shift Δω induced by dHb within and around the vessel is depicted at Figure 1.7. It should be noted that frequency and magnetic field are interchangeable because $\omega = \gamma B$, where γ is the

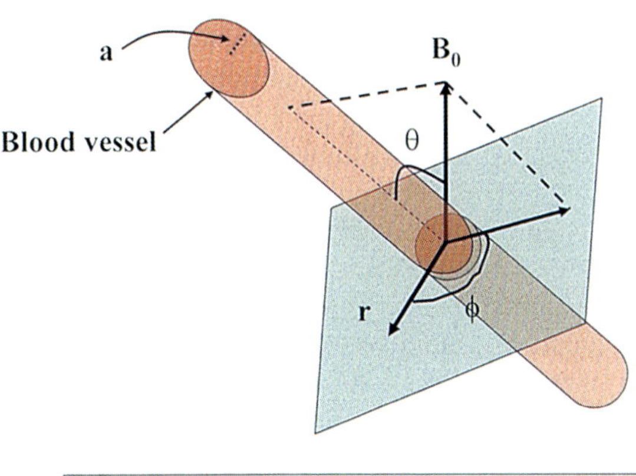


$$\Delta\omega_{in} = 2\pi\, \Delta\chi_0 (1 - Y)\, \omega_0 (\cos^2\theta - 1/3)$$

$$\Delta\omega_{out} = 2\pi\, \Delta\chi_0 (1 - Y)\, \omega_0 (a/r)^2 (\sin^2\theta) (\cos 2\phi)$$

**Figure 1.7.** Diagram of a blood vessel and the parameters that determine the susceptibility effect induced by dHb irons in red blood cells at a distance $r$ from the center of a vessel. The vessel with a radius of $a$ is oriented at angle θ from the main magnetic field $B_o$. ϕ is the angle between $r$ and plane defined by $B_o$ and the vessel axis. Reprinted from *Methods*, Vol. 30, Kim SG, Ugurbil K, High-resolution functional MRI in the animal brain, 28–41. Copyright © 2003, with permission from Elsevier.

gyromagnetic ratio and $B$ is the magnetic field. Inside the blood vessel, the frequency shift is expressed by

$$\Delta\omega_{in} = 2\pi\Delta\chi_o(1-Y)\omega_o(\cos^2\theta - 1/3), \quad (1.5)$$

where $\Delta\chi_o$ is the maximum susceptibility difference between fully oxygenated and fully deoxygenated blood, $Y$ is the fraction of oxygenation in venous blood, $\omega_o$ is the applied magnetic field of magnet in frequency units $\omega_o = \gamma B_o$), and $\theta$ is the angle between the applied magnetic field ($B_o$) and vessel orientation. $\Delta\chi_o$ is dependent on a hematocrit level. Assuming a hematocrit level of 0.38 and the susceptibility difference between 100% oxyhemoglobin and 100% dHb of 0.27 ppm,[8] $\Delta\chi_o$ in whole blood is 0.1 ppm. In a given voxel, many vessels with different orientations exist. Rather than inducing a net phase shift, the random orientations cause a phase dispersion, therefore causing a reduction in $T_2^*$. However, a very large vessel will have its own phase depending on oxygenation level and orientation. Using this property, Haacke and his colleagues determined a venous oxygenation level[43] from a vessel that they determined to be perpendicular to $B_o$.

### Extravascular Component

At any location outside the blood vessel, the frequency shift can be described by

$$\Delta\omega_{out} = 2\pi\Delta\chi_o(1-Y)\omega_o(a/r)^2(\sin^2\theta)(\cos 2\phi), \quad (1.6)$$

where $a$ is the radius of blood vessel, $r$ is the distance from the point of interest to the center of the blood vessel, and $\phi$ is the angle between $r$ and plane defined by $B_o$ and the vessel axis. The dephasing effect is dependent on the orientation of vessel. Vessels running parallel to the magnetic field do not have the EV effect, whereas those orthogonal to $B_o$ will have the maximal effect (see Figure 1.8). At the lumen of vessels ($r = a$), $\Delta\omega_{out}$ is identical and independent of vessel sizes. At $r = 5a$, the susceptibility effect is four percent of the maximally available $\Delta\omega_{out}$. The same frequency shift will be observed at 15 μm around a 3-μm radius capillary and 150 μm around a 30-μm radius venule (see Figure 1.9). This shows that the dephasing effect around a larger vessel is more spatially extensive because of a smaller susceptibility gradient. The EV contribution from large vessels to conventional BOLD signal is significant, regardless of magnetic field strength.[41] During echo time for fMRI studies (e.g., ~50 ms), water molecules diffuse ~17 μm, which covers a space with the entire range of susceptibility effects around the 3-μm radius capillary, but with a small range of static susceptibility effects around the 30-μm radius venule. Thus, tissue water around *capillaries* will be dynamically averaged over the many different fields (i.e., no net phase change like the IV component). However, because tissue water around *large vessels* will be averaged locally during an echo time, the static dephasing effect is dominant (see small circles with dephasing information in Figure 1.9). The dephasing effect around large vessels can be refocused by the 180-degree RF pulse. Therefore, the EV

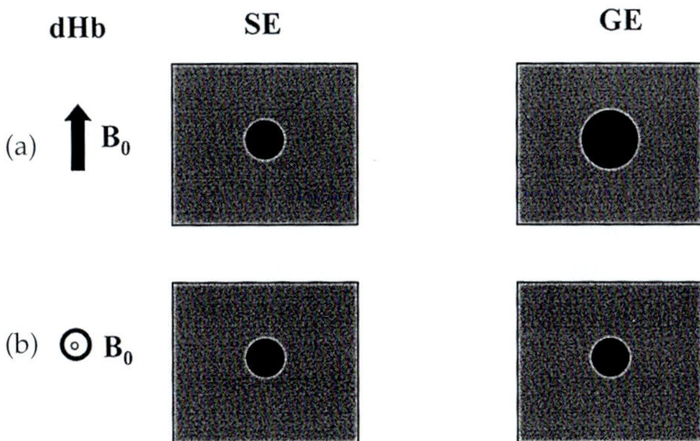


**Figure 1.8.** Spin-echo and gradient-echo image of a capillary filled with blood with deoxyhemoglobin.[7] Two different orientations were used. When vessel orientation is parallel to $B_o$ (b), no signal change outside the capillary was observed. However, when vessel is orthogonal to $B_o$ (a), gradient-echo signal change outside the capillary was detected. Adapted from Ogawa S, Lee T-M. Magnetic resonance imaging of blood vessels at high fields: in vivo and in vitro measurements and image simulation. *Magn Reson Med*. 1990;16:9–18.

contribution of large vessels can be reduced by using the spin-echo technique (see Figure 1.8).

In a given voxel, MRI signal intensity with dephasing effects (i.e., frequency shifts) induced by numerous vessels will be summed, resulting in a decrease in $T_2^*$ and a decrease in MRI signal. Signal in the voxel can be described, according to equation

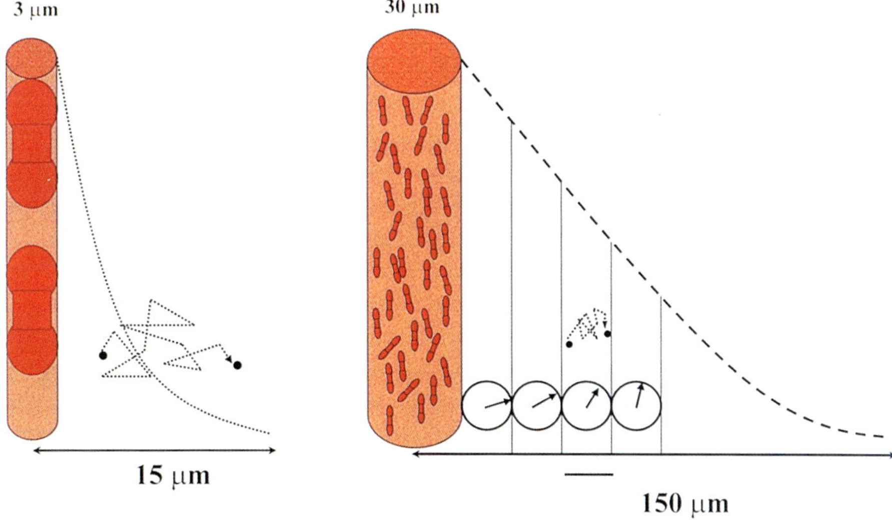


**Figure 1.9.** Extravascular dephasing effects from a 3-μm radius capillary and a 30-μm radius venule. Magnitude of dephasing effect (dashed decay lines from vessels) is shown as a function of distance. Hypothetical displacement of a water molecule is shown. Refocusing RF pulse in the spin-echo sequence cannot refocus dephasing effects around a small vessel because of dynamic averaging, whereas it can refocus static dephasing (shown in averaged phases in circles). Reprinted from *Methods*, Vol. 30, Kim SG, Ugurbil K, High-resolution functional MRI in the animal brain, 28–41. Copyright © 2003, with permission from Elsevier.

$$S(TE) = \sum_i So_i e^{-TE/T_{2i}} e^{-i\omega_i TE}, \quad (1.7)$$

where the summation is performed over the parameter $i$, which designates small volume elements within the voxel (e.g., hypothetically a volume with a small circle with phase shift), the time-averaged magnetic field experienced within these small volume elements. $\omega_i$TE indicates the phase shift of location $i$ at echo time $TE$. This signal loss occurs from *static averaging*. If the variation $\omega_i$ within the voxel is relatively large, the signal will be decayed approximately with a single exponential time constant $T_2^*$. Based on Monte Carlo simulation, the dephasing effect within a voxel can be simplified into $R_2'$ (in order to separate measured $R_2^*$ = intrinsic $R_2 + R_2'$ induced by contrast agent) change as

$$R_2' = \alpha \cdot CBV\{\Delta\chi_O\omega_O(1-Y)\}^\gamma, \quad (1.8)$$

where $\alpha$ and $\gamma$ are constants.[17,44,45] The power term $\gamma$ is 1.0 for static averaging domain and 2.0 for time-irreversible averaging domain.[17,44,45] All venous vessels will have a power term of 1.0 to 2.0; $\gamma$ is 1.0 to 2.0 for the gradient-echo sequence, and 1.5 to 2.0 for spin-echo sequence.[17,44,45] If diffusion-related travel distance of water molecules during echo time is sufficient to effectively average frequency shifts (also related to magnetic field), $\gamma$ will be 2.0. Thus, a longer echo time (i.e., longer diffusion distance) and a higher magnetic field (i.e., large susceptibility gradient) will reduce a vessel size for dynamic averaging. Figure 1.10 shows the $R_2'$ dependency on vessel size and frequency shift, which was obtained from Monte Carlo simulation with CBV of two percent and echo time of 40 milliseconds. $R_2'$ increases linearly with venous CBV.[17] Frequency shift at $Y = 0$ is 40 hertz at 1.5T and 107 hertz at 4T. Let us examine vessels with 3 μm and 30 μm radii. When a frequency shift increases from 32 to 64 hertz (due to an increase in magnetic field and/or a

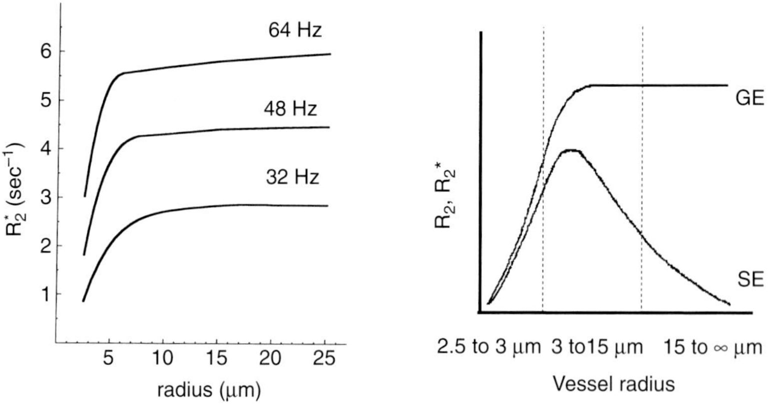


**Figure 1.10.** $R_2^*$ and $R_2$ changes as a function of vessel radius.[17,46] Monte Carlo simulation was performed to calculate $R_2^*$ change induced by three frequency shifts.[17] Reprinted with permission from Ogawa S, Menon RS, Tank DW, Kim SG, Merkle H, Ellermann JM and Ugurbil. Functional brain mapping by blood oxygenation level-dependent contrast magnetic resonance imaging. A comparison of signal characteristics with a biophysical model. *Biophys. J*, 64:803–812;1993.

decrease in oxygenation level), $R_2^*$ values of $3\,\mu m$ and $30\,\mu m$ radius vessels change from 1.2 to $3.5\,sec^{-1}$ and from 2.8 to $6.0\,sec^{-1}$, respectively. A power term $\gamma$ will be 1.5 for a 3-μm vessel and 1.1 for a 30-μm vessel, showing that a smaller size vessel is more sensitive to the frequency shift (such as induced by magnetic field). Spin-echo and gradient-echo BOLD signal changes in a function of vessel size can be seen in Figure 1.10.[46] At capillaries, a change in $R_2$ is similar to that of $R_2^*$. However, when vessel size increases above five- to eight-micrometer radius (which is related to diffusion time and susceptibility gradient), $R_2$ change is reduced, but $R_2^*$ change remains high. Thus, spin-echo BOLD signals predominantly originate from small-size vessels, including capillaries, whereas gradient-echo BOLD signals are contributed from large draining veins.

### Spin Echo versus Gradient Echo BOLD

As has been discussed previously, gradient-echo BOLD signals consist of EV and IV components of venous vessels, regardless of the vessel size (see Figure 1.6). Spin echo refocuses the dephasing effect around large vessels, and thus the spin-echo BOLD image contains the EV effect of vessels with time-irreversible diffusion effect (i.e., small-size vessel) and the IV component of all sizes of vessels. It is important to differentiate parenchyma signals (see a green rectangular box) from large vessel signals because the venous vasculature, including large draining veins, can be distant from the site of elevated neuronal activity (see also Figure 1.6).[32,47–50] Dilution by blood draining from inactive areas should ultimately diminish this non-specific draining-vein effect and thus limit its extent; however, before this occurs, substantial less-specific activation can be generated.[51] Therefore, it is important to minimize draining-vein signals from both intravascular and extravascular contributions for high-resolution studies.

The intravascular component can be reduced by setting an echo time of greater than $3T_2^*$ or $3T_2$ of blood. Thus, at ultrahigh fields, the IV component can be reduced significantly because venous blood $T_2^*$ and $T_2$ decreases faster than tissue $T_2^*/T_2$ when magnetic field increases. The intravascular contribution to the BOLD responses can be examined using bipolar gradients.[52] These gradients induce velocity-dependent phase shifts in the presence of flow and consequently suppress signals from blood because of inhomogeneous velocities within a vessel and the presence of blood vessels of different orientations within a voxel. Based on bipolar gradient studies, the BOLD fMRI signals at 1.5 T originate predominantly from the IV component (70–90%),[44,53,54] whereas those at 7 T and 9.4 T come predominantly from the EV component (see Figure 1.11).[41,55] When bipolar gradients increased to greater than $400\,s/mm^2$, relative percent BOLD signal change maintained constant, even though signal intensity decreased. With relatively high sensitivity of spin-echo BOLD at high fields, high-resolution functional maps can be obtained from human brain at 7 T (see Figure 1.11).

After removing the IV component in the BOLD signal, the EV component remains. In gradient-echo BOLD fMRI, the EV effect around

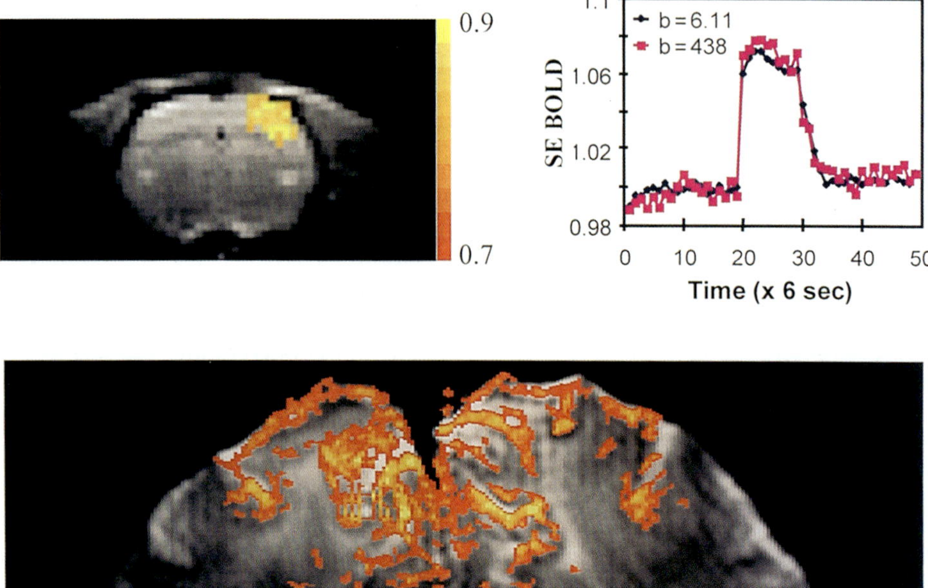


**Figure 1.11.** Spin-echo BOLD-based fMRI at 9.4 T and 7 T.[41,72] (top) An α-chloralse anesthetized rat was used for somatosensory forelimb stimulation. Color indicates a cross-correlation value. Localized activation is observed at the forelimb *S*1. Functional MRI time courses of spin-echo BOLD signal in the primary somatosensory region. To investigate the IV component, flow-crushing gradients (in a unit of *b* value) were used. The higher *b* value will result in the more reduction of the moving blood signal. If the IV component is significant, a much lower BOLD signal change is expected when a larger *b* value is used. However, any reduction of relative BOLD signals was not observed, suggesting that spin-echo BOLD signal does not contain a significant IV component. Somatosensory stimulation was performed during image number 20 to 29. (bottom) High-resolution spin-echo BOLD image was obtained from a human during visual stimulation at 7 T. At high fields, sensitivity of SE BOLD signal is sufficient for high-resolution mapping of human brain. Spatial resolution is $1 \times 1 \times 2\,\text{mm}^3$. Reprinted from Duong TQ, Yacoub E, Adriany G, et al. High-resolution, spin-echo BOLD and CBF fMRI at 4 and 7 T. *Mag Reson Med*. 2002;48:589–593. Copyright © 2002. Reprinted with permission of Wiley-Liss, Inc., a subsidiary of John Wiley & Sons, Inc.

large vessels is linearly dependent on magnetic field, whereas the EV effect around small vessels is supra-linearly dependent on the magnetic field. Even at 9.4 T, the EV effect around large vessels is significant. In spin-echo BOLD fMRI, the EV effect around small vessels is supra-linearly dependent on the magnetic field, whereas that around large vessels is reduced. Thus, the spin-echo technique is more specific to parenchyma than gradient-echo BOLD fMRI. However, because the dephasing effect around vessels is refocused, the sensitivity of spin-echo BOLD signal is reduced significantly. For example, $\Delta R_2/\Delta R_2^*$ is 0.3–0.4 at 1.5 T,[56,57] and also at 9.4 T.[21] Even if respective optimized echo times are used for gradient-echo and spin-echo BOLD fMRI, the gradient-echo BOLD technique provides the higher signal change, even at 9.4 T. For most applications, the gradient-echo BOLD technique is the choice of tools because of high sensitivity, even if its spatial specificity compromises.

## Contrast-to-Noise Ratio

Important consideration of fMRI is contrast-to-noise ratio (neural activity-induced signal change relative to signal fluctuation). Increase of neural activity-induced MRI signal and decrease of noise are important aspects for high-resolution fMRI. Neural activity-induced signal is dependent on both image contrast and imaging techniques used for fMRI. In the $T_2^*$-based measurements, the signal change induced by neural activity ($\Delta S$) can be described by

$$\Delta S = \rho \cdot S_{cont} \cdot \left(e^{-TE \cdot \Delta R_2^*} - 1\right), \tag{1.9}$$

where $\rho$ is the fraction of a voxel that is active, $S_{cont}$ is the signal intensity during the control period, $TE$ is the echo time, and $\Delta R_2^*$ is the change in the apparent transverse relaxation rate in the active partial volume. Signal change is maximal when a gradient echo time is set to $T_2^*$ of tissue at resting conditions. When spin-echo imaging techniques are used, $\Delta R_2^*$ is replaced by $\Delta R_2$. $\Delta R_2^*$ is equivalent to $\Delta R_2 + \Delta R_2'$, where $\Delta R_2'$ is the relaxation rate induced by local inhomogenous magnetic fields. $\Delta S$ for spin-echo BOLD fMRI will be maximal by setting $TE$ of $T_2$ of tissue. In CBF-based techniques, $TE\Delta R_2^*$ is substituted by $TI\Delta R_1^*$, where $TI$ is the spin labeling time (i.e., the inversion time for pulsed labeling methods), and $\Delta R_1^*$ is the change in the apparent longitudinal relaxation rate. $\Delta S$ is maximized by setting $TI$ of $T_1$ of tissue. In any technique, contribution of large vessels increases $\Delta S$. Depending on constraints of spatial specificity for each measurement, the technique with the highest $\Delta S$ should be chosen. Because contribution of small intracortical veins is likely localized within 1.5 millimeters to the site of activation,[58] contribution of small veins can improve SNR for supramillimeter spatial resolution. In typical fMRI studies with supramillimeter spatial resolution, the removal of only large surface arteries and veins may be necessary.

Sources of noise include random white noise, physiological fluctuations, bulk head motion, and system instability if it exists. Random noise is independent between voxels, whereas other noise sources may be coherent among voxels, resulting in spatial and temporal correlation. In fMRI, coherent noises are the major source of signal fluctuation. Bulk head motion can be eliminated by head holders. Physiological motion, which is due mainly to respiration and cardiac pulsation, can be minimized by gating data acquisition and/or reduced by post processing.[59,60]

## Spatial and Temporal Resolution of fMRI

### Spatial Resolution

Spatial resolution of high-resolution fMRI is dependent on signal-to-noise ratio (SNR) and intrinsic hemodynamic response. The intrinsic limit of spatial specificity of hemodynamic-based fMRI can be dependent on how finely CBF is regulated. It has been suggested, based on optical imaging studies, that CBF regulation is widespread beyond neuronally active areas.[61] However, recent studies have suggested that intrinsic CBF changes are specific to sub-millimeter functional domains.[31] The highest CBF change was observed in the middle of the rat somatosensory cortex, cortical layer IV, not at the surface of the cortex during somatosensory stimulation.[21,62] This observation is consistent with invasive 2-DG and $^{14}$C-iodoantipyrine autoradiographic studies in the barrel cortex.[63] To further examine the specificity of CBF response, the perfusion-based FAIR technique has been utilized.[23] From this study, it was found that CBF is regulated to sub-millimeter layer-specific and laminar-specific functional domains.[21,31] Among the available hemodynamic fMRI approaches, the CBF-based signal is the most specific to neuronal active sites because most signals originate from tissues and capillaries. Tissue-specific BOLD signal without large vessel contribution will have a similar spatial specificity to the CBF-weighted signal.[21]

## Temporal Resolution

Because hemodynamic responses are sluggish, it is difficult to obtain very high temporal resolution, even if images can be obtained rapidly. Typically, hemodynamic signal changes are observed at one to two seconds after the onset of neural stimulation and reaches maximum at four to eight seconds (see Figure 1.12). The exact time of neural activ-

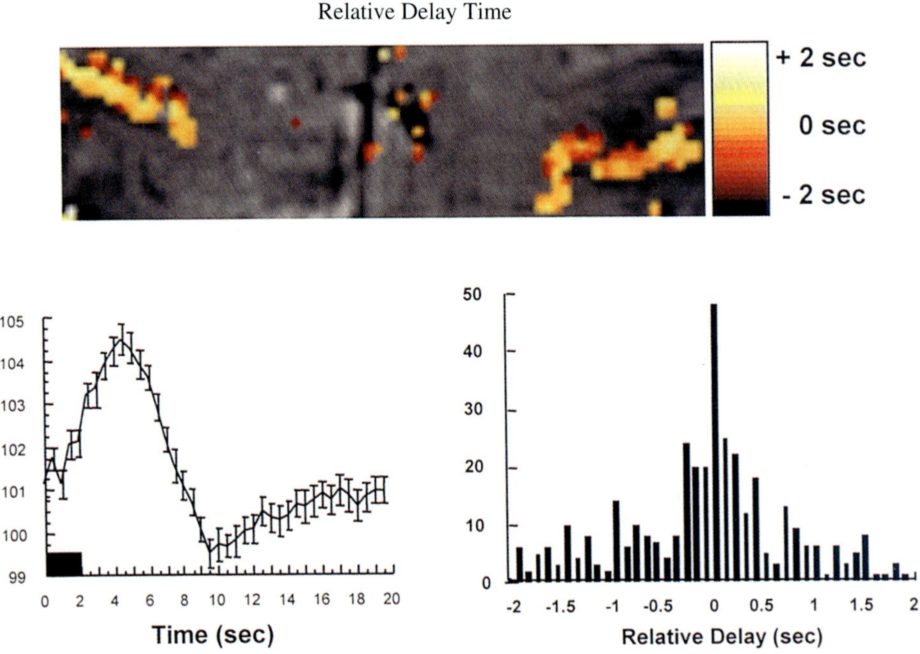


**Figure 1.12.** Heterogeneity of hemodynamic responses.[71] Delay time of $T_2^*$-weighted fMRI signal changes was obtained in the motor cortical areas. Two-second bilateral finger movements were performed at 3T. Although average delay time is approximately one second, there is a large variation in delay time shown in color map, as well as histogram. In histogram and the delay map, relative hemodynamic delay time (not actual delay time) was calculated, which means average of all delay times of zero seconds. Adapted with permission from Bandettini PA. The temporal resolution of Functional MRI. In: Moonen CTW, Bandettini PA, eds. Functional MRI. New York: Springer 1999: 204–220.

ity from hemodynamic responses cannot be obtained easily because hemodynamic response varies depending on vascular structures (see Figure 1.12). The important issue is to determine sequential neural activities of different cortical regions or pixels. If the hemodynamic response times in all regions and in all subjects were the same, neuronal activities could be inferred directly from fMRI time courses. However, this may not be true in all regions and in all subjects (see Figure 1.12); thus, differences in fMRI time courses may be simply related to intrinsic hemodynamic response time differences, hampering temporal studies. Thus, temporal resolution of fMRI is limited. Alternative approaches to overcome these problems have been proposed. To separate intrinsic hemodynamic differences from neural activity differences, a time-resolved event-related fMRI technique can be utilized.[64–67] The idea is to examine how fMRI parameters vary with behavioral correlates and thus requires multiple behavioral outcome measures. Subsequently, temporal characteristics of fMRI responses can be correlated with behavioral data such as response time. Differences in the underlying temporal behavior of neuronal activity can be distinguished from hemodynamic response time variations between subjects and brain areas (see a review article[68]). This approach allows the experimenter to obtain higher temporal resolution. Dynamic fMRI studies can be feasible using standard gradient-echo BOLD fMRI. The issues related to spatial and temporal characteristic is further discussed in detial in chapter 4 of this book.

## Conclusions

Advancement of imaging technologies allows detections of various vascular physiological parameters induced by neural activity. Fortunately, tissue-based hemodynamic response is relatively specific to neuronal active sites. Thus, spatial resolution of fMRI can be achieved up to on an order of a column. Because hemodynamic response is slow, its temporal resolution cannot be reached easily at a level of neural activity time scale. By using an approach with multiple experiments with different stimulus intervals or durations, temporal resolution can be improved up to on the order of 100 milliseconds.

## References

1. Roy CS, Sherrington CS. On the regulation of blood supply of the brain. *J Physiol*. 1890;1:85–108.
2. Raichle ME. Circulatory and metabolic correlates of brain function in normal humans. In: Handbook of Physiology—The Nervous System. Vol. V. Bethesda, MD: American Physiological Society; 1987:643–674.
3. Fox PT, Raichle ME. Focal physiological uncoupling of cerebral blood flow and oxidative metabolism during somatosensory stimulation in human subjects. *Proc Natl Acad Sci USA*. 1986;83:1140–1144.
4. Fox PT, Raichle ME, Mintun MA, Dence C. Nonoxidative glucose consumption during focal physiologic neural activity. *Science*. 1988;241: 462–464.

5. Ogawa S, Lee T-M, Nayak AS, Glynn P. Oxygenation-sensitive contrast in magnetic resonance image of rodent brain at high magnetic fields. *Magn Reson Med*. 1990;14:68–78.
6. Ogawa S, Lee T-M, Kay AR, Tank DW. Brain magnetic resonance imaging with contrast dependent on blood oxygenation. *Proc Natl Acad Sci USA*. 1990;87:9868–9872.
7. Ogawa S, Lee TM. Magnetic resonance imaging of blood vessels at high fields: in vivo and in vitro measurments and image simulation. *Magn Reson Med*. 1990;16:9–18.
8. Pauling L, Coryell CD. The magnetic properties and structure of hemoglobin, oxyhemoglobin and carbonmonoxyhemoglobin. *Proc Natl Acad Sci USA*. 1936;22:210–216.
9. Thulborn KR, Waterton JC, Mattews PM, Radda GK. Oxygenation dependence of the transverse relaxation time of water protons in whole blood at high field. *Biochem Biophys Acta*. 1982;714:265–270.
10. Ogawa S, Tank DW, Menon R, et al. Intrinsic signal changes accompanying sensory stimulation: Functional brain mapping with magnetic resonance imaging. *Proc Natl Acad Sci USA*. 1992;89:5951–5955.
11. Kwong KK, Belliveau JW, Chesler DA, et al. Dynamic magnetic resonance imaging of human brain activity during primary sensory stimulation. *Proc Natl Acad Sci USA*. 1992;89:5675–5679.
12. Bandettini PA, Wong EC, Hinks RS, Rikofsky RS, Hyde JS. Time course EPI of human brain function during task activation. *Magn Reson Med*. 1992; 25:390–397.
13. Ogawa S, Menon RS, Kim S-G, Ugurbil K. On the characteristics of functional magnetic resonance imaging of the brain. *Annu Rev Biophys Biomol Struct*. 1998;27:447–474.
14. Grubb RL, Raichle ME, Eichling JO, Ter-Pogossian MM. The effects of changes in PaCO2 on cerebral blood volume, blood flow, and vascular mean transit time. *Stroke*. 1974;5:630–639.
15. Lee S-P, Duong T, Yang G, Iadecola C, Kim S-G. Relative changes of cerebral arterial and venous blood volumes during increased cerebral blood flow: Implications for BOLD fMRI. *Magn Reson Med*. 2001;45: 791–800.
16. Ito H, Takahashi K, Hatazawa J, Kim S-G, Kanno I. Changes in human regional cerebral blood flow and cerebral blood volume during visual stimulation measured by positron emission tomography. *J Cereb Blood Flow Metab*. 2001;21:608–612.
17. Ogawa S, Menon RS, Tank DW, et al. Functional brain mapping by blood oxygenation level-dependent contrast magnetic resonance imaging. *Biophys J*. 1993;64:800–812.
18. Hoge RD, Atkinson J, Gill B, Crelier GR, Marrett S, G.B.P. Linear coupling between cerebral blood flow and oxygen consumption in activated human cortex. *Proc Natl Acad Sci*. 1999;96:9403–9408.
19. Kim S-G, Rostrup E, Larsson HBW, Ogawa S, Paulson OB. Simultaneous measurements of CBF and $CMRO_2$ changes by fMRI: Significant increase of oxygen consumption rate during visual stimulation. *Magn Reson Med*. 1999;41:1152–1161.
20. Silva A, Lee S-P, Yang C, Iadecola C, Kim S-G. Simultaneous BOLD and perfusion functional MRI during forepaw stimulation in rats. *J Cereb Blood Flow Metab*. 1999;19:871–879.
21. Lee S-P, Silva AC, Kim S-G. Comparison of diffusion-weighted high-resolution CBF and spin-echo BOLD fMRI at 9.4T. *Magn Reson Med*. 2002;47:736–741.

22. Detre JA, Leigh JS, Williams DS, Koretsky AP. Perfusion imaging. Magn Reson Med. 1992;23:37–45.
23. Kim S-G. Quantification of relative cerebral blood flow change by flow-sensitive alternating inversion recovery (FAIR) technique: application to functional mapping. *Magn Reson Med*. 1995;34:293–301.
24. Kwong KK, Chesler DA, Weisskoff RM, et al. MR perfusion studies with T1-weighted echo planar imaging. *Magn Reson Med*. 1995;34:878–887.
25. Schwarzbauer C, Morrissey S, Haase A. Quantitative magnetic resonance imaging of perfusion using magnetic labeling of water proton spins within the detection slice. *Magn Reson Med*. 1996;35:540–546.
26. Edelman RR, Siewert B, Darby DG, et al. Qualitative mapping of cerebral blood flow and functional localization with echo-planar MR imaging and signal targeting with alternating radio frequency. *Radiology*. 1994;192: 513–520.
27. Helpern J, Branch C, Yongbi M, Huong N. Perfusion imaging by un-inverted flow-sensitive alternating inversion recovery (UNFAIR). *Magn Reson Imaging*. 1997;15:135–139.
28. Wong E, Buxton R, Frank L. Qunatitiative imaging of perfusion using a single subtraction (QUIPSS anf QUIPSS II). *Magn Reson Med*. 1998;39: 702–708.
29. Zaini MR, Strother SC, Andersen JR, et al. Comparison of matched BOLD and FAIR 4.0T-fMRI with [$^{15}$O]water PET brain volumes. *Medical Physics*. 1999;26:1559–1567.
30. Lowel S, Freeman B, Singer W. Topographic organization of the orientation column system in large flat-mounts of the cat visual cortex: a 2-deoxyglucose study. *Exp Brain Res*. 1988;71:33–46.
31. Duong TQ, Kim D-S, Ugurbil K, Kim S-G. Localized cerebral blood flow response at submillimeter columnar resolution. *Proc Natl Acad Sci USA*. 2001;98:10904–10909.
32. Duong TQ, Kim D-S, Ugurbil K, Kim S-G. Spatio-temporal Dynamics of the BOLD fMRI Signals: Toward mapping submillimeter columnar structures using the early negative response. *Magn Reson Med*. 2000;44: 231–242.
33. Kim D-S, Duong TQ, Kim S-G. High-resolution mapping of iso-orientation columns by fMRI. *Nature Neurosci*. 2000;3:164–169.
34. Ye FQ, Mattay VS, Jezzard P, Frank JA, Weinberger DR, McLaughlin AC. Correction for vascular artifacts in cerebral blood flow values by using arterial spin tagging techniques. *Magn Reson Med*. 1997;37:226–235.
35. Kim S-G, Tsekos NV. Perfusion imaging by a flow-sensitive alternating inversion recovery (FAIR) technique: Application to functional mapping. *Magn Reson Med*. 1997;37:425–435.
36. Buxton R, Frank L, Wong E, Siewert B, Warach S, Edelman R. A general kinetic model for quantitative perfusion imaging with arterial spin labeling. *Magn Reson Med*. 1998;40:383–396.
37. Weisskoff RM, Zuo CS, Boxerman JL, Rosen BR. Microscopic susceptibility variation and transverse relaxation: Theory and experiment. *Magn Reson Med*. 1994;31:601–610.
38. Wright GA, Hu BS, Macovski A. Estimating oxygen saturation of blood in vivo with MR imaging at 1.5T. *J Magn Reson Imag*. 1991;1:275–283.
39. Ogawa S, Lee TM, Barrere B. Sensitivity of magnetic resonance image signals of a rat brain to changes in the cerebral venous blood oxygenation. *Magn Reson Med*. 1993;29:205–210.
40. Yacoub E, Shmuel A, Pfeuffer J, et al. Imaging brain function in humans at 7 Tesla. *Magn Reson Med*. 2001;45:588–594.

41. Lee S-P, Silva AC, Ugurbil K, Kim S-G. Diffusion-weighted spin-echo fMRI at 9.4T: microvasculuar/tissue contribution to BOLD signal change. *Magn Reson Med*. 1999;42:919–928.
42. Breger RK, Rimm AA, Fischer ME, Papke RA, Haughten VM. $T_1$ and $T_2$ measurements on a 1.5 Tesla commercial imager. *Radiology*. 1989;171: 273–276.
43. Haacke E, Lai S, Yablonskiy D, Lin W. In vivo validation of the BOLD mechanism: A review of signal changes in gradient echo functional MRI in the presence of flow. *Int J Imaging Syst Technol*. 1995;6:153–163.
44. Boxerman JL, Bandettini PA, Kwong KK, et al. The intravascular contribution to fMRI signal change: Monte Carlo modeling and diffusion-weighted studies in vivo. *Magn Reson Med*. 1995;34:4–10.
45. Kennan RP, Zhong J, Gore JC. Intravascular susceptibility contrast mechanisms in tissues. *Magn Reson Med*. 1994;31:9–21.
46. Bandettini PA, Wong EC. Effects of biophysical and physiologic parameters on brain activation-induced R2* and R2 changes: Simulations using a determistic diffusion model. *Int J Imaging Syst Technol*. 1995;6:133–152.
47. Lai S, Hopkins AL, Haacke EM, et al. Identification of vascular structures as a major source of signal contrast in high resolution 2D and 3D functional activation imaging of the motor cortex at 1.5T: preliminary results. *Magn Reson Med*. 1993;30:387–392.
48. Menon RS, Ogawa S, Tank DW, Ugurbil K. 4 Tesla gradient recalled echo characteristics of photic stimulation-induced signal changes in the human primary visual cortex. *Magn Reson Med*. 1993;30:380–386.
49. Kim S-G, Hendrich K, Hu X, Merkle H, Ugurbil K. Potential pitfalls of functional MRI using conventional gradient-recalled echo techniques. *NMR in Biomed*. 1994;7:69–74.
50. Frahm J, Merboldt K-D, Hanicke W, Kleinschmidt A, Boecker H. Brain or vein-oxygenation or flow? On signal physiology in functional MRI of human brain activation. *NMR in Biomed*. 1994;7:45–53.
51. Kim S-G, Ugurbil K. Functional magnetic resonance imaging of the human brain. *J Neurosci Methods*. 1997;74:229–243.
52. Stejskal EO, Tanner JE. Spin diffusion measurements: Spin echoes in the presence of a time-dependent field gradient. *J Chem Physics*. 1965;42: 288–292.
53. Song AW, Wong EC, Tan SG, Hyde JS. Diffusion-weighted fMRI at 1.5T. *Magn Reson Med*. 1996;35:155–158.
54. Zhong J, Kennan RP, Fulbright RK, Gore JC. Quantification of intravascular and extravascular contributions to BOLD. *Magn Reson Med*. 1998;40:526–536.
55. Duong TQ, Yacoub E, Adriany G, Hu X, Ugurbil K, Kim S-G. Microvascular BOLD contribution at 4 and 7 Tesla in the human brain: Diffusion-weighted, gradient-echo and spin-echo fMRI. *Mag Reson Med*. In press.
56. Bandettini PA, Wong EC, Jesmanowicz A, Hinks RS, Hyde JS. Spin-echo and gradient-echo EPI of human brain activation using BOLD contrast: a comparative study at 1.5T. *NMR in Biomed*. 1994;7:12–20.
57. Lowe M, Lurito J, Mattews V, Phillips M, Hutchins G. Quantitative comparison of functional contrast from BOLD-weighted spin-echo and gradient-echo echoplanar imaging at 1.5 Tesla and H215O PET in the whole brain. *J Cereb Blood Flow Metab*. 2000;20:1331–1340.
58. Duvernoy H, Delon S, Vannson J. Cortical blood vessels of the human brain. *Brain Res*. 1981;7:519–579.
59. Hu X, Kim S-G. Reduction of signal fluctuations in functional MRI using navigator echos. *Magn Reson Med*. 1994;31:495–503.

60. Hu X, Le TH, Parrish T, Erhard P. Retrospective estimation and compensation of physiological fluctuation in functional MRI. *Magn Reson Med.* 1995;34:210–221.
61. Malonek D, Grinvald A. Interactions between electrical activity and cortical microcirculation revealed by imaging spectroscopy: Implication for functional brain mapping. *Science.* 1996;272:551–554.
62. Duong TQ, Silva AC, Lee S-P, Kim S-G. Functional MRI of calcium-dependent synaptic activity: Cross correlation with CBF and BOLD measurements. *Magn Reson Med.* 2000;43:383–392.
63. Woolsey TA, Rovainen CM, Cox SB, et al. Neuronal units linked to microvascular modules in cerebral cortex: Response elements for imaging the brain. *Cereb Cortex.* 1996;6:647–660.
64. Kim S-G, Richter W, Ugurbil K. Limitations of temporal resolution in fMRI. *Magn Reson Med.* 1997;37:631–636.
65. Richter W, Andersen PM, Georgopoulos AP, Kim S-G. Sequential activity in human motor areas during a delayed cued movement task studied by time-resolved fMRI. *Neuroreport.* 1997;8:1257–1261.
66. Richter W, Ugurbil K, Georgopoulos AP, Kim S-G. Time-resolved fMRI of mental rotation. *Neuroreport.* 1997;8:3697–3702.
67. Richter W, Somorijai R, Summers R, et al. Motor area activity during mental rotation studied by time-resolved single-trial fMRI. *J Cogn Neurosci.* 2000;12:310–320.
68. Menon R, Kim S-G. Spatial and temporal limits in cognitive neuroimaging with fMRI. *Trends Cogn Sci.* 1999;3:207–215.
69. Duong TQ, Kim S-G. In vivo MR measurements of regional arterial and venous blood volume fractions in intact rat brain. *Magn Reson Med.* 2000;43:393–402.
70. Kim S-G, Tsekos NV, Ashe J. Multi-slice perfusion-based functional MRI using the FAIR technique: Comparison of CBF and BOLD effects. *NMR in Biomed.* 1997;10:191–196.
71. Bandettini PA. The temporal resolution of Functional MRI. In: Moonen CTW, Bandettini PA, eds. Functional MRI. New York: Springer; 1999: 205–220.
72. Duong TQ, Yacoub E, Adriany G, et al. High-resolution, spin-echo BOLD and CBF fMRI at 4 and 7T. *Mag Reson Med.* 2002;48:589–93.

# 2

# fMRI Scanning Methodologies

Alexander B. Pinus and Feroze B. Mohamed

## General Overview

A pervasive and constant challenge in the field of neuroscience is to advance in the understanding of working mechanisms of the human brain and what enacts such complex functions as perception, emotions, and behavior. In areas of clinical psychology, neurophysiology, and neurosciences, it is an ultimate interest to describe neuronal functions quantitatively, as well as qualitatively, under what is considered normal conditions and various disorders, and later use that knowledge for diagnostic purposes.

To investigate these complex concepts, there are a number of techniques developed to detect and characterize neuronal activity of the human brain. In recent years, technical advances in the area of magnetic resonance (MR) research and development tremendously enhanced capabilities of magnetic resonance imaging (MRI) equipment in regard to detection and characterization of minute physiological features, and unprecedentedly widened the number of applications of this modality. Such MRI and nuclear magnetic resonance (NMR) systems with superconducting magnets operating at field strengths of 8 Tesla for human[1] and up to 21 Tesla for animal studies[2,3] have lately become available, allowing extremely fine spatial resolution and considerably improved signal-to-noise ratios (SNRs). The low-noise detection electronics coupled with ultra-fast signal collection algorithms paved the way for new sensitive imaging techniques towards imaging of highly detailed static morphological features, as well as dynamic markers of physiological events and brain functions. The latter may manifest themselves through an intertwined regional changes of such physiological parameters as blood oxygenation and cerebral metabolism, blood flow and volume, and diffusion and perfusion, all of which take place coincidentally.

In the area of the in vivo MRI, various achievements have led to the development of methods of functional MRI (fMRI). Functional MRI is a class of techniques that exploits susceptibility of the magnetic resonance signal to certain physiological properties associated with neuronal activity in general and intrinsic qualities of blood in particular. The most explored and developed fMRI method—Blood Oxygenation Level Dependency (BOLD)—detects tiny changes in magnetic properties of blood caused by metabolic and vascular responses to an elicited neuronal activity.

The brain activity and, in particular, pre-synaptic firings are associated with increased energy demands and are satisfied mainly by way of an oxidative glucose consumption.[4–7] After an onset of a particular brain activity, a nearby feeding arteriole dilates, thus causing the blood flow in downstream capillaries to increase.[8,9] Although during no-stimulus (baseline) conditions, all capillaries are already perfused, brain activity increases the blood flow through the capillaries in an immediate vicinity of active neurons. Because an influx of the blood flow is larger than an increase in oxygen consumption, overall oxygen concentration in blood increases, especially on the venular side of a capillary and further down in venous vessels.[10,11]

Due to such an increase, the blood becomes more oxygenated, which implies that the oxygen dissolved in blood gets bound to partially or fully deoxygenated heme molecules, thus turning deoxyhemoglobin to oxyhemoglobin. In a configuration with bound oxygen, ferrous iron on the heme changes its conformation and becomes more diamagnetic (less paramagnetic) as more oxygen molecules are attached to the heme. Hence, the oxyhemoglobin is more diamagnetic than the deoxyhemoglobin, and, therefore, when placed in the magnetic field of an MR scanner, imparts a different, lesser magnetic susceptibility in regard to the surroundings. The numerical and statistical evaluations of image intensity differences caused by blood magnetic susceptibility during periods of stimulated or spuriously evoked neuronal activity and periods of absence thereof may show neuroanatomical markers of such an activity.

The described phenomenon is the basis of the blood oxygenation level-dependent (BOLD) contrast employed in the fMRI. A quality and an observational value of an MRI study designed to monitor a particular brain function or a number of brain functions involved in a specific physiological or behavioral event depend on assortment of parameters and factors prescribed in a form of MRI pulse sequences.

The imaging pulse sequence is a set of instructions given by a developer to the MR scanner's data acquisition system on how to collect the MR signal and sensitize it to a particular property of the target, which could be of a morphological, functional, or chemical origin. To this end, selectivity of an acquisition protocol usually is accomplished by temporal adjustments of appropriate manipulations with magnitude and phase of the sample's bulk magnetization during the data collection process.

Of particular importance in an MR experiment is to achieve a high SNR and the tissue, or function, or chemical contrast. Higher SNR is achieved by the way of adjusting pulse sequence parameters so that maximum amount of available MR signal returned by a target is captured. Higher contrast is achieved by the way of sensitizing the MR signal to a specific target and, in some cases, suppressing that of the target's surroundings. For instance, in order to perform a routine clinical morphological analysis, MR signal intensities of adjacent tissues have to differ by an amount appreciative to an unaided eye. Similarly, to gain functional information, for instance in a typical BOLD experiment, the nature, structure, and timing of the pulse sequence's manipulations are optimized collect most data when the MR signal related to a studied set of functions is the strongest.

It has been shown that dynamics of the MR signal, especially its decay (relaxation) rates, is dependent on the blood oxygen content.[12,13] In particular, increased magnetic susceptibility caused by the deoxygenation affects $T_2^*$ and $T_2$ relaxation pocesses. Such a dependence may be taken advantage of in fMRI experiments, with pulse sequences purposefully tuned to produce $T_2^*$ or $T_2$ contrast. Such sequences are designed to be sensitive to tiny variations of magnetic fields (microscopic field gradients) induced by changing blood oxygen content. Depending on application objectives, the target's relaxation and MR-related properties, gradient-echo signal formation mechanisms can be used to achieve $T_2^*$ contrast, whereas the spin-echo signal formation algorithms are employed to produce the $T_2$-weighted contrast.

## Spin-Echo and Gradient-Echo Imaging Methods

Conventional single-echo, spin-echo, and gradient-echo signal formation algorithms have been routinely used clinical applications for years, mainly because of their versatility to produce a number of contrasts for various targets. Spin-echo imaging pulse sequences are used in an assortment of anatomical studies to produce $T_1$, $T_2$, and proton density (PD) weighted images; gradient-echo imaging pulse sequences are more likely to be employed in formation of $T_2$ and $T_2^*$ image contrasts, although they are used to render the $T_1$ image contrast, especially in higher-field strength systems. In addition, being sensitive to motion, gradient-echo imaging is used in MR angiography (MRA), volumetric evaluation studies, and those with contrast agents.

Both imaging mechanisms are sensitive to BOLD-associated microscopic field gradients imparted by the neuronal activity. The spin-echo MR signal is susceptible to local gradients due to inflow effects and irreversible diffusion dephasing that introduce $T_2$ weighting. These factors also affect the gradient-echo MR BOLD-coupled signal. Furthermore, the MR signal detected in experiments with gradient-echo pulse sequences reflects conventional reversible $T_2^*$ losses due to the intravoxel field distribution.

### Spin-Echo Formation Mechanism

To generate a spin echo, at least two radio frequency (RF) pulses are required—the first is used to deflect the initial longitudinal magnetization into the transverse plane, and the second is needed to recreate the lost spin phase coherence. Consider the evolution of the transverse

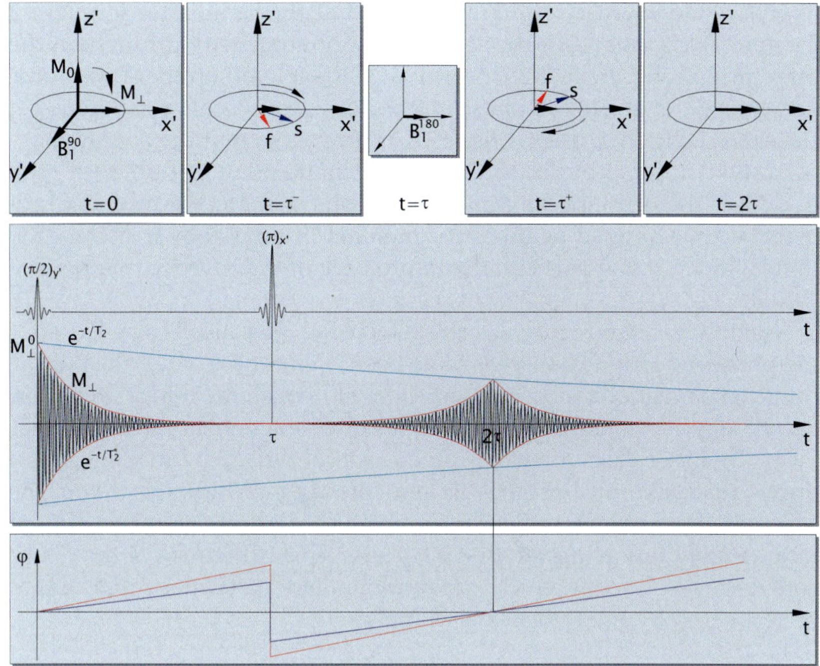


**Figure 2.1.** SE Echo: Evolution, MR Signal, Spin Phase Dynamics.

magnetization and the spin phase in the rotating reference[a] frame, as illustrated in the top portion of the Figure 2.1, and the process of creating the spin echo shown in the laboratory frame[b] in the middle part of the same figure.

At the moment of time $t = 0$, a $\frac{\pi}{2}$-radian RF pulse is applied to the sample along the $y'$ axis, forcing the bulk magnetization into the transverse plane. As the free precession ensues, two isochromats with precessional frequencies $\omega_f > \omega_s > \omega_0$ start to progressively lose coherence and deflect from their original direction along the $x'$ axis. This process lasts until the free precession is somehow disrupted, for instance by another RF pulse applied at the time instance $\tau$. Immediately before time $\tau$ elapses, the isochromats are separated by the phase angle $(\omega_f - \omega_s)\tau^-$; the magnetization has diminished due to the $T_2^*$ relaxation process.

At the moment of time $\tau$, an $x'$-axis–oriented $\pi$-radian pulse is applied that flips both spin isochromats over to the other half of the transverse plane. Consequently, immediately following such an operation, the vector that was ahead is now lagging behind the slower one by the same phase angle that it was leading just prior the $\pi$-radian RF pulse. Because the spin isochromats continue to precess in the same

[a] A precessing frame or reference. Spin isochromats precessing at the Larmor frequency appear stationary.

[b] A stationary frame of reference. All spin isochromats are seen precessing.

direction, clockwise in the graphics, and at the same rates (assuming the spin isochromats see the same field inhomogeneity throughout the echo formation), the faster isochromat starts to gain on the slower one, decreasing the deflection phase angle $-(\omega_f - \omega_s)t$. Because the spins get closer to each other, their coherence improves, so that the overall magnetization starts to build up. After exact same period of time $\tau$ it took to deflect them by the aforementioned phase angle, the two isochromats become aligned again at the moment of time known as the echo time, which, in this particular scenario type of the RF echo, happens at $T_E = 2\tau$.

As shown in the Figure 2.1, the refocusing RF pulse is applied after the phases of individual spins have been "scrambled" and most of the transverse magnetization has vanished. However, the refocusing pulse can be applied even before the transverse magnetization fully fades away. In either case, after the refocusing RF pulse, the magnetization grows gradually and reaches its maximum amplitude. However, the MR signal magnitude at the echo is smaller than the original amplitude immediately following the first RF pulse. This is because of the phase coherence loss encountered from random field fluctuations that cannot be recovered by the refocusing RF pulse.

## Spin-Echo Imaging Pulse Sequence

The pulse sequence that implements the spin-echo measurement is shown in the Figure 2.2. In spin-echo sequences, a $\frac{\pi}{2}$-radian RF pulse typically is applied to excite samples' spin isochromats.

There are generally two excitation regimes, selective and non-selective, with the selectivity referring to a spatial preference of the excitation. The non-selective regime is invoked when no special arrangements are made to associate precessional frequencies of spin isochromats with their positions. Indeed, if all spin isochromats precess at the same frequency, namely the frequency given by the well-known Larmor Equation

$$\omega_0 = \gamma B_0 \tag{2.1}$$

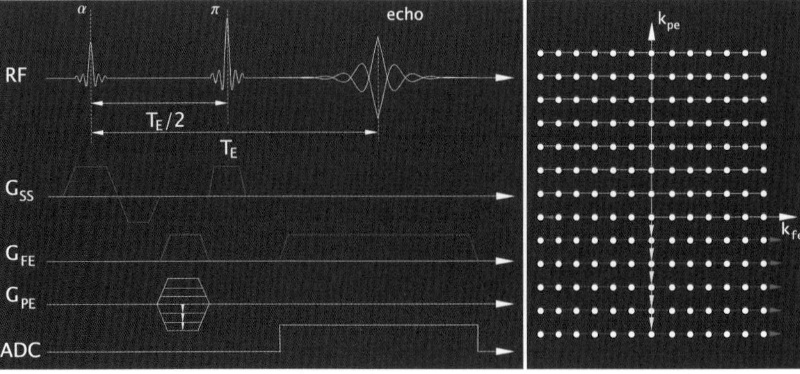


**Figure 2.2.** Spin Echo Timing Diagram.

**Figure 2.3.** The Gradient Field.

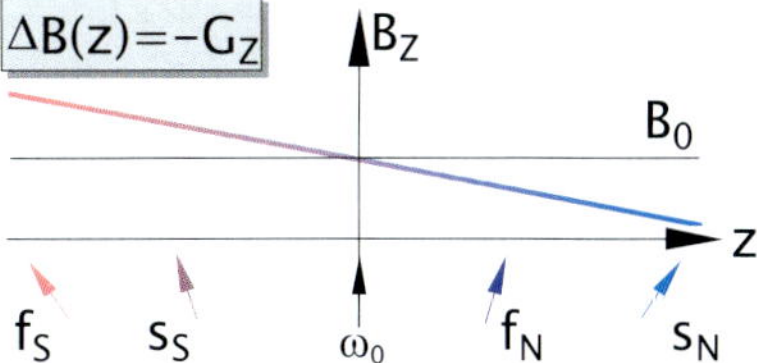


imparted by the static magnetic field $B_0$, it is impossible to tell isochromats apart, and therefore find their position. It also remains infeasible to establish positions of the spin isochromats if precessional rates are affected by local inhomogeneities in a random fashion, or when the inhomogeneity profile is unknown. The RF pulse that affects spins non-selectively is called hard pulse.

In order to spatially differentiate and act on a selected population of spin isochromats, precessional frequencies have to be made a function of position. It typically is achieved by an augmentation of the static magnetic field $B_0$ with a set of supplemental magnetic fields, gradient fields, with known, and usually linear, spatial profiles. Such magnetic fields are a special kind of inhomogeneity that make spin precessional frequency position-dependent in a known fashion.

Indeed, the precessional frequency of the spin isochromat can be evaluated using a slightly modified version of the Equation (2.1), taking into consideration the gradient amplitude. For instance, if the gradient $G_z$ is the field with an amplitude changing along $z$ direction, the precessional frequency of spin isochromats follows the gradient profile, as shown in the Figure 2.3:

$$\omega(z) = \gamma(B_0 + B_{G_z}) = \gamma(B_0 + B_z z) = \gamma\left(B_0 + \frac{\partial B_G}{\partial z} z\right), \tag{2.2}$$

where the amplitude of the applied gradient $G_z$ is given as the spatial partial derivative of the gradient field $B_G$. Similar expressions are valid for the gradients with amplitudes varying along two other axes:

$$\omega(x) = \gamma(B_0 + B_{G_x}) = \gamma(B_0 + G_x x) = \gamma\left(B_0 + \frac{\partial B_G}{\partial x} x\right), \tag{2.3}$$

$$\omega(y) = \gamma(B_0 + B_{G_y}) = \gamma(B_0 + G_y y) = \gamma\left(B_0 + \frac{\partial B_G}{\partial y} y\right). \tag{2.4}$$

The physical magnetic fields $B_{Gx}$, $B_{Gy}$, and $B_{Gz}$ are created by gradient coils, which are current-carrying conductors housed in the MRI system. Because the amplitudes of these fields vary in orthogonal directions, the gradient fields are said to be orthogonal.

When the linear gradient magnetic field

$$B_G = G_x x + G_y y + G_z z \tag{2.5}$$

is added to the static magnetic field $B_0$, precessional frequencies of spin isochromats become varied in all three directions. For a simple case of

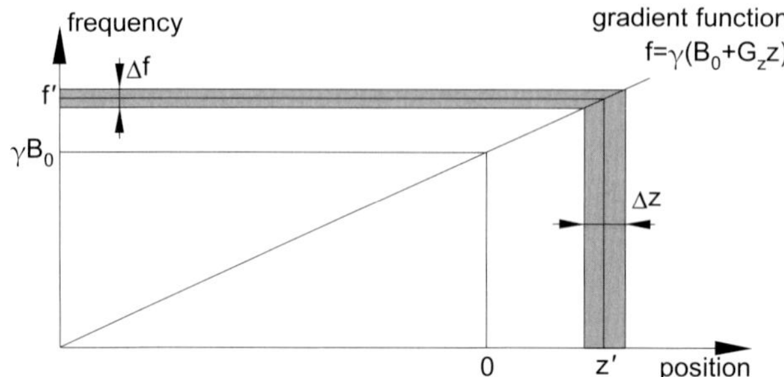


**Figure 2.4.** Position-Frequency Translation.

$$B_G = G_z z = G_{ss} z,$$

the association between the precessional frequency and position of a spin isochromat, as well as the translation of the RF pulse's bandwidth into the slice thickness, is shown in the Figure 2.4. The position of the slice's center $z'$ and its thickness $\Delta z$ can be chosen by varying the central frequency $f'$ and either the gradient's strength $G_z$ (the slope of the line in the graphics) or the bandwidth $\Delta f$ of the RF pulse, respectively. Ultimately, the effect of the gradients on spin isochromats is the separation of their precessional frequencies.

If the RF pulse with a finite bandwidth, and thus a spectrum of frequencies, is applied to a population of spin isochromats frequency-separated by acting gradients fields, only those that are exposed to the pulse and precess at frequencies found within the RF pulse's bandwidth get excited. Such an excitation regime is called selective excitation, and the excitation RF pulse is called a soft pulse.

The arrangement of physical gradients, itself a vector, applied concurrently with RF pulses establishes a direction of the logical gradient called the slice selection gradient, $G_{ss}$. The precessional frequency of spin isochromats follows the shape of the gradient's profile, linearly varying along the gradient's direction.

Because the slice selection gradient makes precessional frequency position-dependent only in the direction of itself, the precessional frequency in two other orthogonal directions is not affected.[c] Therefore, the localization of spin isochromats within the slice remains unfeasible. To that end, the same principle of the position dependency can be applied to localize in-plane spin isochromats.[d]

As the slice selection gradient $G_{ss}$ modulates the precessional frequency of spin isochromats, two similar gradients, frequency encoding ($G_{fe}$) and phase encoding ($G_{pe}$) gradients, are applied to condition spin precessional frequencies in two directions orthogonal to that estab-

[c] An approximation for low gradients, because Maxwell equations demand concomitant fields in orthogonal directions.

[d] That is spin isochromats that lie within the defined slice.

lished by the slice selection gradient. The combination of these gradients defines the spin precessional frequency in the three-dimensional (3D) space. Because each of the gradients defines its own thickness, the trio thus establishes imaging unit volumes—voxels.

The MR signal sample produced by spin isochromats in a particular voxel can be encoded in terms of frequencies varied by the gradient fields. Every such acquired sample of the MR signal comes from spin isochromats precessing at frequencies established by the arrangement of the applied gradients. The entire series of received MR signal samples for all prescribed gradient arrangement, and thus for all necessary precessional frequencies, can be placed conveniently in a matrix. The size of such a matrix and the order in which it gets filled with MR signal samples usually is determined by spatial frequency indices.

Indeed, the precessional frequency of spin isochromats in every voxel within the prescribed slice is defined by an arrangment of in-plane $G_{fe}$ and $G_{pe}$ gradients. Taking into consideration that the gradient field may be a function of time, the indices corresponding to the gradients usually are expressed as integrals of gradient amplitudes over their duration times:

$$k_{ss} = \gamma \int G_{ss} dt, \tag{2.6}$$

$$k_{fe} = \gamma \int G_{fe} dt, \tag{2.7}$$

$$k_{pe} = \gamma \int G_{pe} dt, \tag{2.8}$$

The received MR signal samples are therefore arranged in a form of a matrix, $M(k_{ss}, k_{fe}, k_{pe})$. The location of each spin isochromat is frequency-encoded in such a matrix in terms of spatial frequency $k$ indices, and thus the received MR signal is represented in the spatial frequency space called the $k$-space. The depiction of the MR signal samples that make up the matrix $M(k_{ss}, k_{fe}, k_{pe})$, also known as $k$-space diagram, is shown on the right of the Figure 2.2, where the MR signal samples are represented by solid circles.

A conversion from the frequency-encoded representation of the MR signal, known as the raw MR signal, to its spatially encoded format is performed by a 3D Fourier transformation:

$$m(\mathbf{r}) = \frac{1}{2\pi} \int_{k_{ss}} \int_{k_{fe}} \int_{k_{pe}} M(k_{ss}, k_{fe}, k_{pe}) e^{j(\mathbf{k} \cdot \mathbf{r})} d\mathbf{r}, \tag{2.9}$$

where $\mathbf{r}$ is the basis of the 3D spatial coordinate system. Such a process is known as image reconstruction. This equation implies that the principle prerequisite to the image reconstruction process is the availability of the raw signal matrix, $M(k_{ss}, k_{fe}, k_{pe})$.

After a particular MR signal sample is acquired and recorded into the current element of the raw signal matrix, one or more $k$-indices is incremented and the next MR signal sample is acquired and stored in the successive element of matrix. As the $k$-indices are advanced by changing the amplitudes and timing of the gradients, the current element of the matrix propagates through the *k*-space. This process continues until the entire *k*-space matrix is filled[e] with the MR signal samples. The process of MR signal acquisition and construction of the raw signal matrix often is called the *k*-space coverage.

The *k*-space can be covered in a variety of ways. The most typical coverage path utilized in the majority of conventional pulse sequences is the sequential line-by-line traversal. Its name originates from the appearance of the *k*-space coverage pattern in which the order of placement of the MR signal samples in the *k*-space diagram gives an appearance of the line, as shown by the green arrow on the right of the Figure 2.2.

In order to implement this type of the coverage, one of the in-plane gradients is turned on for a period of time and with the amplitude needed to get the value of the corresponding $k_{pe}$ index advanced to the location of the necessary *k*-space line. Such a move is shown by yellow gradient lobes on the pulse sequence graphics and corresponding arrows in the *k*-space diagram. At the same time, another in-plane gradient, the frequency encoding, is applied to move the index $k_{fe}$ along just-selected *k*-space line to the location of the matrix element that corresponds to a first-to-be-acquired MR signal sample. This advancement is shown by the light blue color. In order to conserve imaging time, these two gradients, respectively called *y*- and *x*-offset gradient pulses, are applied simultaneously and immediately after the slice-selective excitation. The amplitude and duration of these gradients are chosen so that they conclude forwarding corresponding indices to an assigned position in the raw signal matrix before the refocusing π-radian RF pulse is issued, which comes at the moment $t = \tau = \frac{T_E}{2}$ after the initial $\frac{\pi}{2}$-radian excitation RF pulse.

As described in the previous section, the π-radian RF pulse is applied to rephase spins, which were so far dephasing in the transverse plane after the initial excitation pulse. Worth noting again, the effect of such a pulse is the changed character of the precession: faster moving spins now chase slower ones, closing the gap between them. Such a motion causes spins to refocus, hence the refocusing pulse, and regain their in-plane coherence with each other, forming the MR signal echo. The MR signal echo fully develops at $t = 2\tau = T_E$, as indicated in the Figure 2.1. The MR signal acquisition period usually starts immediately after the refocusing pulse, so that the echo would occur in the middle of it. Such an arrangement assures the most efficient imaging conditions with given imaging parameters.

During the signal acquisition period, the detection circuitry and the analog-to-digital converter[f] are turned on to receive and digitize the RF signal from the precessing spin isochromats. Simultaneously, the frequency encoding gradient is turned on in order to encode the preces-

[e] Some pulse sequences fill only a half of the *k*-space, which is then used to compute the other half using a property of the Hermitian complex conjugateness.

[f] Hence the ADC label in the Figure 2.2, and Figure 2.5.

sional frequencies with position. As long as this gradient is applied, the resonance frequency of the spin isochromats is adjusted depending on the gradient's amplitude and moment of time during which a particular sample is acquired. The signal is sampled with the prescribed sampling rate and recorded into the element of the raw MR signal matrix according to the *k*-space indices.

Because the signal sampling takes finite time, the effect of the longitudinal and transverse relaxations on the MR signal has to be taken in to account. That is to say, if the transverse component of the MR signal deteriorates before all samples necessary to reconstruct an image adequately are acquired, the coverage of the *k*-space is performed in several iterations, segments.[g]

In a typical and the most simple *k*-space coverage, such every segment corresponds to a single line. The MR signal acquisition is completed along such a line in a single repetition period,$T_R$. In this case, only one of the *k*-space indices, for instance $k_{fe}$, is incremented, whereas the other in-plane index, $k_{pe}$, is kept constant. When all necessary MR signal samples along the line are acquired, the process moves onto the next iteration, beginning with the next excitation RF pulse. This time, the amplitude of the phase-encoding gradient is incremented between the excitation and refocusing RF pulses so that the corresponding index $k_{pe}$ is advanced to the next *k*-space line. Further on, the detection circuitry is turned on in the presence of the frequency-encoding gradient, and the MR signal is sampled along that *k*-space line.

In the description of the spin-echo formation mechanism and the corresponding pulse sequence, it was presumed that the center of the acquisition window coincides with the center of the *k*-space line. The center of the *k*-space line corresponds to an MR signal sample that has only been encoded partially with spatial information, as one of indices, namely $k_{fe}$, is zero.[h] The center of the acquisition window is taken as a point of time when the phase dispersion created by the offset gradient is compensated fully by the rephasing lobe of the read-out gradient. Only in this case does it become possible to fully eliminate the phase dispersion accrued due to fixed local field inhomogeneities.

Indeed, if the first half of the read-out gradient lasts exactly as long as the *x*-offset gradient and has the same amplitude, the phase of spin isochromats imparted by the gradients is zero in the center of the acquisition window. On the other hand, the phase dispersion developed due to fixed local field inhomogeneities between the excitation and refocusing pulses is nullified by the rephasing following the pulse to form what was described as the spin-echo. Therefore, when the echo time coincides with the center of the *k*-space line, with all other sources of the phase abberations compensated, the overall phase disturbance is imposed only by irreversible random fluctuations due to the $T_2$ relaxation, which are solely responsible for overall image ontrast.

---

[g] In ultra-fast imaging sequences, like echo planar imaging (EPI), the entire *k*-space coverage may be accomplished in a single $T_R$ period.

[h] The center of the *k*-space lacks any spatial information, as both indices, $k_{fe}$ and $k_{pe}$, are zero.

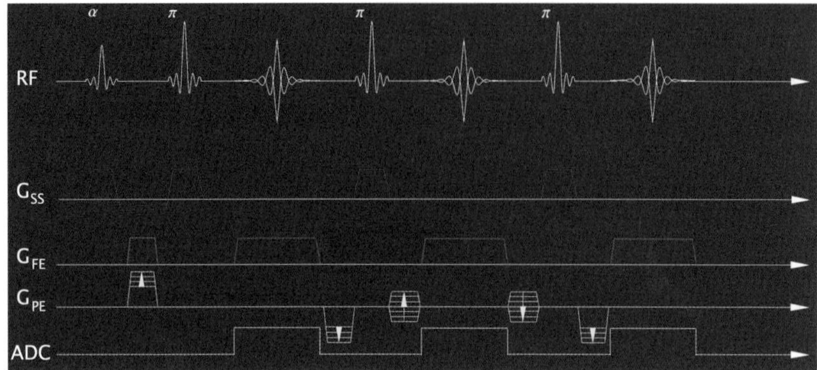


**Figure 2.5.** Fast Spin-Echo Timing Diagram.

However, it is not required for the echo time to match the moment when the *k*-space line's center MR signal sample is acquired along the acquisiton window. The spin-echo can be arranged to occur slightly before or after that particular sample by respectively moving the refocusing pulse toward or away the excitation pulse. The spin-echo is then also moved with it, as it invariably trails the refocusing pulse by exactly the same time as the latter follows the excitation pulse. Therefore, for the spin-echo to occur by a time $\tau$ earlier relative to the center of the *k*-space line, the refocusing pulse has to be transmitted by a time $\frac{\tau}{2}$ earlier than that in the typical symmetrical arrangement. Such an offset spin-echo is referred to as the asymmetric spin-echo (ASE).

No longer in an ASE pulse sequence is the phase dispersion developed out of local inhomogeneities balanced at the moment of passing the *k*-space line's center, thus leaving the MR signal slightly dephased at that time. Because it is the very MR signal sample located in the center of the *k*-space line that contributes the most to the overall image contrast, the magnetic susceptibility effects will be reflected in the final image. Therefore, besides a general $T_2$ contrast, an additional $T_2^*$ weighting is introduced into the MR signal, thus making the ASE pulse sequence more sensitive to the BOLD effect.

It is possible, regardless of the echo position along the acquisition window, to cover several lines in a single iteration. The corresponding pulse sequence diagram is shown in the Figure 2.5.[i] Although there are multiple variations of the multi-echo acquisition scheme, such an arrangement generally is referred to as the fast spin-echo pulse sequence.

In case of such a sequence, a train of echoes is generated after a single excitation pulse by having a manifold of refocusing pulses applied to redirect spin dynamics multiple times. During every formed echo, because the MR signal is sampled along a different line, a distinct phase encoding gradient is needed. The first echo is generated in the same way

---

[i] The $T_R$ has to be adequately short and sampling rate high to allow sufficient amount of the decaying MR signal be detected during the entire acquisition period.

a single spin-echo is formed. However, at the end of the acquisition period, a rewinder gradient is applied in the phase-encoding direction that cancels the effect of the preceding phase-encoding gradient. Such a manipulation is tantamount to a resetting of the $k_{pe}$ index back to zero. Following the first echo, spin isochromats are allowed to continue to dephase. At some point into the dephasing process, another $\pi$-radian pulse is transmitted. The effect of this pulse on spins is exactly the same as that of the original refocusing pulse, namely, it swaps around faster and slower precessing spins. Immediately after the refocusing pulse, another phase-encoding gradient is applied. However, this time its amplitude is set to advance the $k_{pe}$ to a different $k$-space line. The number of formed echoes, and thus the number of covered $k$-space lines, is given as the imaging parameter called echo train length (ETL). A number of echoes can be generated following a single RF excitation pulse, and the total acquisition time is reduced as many times as large as the ETL is.

When the entire raw signal matrix is completed for the selected slice, the process is started anew, either to acquire and average more signal for the same slice or to proceed onto another slice.

## Contrast Characteristics of Spin-Echo Sequences

### *Vascular Effects*

It was briefly mentioned that although the $\pi$-radian pulse refocuses acquired phase offsets by dephasing spin isochromats due to existing inhomogeneities, the phase coherence at the echo time is never restored to the pre-excitation level. Indeed, only in case of a particular spin isochromat seeing a fixed inhomogeneity throughout the acquisition can a phase angle acquired by this spin isochromat before the refocusing pulse be fully balanced out by the phase displacement that the spin isochromat experiences after the refocusing pulse. In other words, in order to fully restore spin coherence, the precessional frequency of a particular spin isochromat has to remain the same throughout the repetition period.

In reality, however, the precessional frequency of spin isochromats constantly experiences tiny aberrations that are largely imparted by the process of diffusion. A diffusing water molecule drifts in a random fashion through inhomogeneity gradients established by various physical factors, including the magnetic susceptibility caused by the BOLD effect. The degree to which the diffusion influences the spin-echo MR signal depends on the spatial range of inhomogeneities in regard to the motion extent a water molecule travels during the acquisition. If inhomogeneities vary significantly only over far larger distances that a wandering water molecule can possibly travel, then it is likely that the spin isochromats experience the same field before and following the refocusing pulse. In this case, the spin-echo is fully refocused and the MR signal does not carry the imprint of inhomogeneities. Conversely, a moving water molecule does change fields if the range of distances it travels is larger than the spatial scale of inhomogeneities. Because water molecules diffuse rather quickly, it is likely that the phase dispersion developed by molecules between two pulses is not refocused by the time of the echo, thus leaving some dephasing to last through the echo and to attenuate the MR signal.

This line of thinking can be used in determining how the vessel size impacts the spin-echo MR signal: Because the spatial extent of inhomogeneities originated from the larger structures such as venulae and arteriola spans further than that of capillaries, the diffusion-related reduction of the MR signal in capillary-rich areas is stronger than in vicinities of larger vessels. Such an argument can be substantiated by assessing the average diffusion-induced displacement a water molecule sustains and comparing it with the average vessel's size.

The average displacement $\langle L \rangle$ over time $t$ of a randomly moving particle can be estimated from the Einstein's diffusion equation:

$$\langle L^2 \rangle = 6\mu kTt = 6Dt, \tag{2.10}$$

where $k \approx 1.38 \cdot 10^{-23} \left[\frac{m^2 kg}{s^2 K}\right]$ – Boltzmann's constant; $T$ is the temperature in Kelvins; the quantity $D = \mu kT$ is called the diffusion coefficient, and $\mu$ is the mobility coefficient that can be expressed through the average time between collisions $\tau_c$ and molecular mass $m$:

$$\mu = \frac{\tau_c}{m}. \tag{2.11}$$

Every particle experiences about $10^{14}$ collisions per second on average, which means that it spends $10^{-14}$ seconds between collisions.[14(p41–48)] The mass of a water molecule is $3 \cdot 10^{-26}$ kilograms. With these values, the diffusion coefficient is on the order of $D \simeq 10^{-9} \left[\frac{m^2}{s}\right]$. It is now possible to estimate the average displacement. Because only the in-plane displacement alters relaxation rates, the corrected expression for the average displacement is now

$$\langle L^2 \rangle = 4Dt. \tag{2.12}$$

Taking $t$ = 100 milliseconds, a typical echo time in case of the spin-echo pulse sequence, the average displacement is estimated at 20 micrometers.

It is therefore expected that the effect of diffusion in areas of venulae larger than 20 micrometers in diameter gradually diminishes reversely proportional to the venule's size. This is due to the fact that the spin-echo is refocused relatively better because the water molecule spends more time in the same field. Consequently, the MR signal is changed ever so slightly. In the areas of smaller venulae and larger capillaries, their diameter being on the order of 10 to 20 micrometers, the water molecule experiences different fields as it wanders in a near vicinity of vessels; hence, the spin-echo is poorly refocused and the MR signal is relatively weaker. For even smaller vessels, mostly capillaries with the lumen's diameter below 10 micrometers, the phase dispersion at the moment of spin-echo is even stronger as water molecules transgress even a larger number of fields. Therefore, it is tempting to expect relaxation rates to increase and the MR signal to lessen further. However, in this case, the average phase dispersion encountered by all water molecules is very similar, as it is more likely that they cross over the same fields. A similar phase dispersion is tantamount to a very little phase dispersion. Therefore, counterintuitively, the spin-echo MR signal coming from areas of very small vessels, namely less than five micrometers in diameter, is in fact comparable to that acquired near the largest vessels.

Thus, the spin-echo MR signal is strongest in areas of very small and very large vessels and dips to its minimum around vessels that measure about 20 micrometers in diameter. Due to such a bell-shaped dependence of the spin-echo MR signal on the vessel's size, the spin-echo sequences are desirable to use in BOLD experiments, as the spin-echo MR signal is sensitized to the BOLD-related oxy/deoxygenated exchanges that occur in capillaries.

### *Flow Effects*

The contrast produced by the spin-echo sequences is sensitive to inflow effects and becomes apparent on $T_2$-weighted images. Implications of the inflow effects on the MR signal are caused primarily by spin isochromats that were brought into the region of the excited imaging volume by the blood flow following the $\frac{\pi}{2}$-radian excitation RF pulse.

It has been discussed earlier that only spin isochromats that initially get excited by the RF excitation pulse can return RF photons and thus contribute to the overall MR signal. Moreover, because the transverse component of the bulk magnetization is solely responsible for production of the MR signal, it is desirable to have initial large longitudinal components of as many spins as possible be transferred to the transverse plane by the excitation RF pulse in order to increase MR signal generation capacity. Finally, the refocusing RF pulse acts to minimize relative phase differences between transverse components of processing spins and to restore the spin coherence in the transverse plane, thus yielding larger bulk magnetization and a stronger MR signal.

Consider fresh, undisturbed spins moving into already excited imaging volume. Because these spins enter between the excitation and refocusing RF pulses, they are exposed only to the $\pi$-radian RF pulse, which is, in effect, an excitation pulse for them, whereas it acts as a refocusing pulse for already excited spins. Unlike the latter, the freshly entered spins are forced into the excited state by the $\pi$-radian RF pulse. As the name of the pulse assumes, a bulk magnetization built out of these spins is rotated by 180 degrees, all the way from being oriented colinearly with the $B_0$ to the opposite direction, thus remaining in the longitudinal plane. Therefore, such a magnetization ends up having a very small transverse component so its contribution to the MR signal generation capacity is greatly reduced. The spins that make up the 180-degree deflected magnetization eventually will return to the unexcited state, contributing little to nothing to the overall MR signal.

In the meantime, a portion of those spins within the blood that were excited along with all other stationary spins were forced to leave the imaging volume by the fresh incoming blood. The spins forced out from the imaging volume before the refocusing pulse was applied to the same imaging volume contribute a negligible amount of the MR signal during the acquisition period because they remained dephased and did not undergo the refocusing. Those excited spins that did experience the refocusing pulse before exiting the imaging volume during the acquisition period do contribute to the MR signal. However, because their space-frequency association is now broken by the blood flow motion, they generate the MR signal that is originated from outside of the selected imaging volume, and therefore can now be regarded as flow artifacts.

The actual number of spins leaving and entering the imaging volume depends on timing characteristics of the sequence, size and position of the excited volume, and the parameters of the flow. If the time between the excitation and refocusing pulses is relatively shorter, a smaller number of excited spins is replaced by fresh ones; therefore, the MR signal would be suppressed to a lesser degree.

From another perspective, the time between the two pulses is equal to $\frac{T_E}{2}$. Therefore, it is optimal to keep the echo time short enough to reduce the inflow suppression, but long enough to collect sufficient amount of the MR signal with BOLD contrast. It was shown that such an optimal echo time is on the order of the $T_2$ relaxation time of the examined tissue.[15]

Because the echo time is usually much shorter than the repetition time for the spin-echo sequences, the inflow suppression would become significant only for relatively high flow velocities, which typically do not occur in the capillaries and small venulae, the primary source of the BOLD contrast.

## Gradient-Echo Formation Mechanism

As has already been shown, the refocusing RF pulse is essential for the spin-echo formation, as it rephases spin isochromats and leads to reappearance of the transverse magnetization. However, the rephasing action and refocusing effect of the RF pulse also can be achieved if gradient fields are employed to modulate spin phase in a controlled fashion. The MR signal is then recovered in the form of a gradient-echo generated only through gradient reversals.

Consider the gradient-echo formation mechanism in an example with a system of four spin isochromats at different locations along the z axis, so that $z_{f_S} = -z_{f_N}$ and $z_{s_S} = -z_{s_N}$[j], as shown in the Figure 2.3. The application of the gradient field makes spins in the North half precess slower than those in the South half. Indeed, because of the additional gradient field, the two South spins experience higher than $B_0$ field, and they precess slightly faster in regard to the spin unaffected by the gradient field, thus precessing at the angular rate of $\omega_0$. Of these two South spins, the one closer to the center of the field, $s_S$, precesses at slower rate because the field deviation at the location of this spin is less and its precessing frequency is closer to the $\omega_0$. Similarly, for the North

[j] The subscripts $_f$ and $_s$ stand for fast and slow. The subsubscripts $_S$ and $_N$ stand for South and North.

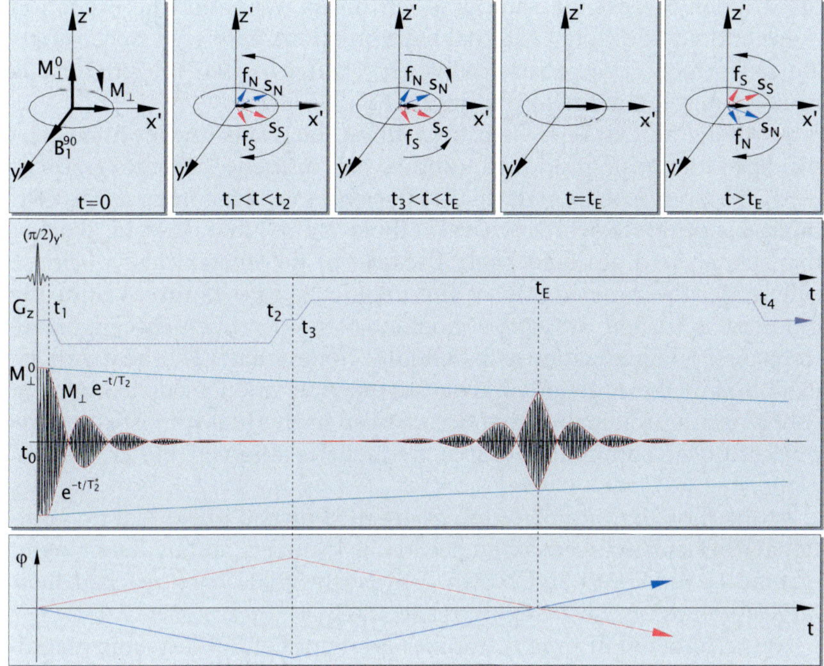


**Figure 2.6.** Gradient-Echo: Evolution, MR Signal, Spin Phase Dynamics.

section where the magnetic field is less that $B_0$, the spins precess generally slower than in the South section, with the one further from the center of the field, $s_N$, precessing slower than the $f_N$ spin.

Therefore, the main effect of the applied gradient field is an introduced spatially depended precessional frequency that makes spin isochromats precess at rates controlled by the amplitude of the applied gradient field. With such a dependence on the gradient field, the generation of the gradient echo can be explained phenomenologically and graphically, as is illustrated in the top of the Figure 2.6.

An excitation $\frac{\pi}{2}$-radian RF pulse[k] is applied at the moment of time $t = 0$, putting the longitudinal magnetization into the transverse plane. Immediately at the end of the excitation pulse, all spin isochromats precess at the same rate. However, naturally occurring spatially varying field inhomogeneities and energy-dissipating interactions between spins[l] change precessional rates, causing spin isochromats to become out of phase with each other. The dephasing is a time-dependent process, increasing linearly with time. The dephasing among individual spin isochromats ultimately leads to decreased aggregate transverse magnetization; therefore, the recoverable MR signal in the process known as *Free Induction Decay* (FID). The FID connotes the MR signal loss due to naturally occurring phenomena taking

[k] In the fast imaging applications, a smaller flip angle can be used, anywhere from $\frac{\pi}{6}$ to $\frac{\pi}{2}$.

[l] $T_2^*$ and $T_2$ types relaxation, respectively.

place when the excited sample is left on its own after the excitation pulse and no additional external manipulations with spin isochromats are performed. The picture, however, changes when the gradient is turned on at the moment of time $t = t_1$.

Applying an extra gradient field along the $z$ axis further intensifies the spin dephasing. Indeed, under the influence of the gradient field, the spin isochromats that experience stronger than usual field rapidly spring forward whereas those spins that sustain weaker than usual field are held back. Because of the general loss of phase coherence, the rapid decay of the magnetization continues until the gradient is turned off at the moment of $t = t_2$, when the aggregate transverse magnetization is essentially nonexistent. The beat pattern exhibited by the aggregate transverse magnetization is due to transient coherence improvements that occur when individual spin isochromats precessing at common multiple frequencies align in the transverse plane.

At the moment of time $t_2$, the gradient is turned off so that no additional gradient-induced coherence loss is incurred, and by the moment of time $t_3$, the South and North spin isochromats have reached their largest values of phase angles, respectively.

At the moment of time $t_3$, another gradient field of the same magnitude and direction, but opposite polarity, is applied to the sample. This gradient field forces previously fast-moving spin isochromats to slow down and assume precessional frequency of the spins that earlier were trailing during the dephasing portion. In a similar manner, the previously slow-moving spins are now chasing those that were moving faster during the dephasing segment. Assuming that the spin isochromats were forced to dephase from the state of full transverse coherence and ignoring the irrecoverable energy-dissipating losses due to interactions between spins[m], the spin isochromats rephase and recreate the transverse coherence exactly after the period of time it took to dephase them, that is, $\tau$. The reinstated coherence is tantamount to a restored aggregate transverse magnetization, and thus newly formed echo; in this case, a gradient-echo.

It can be inferred that the amplitudes of the dephasing and rephasing lobes of the gradient may not be equal, such that the larger amplitude of the rephasing lobe expedites the coherence recovery. However, common to all gradient echo-like signal generation schemes is the combination of the dephasing and rephasing gradient lobes.

### Gradient-Echo Imaging Pulse Sequence

An implementation of a simplest—Fast Low Angle SHot (FLASH)[n]—gradient-echo pulse sequence is shown in Figure 2.7. The design of the gradient sequence includes such components common to all imaging pulse sequences such as the excitation structure, comprised of the RF excitation pulse and the slice selection gradient with the following

[m] As mentioned earlier, such loses are characterized by $T_2$ relaxation time.

[n] Here and further in text the Siemens nomenclature is used.

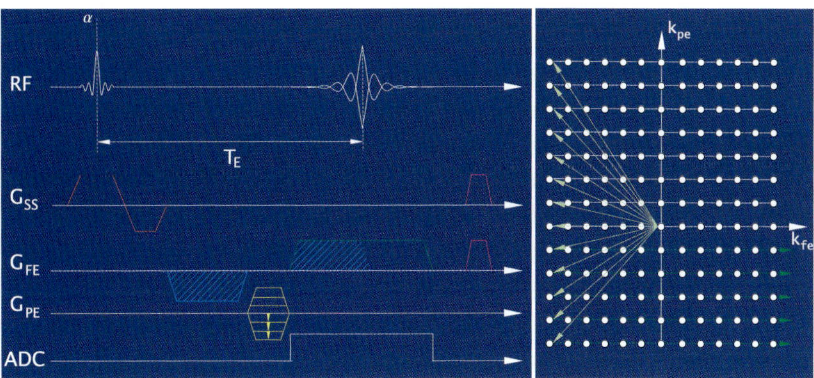


**Figure 2.7.** Gradient-Echo Timing Diagram.

rephasing lobe, and the data collection segment during which the echo is generated and associated MR signal is received. Moreover, it may include additional gradients called spoilers, which are employed to avoid a transverse steady state.

The spatial encoding in a conventional gradient-echo sequence is achieved in the same manner in which it is accomplished for the spin-echo counterpart. In particular, the spatial encoding in one of the directions is performed by conditioning spin isochromats' precessional frequency (the *frequency*-encoding direction), whereas the spatial information in the other direction is encoded by modulating the phase angle of spin isochromats (the phase-encoding direction). During the frequency-encoding period, the scanner's receiver circuitry is turned on and the MR signal returned by spin isochromats is recorded as the raw MR signal.

In the noticeable difference from the spin-echo implementation, the gradient-echo pulse sequence design does not retain a π-radian refocusing pulse. The lack of thereof is rather consequential. First, in the absence of the refocusing pulse, the RF power released by the coil and thus absorbed by tissues is reduced significantly. This factor makes sequences utilizing the gradient-echo signal recovery mechanism safer and more desirable in general. The reduced-energy deposition in the case of the gradient-echo sequence is especially salient when performed in higher field strength scanners (1.5 Tesla and up) because it requires larger amounts of RF energy to disturb a longitudinal equilibrium magnetization. Moreover, with the overall RF energy emission reduced, it is possible to pack more RF pulses closer together and therefore speed up the signal acquisition without a risk of exceeding Specific Absorbtion Rate (SAR) limits established by the U.S. Food and Drug Administration (FDA).

The absence of the refocusing pulse affects the sensitivity of gradient-echo sequences to magnetic field inhomogeneities and, consequently, the type of image contrast. The main effect of the refocusing pulse used in the spin-echo formation mechanism is achieved by nullifying phase angles of spin isochromats and reversing the direction of the dephasing. Therefore, phase angles developed due to constant field inhomogeneities and magnetic susceptibilities are cancelled by the time of the echo.[o] Therefore, the spin-echo sequence has an inherent property to suppress MR signal contributions from large fixed inhomogeneities.

On the contrary, because it lacks the refocusing pulse, the gradient-echo sequence is very much sensitive to field inhomogeneities and magnetic susceptibilities. Indeed, instead of an RF refocusing pulse, the gradient-echo imaging pulse sequence employs a structure that contains alternating gradients to re-establish coherence of spin isochromats and generate the echo, as it is shown in the Figure 2.7. The overall phase change introduced by the gradients by the echo time is zero, as the phase change during the rephase segment is offset by the opposite phase change during the following dephasing segment. However, such a gradient reversal can only compensate for the spin phase gained or lost due to the gradient field itself. Any amount of spin phase advanced or retarded due to factors other than gradients fields, such as effects of sample-related magnetic susceptibilities, remain uncompensated at the echo time. In other words, phase angles, neither refocused nor compensated, continue to develop through the entire echo formation period, and thus are non-zero at the time of an echo, effectively reducing the MR signal.

Because the spin coherence is achieved by having reversal gradients to nullify spin phase changes, thus rendering the refocusing pulse unnecessary, the repetition time $T_R$ now can be made shorter. Having been given less time to die down, the spin coherence at the end of the signal detection period turns out to be higher than that in the spin-echo case,[p] leaving a relatively stronger transverse magnetization to linger before the next excitation pulse.

In addition to the increased transverse coherence, the effects of consecutive RF pulses on the magnetization should be mentioned. It is known that a series of several arbitrary RF pulses is capable of producing spin echoes and so called stimulated echoes.[16] Generally, such echoes are not treated as a primary source of the gradient-echo MR signal, and thus are disregarded in the majority of gradient-echo pulse sequences. However, if allowed to propagate freely and undisturbed throughout subsequent repetition periods, the lingering magnetization responsible for the formation of such echoes may affect the gradient echoes formed later, and is likely to cause imaging artifacts. Moreover, coupled with the aforementioned enhanced transverse magnetization, the artifacts may have very consequential ramifications on the MR signal in pulse sequences where either transverse or longitudinal magnetization is maintained in the steady state.

There are two ways to mitigate the effects of unwanted MR signal echoes—to destroy the lingering transverse magnetization with addi-

[o] The field inhomogeneities and magnetic susceptibilities are assumed constant over the single $T_R$.

[p] It is due to the fact that less transverse magnetization is lost to irreversible $T_2$ relaxation.

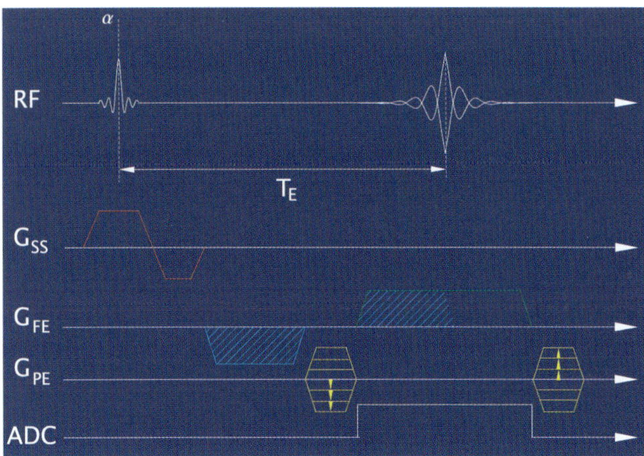


**Figure 2.8.** FISP Pulse Sequence Timing Diagram.

tional gradient fields or RF pulses, or to refocus magnetization components leading to formation of spin and stimulated echoes.

The methods of the first group use either additional gradients alone or coupled with quasi-random flip-angle RF pulses to further and irreversibly[q] dephase spins in the transverse plane, effectively destroying the remnant aggregate transverse magnetization. With the bulk transverse magnetization essentially nonexistent, only longitudinal component of the aggregate magnetization contributes to the fresh bulk transverse magnetization at the next RF pulse, which is during the next $T_R$ period.

Alternative to the mechanism of spoiling of the bulk transverse magnetization is the process of refocusing its components, contributing to formation of spin and stimulated echoes. The first sequence to take advantage of the refocusing was fast imaging with steady precession (FISP).[17] In the most trivial way, it is achieved by adding an extra phase-encoding gradient to the existing FLASH-like pulse sequence, as shown in the Figure 2.8. Its function is to compensate for the phase change introduced by the initial phase-encoding gradient step. For that purpose, the new gradient has the same magnitude as the initial phase-encoding gradient field; however, it is applied in the opposite direction. The partial rephasing of the transverse magnetization allowed an additional $T_2$-weighted signal be recovered from refocused spin and stimulated echoes.

The reversal of gradients just in the direction of the phase encoding does not fully rephase transverse magnetization. Indeed, the phase of spin isochromats is changed by any disturbance, leading to the Larmor frequency variation, regardless of directionality of the such. In order to attain a fully refocused transverse magnetization and the largest

---

[q] So that the transverse magnetization created in this repetition period does not reform sometime later.

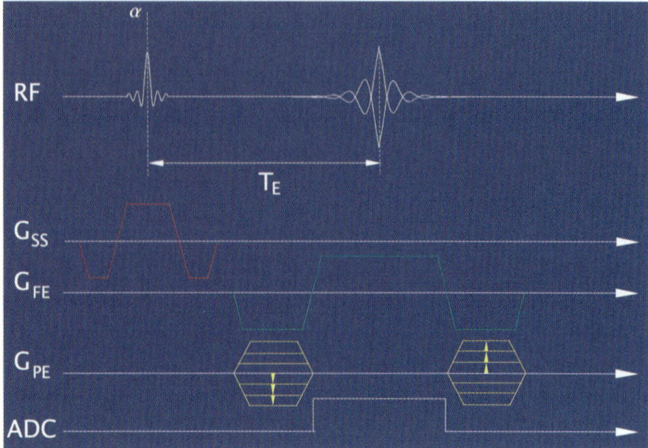


**Figure 2.9.** trueFISP Pulse Sequence Timing Diagram.

possible MR signal, the area under gradient lobes has to be zero in all three directions.

This approach is implemented in the pulse sequence known as trueFISP. The design of the trueFISP sequence (Figure 2.9) contains a train of equally spaced RF pulses and gradient structures balancing the phase in all three directions. Having the phase of the transverse magnetization at the end of the repetition period restored to its prepulse value improves overall transverse coherence, and thus the SNR while maintaining a relatively short $T_R$ and higher receiver bandwidth. The recent studies showed that the trueFISP sequences are capable of recovering a relatively strong BOLD signal.[18]

### Contrast Characteristics of Gradient-Echo Sequences

#### *Vascular Effects*

As in the case with the spin-echo pulse sequences, the diffusing motion of water molecules is a crucial and defining factor in the development of the gradient-echo contrast. The nature of diffusion effects is again due to microscopic phase variations that the water molecule experiences as it traverses through magnetic field gradients established by nearby vessels. However, although identical by nature, the diffusion effects are exhibited somewhat differently in case of the gradient-echo pulse sequences.

If the spatial extent of field variations created by larger venule vessels spans over distances larger than a diffusing molecule travels on average, it experiences a very similar field at any point of its trajectory. Without a refocusing pulse, the average phase displacement acquired by molecules due to these offset fields is increased linearly as a function of time and is not compensated at the end of the acquisition period. Consequently, due to the procured dephasing, the relaxation rate increases and the MR signal is weakened to a relatively higher degree.

When water molecules traverse several fields over their trajectory's average length, the phase offsets gained by water molecules are very similar; therefore, the range of phase offsets is minimal, as is the overall dephasing. The $T_2$ relaxation rate, and thus the MR signal, remain largely unaffected. Such an attenuation regime is identical to that achieved with the spin-echo formation mechanism for vessels up to six micrometers in diameter.

The extent to which the MR signal is attenuated depends on the amount of the phase offset that spin isochromats accumulate during their traversal through field gradients over a specific time, usually the echo time $T_E$. Therefore, it can be inferred that the relaxation rate increases with the vessel's size.

It is noteworthy to compare the sensitivity of spin- and gradient-echo formation mechanisms to the BOLD-related changes as a function of vessel's size. It has been mentioned previously in this chapter that the spin-echo pulse sequences appears to be most sensitive to diffusion effects occurring in capillaries. In contrast, the sensitivity of the gradient-echo sequence reaches its maximum towards larger structures, like venulae and small veins.

*Inflow Effects*

The impact that the blood inflow has on the gradient-echo MR signal mechanism is quite different from that on the MR signal recovered in a spin-echo. In the case of the spin-echo sequence, contrary to the MR signal reduction caused by unexcited spins flowing into a region partially saturated after a series of closely following excitation pulses, the inflow of unsaturated spins leads to the increase of the MR signal collected by the gradient-echo sequence.

Consider an imaging slice with a vessel carrying flowing blood surrounded by stationary tissues. Continuous application of RF excitation pulses designed to nutate the longitudinal magnetization into the transverse plane by partial flip angles[r] may cause a condition called saturation. The spin ensemble within stationary tissues becomes saturated after a considerable number of RF pulses are transmitted in a rapid succession, each released before the longitudinal magnetization is allowed to recover fully to its equilibrium value, $M_0$. During the allotted time, $T_R$, only so much of the longitudinal magnetization gets restored so that at the end of current $T_R$ period

$$M_z < M_0.$$

This implies that not all spins excited by the last excitation pulse have radiated RF photons and are returned to their stable state, and the next RF excitation pulse acts on the longitudinal magnetization $M_z$, which is restored only partially. Similarly, at the end of the next repetition interval, the longitudinal magnetization is not given to relax to its pre-pulse value, $M_z$, so that even less of the fresh longitudinal magnetization is available to be acted upon by the following excitation pulse.

---

[r] Partial is any flip angle which causes less than $\frac{\pi}{2}$-radian nutation.

Thus, each following RF pulse acts on smaller longitudinal magnetization than the previous one.

On the other hand, each RF pulse brings a magnitude of the longitudinal magnetization to the same value, since the RF pulse's flip angle is kept constant.[s] Because the magnitude of the pre-pulse longitudinal magnetization is falling and its post-pulse magnitude is maintained, it can be inferred that the reduction of the longitudinal magnetization gradually[t] ceases after a certain number of RF pulses. Such dynamics imply that the magnitude of the longitudinal magnetization becomes confined between its pre- and post-pulse values throughout the entire $T_R$ interval. This happens when the number of excited spins returned to their stable state is equal to the number of spins excited by the following RF pulse.

Because few spins get excited by a new RF pulse and consequently return the signal at the end of the $T_R$ interval, the pre-pulse magnitude of the longitudinal magnetization is only slightly different from its post-pulse value; thus, the amount of available MR signal from stationary tissues is reduced. On the other hand, fresh spins contained in the blood entering the imaging slice are not saturated at all because they did not experience all previous excitations. The spins from the flowing blood enter the imaging slice and become slightly saturated as they pass through it. Since less saturated spins are capable of returning higher MR signal than the more saturated, such a dynamic leads to an intense MR signal coming from the blood. The differences between sufficiently saturated stationary tissues and partially saturated moving blood can therefore be identified in the image contrast.

The degree of saturation sustained by the blood spins largely depends on the blood flow velocity, the $T_R$ interval, and the amount of the RF energy transferred to the spins, which is tantamount to the flip angle. The increase of the MR signal occurs when the sufficient number of unsaturated spins enter the imaging slice over several $T_R$ periods. In case of the relatively short $T_R$ or a fast blood flow, the MR signal increases due to the partial desaturation by the fresh spins. However, with the longer $T_R$ period, a larger number of the saturated spins may have sufficient time to return to the equilibrium so that the signal from stationary tissues increases and the contrast with the blood MR signal diminishes. In case of a relatively slower blood flow, for instance capillary flux, it may take a few more $T_R$ intervals for entered spins to pass through the imaging slice. Experiencing more RF pulses, blood spin isochromats become more saturated, which also equalizes the contrast between MR signals from stationary tissues and blood.

In addition to their inflow sensitivity, the gradient-echo methods are likely—more so than those of a spin-echo variety—to produce an MR signal that reflects sample-induced magnetic susceptibilities and

---

[s] Of course, variable flip angles are possible,[19] however consideration of such is beyond of this chapter's scope.

[t] As a matter of fact, exponentially, with the exponent's power being negative.[20,p127]

scanner-related field inhomogeneities. Generally, the increased sensitivity of the gradient-echo methods to such perturbations originates from uncompensated spin phase contributions developed during an MR signal echo's formation.

Indeed, a spatially dependent field distribution gives rise to a corresponding spatially varying distribution of the Larmor frequency. In this case, even adjacent spin isochromats may happen to precess at slightly different frequencies, leading to the phase dispersion and loss of the aggregate transverse magnetization. As was pointed out in the previous section, it is due to the absence of a refocusing pulse that the phases acquired by spin isochromats due to sustained inhomogeneities other than gradient fields do not get cancelled, but rather continue to develop until the echo time. On top of a distribution of fixed Larmor frequency-affecting factors, there are various effects that further modulate local field: random motion of water molecules (diffusion), varying magnetic properties of blood and tissues (oxygenation/deoxygenation), and eddy currents.

Sample-induced susceptibilities alter local magnetic fields, thus causing inhomogeneities. The effects created by sample-related susceptibilities usually can be seen as signal enhancement/reduction near tissue–tissue and, even to a larger degree, tissue–air interfaces. Furthermore, image distortions may be observed in or near regions with cavities and sinuses, where the inhomogeneities are high.

Only in part does the severity of image distortions depend on the degree of the inhomogeneity. Equally consequential are the imaging parameters, such as receiver bandwidth, direction of phase encoding, image resolution, and others. The imaging parameters have to be changed with caution and with the understanding of the implications of such changes. For instance, raising the receiver bandwidth mitigates image distortions, especially so in the phase-encoding directions. However, it also would decrease the SNR.

## Echo Planar Imaging Methods

The generic gradient-echo sequence displayed in the Figure 2.7 acquires $n$ MR signal samples sequentially, one by one, along a single chose $k$-space line per an excitation period. Therefore, it has to be repeated $n$ times in order to create a $n \times n$-pixel image.[u] The acquisition time is reduced in the steady-state sequences, for their $T_R$ values usually are shorter than that of a conventional FLASH-like gradient-echo methods. Although either of these sequences can be used to detect gross BOLD-related MR signal variations originated in areas that are capable of producing a relatively robust signal, such as visual or motor cortices, they are proved to be unfittingly sluggish to adequately resolve rather fine BOLD effects elicited by swift subtle cognitive and behavioral processes.

---

[u] A trivial case is considered here, as the $n \times n$ pixel image also can be created from the undersampled MR signal pool using various reconstruction tricks.

The pulse sequence tailored for imaging of physiological markers of transient events and processes would acquire the MR signal needed to reconstruct the entire image in the shortest time possible, at the same time lasting sufficiently long enough for BOLD-inducing factors influencing the MR signal to develop. The demand for higher temporal resolution necessitates more rapid MR signal sampling. Certainly, the shortest acquisition time is attained when the entire *k*-space is covered after a single excitation pulse. The group of imaging methods that traverse the *k*-space in a single passing shot, or in a series of multiple shots or segments, make up a class of Echo Planar Imaging (EPI) techniques.

It is noteworthy to mention that although the EPI methods belong to the distinct class of imaging techniques, they are not based on nor do they establish entirely new acquisition principles. As a matter of fact, EPI pulse sequences use the same echo-formation mechanisms as spin- or gradient-echo methods, with an exception that they are very quick to traverse the entire *k*-space, and thus offer a drastic improvement in acquisition time.

## Echo Planar Imaging Pulse Sequences

As implied above, unlike the collection strategy employed in the conventional imaging that repeats excitation-sampling pair over every *k*-space line, a typical EPI pulse sequence collects and spatially encodes all MR signal samples necessary for a subsequent reconstruction of the entire image in a single acquisition period following an excitation pulse.

The schematics of a generic EPI pulse sequence is shown in Figure 2.10. Initially, a pair of gradients is applied in both the phase- and frequency-encoding directions in order to advance to the first sample point of the first *k*-space line. Then an oscillatory gradient is applied along the frequency-encoding direction so that the train of echoes is generated, each for every gradient lobe, positive or negative.

Such a waveform of the read-out gradient establishes alternating directions of traversing the read-out lines, whereas brief blip phase-encoding gradient pulses shift the current *k*-space location from one line to another in the phase-encoding direction. Such waveforms of the phase- and frequency-encoding gradients draw the zig-zag *k*-space trajectory shown in the right of Figure 2.10. As it can be seen on the *k*-space diagram, each line comes through the point of $k_x = 0$. This is the moment of time when the line-echo is formed. Each echo is produced in the same fashion as the gradient-echo, that is via an application of the bipolar dephasing–rephasing gradient structure. After every echo, the phase-encoding gradient advances the trajectory to the next line, and so on until the entire *k*-space is traversed.

It should be taken into account that although every gradient forms its own echo, only the echo that coincides with the *k*-space center, the so-called primary-echo where the net gradient encoding is zero, is taken to calculate the echo time. Because the effect of gradients on spins during the formation of this echo is minimal so that their precessional frequencies are very near the Larmor frequency established by the main

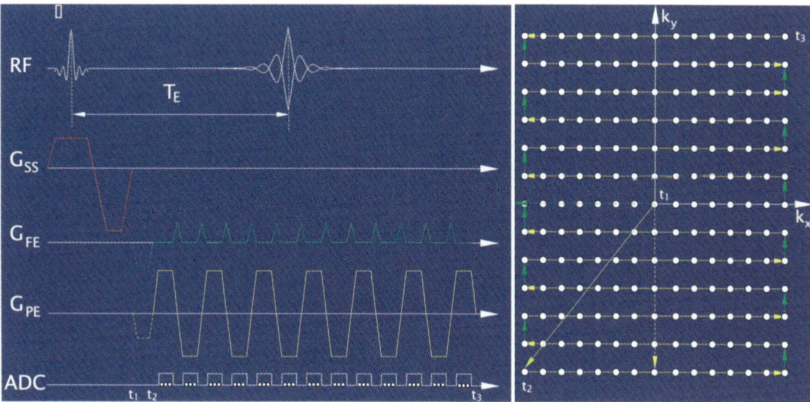


**Figure 2.10.** EPI Pulse Sequence Timing Diagram.

magnetic field $B_0$, the MR signal gain during this echo is the largest and determines the image contrast.

The implementation of the acquisition mechanism that allows a rapid collection of data to complete an entire image does not come without a few principle obstacles and challenges along the way. The accelerated sampling and shortened acquisition time that becomes comparable with such characteristic relaxation time $T_2^*$ and $T_2$ put additional demands on the scanner's gradient hardware, and the relaxation effects that influence the collected MR signal become more pronounced. In fact, the greatest challenge in the design of EPI sequences is imposed by the effect of the intrinsic decay owing to the $T_2^*$ relaxation. Such an effect is twofold.

The $T_2^*$ relaxation accounts for the global MR signal dropout across the entire image. Indeed, every $k$-space sample is attenuated by the signal decay during the acquisition, including the one located at the $k$-space center $k_x = k_y = 0$. Because this MR signal sample coincides with the primary and the strongest echo, the overall signal dropout is determined by the amount of the MR signal lost to the $T_2^*$ relaxation at the time of passing through the $k$-space center. Thus, the effective $T_E$ assigned to the time of the primary echo defines the overall loss of the MR signal.

Whereas the extent of the MR signal dropout depends on the position of the primary echo in respect to the $T_2^*$-relaxation decay profile, the length of the acquisition window determines the amount of the image blurring accounted to the $T_2^*$ relaxation. Because the sampling through the entire $k$-space is performed within a single acquisition window, the MR signal may experience the $T_2^*$ decay modulation large enough to cause a significant difference between the magnitude of MR signal samples acquired at the beginning and at the end of the acquisition window. In the zig-zag trajectory, it is high spatial frequencies ascribed by the peripheral $k$-space samples that get covered at the edges of the acquisition window. To this end, the substantial drop of the MR signal's amplitude over the acquisition window amounts to the image blurring.

Both caused by a decay due to the $T_2^*$ relaxation, these effects are related, but somewhat separable. Consider an MR signal collected during a 20-millisecond long acquisition window with its primary echo located around $T_E = 100$ milliseconds. If the shortest $T_2^*$ is 40 milliseconds, only minimal blurring occurs because the amplitude of *k*-space samples acquired in the beginning of the window does not differ substantially from that acquired at the window's rear. On the other hand, the signal decays considerably by the time of the primary echo. Therefore, the image reflects the overall attenuation rather than the blurring effects. Alternatively, the blurring in the image made with the acquisition window of 100 milliseconds long and centered around $T_E = 50$ milliseconds dominates over global attenuation effects.

Therefore, in order to mitigate the blurring, the length of the acquisition window has to be shortened. Usually, it is realized by increasing the reception bandwidth that allows faster MR signal sampling. The contrariety of the raised bandwidth is reduced image SNR. The length of the acquisition window also can be abridged by lowering the image resolution and thus the number of acquired *k*-space samples, for instance, from the image matrix of 128 × 128 pixels to one comprised of 64 × 64 pixels. In this case, in order to preserve the same coverage, the in-plane size of voxels is increased twofold. Having more spins in each voxel provides a larger per-voxel MR signal, and thus the SNR. However, it is more likely for a larger voxel to span intrinsic gradients caused by local inhomogeneities. To that end, the degree of the intravoxel inhomogeneity is also higher because it includes a wider range of frequencies; it inevitably shortens the $T_2^*$ and decreases the SNR. The shorter $T_2^*$ forces the $T_E$ to decrease accordingly in order to maintain sufficient SNR, per global attenuation effect described above. On the other hand, the $T_E$ has to be long enough to let the BOLD effect sufficiently modulate the MR signal.

Another aspect of the sampling process performed by an EPI pulse sequence is associated with characteristics of gradient coils. Implementation of EPI pulse sequences requires rather high gradient strength and switching rates in order to accomplish the rapid sampling. Based on the chosen field-of-view (FoV) and the resolution (image matrix), a size of the *k*-space grid that must be covered during the acquisition and the spacing between adjacent samples $\Delta k$ are prescribed. From Equations (2.6–2.8), simplified for the case of a constant gradient, the distance between adjacent *k*-space samples is:

$$\Delta k = \gamma G \Delta t, \tag{2.13}$$

where $\Delta t$ is the sampling rate. The FoV and $\Delta k$ are directly connected as

$$\text{FoV} = \Delta k^{-1}. \tag{2.14}$$

The sampling rate can be found if the resolution $N_{fe}$, $N_{pe}$ and the duration of the acquisition window $T$ are known:

$$\Delta t \approx \frac{T}{N_{fe} \cdot N_{pe}}. \tag{2.15}$$

In the most favorable case, when the duration of the excitation RF pulse[v] and the gap between its end and the beginning of the gradient waveform are neglected, the duration of the acquisition window is almost equal to the total acquisition time. The sampling rate can be readily found under such approximation conditions. If the pulse sequence is designed so that its primary echo occurs in the center of the acquisition window, then the total time is about twice the echo time, $T = 2T_E$. The estimated gradient amplitude can now be expressed through conventional imaging parameters:

$$G \approx \frac{N_{fe} \cdot N_{pe}}{2\gamma \cdot \mathrm{FoV} \cdot T_E}. \tag{2.16}$$

Therefore, to acquire a 128-square-pixel image with the FoV of 220 millimeters and the echo time of 30 milliseconds, the highest gradient amplitude should be on the order of 30 milliTesla per meter (mT/m). Technically challenging to implement a mere five years ago, gradient fields of such magnitude are now considered typical, and they become increasingly available for research and clinical applications. Following recent FDA approval of operating MR scanners equipped with gradient coils capable of reaching gradient field magnitudes as high as 40 mT/m, such imaging techniques as EPI-based diffusion and perfusion and *f*MRI are now actively employed in clinical studies. Even higher gradient strengths, up to 1000 mT/m, are available on experimental human and animal scanners.

Another essential characteristic of gradient field hardware and coil is the slew rate that describes how fast the gradient field can be changed. It is defined as a ratio

$$\text{Slew rate} = \frac{\text{Gradient magnitude}}{\text{Rise time}},$$

where the rise time is the time required to advance the gradient amplitude from 0 to its maximum. Typical for clinical scanners, rise times may vary from 100 to 600 microseconds. The gradient ramping, the period of time during which the gradient's amplitude changes between its extrema is thus twice as long, if the rise time is constant. Therefore, the slew rate is on the order of few hundred Tesla per meter per second, with the most prevalent values being 100 to 200 T/m·s.

As the EPI pulse sequences are in essence a special way to traverse *k*-space and do not introduce fundamentally new echo formation principles, the same contrast mechanisms can be implemented using the EPI spatial encoding scheme.

### *Gradient Echo-Recalled EPI Sequence*

The gradient echo-recalled EPI acquisition is the most commonly used imaging method in functional neuroimaging applications and research due to several reasons. First and foremost, although some amount of the $T_2$ weighting is inevitably present because of the overall irreversible

[v] The duration of the excitation RF pulse ranges from two to five milliseconds.

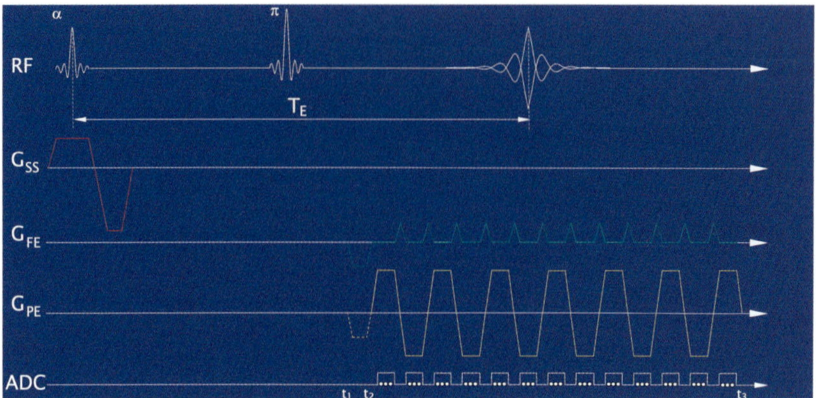


**Figure 2.11.** Spin-Echo EPI Pulse Sequence Timing Diagram.

transverse decay through the acquisition, the MR signal generated by this type of the EPI sequence carries a robust $T_2^*$ contrast. The prevailing $T_2^*$-weighted contrast component comes from the sensitivity of the sequence's echo-formation mechanism to local field inhomogeneities. Because the nature of the BOLD contrast is exactly rooted in tiny field inhomogeneities imparted by variations in oxy/deoxyhemoglobin-induced blood susceptibility, the gradient-recalled EPI sequences are very appropriate for collection of BOLD-related MR signal changes sought in the functional imaging.

As in generic gradient-echo sequences, a smaller flip angle can be employed in gradient-recalled EPI designs without suffering large MR signal losses. The smaller flip angle makes it possible to decrease the $T_R$ period, as less time is needed to restore the original longitudinal relaxation. Alternatively, a larger number of slices can be covered over the same $T_R$ period. The optimal flip angle at which the gradient-echo–generated MR signal reaches its maximum, the Ernst angle, can be calculated to provide the best possible contrast.[21]

***Spin-Echo Recalled EPI Sequence***

When the EPI spatial encoding mechanism itself is not a subject of interest but rather is taken as a component of a pulse sequence in whole, it can be considered as a black box that is designed to properly encode recovered MR signal and fill the *k*-space matrix. In case of a spin-echo pulse sequence, it is positioned following the excitation and refocusing RF pulses and all necessary gradient structures that define the image contrast, as is shown in the Figure 2.11.

The contrast-defining properties of the spin-echo–recalled EPI are similar to those of a regular spin-echo pulse sequence. In particular, although the spin-echo pulse sequence appears to be most susceptible to inhomogeneities imparted by capillaries, overall image contrast generated by this pulse sequence shows relatively little sensitivity to field inhomogeneities.

Somewhat more sensitive to BOLD-related changes in the $T_2^*$ relaxation is the asymmetric spin-echo. As discussed earlier, a key feature that differentiates it from the typical spin-echo pulse sequence is temporal misalignment between the center of the *k*-space (no spatial encoding condition) and the echo time. Such a mismatch usually is achieved by advancing the refocusing pulse and, consequently, the EPI spatial collection module towards the excitation pulse. In this case, there is a certain amount of $T_2^*$ dephasing present at the moment of the contrast-defining central echo of the EPI read-out echo train, thus bringing about the imprint of BOLD-related inhomogeneities.

The benefit from using the ASE pulse sequence may become greater in higher field strengths, where the effects of constant inhomogeneities are amplified, and thus present an increasingly bothersome factor in SNR and overall image quality.

## Spiral-Echo Planar Imaging Methods

Because the EPI is just a clever trick to cover the entire *k*-space fast, there is no restriction on the trajectory along which the *k*-space is traversed. In fact, it can be quite arbitrary, as suggested by Dale and colleagues.[22] One of trajectories that has been proven effective to implement fast scanning technique while producing relatively high BOLD-related SNR resembles a spiral. Thus, the pulse sequence that utilizes such a trajectory is called spiral EPI pulse sequence. These sequences have been found effective in cardiovascular, renal,[23,24] and multiple functional brain imaging studies.[25,26] The imaging with spiral algorithms excels in these application because of its relatively low sensitivity to motion and flow and an efficient use of the gradient power.[27]

The term spiral refers to the method of the *k*-space traverse. In particular, the *k*-space trajectory is indeed a spiral, as shown in Figure 2.12. The spiral sequences do not constitute a whole new class of imaging

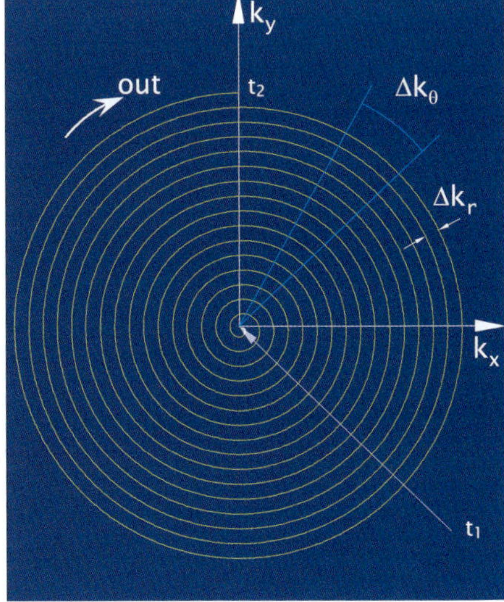


**Figure 2.12.** *k*-Space Diagram for Spiral EPI.

methods. Rather, they should be considered as a subset of EPI techniques because of many similarities between their designs, including collection of the MR signal corresponding to a large portion of the $k$-space with time-varying gradients following a single excitation pulse.

The design of a spiral pulse sequence involves two aspects. First, based on the mathematical expressions for a particular spiral trajectory and system-specific hardware characteristics, the gradient waveforms are calculated. The simplest type of the spiral trajectory, a so-called Archimedean spiral, is described by a running angle $\theta$ as a function of the trajectory radius at a particular point along the spiral, as shown in the right portion of Figure 2.12:

$$k(t) = A\theta(t)e^{i\theta(t)}, \tag{2.17}$$

where the azimuthal angle $\theta(t) = \omega_0 t$, with $\omega_0$ being a constant angular velocity. The gradient waveforms that implement the spiral traversal starting in the center and ending on the periphery of the $k$-space are shown on the pulse sequence diagram in Figure 2.13.

Other shapes of spiral trajectories are possible and widely used. For instance, in order to reduce physiologic noise effects that typically contaminate lower spatial frequencies, the vicinity of the $k$-space center often is oversampled by making more winds around the $k$-space's center, thus increasing the coverage density. To achieve an optimal density throughout the $k$-space and keep acquisition time from growing overly long, the varying sampling density spiral trajectory was proposed by Spielman and colleagues.[28] In this case, the image contrast improves because more MR signal samples are obtained around the center of the $k$-space and the contribution by physiological noise becomes limited.

Following the signal acquisition, a complementary image-reconstruction algorithm has to be applied to the raw signal data. The

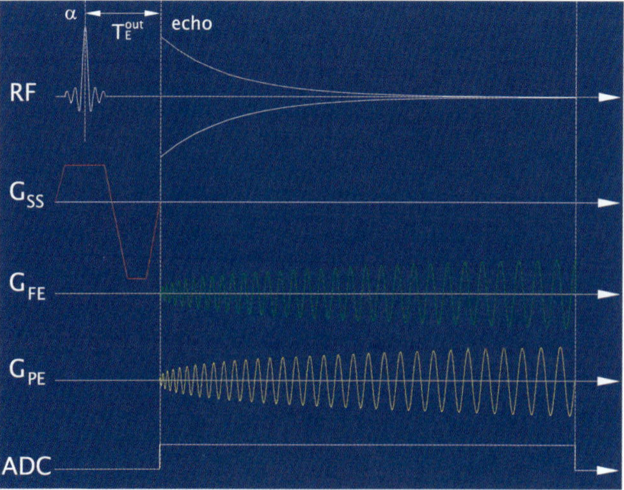


**Figure 2.13.** Spiral-Out Pulse Sequence Timing Diagram.

need for a gradient-specific reconstruction algorithm implementation is justified by limitations related to fast Fourier transformation (FFT) used to reconstruct the image from the raw MR signal. The regular FFT operation relies on a symmetrical and uniformly sampled rectilinear distribution of *k*-samples. This is not true for spiral-like traversals—not only do the collected data points not fall on the two-dimensional (2D) grid, but also their distribution is often nonuniform, as in case of the trajectory with the varying sampling density. Therefore, an operation that regrids the distribution of the *k*-samples into a rectilinear array and approximates the actual trajectory has to be applied before the data is submitted for the FFT.

There are seemingly two key ways to follow the spiral—namely, from the center to the periphery of the *k*-space and in the opposite direction. The spiral-out pulse sequence traverses the center of the *k*-space in the beginning of the acquisition period, and therefore obtains the contrast-defining echo immediately following the excitation pulse. In such a design, there is very little time to develop any appreciable $T_2^*$ relaxation; the FID signal is strong and any motion did not have enough time to have an impact on the spatial encoding. On the contrary, the traverse in the opposite direction, from the periphery to the *k*-space center, leads to accumulation of $T_2^*$-related phase offsets that sensitizes the image contrast to the field inhomogeneities.

Each of these traversals has benefits and limitations that should be considered in the context of a specific application. In cardiac imaging, where motion and flow artifacts could be severe, the pulse sequence that is capable to limit contributions thereof to the MR signal is advantageous. Therefore, the spiral-out design is more desirable in cardiac and abdominal studies. On the other hand, in order to detect BOLD-related MR signal changes, the inhomogeneities have to be allowed to influence the MR signal. If the contrast-defining echo comes too soon after the excitation pulse, the phase offsets are negligible, thus limiting their effect on the MR signal. Therefore, in BOLD studies, the spiral-in pulse sequence is preferred.

There is, however a significant drawback associated with such a design. Namely, if the entire *k*-space is sampled over the single trajectory, the overall MR signal may experience a considerable $T_2^*$ decay, leading to the decreased SNR. The solution to this particular predicament is to split the acquisition into several parts, covering the *k*-space in segments, so that the last echo appears earlier, but still at the end of the acquisition period. This approach reduces nonuniformity effects and eventually increases the SNR. However, the cardiac motion and respiration gives rise to undesirable image-to-image variations.

Several pulse sequence designs were proposed to accommodate the best of two traversals. For instance, one of designs is a two-segment acquisition that includes the spiral-in segment, followed by the spiral-out portion. In this case, both echoes, at the end of the spiral-in segment and at the beginning of the spiral-out portion, occur one after the other. Because the center of the *k*-space in each segment was acquired virtually at the same time, the two echoes have identical contrast. The MR signal collected during the leading spiral-in section is not severely decayed, which reflects an inhomogeneity modulation. The MR signal recovered in the consecutive spiral-out segment does not experience any substantial inhomogeneity effects and does not suffer from ongoing $T_2^*$ decay. Two $k$-space samples covered in both segments are later combined into a single $k$-space and the image is formed through the FFT. As expected, such an image can be sufficiently BOLD-modulated while sustaining sufficient MR signal magnitude and avoiding being degraded by $T_2^*$ relaxation.

By default, the spiral sequences are GE, but they can be turned into SE, and also can be united to produce double-contrast sequences.

In summary, this chapter gives an overview of the various pulse sequences that currently are used today in fMRI BOLD imaging, as well as their characteristics. The appropriate choice of the pulse sequence and its optimal parameters are key factors in maximizing the BOLD signal for every fMRI experiment performed.

## References

1. Robitaille PM, Abduljali AM, Kangarlu A. Ultra high resolution imaging of the human head at 8 tesla: 2K × 2K for Y2K. *J Comput Assist Tomogr.* 2000; 24(1):2–8.
2. Guinnessy P. Powerful NMR mashines debut in USA. *Physics Today.* 2002;55(3):30–31.
3. Constans A. NMR hits the big time. *The Scientist.* 2003;17(7):45–47.
4. Clark DD, Sokoloff L. Basic neurochemistry. In: *Circulation and Energy Metabolism of the Brain,* New York: Raven; 1994:645–680.
5. Hasselbalch SG, Knudsen GM, Jakobsen J, Hagenman LP, Holm S, Paulason OB. Brain metabolism during short term starvation in humans. *J Cereb Blood Flow Metab.* 1994;14:125–131.
6. Schwartz WJ, Smith CB, Davidsen L, Savaki H, Sokoloff L, Mata M, Fink DJ, Gainer H. Metabolic mapping of functional activity in the hypothalamo-neurohypophysial system of the rat. *Science.* 1979;205:723–725.
7. Hyder F, Rothman DL, Mason GF, Rangarajan A, Shulman KL. Oxidative glucose metabolism in rat brain during single forepaw stimulation: A spatially localized $^1$H[$^{13}$C nuclear magnetic resonance study]. *J Cereb Blood Flow Metab.* 1997;17:1040–1047.
8. Gross PM, Sposito NM, Pettersen SE, Panton DG, Fenstermacher JD. Topography of capillary density, glucose metabolism, and microvascular function within the rat inferior colliculus. *J Cereb Blood Flow Metab.* 1987;7:154–160.
9. Klein B, Kuschinsky W, Schrock H, Vetterlein F. Interdependency of local capillary density, blood flow, and metabolism in rat brains. *Am J Physiol.* 1986;251:H1333–H1340.
10. Fox PT, Raichle ME, Mintun MA, Dence C. Nonoxidative glucose cosumption during focal physiologic neuronal activity. *Science.* 1988;241: 462–464.
11. Davis TL, Kwong KK, Weisskoff RM, Rosen BR. Calibrated functional MRI: Mapping the dynamics of oxidative metabolism. *Proc Nat Acad Sci USA.* 1998;95:1834–1839.
12. Thulborn KR, Waterton JC, Mattews PM, Padda GK. Oxygenation dependence of the transverse relaxation time of water protons in while blood at high field. *Biochem Biophys Acta.* 1982;714:265–270.

13. Turner R, Le Bihan D, Moonen CT, Despres D, Frank D. Echo-planar time course MRI of cat brain oxygenation changes. *Magn Resón Med.* 1991;22: 159–166.
14. Feynman RP, Leighton RB, Sands M. *The Feynman Lectures on Physics*, vol. 1. Addison-Wesley Publishing Company; 1964.
15. Bandettini PA, Wong EC, Jesmanowicz A, Hinks RS, Hyde JS. Spin-echo and Gradient-echo EPI of human brain activation using BOLD contrast. A comparative study at 1.5T. *NMR Biomed.* 1994;7:12–20.
16. Hahn EL. Spin echoes. *Physical Rev.* 1950;80:580–594.
17. Oppelt A, Graumann R, Barfuss H. FISP: A new fast MRI sequence. *Electromedica.* 1986;54:15–18.
18. Scheffler K, Seifritz E, Bilecen D, Venkatesan R, Hennig J, Deimling M, Haacke EM. Detection of BOLD changes by means of a frequency-sensitive trueFISP technique: Preliminary results. *NMR Biomed.* 2001;14(7–8): 490–496.
19. Scheffler K, Hennig J. TIDE (transition into driven equilibrium)-sequences for brain imaging with improved signal and contrast behaviour. In: *Proceedings of ISMRM. 11th Scientific Meeting and Exhibition.* Toronto, Ontario, Canada: 2003:973.
20. Haake EM, Brown RE, Thompson MR, Venkatesan R. *Magnetic Resonance Imaging: Physical Principles and Sequence Design.* New-York: John Wiley & Sons Inc.; 1999.
21. Ernst R, Anderson W. Application of Fourier transform spectroscopy to magnetic resonance. *Rev Sci Instrum.* 1966;37:93–102.
22. Dale B, Wendt M, Duerk JL. A rapid look-up table method for reconstructing MR images from arbitrary *k*-space trajectories. *IEEE Trans Med Imaging.* 2001;20(3):207–217.
23. Meyer C, Hu B, Nishimura DG, Macovshi A. Fast coronary artery imaging. *Magn Reson Imaging.* 1992;28:202–213.
24. Yacoe ME, Li KC, Cheung L, Meyer CH. Spiral spin-echo magnetic resonance imaging of the pelvis with spectrally and spatially selective radiofrequency excitation: Comparison with fat-saturated fast spin-echo imaging. *Can Assoc Radiol J.* 1996;48:247–251.
25. Noll DC, Cohen JD, Meyer CH, Schneider W. Spiral *k*-space MR imaging of cortical activation. *J Magn Reson Imaging.* 1995;5(1):49–56.
26. Cohen JD, Perlstein WM, Braver TS, Nystrom LE, Noll DC, Jonides J, Smith EE. Temporal dynamics of brain activation during a working memory task. *Nature.* 1997;386:604–608.
27. Nishimura DG, Irarrazabal P, Meyer CH. A velocity *k*-space analysis of flow effects in echo-planar and spiral imaging. *Magn Reson Med.* 1995;33: 549–556.
28. Spielman DM, Pauly JM, Meyer CH. Magnetic resonance fluoroscopy using spirals with variable sampling densities. *Magn Reson Med.* 1995;34:388–394.

# 3

# Experimental Design and Data Analysis for fMRI

Geoffrey K. Aguirre

## Introduction

Functional magnetic resonance imaging (fMRI) methods have evolved rapidly over the last decade. Ever more subtle experimental designs have been joined by ever more powerful data analysis methods to detect evoked changes in neural activity. Despite constant developments, there are several core principles of fMRI methodology that can be used as a guide to understand the current state of the field, as well as whatever advances await tomorrow. Here, the primary concern will be with this core understanding, but several specific aspects of fMRI experiments also will be considered. Along the way, some of the specific challenges that face fMRI studies of clinical populations will be noted, although a detailed consideration of these issues is contained in Chapter 5.

Topics will be raised roughly as they present in the course of the conception and completion of an fMRI experiment. This order of presentation will also move us from general issues in neuroimaging inference to more specific aspects of fMRI, and finally to the idiosyncratic properties of blood oxygenation level-dependent (BOLD) fMRI and their implication for experimental design and analysis. To start, three general categories of neuroimaging experiments will be considered, each of which probes a slightly different aspect of the relationship between the brain and behavior. Next, different techniques of isolating and manipulating mental operations that might be used in the service of these experimental designs will be discussed. Rounding out experimental design, the possible temporal ordering of stimuli within an fMRI experiment will be considered, including the paradigmatic blocked and event-related designs. This section will require us to grapple with two critical properties of BOLD fMRI data: the hemodynamic response function and the temporal autocorrelation of the noise. Attention will then be turned to related analysis issues. The steps of data preprocessing that prepare fMRI data for statistical analysis will be reviewed, followed by a consideration of univariate analysis of fMRI data.

## Basic Types of Neuroimaging Inference

Regardless of the particular neuroimaging methodology employed [e.g., fMRI, positron emission tomography (PET), event-related potential (ERP)], there are a few broad categories of experimental question that might be asked. Each category probes a different aspect of the relationship between the brain and behavior, and each makes different assumptions for valid inference. Although not an exhaustive classification, these categories can help organize one's thinking about the assumptions that underlie a particular experiment.

In the past, neuroimaging techniques have been applied mostly to *localization* questions that asked: what are the anatomical neural correlates of a given mental operation? For example, does perception of a face activate a particular area of the brain different from that evoked by perception of other stimuli? Does the cognitive process of working memory evoke neural activity within the frontal lobe or somewhere else? In general, these designs present a subject with a task designed to selectively evoke a particular cognitive state of interest, and the neuroimaging method identifies if and where changes in neural activity accompany that cognitive process. Clearly, this type of experiment requires a way to manipulate the mental state of the subject, isolating the mental operation of interest from the other processes that invariably are present (e.g., button pushing, preparing responses, etc.). In the next section, several methods are considered that might be used to do so.

If successful, a localization study allows one to conclude that a particular area of the brain is activated by a particular cognitive operation. Importantly, neuroimaging methods in general are severely restricted in their ability to make conclusions regarding the necessity of a region for a cognitive operation. In other words, the presence of focal activation for a particular mental operation does not imply that a lesion to that area of the brain would impair the subject's ability to perform that mental operation. The reasons for this are manifold; for example, multiple areas of activity might be found, any one of which (perhaps working in parallel, or one serving as a backup for the other) would be capable of supporting the process of interest. In this case, the region still plays an interesting role in the cognitive process, although it is not strictly necessary. A second challenge is that we do not have perfect control over the mental states of the subject we seek to study. Although stimuli and instructions designed to evoke a particular cognitive process can be pesented, there are no guarantees that the subject has entered that cognitive state and no other. The subject may unwittingly engage in confounding cognitive processes in addition to that intended by the experimenter, or alternatively, may fail to differentially engage the process. This is the central challenge of interpretation of most neuroimaging studies of localization—it is difficult to be certain that the experimental variable of interest has been properly manipulated.

Several applications of localization-type neuroimaging studies of patient populations can be conceived. The use of fMRI to identify the eloquent (or otherwise functionally important) cortex for neurosurgical planning is one example. Importantly, the caveats expressed above regarding the conclusion of necessity using a neuroimaging study are particularly relevant for this application (see Chapter 7 for further details). Localization studies also can be used in the study of rehabilitation and brain-damaged patients. Consider a patient with a focal lesion within a cortical area that previously has been demonstrated to be activated by a given mental operation. If the patient can still perform that mental operation despite the lesion, it could be presumed that some other back-up cortical area is now mediating this ability. A localization study could be used to identify the other cortical areas that are involved in the cognitive process.

In contrast, implementation studies ask about the computational mechanisms of a cognitive process within a cortical region. This type of study begins with the assumption that a cortical region engages in computations that support a particular cognitive process. The purpose of the study is then to determine the parameters of neural activity that mediate the area's participation in that process; for example, does an area of the prefrontal cortex change its bulk level of neural activity as a function of increasing working memory load (i.e., remember four items instead of two)? Is speed of motion encoded differently from direction of motion within area MT? As the field of cognitive neuroscience has moved beyond brain mapping, implementation experiments have become more prevalent. Patient studies might apply an implementation design to understand how altered performance in a clinical population is reflected in regional neuro-computational processing; for example, autistic patients are known to have impaired face recognition ability. Within an area of the fusiform gyrus that responds maximally to faces, do autistic patients have a blunted (or exaggerated?) response to changes in some properties of face perception, but not others; for example facial identity, emotional expression, or direction of gaze? Such a study might identify the specific processing impairment in autistics that is manifest clinically as impaired facial perception.

Finally, an evocation design reverses the typical direction of neuroimaging inference and asks: What cognitive process does a given task evoke? This type of experiment leverages knowledge about the neural correlates of particular mental states to learn something about an imperfectly understood behavior. One begins by assuming that neural activity in a particular area of the brain is a marker of the presence of a particular mental state and no other; for example, neural activity of a certain magnitude at a certain spot in the fusiform gyrus indicates that the subject has the visual perception of a face. The subject then performs a task that may or may not evoke the cognitive process of interest; for example, ambiguous stimuli are presented that can be perceived as a face or a vase. If the specified neural activity is seen, the conclusion is drawn that the subject saw a face at that moment in time. Therefore, this type of design may be used to test hypotheses regarding the engagement of cognitive processes during a behavioral state in which the cognitive processes need not be under experimental control. Within the clinical realm, this type of design could be used, for example, to reveal intact visual pathway responses in patients with functional impairments from the psychiatric diagnosis of conversion disorder. The extent of depression might be inferred from the functional responses of the amygdala to sad stimuli. Alternatively, the level of consciousness or pain perception of a patient who is in a locked-in state might be assessed.

Usually, experiments from these three categories concern changes in the bulk neural activity measured by neuroimaging methods. However, other types of inference are also possible; for example, methods exist to measure the degree of effective connectivity between different cortical regions—the extent that one cortical region influences neural activity in another region.[1] Such a metric could be used with any of these three categories of inference. One might hypothesize within an implementation framework that retrieval of semantic information about living things increases the effective connectivity between inferior frontal and ventral temporal regions, whereas retrieval of semantic information about tools is associated with similar connections between inferior frontal and premotor cortical areas.

## Manipulation of the Cognitive Process

As was discussed previously, many neuroimaging experiments depend upon the isolated manipulation of a cognitive process for study. In particular, localization experiments require that a cognitive process of interest be isolated from other mental operations so that the neural correlates of that solitary process can be observed. In implementation experiments, some aspect of the stimulus or mental operation must be varied so that the neuro-computational correlate of its processing can be studied. Here, several broad classes of experimental manipulation of a cognitive operation are considered. Note that any of these techniques can be coupled with a particular temporal structure of design (e.g., event-related or blocked), which is described in the next section.

Cognitive subtraction is the prototypical method of isolation of a cognitive processes, and it is the most problematic. Typically, one condition of an experiment is designed to engage a particular cognitive process, such as face perception, episodic encoding, or semantic recall. This experimental condition is contrasted with a control condition designed to evoke all of the cognitive processes present in the experimental period except for the cognitive process of interest. Differences in neural activity between the two conditions are attributed to the cognitive process of interest. In essence, a cognitive process is isolated in an all-or-none fashion. As was discussed previously, we do not have direct control over the mental states of the subject, so the danger is always present that the subject might engage in a confounding mental operation in addition to the one of interest. Additionally, cognitive subtraction relies upon the assumption that a cognitive process can be added to a pre-existing set of cognitive processes without affecting them (an assumption termed pure insertion). This might fail if, for

experimental designs can work is that some patterns of events that occur rapidly or switch rapidly create a low-frequency envelope—a larger structure of pattern of alternation that can pass through the hemodynamic response function. In the next section, several types of temporal structures for BOLD fMRI experiments will be discussed, and how the shape of the HRF dictates the properties of these designs will be considered.

Another important property of BOLD fMRI data is that greater power is present at some temporal frequencies as compared to others under the null hypothesis (i.e., data collected without any experimental intervention). The power spectrum (a frequency representation) of data composed of independent observations (i.e., white noise), should be flat, with equal power at all frequencies. When calculated for BOLD fMRI, the average power spectrum is found to contain ever-increasing power at ever-lower frequencies, often termed a 1/frequency distribution. This pattern of noise also can be called pink, named for the color of light that would result if the corresponding amounts of red, orange, yellow, etc., of the visible light-frequency spectrum were combined. The presence of noise of this type within BOLD fMRI data has two primary consequences. First, traditional parametric and nonparametric statistical tests are invalid for the analysis of BOLD fMRI data, which is why much of the analysis of BOLD fMRI data is conducted using Keith Worsley and Karl Friston's "modified" general linear model[7] and its heirs, as instantiated in SPM and other statistical packages. The second impact is upon experimental design. Because of the greater noise at lower frequencies, slow changes in neural activity are more difficult to distinguish from noise.

Interestingly, the consequences for experimental design of the shape of the HRF and the noise properties of BOLD fMRI are at odds. Specifically, the shape of the HRF would tend to favor experimental designs that induce slow changes in neural activity, whereas the presence of low-frequency noise would argue for experimental designs that produce more rapid alterations in neural activity. As it happens, knowledge of the shape of the HRF and the distribution of the noise is sufficient to provide a principled answer as to how best balance these two conflicting forces.

It is worth noting that other neuroimaging methods have different data characteristics, with different consequences for experimental design; for example, perfusion fMRI is a relatively new approach that provides a non-invasive, quantifiable measure of local cerebral tissue perfusion.[8] Perfusion data do not suffer from the elevated low-frequency noise present in BOLD; consequently, perfusion fMRI can be used to detect extremely long time-scale changes in neural activity (over minutes to hours to days) that would simply be indistinguishable from noise using BOLD fMRI.[9] This may prove to be very advantageous in studies of clinical populations. Functional changes in patient cognition, either improvement by functional recovery following focal lesions or decline in neurodegenerative disease, evolve over long time scales as well. Perfusion fMRI can be used to obtain stable measurements of evoked neural activity from this dynamic system.

## Different Temporal Structures of BOLD fMRI Experiments

As BOLD fMRI experiments by necessity include multiple task conditions (prototypically, an experimental and control period), several ways of ordering the presentation of these conditions exist. Different terms are used to describe the pattern of alternation between experimental conditions over time and include such familiar labels as blocked or event-related. Whereas these often are perceived as rather concrete categories, the distinction between blocked, event-related, and other sorts of designs is fairly arbitrary. These may be better considered as extremes along a continuum of arrangements of stimulus order. Consider every period of time during an experiment as a particular experimental condition. This includes the inter-trial–interval or baseline periods between stimulus presentations. In this setting, blocked and event-related designs are viewed simply as different ways of arranging periods of rest (or no stimulus) with respect to other sorts of conditions. (For a more complete exploration of these concepts, see Friston[10]).

The prototypical fMRI experimental is a blocked approach in which two conditions alternate over the course of a scan. For most hypotheses of interest, these periods of time will not be utterly homogeneous, but will consist of several trials of some kind presented together. For example, a given block might present a series of faces to be passively perceived, a sequence of words to be remembered, or a series of pictures to which the subject must make a living/nonliving judgment and press a button to indicate his response. Blocked designs have the obvious difficulty that the subject can anticipate trial types, which may be undesirable in some settings (e.g., studies of recognition of novel versus previously learned words). On the other hand, blocked designs have superior statistical power compared to all other experimental designs. This is because the fundamental frequency of the boxcar can be positioned at an optimal location with respect to the filtering properties of the hemodynamic response function and the low-frequency noise. For typical shapes of the HRF and distributions of temporal noise, this ideal balancing point occurs with epochs of about 20 to 30 seconds in duration.

Event-related designs model signal changes associated with individual trials, as opposed to blocks of trials. This makes it possible to ascribe changes in signal to particular events, allowing one to randomize stimuli, assess relationships between behavior and neural responses, and engage in retrospective assignment of trials. Conceptually, the simplest type of event-related design to consider is one that uses only a single stimulus type and uses sufficient temporal spacing of trials to permit the complete rise and fall of the hemodynamic response to each trial; a briefly presented picture of a face once every sixteen seconds for example. This is frequently termed a sparse event-related design. Importantly, while this prototypical experiment has only one stimulus, it has *two* experimental conditions (the stimulus and the inter-trial–interval). If one is willing to abandon the fixed ordering and spacing of these conditions, more complex designs become possible. For example, randomly ordered picture presentations and rest periods could be presented as rapidly as once a second. The ability to present rapid alternations between conditions initially seems counterintuitive, given the temporal smoothing effects of the hemodynamic response function. Whereas BOLD fMRI is insensitive to the particular high-frequency alternation between one trial and the next, it is still sensitive to the low-frequency envelope of the design. In effect, with closely spaced, randomly ordered trials, one is detecting the low-frequency consequences of the random assortment of trial types. These rapid event-related designs are fairly sensitive to the accurate specification of the HRF for their success (unless a basis set is used for analysis; see below).

For experimental settings in which one has an unlimited number of trials to present (e.g., flashes of light) but a limited period of scanning time, then rapid randomly ordered designs are more statistically powerful than sparse designs. Alternatively, when the experiment is limited by the number of available trials (e.g., pictures of flightless birds), then maximal statistical power is obtained by presenting the available trials in a sparse manner and stretching the scanning period out as long as possible.

The discussion thus far regarding event-related designs has assumed an ability to randomize perfectly the order of presentation of different event types. There are certain types of behavioral paradigms, however, that do not permit a random ordering of the events. For example, the delay period of a working memory experiment always follows the presentation of a stimulus to be remembered. In this case, the different events of the trial cannot be placed arbitrarily close together without risking the possibility of false-positive results that accrue from the hemodynamic response to one trial event (e.g., the stimulus presentation) being interpreted as resulting from neural activity in response to another event (e.g., the delay period). It turns out that, given the shape typically observed for hemodynamic responses, events within a trial as close together as four seconds can be reliably discriminated.[11] Thus, event-related designs can be used to examine directly, for example, the hypothesis that certain cortical areas increase their activity during the delay period of a working memory paradigm without requiring the problematic assumptions traditionally employed in blocked subtractive designs.

There is a multiplicity of further designs that might be considered that do not fall strictly within blocked or event-related categories. Neural-onset asynchrony designs[12,13] are used to detect differences in the timing of neural activity evoked by different stimuli. Here, a sparse event-related design is used, along with exquisite coupling of the timing of stimulus presentation to image acquisition. A difference in the time of onset of the smooth BOLD hemodynamic response evoked by two different stimuli within a cortical region is sought. Traveling wave stimuli are used to define topographic maps of cortical responses, the most familiar being the retinotopic organization of early visual areas.[14] These designs use stimuli that vary continuously across some sensory space (e.g., retinal eccentricity), and identify for any point within a cortical area what was the optimal position of the stimulus within the sensory space for the evocation of neural activity. These designs often are combined with cortical flat-map techniques for the display of results.[15]

## Data Preprocessing

In a perfect world, BOLD fMRI images would be acquired instantaneously from a stationary brain of uniform shape. Unfortunately, this is not the case, and a number of processing steps must be performed prior to the statistical analysis of fMRI data. These steps have two primary goals: 1) to reverse displacements of the data in time or space that may have occurred during acquisition, 2) to enhance the ability to detect spatially extended signals within or across subjects. In this section several preprocessing steps will be discussed that are commonplace in the analysis of BOLD fMRI data.

### Distortion Correction

Blood oxygenation level-dependent fMRI data typically are acquired as echoplanar images, and as such are likely to be distorted (stretched and pulled) in space to some extent as a result of static magnetic field inhomogeneities produced by concentration of magnetic field lines at (for example) air tissue interfaces. There are several methods to correct for this spatial distortion; in most cases, they use a map of the magnetic field within the bore of the magnet to correct distortion. Additionally, in most cases, this correction is performed by the scanning system itself prior to writing out image data for analysis and does not enter into the routine preprocessing of fMRI data at most institutions.

### Slice Acquisition Correction

A single volume of BOLD fMRI data, collected during one TR, is assembled from multiple planar acquisitions (slices). One slice is collected at a time, either sequentially or in an interleaved fashion, with the result that each slice samples a slightly different point in time. For a repetition time (TR) of two seconds and 20 axial slices, this would mean that one slice of the brain would be obtained 1.8 seconds later than another spatially adjacent slice within the same TR. Consequently, a neural event that occurs simultaneously on multiple slices within the brain will appear as different time-delayed BOLD fMRI responses in the data from different slices. Slice-acquisition correction compensates for this staggered order of slice acquisition. The correction works by calculating (using sinc-interpolation) the BOLD fMRI signal that would have been obtained for a given slice had that slice been acquired instead at the beginning of the TR. While not of great importance for low-temporal-frequency blocked designs, this preprocessing step is quite important for even-related designs.

## Motion Correction

A variety of methods are used to minimize head motion during scanning. These include foam padding around the head; bite bars; custom-designed, thermo-plastic face masks; and so on. Despite these efforts, subjects nonetheless move their heads during scanning. Therefore, a common data preprocessing step is to attempt to correct for the effects of this motion. This generally is done by realigning the image of the brain obtained at each point in time back to the first image acquired at the start of the scanning session. Several methods exist to do so, but most use a six-parameter motion correction in which the brain is treated as a rigid body and the six possible movements (three translations and three rotations) are calculated at each point in time to minimize the image difference between the realigned brain and the brain in its original position. Importantly, motion correction of this kind does not completely remove the effects of movement upon the BOLD fMRI signal. This is because movement of the brain within the exquisitely defined magnetic field gradients created during scanning alters the signal obtained at different points in the slice acquisition. As a result, even after realigning the brain to its original position, movement-induced signal artifacts can remain. Consequently, statistical analysis of BOLD data often will include nuisance covariates that are themselves the six movement parameters measured during realignment. These covariates serve to account for changes in the signal within voxels that are correlated with the movement of the head (see below for a further description of nuisance covariates).

## Spatial Normalization

If one wishes to test a hypothesis regarding a certain area of the brain within a population, then it is first necessary to identify that same area of the brain across subjects. This is frequently done by computationally warping the anatomical structure of the brain of one subject to match a template brain within a standard defined space. While there are a variety of sophisticated methods available for registering and aligning the brains of different subjects into a standard space, there are theoretical limits to what such an alignment can achieve. First, there may be intersubject variability in anatomy that cannot be overcome by warping brains to a standard space. For example, the arrangement of the sulci may vary between subjects. Thus, while two subjects may have neural responses at the same true cyto-architectonic location, the position of this site with respect to other landmarks in the brain may differ between subjects, leading to spread of these locations when data are converted to a standard space. Second, even given rigid alignment of anatomy across subjects, there may be variability in the structure to function relationships between subjects. For example, two subjects may truly have distinct face-selective neural regions, but these may be located in different sections of a cortical area as a consequence of differences in experience. Again, when normalized to a standard space, this variability in location will obscure functional dissociations. An alternative to anatomical registration is functional identification. The approach here is first to identify a region across subjects by its functional responses. For example, one might identify a region that responds more to pictures of faces than to general objects. Then hypotheses regarding the response of this functionally defined region to other types of stimuli can be tested independently across subjects within this area. This powerful approach allows one to make inferences across subjects regarding the responses of some functional area (e.g., the fusiform face area) at the expense of making statements regarding some particular position in a standardized anatomical space.

### Spatial Smoothing

It is a common practice to digitally smooth BOLD fMRI data in space prior to statistical analysis. There are several reasons for this. First, BOLD fMRI data typically are composed of time-series information from many thousands of individual voxels. Statistical analysis of this data involves application of a statistical test (e.g., $t$ test) at each of these voxels. Because there are thousands of individual statistical tests being performed, control of the false-positive rate requires a fairly large $t$ result to exceed the chance that random noise will produce a significant result in one or more of those thousands of voxels. By smoothing the data in space, one reduces the number of independent statistical tests that are being performed, thus allowing less-stringent control over what $t$ value is considered a significant result. Another motivation for smoothing is that, when analyzing data across a population, spatial smoothing helps to overcome residual differences in anatomy between subjects that might otherwise render common areas of activation nonoverlapping. The amount of spatial smoothing to perform can be difficult to determine, as smoothing too much will decrease statistical sensitivity for small focal areas of activation, whereas smoothing too little will have the same deleterious effects upon large areas of signal change. A reasonable balance between these two extremes can be obtained by smoothing data with a filter that has a width roughly equal to the size (in voxels) of predicted areas of activity.

## Statistical Analysis

Several methods exist to analyze BOLD fMRI data. Some of these are described as multivariate techniques, in which latent patterns of spatially coherent activity are identified automatically by the method (e.g., Partial Least Squares[16]). The more commonly implemented univariate techniques will be focused upon here, in which a statistical model is applied to each voxel independently within a data set. The discussion concerns in particular the details of the creation of a statistical model for analysis. In many software packages, such as statistical parametric mapping (SPM), some of these details are handled automatically. The purpose of this section is to provide an understanding of what is going on under the hood.

The centerpiece of the analysis of neuroimaging data is the construction of a model that is composed of one or more covariates. In general, covariates are predictions regarding patterns of variability in the data expressed as changes in the BOLD fMRI signal over time within a single voxel. The better the predictions, the more valid and powerful the statistical model becomes. Covariates can be divided broadly into two categories. Covariates of interest describe changes in the signal that typically are the result of experimental manipulations and are the subject of hypothesis testing. Covariates of no interest instead describe changes in the signal that are unintended or undesired; thay are not typically the focus of a hypothesis test.

Covariates of interest might be generated in one of two ways. First, covariates might be created to model the expected shape in time of evoked BOLD fMRI signal changes. A principled way to create covariates of this kind is to begin with a prediction regarding the pattern of neural activity that might be evoked by the experiment in a single voxel. For example, a simple blocked experimental design might be predicted to produce a uniformly greater amount of bulk neural activity during an experimental condition as compared to a control condition. The anticipated BOLD fMRI signal under these circumstances can be obtained by applying a model of the HRF to the predicted pattern of neural activity. As was mentioned previously, knowledge of the HRF is sufficient to predict the BOLD fMRI signal that will result from any arbitrary pattern of neural activity through the mathematical process of convolution. This prediction of BOLD fMRI signal change is then suitable for use as a covariate of interest. The model of the HRF that is used might be obtained from the subject himself during a preliminary experiment,[5] or an average representation of an HRF across subjects might be employed, as is the case in the SPM and other analysis packages.

Alternatively, covariates of interest can represent not a specific pattern of BOLD fMRI response, but instead have the property of flexibly fitting a family of possible responses that might occur. This approach uses a basis set, which is a collection of covariates that can be scaled and combined to fit any pattern of BOLD fMRI response that might be evoked within a set period of time by a particular experimental condition. In general, the basis set will be composed of multiple covariates, with as many elements as there are points in time to be modeled. For example, in a sparse event-related experiment in which a stimulus is presented every 8 TRs (16 seconds at a TR of 2), then a basis set of eight covariates will be needed to model, in effect, the average evoked BOLD fMRI response across trials. Typically, there is no clear interpretation of any one element of a basis set. Instead, one interprets the explanatory power of the set en mass using an *F* test. Basis set approaches provide the advantage of flexibility in that one is sensitive to any pattern of response (or difference between two trial types) that might take place. The price of this flexibility is reduced inferential power. One can no longer say, for example, that a given response was greater in amplitude than another, or longer in duration. Instead, one can only say that some consistent response was present.

As was mentioned earlier, covariates of no interest model changes in the BOLD fMRI signal that are not thought to be the result of experimental influence. For example, if one was aware of an influence of the room temperature upon the BOLD fMRI signal, and if the pattern of fluctuations of the room temperature were known, a representation of temperature could be included as a covariate to explain variations in the signal that are attributable to temperature fluctuations. Note that some covariates that are not of interest model changes in neural activity and some do not. For example, the experiment occasionally may present instruction screens, which would be expected to elicit transient changes in neural activity that are not the subject of any hypothesis. For these types of covariates that model expected neural effects of no interest, one would want to convolve the representation of neural change by the HRF. For other covariates that are not derived from neural activity (e.g., a measure of subject head motion), then convolution is not indicated.

One can further classify covariates of no interest as nuisance covariates or confounds. A nuisance covariate is defined as a covariate, the inclusion of which is expected to alter only the magnitude of the error term, but not the relationship between the data and covariates of interest. When covariates of no interest are correlated with covariates about which one wishes to test a hypothesis, they are termed confounds, and their inclusion will be expected to alter the behavior of the covariates of interest. Under some circumstances, the sign of the relationship between the covariate of interest and the data can be reversed. An example of a covariate that frequently acts as a confound is a global signal covariate. A global signal is average signal change over time across the entire brain, obtained by taking a simple average of the voxel-wise time series. It is common to included a measure of the global signal as a covariate of no interest (or to scale the data prior to analysis by this measure) to remove changes in blood oxygenation that impact the entire brain (resulting from changes in heart rate or respiration) that otherwise would obscure regional changes in neural activity. Because of the way in which it is measured, however, the global signal is expected to have some positive correlation with any experimentally evoked signal changes (as the average of all brain voxels will include those voxels responding to the task). As a result, correction for global signal changes can have a confounding effect upon covariates of interest and greatly change the interpretation of evoked signal changes.[17]

The resulting statistical model, composed of covariates of interest and those of no interest, is then used to evaluate the time-series data from each voxel within the brain. The resulting weights upon the covariates (termed beta values) then can be evaluated alone or in combinations using $t$ and $F$ statistics. The product is a statistical map in which every voxel in the brain contains a corresponding statistical value for the contrast of the covariates of interest. The final step of analysis involves assigning a level of statistical significance to those values. If the data set was composed of a single voxel, then this would be a straightforward enterprise: a $t$ value of greater than 1.96 would be significant at a $p = 0.05$ level (presuming many degrees of freedom and a two-tailed test). Because there are many voxels, however, the likelihood that noise alone might render one $t$ value significant if many are tested must be corrected. Such a correction attempts to control the false-positive rate at a *map-wise* level, meaning that if twenty statistical maps were produced under null-hypothesis conditions (i.e., in the absence of any actual experimental treatment), only one, on average, would be expected to contain even a single false-positive voxel. Solutions to perform this correction in the face of spatial smoothness within the statistical map (which yields statistical test in adjacent voxels that are not fully independent) exist within Gaussian Random Field Theory.[7]

Performing the appropriate map-wise correction to control the false-positive rate frequently can yield a rather stringent statistical value necessary to label any result significant. In turn, this raises concerns about false-negative results in which true experimental effects might be missed because the experiment is underpowered. There are several responses to this concern. Beyond the flippant call for more data, one might choose to relax the $p$ value that will be accepted as significant. Note that stating that the data were evaluated at a $p = 0.1$ level (corrected for multiple comparisons) is more intellectually honest than reporting results at a $p = 0.00023$ level (uncorrected), the latter tending to lull statistically naïve readers into a false sense of security. It also is preferable, whenever possible, to anatomically narrow one's hypothesis test. Using a predefined region of interest within which to test hypotheses can greatly reduce the number of independent statistical tests for which correction is required improves power. In the limit, the number of tests can be reduced to one by taking the average signal within a region and performing the statistical test upon this representative data. Several methods are available for the definition of regions of interest. They might be defined anatomically based upon gyral or cyto-architectonic boundaries, or on the basis of previously reported lesion or functional neuroimaging studies. Regions of interest also might be defined functionally; for example, subjects might participate in an initial scan, the purpose of which is to define a region of cortex that is maximally responsive to faces. Data obtained from this putative face region in subsequent experiments could then be studied with the benefits of having focused the hypothesis test. Finally, regions might be defined using a main effect contrast, with subsequent orthogonal interaction contrasts tested within the region. For example, an experiment might present pictures of upright faces and inverted faces. A region would be defined as the area that responds more to pictures of faces, in either orientation, as compared to a third baseline condition. Within the defined region, the difference in response between upright and inverted faces could be assessed without loss of statistical rigor, as the result of the test used to define the region does not prejudice the result of the subsequent orthogonal test of the effect of orientation of the stimulus. Of course, there are inferential consequences (such as loss of generality) of testing hypotheses only within predefined regions of interest. This might be countered by performing in the same experiment-focused hypothesis tests within regions of interest, followed by more exploratory analyses that evaluate the data from the remainder of the brain using appropriate map-wise correction for the increased number of voxels.

Yet another approach that has gained popularity is the use of a false-discovery rate statistical threshold.[18] Instead of controlling the false-positive rate at a map-wise level (allowing, for example, only one in twenty maps to have a single false-positive voxel), the FDR method controls the proportion of false-positive voxels present within a single map. For example, an FDR threshold of five percent implies that, of the voxels identified as significant within a statistical map, five percent of them are, on average, expected to be false positives. This is neither better nor worse than traditional map-wise control of the statistical significance, but is instead a different stance with regard to inference. FDR methods will likely be of considerable use in clinical applications; for example, it may be desirable to express the confidence of results of functional mapping for surgical planning in terms of the specificity of the population of voxels identified.

Another approach for estimating a collection of unobservable signals from observation of their mixtures uses independent component analysis (ICA). Several researchers have demonstrated that ICA identifies task-related loci of activation with accuracy comparable to that of established techniques (see the Appendix for details on ICA).

## References

1. Buchel C, Friston KJ. Assessing interactions among neuronal systems using functional neuroimaging. *Neural Netw.* 2000;13:871–882.
2. Price CJ, Friston KJ. Cognitive conjunctions: a new experimental design for fMRI. *Neuroimage.* 1997;5:261–270.
3. Sternberg S. Separate modifiability, mental modules, and the use of pure and composite measures to reveal them. *Acta Psychol.* 2001;106:147–246.
4. Grill-Spector K, Malach R. fMR-adaptation: a tool for studying the functional properties of human cortical neurons. *Acta Psychol.* 2001;107:293–321.
5. Aguirre GK, Zarahn E, et al. The variability of human BOLD hemodynamic responses. NeuroImage 1998;8:360–369.
6. D'Esposito M, Zarahn E, et al. The effect of normal aging on coupling of neural activity to the BOLD hemodynamic response. *Neuroimage.* 1999; 10(1):6–14.
7. Worsley KJ, Friston KJ. The analysis of fMRI time-series revisted-again. *Neuroimage.* 1995;2:173–182.
8. Detre JA, Alsop DC. Perfusion fMRI with arterial spin labeling. In: Bandettini PA, Moonen C, eds. *Functional MRI.* Berlin: Springer Verlag; 1999:47–62.
9. Aguirre GK, Detre JA, et al. Experimental design and the relative sensitivity of BOLD and perfusion fMRI. *Neuroimage.* In press.
10. Friston KJ, Zarahn E, et al. Stochastic designs in event-related fMRI. *Neuroimage.* 1999;10:607–619.
11. Zarahn E, Aguirre GK, et al. A trial-based experimental design for fMRI. *Neuroimage.* 1997;6(2):122–138.
12. Menon RS, Luknowsky DC, et al. Mental chronometry using latency-resolved functional MRI. *Proc Nat Acad Science U S A.* 1998;95:10902–10907.

13. Henson RNA, Price CJ, et al. Detecting latency differences in event-related BOLD responses: application to words versus nonwords and initial versus repeated face presentations. *Neuroimage.* 2002;15:83–97.
14. Engel SA, Rumelhart DE, et al. fMRI of human visual cortex [letter] [published erratum appears in Nature 1994 Jul 14;370(6485):106]. *Nature.* 1994;369(6481):525.
15. Sereno MI, Dale AM, et al. Borders of multiple visual areas in humans revealed by functional magnetic resonance imaging [see comments]. *Science.* 1995;268(5212):889–893.
16. McIntosh AR, Bookstein FL, et al. Spatial pattern analysis of functional brain images using partial least squares. *Neuroimage.* 1996;3:143–157.
17. Aguirre GK, Zarahn E, et al. The inferential impact of global signal covariates in functional neuroimaging analyses. *Neuroimage.* 1998;8(3):302–306.
18. Nichols T, Hayasaka K. Controlling the familywise error rate in functional neuroimaging: A comparative review. *Stat Methods Med Res.* 2003;12(5): 419–446.

# 4

# Challenges in fMRI and Its Limitations

R. Todd Constable

## Introduction

This chapter will explore some of the challenges of functional magnetic resonance imaging (fMRI), particularly the constraints encountered in terms of spatial and temporal resolution, as well as the factors that limit the ability of MRI to detect functional activation. These issues of sensitivity and resolution are intimately related and not easily separable; for example, increasing spatial resolution usually can only be achieved at the expense of temporal resolution and sensitivity loss. In addition to examining the factors limiting the sensitivity and resolution of fMRI, this chapter will explore some of the trade-offs involved in optimizing one or more of these variables.

There are a number of characteristics that the ideal functional MRI experiment would exhibit. Chief among them is the ability to acquire reliable data in a short period of time with high spatial and temporal resolution. It is currently an open question as to what the ultimate spatial and temporal limits should be. Generally, if investigators had the flexibility of choosing from a range of spatial and temporal resolutions, the choice would need to be tailored to the specific application. The challenges in obtaining reduced acquisition times with high spatial and temporal resolution will be discussed in detail in the sections that follow.

As fMRI experiments are performed at higher fields, the limits of temporal and spatial resolution continue to be pushed. Recent experiments have shown that fMRI is capable of sufficient resolution to examine cortical columns in the visual cortex, and that activation maps have been presented demonstrating differential activation across cortical layers. It is unlikely, for reasons explained below, that ultimately all experiments will be performed at very high spatial resolution (at the layer of columns), but continued improvements in fMRI acquisition strategies are bringing this goal closer. Clearly, much more needs to be understood about brain function at the systems level, at the level of the cortical layers, and ultimately at the neuronal level. Much research is underway examining brain function at all of these levels, and as these systems become better understood, the required spatial and temporal resolution for specific fMRI investigations will become more clear.

Most cognitive and many sensory/motor fMRI experiments are limited in terms of spatial and temporal resolution by a range of factors. Some of the limitations are imposed by the physics of magnetic resonance (MR), some are physiological, and others are neuronal systems based. The sections that follow discuss these issues in detail.

## MR Physics-Based Limitations in fMRI

As explained in Chapter 1, the reader should keep in mind that magnetic resonance imaging (MRI) is based primarily on measuring signals from protons (H) on water molecules ($H_2O$). The local magnetic environment that these protons experience determines in part the signal strength obtained from a given tissue region. The magnetic properties of blood are different depending on the oxygenation state of the hemoglobin (Hb), with deoxyhemoglobin (diamagnetic) introducing small local field inhomogenenities and oxyhemoglobin (paramagnetic) producing a more uniform microscopic field homogeneity. During the echo time (TE), the protons (water molecules) diffuse in and around these Hb molecules. Protons diffusing near deoxyhemoglobin will experience a range of local magnetic fields, leading to rapid dephasing of the signal, and hence, signal loss. This state typically represents the baseline or control condition in an fMRI experiment. As deoxygenated blood is replaced by oxygenated blood upon neuronal activation, the amount of dephasing is reduced as the local field inhomogeneities are reduced and the water protons experience a more uniform field as they diffuse. Therefore, the signal in the presence of oxygenated blood decays more slowly, and thus, at the echo time, TE, there will be more signal remaining in the oxygenated state than in the deoxygenated state. Comparing the signal obtained in the activation state with the control state, a small increase in signal intensity is observed of the order of four percent or less (at 1.5T), with the actual amount dependent upon a range of factors. This slight change in signal is the chief mechanism exploited in fMRI and forms the basis of blood oxygenation level-dependent (BOLD) contrast.

### Physics-Based Limitations on Spatial Resolution

Two parameters are of interest in determining the optimum spatial resolution of MRI; these are image signal and noise. Signal is the signal intensity recorded by the coil for any given tissue. It is dependent upon the amount of magnetization present at the time of the echo. The amount of magnetization present is dependent upon field strength (higher field strength results in higher spin polarization, leading to greater initial magnetization), relaxation times (signal decays with two different relation times T1, T2, and in the case of gradient echo imaging, a third time, T2*), proton density, and the imaging parameters and magnetization history. Proton density refers to how much water is present in a given volume of tissue.

Holding all other imaging parameters constant, the signal varies in direct proportion to the voxel volume. The voxel volume, of course, is directly related to the spatial resolution, and it is typically changed by changing the spatial encoding gradient strength (and hence the field of view) and/or by increasing the acquisition matrix size. The relationship between spatial resolution and the signal-to-noise ratio (SNR) is given by: $SNR \propto \Delta x \Delta y \Delta z \sqrt{N_x}\sqrt{N_y}\sqrt{N_{ave}}/\sqrt{\upsilon}$, where $\Delta x$ and $\Delta y$ represent the voxel dimensions in $x$ and $y$, $\Delta z$ is the slice thickness, $N_x$, $N_y$ represent the sampling matrix size in the $x$ and $y$ directions, $N_{ave}$ is the number of averages, and $\upsilon$ represents the acquisition bandwidth (one over the sampling rate of the data acquisition).

In general, the noise is unaffected by changes in voxel volume, but the signal intensity is directly proportional to the voxel volume. Voxel volume is determined by the product of slice thickness times the in-plane spatial resolution (volume = $\Delta x \Delta y \Delta z$). The in-plane resolution is determined by dividing the field of view (FOV) in the $x$- and $y$-directions by the acquisition matrix size in these directions. Consider some typical imaging parameters—For a 200 × 200 millimeter (mm) FOV and an acquisition matrix of $(N_x = 64) \times (N_y = 64)$ the in-plane voxel size is 3.125 × 3.125 millimeter (dividing 200 mm/64). A slice thickness of $\Delta z = 5$ mm will then result in a voxel volume of $3.125 \times 3.125 \times 5 = 48.8\,\text{mm}^3$. Changing any of these dimensions can have a dramatic effect on SNR. Decreasing the slice thickness by a factor of two will reduce the volume by half; thus, the SNR will be reduced by a factor of two. Similarly, doubling the in-plane resolution in the $x$ and $y$ directions simultaneously (which will reduce the voxel size in the above example to $1.56 \times 1.56\,\text{mm}^2$) will reduce the voxel volume, and hence the SNR, by a factor of four. Clearly, the choice of imaging resolution has a significant impact on the SNR of the images.

If sufficient SNR is present in the raw images of an fMRI experiment, the spatial resolution may be increased by increasing the matrix size, or decreasing the FOV, or both. Ultra-high resolution MR images have been obtained with in-plane resolutions of the order of tens of micrometers, which is easily the size of individual neurons. The ultimate constraints on the spatial resolution in MR arise from two phenomena. First, most imaging is performed by collecting an echo, and while this echo is being collected, the signal is decaying across the echo with a relaxation time of T2 in a spin echo sequence, or T2* in a gradient echo sequence. In most fMRI experiments, the effects of this T2 decay across the echo are minimal, but as the resolution becomes very high, the blurring caused by T2 decay can begin to dominate and limit the resolution achievable. At this extreme, tissues with long T2 will be sharper than tissues with shorter T2; thus, the resolution throughout the image may vary as a function of tissue T2. The second limiting factor is the diffusion rate of water. Because MR images rely on the signal obtained from freely diffusing water, if the water molecules move a significant amount during data acquisition, this will lead to a blurring, reducing the ability to localize the signal. The localization of this signal is limited to the mean square diffusion distance of water in the amount of time required to spatially localize the signal.

At the extremes of spatial resolution in MR, water diffusion is the ultimate limiting factor (see Callaghan PT, Principles of Nuclear Magnetic Resonance Microscopy, Oxford Science Publications, 1993). To date, MRI experiments are in a regime well removed from this diffusion effect; therefore, this is not a primary limiting factor in fMRI. As will be seen below, there are a number of other considerations—such as the number of slices acquired, temporal resolution, image distortion, and brain coverage—that can influence the choice of spatial resolution. Most studies to date that have used very high spatial resolution tend to focus on one specific cortical area, and studies involving whole brain coverage typically are performed at much more modest spatial resolutions.

### SNR and Field Strength

Increasing field strength leads to increased polarization of spin populations, and therefore to a larger initial magnetization vector. This holds true in fMRI with the added benefit that the measured change in BOLD amplitude also is larger at higher field.[1,2] This increase in BOLD signal change, and the increase in image SNR, can allow for imaging at higher spatial resolutions at higher fields, allowing for imaging at higher temporal resolution [repetition time (shorter TR)], and/or allow shorter imaging sessions. T1s are longer at higher field strength; thus, smaller flip angles or longer TRs must be used to ensure maximal signal amplitude. In contrast, T2s, and T2* in particular, are shorter at higher field strength; thus, the optimum TE for BOLD imaging is shorter than at lower field strength.

Noise in MRI is the term given to any unwanted signal, and these unwanted signals may arise from multiple sources. Thermal noise (random fluctuations of spins aligned with the field) is always present in MRI and can only be eliminated by reducing the sample temperature to absolute zero, which usually is not practical in fMRI. Some noise also is generated in the electronics of the MR scanner, and if other electronic equipments, such as projectors for presenting visual stimuli, are present in the room, these devices may emit radiofrequency (rf) radiation at a frequency that the head coil could pick up, also leading to significant noise. If the noise from a projector is at a particular frequency, then a streak artifact, a line of bright intensity, in the phase-encoded direction will be clearly visible, whereas if the rf noise is of a broader bandwidth, it will simply decrease the overall SNR of the images (and thus decrease the significance of any activations) without obvious artifacts.

### Static Field Inhomogeneities

Also amplified at higher field strengths are the problems of field inhomogeneities that result in signal loss and image distortion. Thus, without compensation methods for BOLD imaging in the presence of field inhomogeneities, moving to higher field strengths may not always be advantageous. Medial frontal and medial temporal areas are particularly affected by the amplification of susceptibility effects.

A number of methods have been investigated to attempt to reduce the impact of macroscopic field inhomogeneities. These are the local field inhomogeneities that arise at air/tissue junctions and, in particular, in brain regions near sinuses.[3] These are referred to as macroscopic static field inhomogeneities because they alter the main magnetic field in relatively large areas. The challenge in solving this problem is that the BOLD mechanism relies upon differences in local microscopic field inhomogeneities between paramagnetic oxygenated and diamagnetic deoxygenated blood; therefore, a method that removes the pulse sequence sensitivity to field inhomogeneities will solve the signal-loss problem due to static field effects, but also will remove sensitivity to BOLD signal changes.

Static field effects are more pronounced along the largest dimension of a voxel, and the source of signal loss is dephasing across this dimension. In most cases, the slice thickness ($\Delta z$) represents the largest dimension of a voxel, and because the largest dimension is the most sensitive to signal loss through dephasing, all the methods developed to date have focused on reducing this through-plane dephasing. It should be noted, however, that most of the methods developed are general and can be applied in any direction. Decreasing the voxel size in any dimension ($\Delta x$, $\Delta y$, $\Delta z$) will reduce the dephasing across that dimension. The simplest approach to reducing macroscopic susceptibility loss is to move to thinner slices and higher spatial resolution.[4,5] This involves a significant cost, however, in terms of absolute number of images collected and the necessarily longer TR required to accommodate the additional slices need to cover the same brain region. Increasing the TR to accommodate these additional slices leads to a decrease in statistical power[6] and decreases temporal resolution.

Other approaches to solving this problem include $z$-shimming[7–9,73,74] based on original work by Frahm,[10] in which multiple acquisitions are collected with different $z$-refocusing gradient lobes, wherein these gradients are designed to cancel the gradients created by macroscopic susceptibility effects in the body. A minimum of two acquisitions are required (thereby effectively doubling TR), with more acquisitions leading to better compensation. An alternative approach is to design tailored rf pulses[11,12] such that the rf imposes a phase gradient across the slice, which compensates the phase shifts introduced by the local field gradients. Theoretically, such pulses can be designed, but in practice it is very difficult to play out these pulses in a reasonable amount of time, and the rf power deposition can be a limiting factor.

Many of these approaches are multi-shot approaches, requiring 2 or more acquisitions, and thus incur penalties in temporal resolution and statistical power. Two single-shot z-shimming approaches have been presented. Song and colleagues[13] showed results in which two gradient echo images were collected with different $z$-shim gradients on each side of a 180-degree rf pulse. More recently, Yang[14] published a single-shot approach in which the even echoes in an echo train had one $z$-shim value, whereas the odd $k$-space line acquisitions had a second $z$-shim value and the phase-encoded gradient was only incremented on every other echo rather than on each echo. Such an approach produces two exactly registered (except for distortion effects in the $x$-direction) $z$-shim images with equal T2* weighting in a single shot, and therefore without the usual penalty in TR. This approach, however, doubles the width of the acquisition window, which in turn increases the geometric image distortion in the $y$ direction by a factor of two. Because these single-shot approaches also at least double the acquisition window width, fewer slices may be obtained within a given TR, or increased TR is required to collect the same number of slices as a conventional single-shot acquisition. Thus, the ideal solution remains to be found for compensating for these field inhomogeneities while maintaining BOLD sensitivity and temporal resolution.

Moving to higher field strengths, such as 3T or greater, provides sufficient BOLD contrast using spin echo techniques or asymmetric spin-echo methods wherein microscopic field effects are not refocused by the spin echo, but macroscopic effects are refocused. Spin echo–based BOLD imaging has been shown at 1.5T[15], but the sensitivity at this relatively low field strength is insufficient for most fMRI applications. Sensitivity increases with field strength, and using an asymmetric spin echo echo planar imaging (EPI) acquisition, it is possible to tune the sensitivity to field inhomogeneities at different scales.[16–18]

### Effect of Acquisition TR

If functional imaging is to be performed in a small, localized brain region, and if subject motion is minimal, then scanning with short TR of the order of one second or less provides excellent statistical power relative to the same study performed with a much longer TR.[6] In the limit of decreasing TR, the temporal correlations in the data leads to redundant data collection, and thus the gain in statistical power as TR is decreased diminishes at very short TR. However, if subject motion is a problem, moving to a longer TR with maximal spatial coverage and very high resolution (both in-plane and through-plane) maximizes the ability of motion-correction algorithms to re-register the brain volumes collected over time. In this case then, moving to a longer TR and increasing through-plane resolution and coverage can improve the statistical power in the data. The reader is clearly learning at this point that there are no easy trade-offs in fMRI and many factors must be considered in designing a study and choosing the imaging pulse sequence and parameters. While the discussion above has focused primarily on MR physics-based challenges in fMRI, the next section discusses a number of physiological phenomena that tend to be the dominant factors limiting the resolution of fMRI.

## Physiological Factors Influencing Spatial Resolution

In addition to the standard physics-based factors of signal and noise influencing the spatial resolution of the underlying MR images, a number of physiological factors also impact the resolution that can be obtained with functional MRI.

### Physiological-Based Limitations/Constraints in fMRI

Physiological noise refers to the introduction of unwanted signal changes to the fMRI time-course data as a function of various physiological processes not directly associated with the functional region of the brain that is of interest. The two dominant sources of this noise include signal changes as a function of pulsatile flow through the brain associated with the cardiac cycle and signal changes associated with respiration. These two primary sources of noise contribute substantially to the need for collecting multiple images per task condition in order to reliably detect brain activation. In the case of the cardiac cycle, the entire brain pulsates with each beat of the heart, introducing both very small motions and variable vessel flow conditions that must be averaged out of the data. Respiration changes the susceptibility in the chest as deoxygenated air in the chest is replaced with oxygenated air, and while the chest is obviously some distance from the brain, these changes in susceptibility are detectable in the brain.[19]

### Blood Oxygenation Changes and Localization

A local change in blood oxygenation in the capillaries does not simply produce a local change in the magnetic field in the capillary. Magnetic field changes are always locally smooth (there are never discontinuities in magnetic field gradients); thus, the field inhomogeneity produced by deoxyhemoglobin extends beyond the wall of the capillary containing the blood. Furthermore, the water, which, as was seen above, produces the signal that is recorded, diffuses some distance past these inhomogeneities and also can broaden the effective spatial extent of the field perturbation. Together these factors tend to increase the area in which the signal changes are detectable and lead to signal changes in the cortical tissue, not just the individual capillaries.

The density of the local vasculature also may impact the amplitude of the signal change detected. A change in oxygenation of blood in a capillary-dense region (high blood volume) will have a bigger impact on the BOLD signal intensity than the same relative change in oxygenated blood in a region with a sparse capillary network. Work in animal models has demonstrated variable cortical and subcortical capillary densities in several brain regions.[20]

The change in blood oxygenation that occurs with activation is over and above the increase in demand for oxygenated blood, and the extent of the region in which a vasculature response is initiated may be larger than the local region where function is increased. This also may contribute to an over estimation of the functional area under investigation. It is currently unclear as to what is the exact relationship between the spatial extent of the cortical tissue activated (and the number or fraction of neurons in that region that are activated) and the spatial extent of the region experiencing a blood-flow response.

### Functional Spatial Limitations

The question of maximal resolution obtainable with fMRI may be turned around, and the question might be posed in terms of the minimum functional unit that can cause a blood-flow response upon activation. In fMRI, typically hundreds of thousands of neurons are included in a voxel, and it is the mean activity of some part of those neurons that leads to a blood-flow response. The relationship between the number of neurons that fire and the BOLD response associated with that number is unclear. However, it is clear that there is a tight coupling between glucose utilization and neuronal spike activity, at least in the sensory/motor cortex. It is not currently feasible to measure by independent methods a significant fraction of the neurons involved in a particular task; thus, to date, investigators have either examined gross EEG-based signals or recorded single neuron spike activity and related magnitude changes in these measures (using either the change in power at a particular frequency in the case of EEG, or the spike rate in the case of single unit recordings) to the BOLD signal change detected.[21–25] Better spike recording methods must be developed before the relationship between the fraction of neurons firing in a voxel can be directly related to a change in oxygenation and/or blood-flow.

### Brain System Dependent Limitations

As cognitive tasks become more sophisticated in design and more subtle cognitive functions are examined, it will be important to relate the BOLD activation signal to specific networks involved in a task; for example, in a region such as the primary motor cortex wherein the neurons for the digits in the hand are highly interleaved, it is not currently possible to distinguish activation patterns for the individual digits. There may be many other brain systems that are wired in this interleaved fashion, in which case it could be very difficult to distinguish between different functional roles for these interleave neurons. Clearly, if neurons are highly interleaved in the cortex, then different groups of neurons may be activated by different tasks within a single voxel, but if the same number are activated by different tasks, no difference in activation will be detectable. This also is related to the issue of the modularity of the brain. To what extent can brain functions be divided into separate modules and what are the neuronal components that make up these modules? Higher resolution fMRI studies may someday answer such questions, and this issue will ultimately determine the spatial resolution required for fMRI.

### Draining Vein Problem

A problem that has been discussed since the advent of fMRI is the potential spatial misregistration of functional activity that may occur as a function of the microvasculature. The capillaries, in which the small changes in oxygenation take place upon activation, drain into larger veins downstream from the activation site. Because the amount of blood in a draining vein may be larger than in the upstream capillaries, and because the small changes that occur in each capillary may add up to larger BOLD signal changes in the draining veins, this effect could contribute to spatial misregistration of the activation some distance downstream from the true area of cortical activity. A recent study by Turner[26] used a quantitative analysis of the geometry of the venous vasculature together with hydrodynamic considerations to calculate upper bounds on the extent of this problem. These calculations revealed that an activated cortical area of 100 square millimeters could generate an oxygenation change in venous blood that extends no more than 4.2 millimeters beyond the edge of the activated area. While the venous blood obviously drains much greater distances beyond this limit, the oxygenation effect is sufficiently diluted as to be undetectable.

In an attempt to reduce the draining-vein problem and produce highly localized functional maps, Menon and Goodyear[27] used the initial increase in the BOLD signal intensity to image ocular dominance columns in the human visual cortex and demonstrated that this use of the initial slope of the BOLD signal increase was effective.

Field strength also influences the relative signal change with changes in oxygenation for both tissue and vessels. It has been shown, for example[28], that increasing field strength increases the BOLD sensitivity to tissue changes in oxygenation faster than the increase in vessels. Thus, moving to higher field strengths reduces the relative contribution of the venous signal changes compared to the true tissue signal changes.

The reader should keep in mind that the draining-vein problem does not preclude true BOLD activation in the cortical region activated, but can produce additional, potentially stronger activations further downstream. The fact that the BOLD response in draining veins can be large allows them to be identified by the large percent signal change measured. Excluding signal changes above a certain threshold (in terms of percent signal change), it is possible to produce high-resolution maps of cortical function free of this draining-vein problem. Cheng and colleagues,[29] for example, produced maps of the cortical columns in the visual cortex adapting this approach to sustained stimulus presentations. But caution is required with this activation amplitude threshold approach because the signal in draining veins does not necessarily have to be large and the signal does gradually decrease with distance from the activation site so at some point the threshold approach will fail—and this point is unfortunately at maximal distance from the activation site.

Spin-echo imaging is sensitive to microscopic but not macroscopic susceptibility effects.[16–18] At high field strengths (3T and greater), this approach can achieve sufficient sensitivity for fMRI experiments and can mostly eliminate the draining-vein problem. It is well known that spin echo sequences are much less sensitive to the draining-vein problem. While most investigators do not like to admit it, the additional relatively large signal changes associated with larger veins can aid in detecting activation. The sensitivity of gradient echo and spin echo sequences to microscopic susceptibility changes is essentially equal; thus, the choice of gradient echo imaging over spin echo imaging is made to allow the contribution of larger vessels to the BOLD signal change to get an added boost from the bigger signal changes associated with these vessels.

Diffusion gradients also can be applied to BOLD imaging sequences to reduce contributions from large vessels[30,31]; in fact, it is possible to use maps of apparent diffusion coefficients to detect activation.[32–34]

## Initial Dip

Another method to eliminate the draining-vein problem and to possibly provide more precise spatial localization of fMRI activity is to localize activation based on finding regions that exhibit an initial dip in BOLD signal intensity prior to the main signal-intensity increase. Following the presentation of a stimulation event, the blood-flow response in the cortical region involved in detecting or responding to the event often leads to a complicated pattern of signal changes. Some experiments have shown that there is first a decrease in signal intensity prior to the increased signal intensity typically observed in BOLD experiments. The initial dip was first observed using optical measures of oxy- and deoxyhemoglobin[35,36] and has more recently been demonstrated using BOLD-sensitive fMRI methods in the visual[37–40] and in the sensory/motor cortex.[75,76] Because the increased oxygen consumption occurs before the blood-flow response has had a chance to compensate, there is a brief decrease in the ratio of oxygenated to deoxygenated blood, leading to an initial dip in signal intensity. This initial dip is followed by a signal-intensity increase as the blood-flow response kicks in and overcompensates for the increased oxygen consumption, leading to an increase in the ratio of oxyhemoglobin to deoxyhemoglobin in the blood and the increase in BOLD contrast that most fMRI experiments typically rely upon. As the blood flow returns to baseline levels after these events, an under-shoot of the signal intensity is also often observed before the intensity finally returns to pre-stimulus levels.

Theoretically, the initial dip could provide extremely good localization of the activated regions because there is no draining-vein problem with this phenomenon, and it directly reflects increased oxygen consumption.[40] Kim and colleagues[41] exploited this phenomenon to map iso-orientation columns in the rat visual cortex. The initial dip also may be important in understanding the link between changes in cerebral blood flow (CBF), cerebral blood volume (CBV), partial pressure of oxygen ($PO_2$), and oxygen metabolism under dynamic conditions. However, there are two difficulties associated with the initial dip phenomenon. First, it is controversial in that it is not always observed. As Buxton[42] pointed out in a commentary on this issue, two recent studies using optical imaging techniques and whisker barrel stimulation paradigms in a rat model came to opposite conclusions regarding this phenomenon. Lindauer and colleagues[43] found no evidence for this initial decrease in tissue oxygenation, whereas Jones and colleagues[44] did find a reproducible initial increase in deoxyhemoglobin. Many fMRI experiments have failed to detect the initial dip. However, when dealing with such a small signal change in the presence of significant physiological noise, a negative result does not necessarily mean the phenomena does not exist. Secondly, the BOLD signal change associated with the initial dip is approximately one-tenth that observed with the later BOLD signal increases; thus, it is very difficult to measure with fMRI and not practical with current methods for the majority fMRI studies. Thus, while the initial dip may have the potential to provide excellent localization, it has so far proved elusive and the signal changes are much too small to yield reliable results.

### Subject Movement

Subject movement is also a constant problem in fMRI experiments, and if human experiments are to move to considerably higher spatial resolution, improved motion-correction methods and motion-limiting devices will need to be developed. The trade-off in limiting subject motion is the tension between subject comfort and ability to move. It is possible to position a subject with sufficient padding, tape, and bite bars, such that they cannot move—however, it is not possible to keep such a subject in the magnet for very long time due to the discomfort associated with these restraints. Systems designed to track motion and algorithms that allow image registration incorporating geometric distortion-correction methods may ultimately improve the ability to correct for any motion, thereby eliminating the need for uncomfortable constraints to be placed on the subjects. Moving to higher field strengths may allow for reductions in the overall study time, and therefore may also allow more restraining devices to be used, particularly if the subject is made aware of the fact that the discomfort is only for a brief period of time. In most cases, however, the gain in SNR in moving to higher field strengths is used to increase the spatial resolution or add more tasks, both of which are good choices, but with the result that study time remains fixed.

### Other Physiological Changes Associated with Brain Activation

As discussed above, if cerebral metabolic rate of oxygen consumption ($CMRO_2$) could be directly measured, or if a BOLD measure of the initial dip does indeed reflect the initial consumption of oxygen, then these approaches would likely provide the maximal spatial resolution. It is unlikely that other MR measures of neural activity, such as changes in CBV and CBF, will provide higher spatial resolution than the BOLD effect, as these changes also represent rather gross brain responses to increased oxygen demand.

### Threshold Effects and Localization

All functional maps are statistical maps of some sort and therefore involve the use of a statistical threshold to be chosen in order to classify some tissue(s) as activated and some tissue(s) as unactivated. However, the actual threshold chosen is arbitrary and the spatial extent of activation varies significantly as a function of this arbitrary statistical threshold. In order to reduce the multiple comparisons problem and reduce the occurrence of spurious single voxel activations arising by chance alone, spatial filtering is also often preformed in the form of a median or cluster filter of some sort. The definition of the size of these filters is also arbitrary and can significantly influence the extent of the activation measured. Thus, spatial resolution of the final activation maps can be significantly influenced by the statistical parameters chosen in the analysis/display software.

## Temporal Resolution of the BOLD Response

The above sections have focused on the issue of spatial resolution in fMRI, but in some cases it may be important to examine the time-course of activation for individual events. Action potentials are recorded as electrical spike activity, and these spikes fire over the course of milliseconds. Electrical recordings of ensembles of firing neurons record characteristic peaks and troughs in the form of evoked response potentials in time-scales of the order of hundreds of milliseconds. Functional MR imaging relies on the blood-flow response to such neuronal activity, which itself is much, much slower than the activity of individual neurons. From a single event, say, for example, a flash of a bright light lasting only 100 milliseconds, the blood-flow response in the primary visual cortex may start to increase some two seconds after the event, it may peak between six to eight seconds and return to baseline by 16 to 20 seconds after this single 100-millisecond flash of light. Because fMRI usually is focused on measuring the response of ensembles of neurons to particular stimuli, it may not be necessary to measure activity with extremely high temporal resolution. However, many interesting questions may be probed by examining even this slow blood-flow response with high temporal resolution, and recent work by Qgawa et al.[77] demonstrates BOLD sensitivity to neuronal system interaction that occur on the millisecond timescale.

There is little evidence to date that within the gross blood-flow response typically measured in fMRI there is detailed information reflecting evoked response potential patterns or specific spike timings. To investigate this further, fMRI experiments will need to be performed with very high temporal resolutions of the order of tens of milliseconds, and such acquisitions are possible—albeit with a very limited number of slices—with the current technology. The mechanism prompting the blood-flow response in the brain is not well understood, nor is the spatial extent of this mechanism clear relative to the actual neuronal activity, and it remains to be seen if there is a meaningful fine-grained modulation of this response with neuronal activity.

Most early fMRI experiments relied upon block designs wherein an activation condition was presented for 30 seconds or more at a time, and this was alternated with a control condition of equal duration many times over the course of a study. In such experimental designs, many images could be collected over the course of a condition and high temporal resolution was not all that important. (Although, as discussed above, shorter TR acquisitions can have significant benefits in terms of statistical power in the activation maps.) Many experiments are still performed using block-designed paradigms because these studies do not require precise timing between the image acquisition and the stimulus presentation, and because the statistical power in such studies is maximized and usually considerably greater than that obtained in event-related designs. Cognitively, however, block-design experiments can be of limited value if habituation effects or changes in strategy occur over the course of a long block of similar stimuli, or if the goal is to separate responses to individual stimuli according to some behavioral measure.

To make for much more natural stimulus presentations and to examine the blood-flow response to specific stimuli, many experimental designs have moved towards event-related studies. Despite the slow blood-flow and oxygenation responses to neuronal activity, many interesting phenomena can be investigated with event-related experimental designs; for example, it is possible to examine the temporal response in a specific region to a wide range of stimuli and quantitatively assess parameters such as time-to-peak, width of response, peak height, and other such factors. For a given brain region, it is possible to examine the linearity of the response as stimulus presentation rate is modified; such studies can provide insight into the coupling of blood-flow, oxygenation, and neuronal activity changes.

To properly sample this blood-flow response function, short TR acquisitions should be used. The TR should be of the order of two seconds or less, with shorter TR again being better, or a technique whereby the time-lock between stimuli presentation and image acquisition is varied such that over the course of many events, the blood-flow response is sampled with high temporal resolution.[78] Increasing the temporal resolution by decreasing the TR necessitates reducing the flip angle of the rf excitation pulse in order to maintain optimum signal. This reduced flip angle in turn leads to decreased SNR in the individual images, but the gain in statistical power associated with more of these noisier images being collected in a fixed imaging time, more than compensates for the slight decrease in SNR of the individual images.

It is very difficult, however, to compare the blood-flow responses across different brain regions, as local differences in the structure of the microvasculature may account for differences in the time-courses observed. It would be desirable to observe temporal progression of activation patterns moving from one region of the brain to another, thereby obtaining a sense of the communication between different brain areas. This is not possible, however, without first characterizing the local variations in the structure of the microvasculature in different cortical regions. Thus, while it is difficult to make claims about the progression of activation from region A to B to C as a single task progresses, it is possible to observe differences in the order of this progression across two or more different tasks, assuming the plumbing remains constant and independent of the task. Event-related paradigms combined with high temporal resolution fMRI acquisition techniques are still in their infancy, and much more will be learned from such studies as the field progresses. A detailed review of such experimental designs for use in fMRI is given in the previous chapter.

Temporal resolution as defined by TR also impacts the ability to filter out or remove periodic noise such as that arising from the cardiac or respiratory cycle. Most acquisition strategies sample at a high enough rate to remove some noise from respiratory effects, but a close look at the noise power spectrum in fMRI revealed that components associated with the cardiac cycle aliased at many different (lower) frequencies due to the relatively low sampling rate of the fMRI data. By low sampling rate, it is meant that a slice acquisition is repeated say every second or more, rather than the required sampling rate of at least 500 milliseconds relative to the cardiac cycle, which has a period of approximately 1,000 milliseconds. Sampling at rates that are at least double the periodicity avoids aliasing of noise components to lower frequencies and makes removal of these components much easier in postprocessing.

## Pulse Sequences for fMRI: Spatial/Temporal Resolution

The most common pulse sequences used in fMRI, EPI, and spiral imaging are discussed in detail in Chapter 2. This section will discuss briefly some aspects of these two sequences and alternative strategies that have been investigated to date. If high temporal resolution is desired, most MR imagers are now equipped with the gradient hardware to provide this information with image acquisition times of the order of 40 milliseconds or less. Echo planar imaging and single-shot spiral methods acquire the entire data set for an image from a single excitation pulse, and thus within a single TR. In conventional MRI, a separate excitation pulse is used for each line of data acquired, allowing a time, TR, to elapse for the magnetization to recover before the next excitation pulse. Thus, in conventional scanning, an image with 64 phase-encoding steps would require $64 \times$ TR seconds to acquire the entire dataset. With a TR of 1.5 seconds, this represents an acquisition time of over one minute. Echo planar imaging methods, on the other hand, can collect the data for an entire image in as little as 40 milliseconds. Collecting the data in such a rapid manner does have drawbacks. There is a significant decrease in SNR due to the high bandwidth of the data acquisition, which is needed to collect the data rapidly, and there are also significant distortion effects arising from the accumulation of phase errors over the sampling window. These distortion effects arise in the phase-encoded direction in EPI, and they are projected in all directions in spiral scanning. This distortion is not present in the conventionally acquired anatomic scans, upon which the activation is usually highlighted. Thus, caution must be used in high-resolution work to ensure that the distorted functional image is registered appropriately to the undistorted anatomic image. This is a difficult problem, as the distortion in the functional images is locally variable; thus, simple rigid body fitting of the two different acquisitions is not sufficient to avoid this problem.[45]

Methods for reducing the image distortion include moving to multishot methods, which of course involves a penalty in temporal resolution. Another approach is to measure in vivo the image distortion, and then use a map of the distortion to correct the final image. Two approaches have been devised to perform this measure; these are field mapping (the image distortion is directly proportional to the distortion in the static magnetic B-field)[46–48] and point spread function mapping (PSF).[49,50] The field map approach can provide a relatively simple method for correcting image distortions, but it contains no knowledge of the initial distribution of image intensities. This limitation makes it difficult to assign the correct image intensity—and hence functional activation—to the undistorted voxels. The PSF approach can correctly assign the appropriate image intensities to each voxel in addition to correctly locating each voxel in space.

A field map can be obtained using EPI with only two EPI data acquisitions. However, because the field map is calculated from the phase difference between these two images, phase wrap can be a problem. This problem can be reduced by collecting several acquisitions with different phase-offsets, thereby making unwrapping of the phase errors much easier. Point spread function maps require a minimum of 16 acquisitions to obtain the PSF in a single direction, but more acquisitions yield higher-resolution PSF maps, and thus better correction of the image distortion. In summary, with acquisition times of one minute or less, field maps or PSF maps can be obtained at some point in an fMRI study, allowing correction of the geometric image distortion.

Despite this problem of image distortion, the gain in statistical power in collecting multiple images in a short period of time and the need for activation/control intervals to be short for cognitive reasons necessitates the use of EPI or spiral pulses sequences. Echo planar imaging scans the data space using a raster scan approach and requires state-of-the-art gradients in order to produce high-quality images with minimal image distortion. Spiral scanning, as the name implies, spirals, either in- or out-, from the center of the data space and can be less demanding on the gradient hardware. Most modern magnets now have gradients, which easily ramp as fast as allowed by the United States Food and Drug Administration (US-FDA). The limitations currently encountered are not hardware limitations, but are based on subject safety issues. The US-FDA mandates limitations in dB/dt (the rate at which the gradient can be ramped) because ramping gradients can very rapidly induce current loops in the body that could result in stimulation of muscle groups such as the heart. Small gradient insert coils have been developed that may allow even faster ramping of the gradients, as the active length of the gradients may be short enough to minimize the current loops. These gradient insert systems, however, can be physically restricting, limited in terms of FOV, and are not easily moved in and out of the magnet due to the heavy weight of the combined gradients and cooling system. Manufacturers have been reluctant to develop such gradient inserts because the coils are awkward to move, weighing several hundred pounds, and they must be properly fastened down each time they are moved lest they torque in the magnet and seriously injure the subject. Going faster also requires faster sampling along the readout gradient, which increases the bandwidth of the data acquisition and negatively impacts the SNR, but with the advantage of decreased geometric distortion.

While EPI and spiral gradient echo acquisitions in their many forms are by far the most commonly used approaches, these sequences are sometimes implemented in three-dimensional (3D) acquisition mode,[1,9] and besides EPI and spiral scanning, there are many other acquisition strategies that can be adapted to fMRI. Other pulse sequences include asymmetric spin echo imaging[51], which combines some gradient echo (T2*) contrast with spin echo (T2) contrast in order to reduce the signal-loss problem associated with static field inhomogeneities and to reduce the contribution of large vessels while maintaining sensitivity to the BOLD affect. Inversion recovery asymmetric spin echo[52] has been used to reduce the contribution of CSF to the functional images, reducing the chance of spurious activations arising from pulsatile movement of the CSF.

Fast spin echo imaging[15] has been used in MRI, but its sensitivity at 1.5T is too low for most cognitive studies. Variations on the fast spin echo imaging approach include techniques such as GRASE imaging[79] and ultra-fast low-angle RARE imaging (UFLARE),[80] both of which have similar performance to FSE, but with reduced power deposition that can be particularly important as one moves to higher field strength. These sequences can be applied with or without inversion recovery pulses to reduce the contribution of CSF. FSE, GRASE and UFLARE can all be applied in single-shot mode, but because of the large number of additional rf pulses included in these sequences relative to EPI or spiral imaging, the acquisition window can be long. Longer acquisition windows mean fewer slices can be acquired in a TR interval.

A novel technique by Scheffler and colleagues[53] uses true fast imaging with steady precession (FISP) imaging and detects signal changes that occur upon activation due to a slight frequency shift associated with local changes in tissue oxygenation. However, this approach requires long TR and a highly uniform static field to be useful.

Single-shot techniques by definition are fast, but there are also methods for accelerating multi-shot techniques. Multi-shot acquisitions are particularly amenable to multi-coil acquisition strategies and the use of sensitivity-encoded (SENSE) reconstruction techniques. In this approach, fewer phase-encoded lines are collected (thereby saving time), but in order to maintain resolution, the FOV is reduced in direct proportion with the number of phase-encoded lines. Reducing the FOV below approximately 20 centimeters when imaging the brain usually results in FOV wrap artifacts wherein the structures that extend beyond the FOV are folded back over into the image. With multi-coil imaging and SENSE reconstruction, however, the sensitivity profiles of the individual coils making up the multi-coil array are used to unwrap the fold-over artifacts and yield high-quality images in reduced imaging times. Some decrease in SNR occurs, and as the reduction in the number of phase-encoded steps increases, the reconstruction begins to deteriorate, limiting the reductions to factors of two or three. Collecting fewer phase-encoded steps with this approach can be used reduce the imaging time, or it may allow for more slices to be collected within the TR window, thereby increasing spatial coverage without a sacrifice in temporal resolution.

As described above in the discussion on geometric image distortion, increasing the acquisition bandwidth also can allow an extra slice or two to be acquired within a given TR because increased bandwidth leads to shorter acquisition windows. However, this shorter readout time will reduce image distortion and SNR; for example, an acquisition with a bandwidth of 64 kilohertz may have a SNR of 50. Doubling the acquisition bandwidth to 128 kilohertz will reduce the image distortion by a factor of two and reduce the SNR by $\sqrt{2}$ and allow a few more slices to be squeezed into the TR interval.

## Imaging Approaches to Other Physiological Measurements

Rather than measuring changes in signal intensity related to relative changes in blood oxygenation as the BOLD contrast mechanism does, it is possible to directly measure changes in cerebral blood flow with neuronal activity. As pointed out by Calamante and colleagues[54] in a review of cerebral blood flow (CBF) methods, the sensitivity of MRI to moving spins was noted in the earliest days of nuclear magnetic resonance (NMR).[55] Today, this approach is exploited in imaging applications using both single-slice and multi-slice acquisition strategies. It is now possible using these MRI approaches to measure absolute CBF, or, more simply, relative changes in CBF with activation. The techniques for performing such measurements generally are referred to as arterial spin labeling methods.

## Arterial Spin Labeling

Arterial spin labeling (ASL) incorporates magnetic labeling of blood flowing into the imaging slice in order to obtain quantitative information on CBF. The basic strategy of ASL is to acquire two acquisitions, one with and one without labeling of flowing blood, such that subtraction of these acquisitions can yield quantitative perfusion information. This approach makes use of the properties of spins in flowing blood and does not require an exogenous contrast agent. Several studies have been published describing the application of ASL techniques in functional brain imaging.[56–61] For an excellent review, see Yang.[62]

There are two categories of methods for approaching spin labeling, and these include continuous ASL and pulsed ASL. Continuous ASL uses a train of rf pulses to continuously saturate protons in the blood upstream from the imaging slice.[63,64] The saturated spins flow into the imaging slice and establish a steady-state exchange of magnetization with the brain-tissue water such that the magnetization measured can be related to the CBF. Pulsed ASL applies a single inversion pulse prior to image acquisition and varies the selectivity of the inversion pulse in successive acquisitions. In pulsed ASL, the inversion pulse is placed upstream of the imaging slice and difference images are obtained from acquisitions with and without this labeling pulse.

In both approaches, there are many factors that can influence the quantification of the CBF. These include slice profile effects, wherein a blurred slice profile can make determination of the arrival time of the tagged spins more difficult to determine. These effects can be minimized with well-designed inversion pulses, which produce very sharp slice profiles, such as some of the longer adiabatic FOCI inversion pulses.[65] Transit time or path-length effects also can introduce quantification difficulties.[66] Most CBF analysis approaches assume a straight-line trajectory from the tagging plane to the imaging plane; however, this is not necessarily true. Tagged spins can flow obliquely between the two planes and the spins likely will not flow along a straight line, thereby increasing the path length and transit time to the imaging slice. Knowledge of these pathways for all slices and all locations is usually very limited, making it difficult to take this issue into account in quantifying the CBF. Minimizing the distance between the labeling slice and the imaging slice can reduce these path-length effects simply by reducing the path-length, and therefore the time allowed for these errors to accumulate. Magnetization transfer (MT) effects also can cause changes in signal intensity in the imaging slice, leading to spurious CBF measures. The MT effect leads to direct signal changes in the imaging slice, even in the absence of perfusion. Magnetization transfer effects also can lead to decreases in the apparent T1, which must be taken into account if absolute CBF is to be determined.[67] To avoid such effects, labeling pulses can be applied in a second acquisition, on the opposite downstream side of the slice equidistant from where these pulses were applied on the upstream side. Both acquisitions then will have the same MT effect, and thus, subtraction will eliminate this as a variable.

A final complicating issue in the application of ASL in fMRI is the need for multi-slice acquisitions. Because all the slices cannot be obtained simultaneously, different slices will have different transit times and different distances from the labeling pool. This can lead to erroneous differences in the apparent CBF between slices, when in fact there may be none. Applying ASL techniques with very fast imaging approaches, and taking the different transit time and path-length effects into consideration, can make multi-slice imaging more practical.[68,69]

Most ASL approaches used in fMRI have used fast imaging pulse sequences such as EPI[37,70] or spiral imaging, although modified single-shot RARE and GRASE pulse sequences have been adapted to ASL for fMRI.[61] The advantage of these multi-shot approaches lies in their reduced sensitivity to field inhomogeneities and, in particular, to the image-distortion effect, which can be large in EPI and lead to significant blurring in spiral scanning and in increased SNR due to the short effective TEs that can be used (although it should be noted that spiral out sequences also can have very short TEs). These sequences, however, require multiple shots, which increases imaging time, and the imaging time can only be reduced by increasing the echo train length and decreasing the number of slices acquired. As in BOLD imaging, these CBF imaging sequences may be combined with the parallel imaging approaches (multi-coil SENSE), but to date, that has not been done. Other approaches have been designed to measure both BOLD and CBF in an interleaved fashion in order to better characterize the activation observed.[14,60,71] Finally, just as in BOLD imaging, moving to higher fields with ASL techniques also has its advantages. The SNR is generally higher, and because T1 is longer at high field labeling, it is better and transit time effects are less significant.[14]

## Sensitivity

By far the most commonly used measure of neuronal activation is the BOLD contrast mechanism. There are, however, other contrast mechanisms that can be exploited. Changes in both cerebral blood volume (CBV) and CBF can be measured with MR using a contrast agent for the former measure and a technique such as arterial spin labeling as described above for the latter. The change in CBV with activation can be quite large and has been reported to be of the order of 30%. In fact, one of the first functional studies in humans was performed using CBV as the measure of activation.[72] Cerebral blood volume typically is not measured in most experiments, however, as it requires the injection intravenously of a contrast agent that entails a small risk and some discomfort on the subjects part.

As discussed above, CBF can be measured using arterial spin labeling, but this requires extra hardware and/or pulse sequences that usually are not found as standard equipment on most imagers. This approach is most effective in cases where only a very limited number of slices need to be acquired (one) and in cases where it is acceptable to define the slice orientation based on the anatomy of the arterial vasculature. The sensitivity of this approach, however, can be high, as the change in CBF as a function of activation is of the order of 20% or more, with some investigators reporting changes in CBF as high as 100% in animal experiments.

## Summary

It is hoped that this chapter has shed some light on the issues associated with defining the spatial and temporal resolution limits and the sensitivity in fMRI. New pulse sequences and new imaging hardware are being developed constantly and, combined with a better understanding of the physiological changes that occur with brain activation, the ability to obtain high resolution fMRI studies in short exam times will continue to improve. There are many trade-offs to be made in deciding on the imaging sequence and parameters to use, and it is hoped that this brief overview will shed some light on the issues involved. Clearly, because many trade-offs must be made, an understanding of these issues will help the investigator to tailor some of these parameters to the specific brain region or study design of interest.

## References


1. Yang Y, Wen H, Mattay VS, Balaban RS, Frank JA, Duyn JH. Comparison of 3D BOLD functional MRI with spiral acquisition at 1.5T and 4.0T. *Neuroimage.* 1999;9:446–451.
2. Yacoub E, Shmuel A, Pfeuffer J, Van De Moortele PF, Adriany G, Andersen P, Vaughan JT, Merkle H, Ugurbil K, Hu X. Imaging brain function in humans at 7 Tesla. *Magn Reson Med.* 2001;45(4):588–594.
3. Ojemann JG, Akbudak E, Snyder AZ, McKinstry RC, Raichle ME, Conturo TE. Anatomic localization and quantitative analysis of gradient refocused echo-planar fMRI susceptibility artifacts. *Neuroimage.* 1997;6: 156–167.
4. Merboldt KD, Finsterbusch J, Frahm J. Reducing inhomogeneity artifacts in functional MRI of human brain activation—thin sections versus gradient compensation. *J Magn Reson.* 2000;145(2):184–191.
5. Wadghiri YZ, Johnson G, Turnbull DH. Sensitivity and performance time in MRI dephasing artifact reduction methods. *Magn Reson Med.* 2001; 45:470–476.
6. Constable RT, Spencer DD. Repetition time in echo planar functional MR imaging. *Magn Reson Med.* 2001;46(4):748–755.
7. Constable RT. Functional MR imaging using gradient echo EPI in the presence of large static field inhomogeneities. *J Magn Reson Imaging.* 1995;5(6):746–752.
8. Yang QX, Dardzinski BJ, Li S, Smith MB. Multi-gradient echo with susceptibility inhomogeneity compensation (MGESIC): demonstration of fMRI in the olfactory cortex at 3.0T. *Magn Reson Med.* 1997;37:331–335.
9. Glover GH. 3D z-shim method for reduction of susceptibility effects in BOLD fMRI. *Magn Reson Med.* 1999;42(2):290–299.
10. Frahm J, Merboldt JD, Hanicke W. Direct flash MR imaging of magnetic field inhomogeneities by gradient compensation. *Magn Reson Med.* 1988;6:474–480.
11. Cho ZH, Ro YM. Reduction of susceptibility artifact in gradient-echo imaging, *Magn Reson Med.* 1992;23:193–200.
12. Stenger VA, Boada FE, Noll DC. Multishot 3D slice-select tailored RF pulses for MRI. *Magn Reson Med.* 2002;48(1):157–165.
13. Song AW. Single-shot EPI with signal recovery from susceptibility induced losses. *Magn Reson Med.* 2001;46:407–411.
14. Yang Y. Perfusion MR Imaging with pulsed arterial spin-labeling: Basic principles and applications in functional brain imaging. *Concepts Magn Reson.* 2002;14:347–357.
15. Constable RT, Kennan RP, Puce A, McCarthy G, Gore JC. Functional MR imaging using fast spin echo at 1.5T. *Magn Reson Med.* 1994;31: 686–690.
16. Boxerman JL, Hamberg LM, Rosen BR, Weisskoff RM. MR contrast due to intravascular magnetic-susceptibility perturbations. *Magn Reson Med.* 1995; 34:555–566.
17. Weisskoff RM, Zuo CS, Boxerman JL, Rosen BR. Microscopic susceptibility variation and transverse relaxation: theory and experiment. *Magn Reson Med.* 1994;31:601–610.
18. Kennan RP, Zhong JH, Gore JC. Intravascular susceptibility contrast mechanisms in tissues. *Magn Reson Med.* 1994;31:9–21.
19. Raj D, Anderson AW, Gore JC. Respiratory effects in human functional magnetic resonance imaging due to bulk susceptibility changes. *Phys Med Biol.* 2001;46(12):3331–3340.

20. Cavaglia M, Dombrowski SM, Drazba J, Vasanji A, Bokesch PM, Janigro D. Regional variation in brain capillary density and vascular response to ischemia. *Brain Res.* 2001;910(1–2):81–93.
21. Heeger DJ, Huk AC, Geisler WS, Albrecht DG. Spike versus BOLD: What does neuroimaging tell us about neuronal activity? *Nat Neurosci.* 2000; 3(7):631–633.
22. Rees G, Friston K, Koch C. A direct quantitative relationship between functional properties of human and macaque V5. *Nat Neurosci.* 2000;3:716–723.
23. Logothetis NK, Guggenberger H, Peled S, Pauls J. Neurophysiological investigation of the basis of the fMRI signal change. *Nat Neurosci.* 1999;2: 555–562.
24. Hyder F, Rothman DL, Shulman RG. Total neuroenergetics support localized brain activity: implications for the interpretation of fMRI. *Proc Natl Acad Sci* USA. 2002;99(16):10771–10776.
25. Smith AJ, Blumenfeld H, Behar KL, Rothman DL, Shulman RG, Hyder F. Cerebrla energetics and spiking frequency: the neurophysiological basis of fMRI. *Proc Natl Acad Sci USA.* 2002;99(16):10765–19770.
26. Turner R. How much cortex can a vein drain? Downstream dilution of activation-related cerebral blood oxygenation changes. *Neuroimage.* 2002; 16:1062–1067.
27. Menon RS, Goodyear BG. Submillimeter functional localization in human striate cortex using BOLD contrast at 4 Tesla: Implications for the vascular point spread function. *Magn Reson Med.* 1999;41:230–235.
28. Gati JS, Menon RS, Ugurbil K, Rutt BK. Experimental determination of the BOLD field strength dependence in vessels and tissue. *Magn Reson Med.* 1997;38:296–302.
29. Cheng K, Waggoner RA, Tanaka K. Mapping human ocular dominance columns with high field (4 T) functional magnetic resonance imaging. *Proc Intl Soc Magn Reson Med.* 2000;8:978.
30. Song AW, Wong EC, Tan SG, Hyde JS. Diffusion weighted fMRI at 1.5 T. *Magn Reson Med.* 1996;35:155–158.
31. Andersson L, Bolling M, Wirestam R, Holtas S, Stahlberg F. Combined diffusion weighting and CSF suppression in functional MRI. *NMR Biomed.* 2002;15:235–240.
32. Zhong J, Kennan RP, Gore JC. Effects of susceptibility variations on NMR measurements of diffusion. *J Magn Reson.* 1991;95:267–280.
33. Lee SP, Silva AC, Ugurbil K, Kim SG. Diffusion-weighted spin-echo fMRI at 9.4 T: microvascular/tissue contribution to BOLD signal changes. *Magn Reson Med.* 1999;42(5):919–928.
34. Song AW, Woldorff MG, Gangstead S, Mangun GR, McCarthy G. Enhanced spatial localization of neuronal activation using simultaneous apparent-diffusion-coefficient and blood-oxygenation functional magnetic resonance imaging. *Neuroimage.* 2002;17:742–750.
35. Frostig RD, Lieke EE, Ts'o DY, Grinvald A. Cortical functional architecture and local coupling between neuronal activity and the microcirculation revealed by in vivo high-resolution imaging of intrinsic signals. *Proc Natl Acad Sci* USA. 1990;87:6082–6086.
36. Malonek D, Grinvald A. Interactions between electrical activity and cortical microcirculation revealed by imaging spectroscopy: Implications for functional brain mapping. *Science.* 1996;272:551–554.
37. Ernst T, Hennig J. Observation of a fast response in functional MR. *Magn Reson Med.* 1994;32:146–149.
38. Menon RS, Ogawa S, Strupp JP, Anderson P, Ugurbil K. BOLD based functional MRI at 4 Tesla includes capillary bed contribution: Echo-planar

imaging correlates with previous optical imaging using intrinsic signals. *Magn Reson Med.* 1995;33:453–459.
39. Hu X, Le TH, Ugurbil K. Evaluation of the early response in fMRI in individual subjects using short stimulus duration. *Magn Reson Med.* 1997;37: 877–884.
40. Duong TQ, Kim DS, Ugurbil K, Kim SG. Spatiotemporal dynamics of the BOLD fMRI signals: towards mapping submillimeter cortical columns using the early negative response. *Magn Reson Med.* 2000;44(2): 231–242.
41. Kim DS, Duong DQ, Kim S-G. High resolution mapping of iso-orientation columns by fMRI. *Nat Neurosci.* 2000;3:164–169.
42. Buxton RB. The elusive initial dip. *Neuroimage.* 2001;13:953–958.
43. Lindauer U, Royl G, Leithner C, Kuhl M, Gold L, Gethmann J, Kohl-Bareis M, Villringer A, Diirnagl U. No evidence for early decrease in blood oxygenation in rat whisker cortex in response to functional activation. *Neuroimage.* 2001;13:986–999.
44. Jones M, Berwick J, Johnston D, Mayhew J. Concurrent optical imaging spectroscopy and laser-doppler flowmetry: The relationship between blood flow, oxygenation, and volume in rodent barrel cortex. *Neuroimage.* 2001;13:1000–1013.
45. Studholme C, Constable RT, Duncan JS. Accurate alignment of functional EPI data to anatomical MRI physics based distortion model. *IEEE Trans Med Imaging.* 2001;19(11):1115–1127.
46. Jezzard P, Balaban RS. Correction for geometric distortion in EPI from $B_o$ variations. *Magn Reson Med.* 1995;34:65–73.
47. Jezzard P, Clare S. Sources of distortion in functional MRI data. *Hum Brain Mapp.* 1999;8(2–3):80–85.
48. Reber PJ, Wong EC, Buxton RB, Frank LR. Correction of off resonance related distortion in echo planar images from Bo field variations. *Magn Reson Med.* 1995;34:65–73.
49. Robson MD, Gore JC, Constable RT. Measurement of the point spread function in MRI using constant time imaging. *Magn Reson Med.* 1997;38(5): 733–740.
50. Zeng H, Constable RT. Image distortion correction in EPI: Comparison of field mapping with point spread function mapping. *Magn Reson Med.* 2002;48:137–146.
51. Houston GC, Papadakis NG, Carpenter A, Hall LD, Mukherjee B, James MF, Huang CLH. Mapping of the cerebral response to hypoxia measured using graded asymmetric spin echo. *Magn Reson Imag.* 2000;18: 1043–1054.
52. Zheng J, Ehrhardt JC, Cizadlo T, Yuh WTC. Comparison of inversion-recovery asymmetric spin-echo EPI and gradient-echo EPI for brain motor activation study. *J Magn Reson Imaging.* 1997;7:843–847.
53. Scheffler K, Seifritz E, Bilecen D, Venkatesan R, Hennig J, Deimling M, Haacke EM. Detection of BOLD changes by means of a frequency-sensitive trueFISP technique: preliminary results. *NMR Biomed.* 2001;14: 490–496.
54. Calamante F, Thomas DL, Pell GS, Wiersma J, Turner R. Measuring cerebral blood flow using magnetic resonance imaging techniques. *J Cereb Blood Flow Metab.* 1999;19:701–735.
55. Singer JR. Blood flow rates by nuclear magnetic resonance measurements. *Science.* 1959;130;1652–1653.
56. Edelman RR, Siewert B, Darby DG, Thangaraj V, Nobre AC, Mesulam MM, Warrash S. Quanlitative mapping of cerebral blood flow and functional

localization with echo-planar MR imaging and signal targeting with alternating radio frequency. *Radiology.* 1994;192:513–520.

57. Edelman RR, Chen Q. EPISTAR MRI: Multislice mapping of cerebral blood flow. *Magn Reson Med.* 1998;40:800–805.
58. Kim SG. Quantification of relative cerebral blood flow change by flow-sensitive alternating inversion recovery (FAIR) technique: application to functional mapping. *Magn Reson Med.* 1995;34:293–301.
59. Yang Y, Frank JA, Hou L, Ye FQ, McLaughlin AC, Duyn JH. Multislice imaging of quantitative cerebral perfusion with pulsed arterial spin-labeling. *Magn Reson Med.* 1998;39:825–832.
60. Hoge RD, Atkinson J, Gill B, Crelier GR, Marrett S, Pike GB. Investigation of BOLD signal dependence on cerebral blood flow and oxygen consumption: the deoxyhemoglobin dilution model. *Magn Reson Med.* 1999;42: 849–863.
61. Crelier GR, Hoge RD, Munger P, Pike GB. Perfusion based functional magnetic resonance imaging with single shot RARE and GRASE acquisitions. *Magn Reson Med.* 1999;41:132–136.
62. Yang Y, Gu H, Zhan W, Xu S, Silbersweig DA, Stern E. Simultaneous perfusion and BOLD imaging using reverse spiral scanning at 3T: characterization of functional contrast and susceptibility artifacts. *Magn Reson Med.* 2002;48(2):278–289.
63. Detre JA, Leigh JS, Williams DS, Koretsky AP. Perfusion imaging. *Magn Reson Med.* 1992;23:37–45.
64. Gonzalez-At JB, Alsop DC, Detre JA. Cerebral perfusion and arterial transit time changes during task activation determined with continuous arterial spin labeling. *Magn Reson Med.* 2000;43:739–746.
65. Yongbi MN, Yang Y, Frank JA, Duyn JH. Multislice perfusion imaging in human brain using the C-FOCI inversion pulse: comparison with hyperbolic secant. *Magn Reson Med.* 1999;42:1098–1105.
66. Alsop DC, Detre JA. Reduced transit-time sensitivity in noninvasive magnetic resonance imaging of human cerebral blood flow. *J Cereb Blood Flow Metab.* 1996;16:1236–1249.
67. Zhang W, Williams DS, Koretsky AP. Measurement of brain perfusion by volume-localized NMR spectroscopy using inversion of arterial water spins: accounting for transit time and cross-relaxation. *Magn Reson Med.* 1992;25:362–371.
68. Wong EC, Buxton RB, Frank LR. Implementation of quantitative perfusion imaging techniques for functional brain mapping using pulsed arterial spin labeling. *NMR Biomed.* 1997;10(4–5):237–249.
69. Ye FQ, Yang Y, Duyn J, Mattay VS, Frank JA, Weinberger DR, McLaughlin AC. Quantitation of regional cerebral blood flow increases during motor activation: A multislice, steady-state, arterial spin tagging study. *Magn Reson Med.* 1999;42:404–407.
70. Darby DG, Nobre AC, Thangaraj V, Edelman R, Mesulam MM, Warach S. Cortical activation in the human brain during lateral saccades using EPISTAR functional magnetic resonance imaging. *Neuroimage.* 1996;3: 53–62.
71. Lai S, Wang J, Jahng G-H. FAIR exempting separate T1 measurement (FAIREST): a novel technique for online quantitative perfusion imaging and multi-contrast fMRI. *NMR Biomed.* 2001;14:507–516.
72. Belliveau JW, Kennedy DN, McKinstry RC, Buchbinder BR. Weisskoff RM, Cohen MS, Vevea JM, Brady TJ, Rosen BR. Functional mapping of the human visual cortex by magnetic resonance imaging. *Science.* 1991;254(4): 716.

73. Constable RT, Carpentier A, Pugh K, Westerveld M, Oszunar Y, Spencer DD. Investigation of the human hippocampal formation using a randomized-event-related paradigm and z-shimmed functional MRI. *Neuroimage*. 2000;12:55–62.
74. Constable RT, Spencer DD. Composite image formation in z-shimmed functional MR imaging. *Magn Reson Med*. 1999;42(1):110–117.
75. Yacoub E, Shmuel A, Pfeuffer J, Van De Moortele PF, Adriany G, Ugurbil K, Hu X. Investigation of the initial dip in fMRI at 7 Tesla. *NMR Biomed*. 2001;14(7–8):408–412.
76. Yacoub E, Hu X. Detection of the early decrease in fMRI signal in the motorarea. *Magn Reson Med*. 2001;45:184–190.
77. Ogawa S, Lee T-M, Stepnoski R, Chen W, Zhu X-H, Ugurbil K. An approachto probes some neural systems interaction by functional MRI at neural timescale down to milliseconds. *Proc Natl Acad Sci USA*. 2000;97(20): 11026–11031.
78. Miezin FM, Maccotta L, Ollinger JM, Petersen SE, Buckner RL. Characterizing the hemodynamic response: effects of presentation rate, sampling procedure, and the possibility of ordering brain activity based on relative timing. *Neuroimage*. 2000;11:735–759.
79. Jovicich J, Norris DG. Functional MRI of the human brain with GRASE-basedBOLD contrast. *Magn Reson Med*. 1999;41:871–876.
80. Niendorf T. On the application of susceptibility-weighted ultra-fast low-angle RARE experiments in functional MR imaging, *Magn Reson Med*. 1999;41:1189–1198.

# 5

# Clinical Challenges of fMRI

Nader Pouratian and Susan Y. Bookheimer

## Introduction

Functional magnetic resonance imaging (fMRI) has revolutionized clinical brain mapping and has become the predominant functional neuroimaging technique since its original report by Belliveau and colleagues.[1] The appeal of fMRI is attributable to several advantages that it offers over other functional neuroimaging techniques. Functional MRI is non-invasive; it is a rapid technique that offers the opportunity for repeated measurements of the same task to investigate response consistency, to compare activations across tasks, and to measure change over time.

Despite its advantages, fMRI presents several unique challenges, especially in the clinical setting (Table 5.1). Many of these challenges arise from the fact that fMRI does not directly measure neuronal activity. Instead, fMRI detects perfusion-related signals that are coupled to neuronal activity. Many studies make assumptions about the characteristics of neurovascular coupling, and therefore the significance of fMRI activations; these assumptions are more suspect in a clinical setting when pathology may alter normal coupling mechanisms; for example, the presence of intracerebral pathologies [e.g., arteriovenous malformations (AVMs)] can induce field inhomogeneities and also may alter neurovascular coupling mechanisms, both of which may hamper measurement of reliable hemodynamic-based fMRI signals. Another challenge of clinical fMRI includes the inability of patients to comply with imaging protocols. One study[2] showed that nearly 30% of subjects with intracranial masses were excluded from the final analysis due to gross motion artifact. This may be a particularly difficult problem if one wishes to study patients with known movement disorders. Impairments in cognition also may alter patients abilities to complete tasks, both with respect to motivation and task difficulty.

Finally, clinical brain mapping emphasizes results for an individual rather than for a group, impacting strongly on choice of analysis methods. Moreover, altered anatomy due to intracerebral lesions may prohibit spatial registration and normalization tools commonly used in

**Table 5.1. Potential Limitations of fMRI in Clinical Populations**

| |
|---|
| Field inhomogeneities in ROI |
| Movement artifacts |
| Altered baseline intelligence |
| Impaired task compliance |
| Impaired motivation |
| Sensitivity to certain stimuli (e.g., flickering lights) |

group statistics, making it difficult to directly compare results from patients with those from a normative sample.[3] This chapter will elaborate on the challenges of fMRI in clinical populations, including issues of field strength and sequence selection, study and task design, and data analysis.

## A Brief History of Clinical Brain Mapping

Until the advent of fMRI and other perfusion-based brain mapping techniques, such as positron emission tomography (PET),[4] optical imaging of intrinsic signals (OIS),[5] and near-infrared spectroscopy (NIRS),[6] our understanding of the functional organization of the brain largely stemmed from studying the effects of brain lesions. Although brain lesions initially were limited to strokes and other accidents of nature. Penfield recognized in 1937 that temporary brain lesions also could be induced to study brain function by applying electrical stimulations directly on the cortex.[7] Most recently, transcranial magnetic stimulation (TMS) has been introduced as a means of inducing temporary lesions non-invasively.[8] By mapping the effects of lesions, these disruption-based techniques identify parts of the brain that are essential and critical for executing a given task. These disruption-based techniques of mapping the brain have emerged as the gold standard of clinical brain mapping, especially in the neurosurgical arena.

Functional MRI differs fundamentally from the classic lesion-based approach to clinical brain mapping in that, instead of only identifying areas of the brain that are essential for performing a task, fMRI indicates all brain areas that demonstrate activity-related changes during a given task, regardless of whether a given brain area is, in fact, critical for task performance (i.e., both essential and supplementary cortical areas). Because of the differences in methodology, fMRI maps and lesion maps will inevitably differ. Both maps are probably clinically relevant, but one must be aware of the different data produced, their implications, and the types of conclusions that can be drawn from each.

## Hemodynamic Basis of fMRI Maps

As discussed in earlier chapters, fMRI offers an indirect measure of brain function: instead of directly measuring neuronal activity, fMRI maps the brain by detecting functional hemodynamic responses that are coupled to neuronal activity. The clinical challenges of fMRI stem, in part, from the fact that the fMRI map is an indirect measure of brain activity. To establish clinical validity of the instrument assumes both that MRI signal changes reflect underlying neural activity, and assuming we accept this relationship, that a particular patient has a normal fMRI response (e.g., the blood-flow response is unaffected by their clinical condition). This complexity can be illustrated by conceptualizing brain mapping as a series of mathematical functions (Figure 5.1).[9]

Given a stimuluxs $x$, there is a given neuronal response $f(x)$, which represents the true brain map. The neuronal response is coupled to a functional hemodynamic response by a neurovascular coupling function, $p$. The uncertainty of this neurovascular coupling function introduces one of the biggest challenges and one of the most significant sources of error in interpreting clinical fMRI studies. What ultimately matters about the neurovascular relationship is the degree and precision of spatial coupling between neuronal activity. As discussed below, the spatial coupling between fMRI activation signals and electrophysiologically active cortices may not be as precise as most would like.

Several recent studies have indicated that hemodynamic responses can be significantly different across brain regions, especially when adjacent to major pathology. In a study of 98 patients, Krings and colleagues showed that the distance of a central mass from the motor region significantly influenced the magnitude of activation, even within patients without paresis.[10] Other studies have found similar suppression of the hemodynamic response adjacent to pathology.[11,12] Conversely, in a study of 14 patients, Schlosser and colleagues suggested that fMRI activation patterns within patients with frontal lobe tumors, when mapped using a verbal fluency paradigm, were comparable to signals in normal controls.[13] Similarly, Righini and colleagues studied 17 patients with frontoparietal masses and found little difference in motor activations between the affected and unaffected hemispheres.[2] The contradiction in these studies highlight the need to be aware of the possibility that adjacent pathologies may alter cerebral hemodynamics, but that this alteration is most likely pathology and location dependent and, possibly, task dependent. Finally, different physiological states (e.g., hypercapnia, hypoxia, hypertension) and different disease states (e.g., vasculitis, angiopathies) can impact differentially the relationship between neuronal activity and functional perfusion. Schmidt and

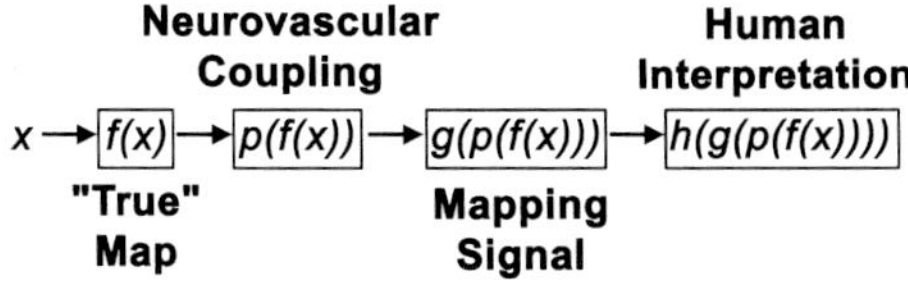


**Figure 5.1.** Cascade of functional brain mapping functions. The mapping signal observed and reported is actually not a true map of neuronal activity. Rather, it is a product of a series of complex functions, including, for example, the coupling of neuronal activity and local cerebral perfusion, or neurovascular coupling ($p$). In order to better understand how functional brain maps relate to underlying true maps it is critical to characterize the robustness of neurovascular coupling under different stimulus conditions, in different cortices, and in the presence of different pathologies.

colleagues have shown in a rodent model that brief exposure to hypercapnia may potentiate the hemodynamic response without affecting the underlying electrophysiological response.[14,15] In fact, highlighting the effect that hypercapnia may have on signals in normal subjects, hypercapnia can be used in normal subject as a means of contrast enhancement.[16] The age of the subject also may affect the magnitude of the hemodynamic response and the coupling mechanism itself.[10] Understanding the underlying coupling dynamics is essential to interpreting fMRI results. It is this uncertainty that continues to motivate continued investigation of neurovascular coupling dynamics.

Assuming neurovascular coupling is intact, several more functions are still applied before arriving at any conclusions from fMRI data. The functional perfusion response produces a brain mapping signal, $g$: $g(p(f(x)))$. The function $g$ is determined not only by the physics behind fMRI signals sources (i.e., field strengths, scan sequences), but also by the recording capabilities of the particular scanner. This includes, but is not limited to, resolution limitations, data filtering, and artifacts that may be introduced by different disease processes or medical interventions (e.g., coils, clips, arteriovenous malformations, air cavities after neurosurgical resections).

Finally, yet another function is introduced into the formula, $h$, for the introduction of human study design, human interpretation, and statistics. Human interpretation of mapping signals, when not quantitative, is always susceptible to bias. The bias may be inadvertent and may be as subtle as in selecting an inappropriate control for comparison or measuring inappropriate signal parameters from which to draw conclusions. The statistics commonly used in fMRI also introduce error and misinterpretations, presenting yet another challenge to clinical interpretation scans.

Although many studies compare blobs across groups, there are a number of assumptions that underlie those blobs. To better understand the underlying map, or $f(x)$, this complex function must be deconvolved by characterizing the factors that influence all of these functions. Alternatively, the investigator can pay special attention to study design and analysis in order to minimize assumptions and to strengthen their conclusions. Many of these issues of study design and analysis are discussed below.

## Technical Considerations

### Field Strength

Magnetic field strength is an important consideration in clinical fMRI study design. Increasing field strength provides a greater dynamic range of data collection and, ultimately, a greater signal-to-noise ratio (SNR) and contrast-to-noise ratio (CNR).[17] Increased SNR and CNR improve study power and decrease Type II errors. Presumably, increased CNR can reduce the scanning time needed to obtain significant results, or make it possible to scan in multiple paradigms in the same amount of time.

Another advantage of increased field strength is the potential for increased spatial resolution (smaller voxel size) with greater SNR given the same acquisition time than at lower fields. Increasing spatial resolution can enhance the sensitivity of the mapping technique, particularly where small differences in localization of function are crucial to the clinical decision or outcome. Large voxel size limits fMRI sensitivity because functional changes at cortical capillaries, which are orders of magnitude smaller than voxel size and represent only a small fraction of total voxel size, are drowned out at the level of the voxel. This partial-volume effect is reduced with smaller voxel sizes. Ultimately, if voxel sizes are too large, a lack of difference between subjects or groups may not actually mean there is no difference. Rather, this may represent a sensitivity limitation of the technique.

However, higher field strengths also pose problems that, in some brain regions or in some clinical conditions, may prove insurmountable. The most difficult complication arising from increased field strength is the associated increase in susceptibility artifact, especially near air–tissue interfaces. This is a particular problem in the inferior temporal lobes and the inferior medial frontal lobes, which are adjacent to the air-filled sinuses. These areas of susceptibility artifact produce both spatial distortion and MR signal loss, which make it difficult or impossible to identify activity-related changes in fMR images. This is of particular importance for language mapping, in which investigators expect to find several temporal lobe language areas.[18] Lack of signal in these regions does not indicate lack of activity, but may be due to lack of sensitivity to identify appropriate signals. Devlin and colleagues have proposed alternate strategies when imaging these regions of high susceptibility, but they also acknowledge that these artifacts can only be partially overcome and that alternative data acquisition paradigms are necessary to address this issue.[19] In some cases, appropriate selection of scan sequence may help overcome some susceptibility artifacts, especially when imaging adjacent to pathology.

### Scan Sequence and Susceptibility

The most commonly used fMRI pulse sequence is the gradient echo echo planar imaging (EPI) sequence. Echo planar imaging is the fast scanning technique that acquires all slice locations with a single response time (TR), and which has made fMRI practical.[20] The gradient echo sequence is optimized to maximize susceptibility due to blood oxygenation level-dependent (BOLD) contrast. An unfortunate but necessary side effect is that it also maximizes unwanted susceptibility artifacts at tissue interfaces, especially at high field. In certain brain regions—particularly the amygdala, basal temporal region, and orbitofrontal cortex—the susceptibility artifacts may make imaging these regions impossible.

Clinical fMRI within patients who have had prior brain surgery may be complicated by the presence of implanted devices, such as plates and screws. Whereas most of these devices are considered magnet compatible, that is, they are not ferromagnetic and do not pose a safety concern, susceptibility artifacts can generate profound distortions around these objects that include massive signal loss and spatial distortion. It also should be noted that many of these devices have not been tested at high field and could pose a safety risk that does not exist at lower field strength. Typically, these objects will be implanted close to or on top of the precise regions the clinician would like to have mapped.

There are a variety of simple approaches to reducing susceptibility artifacts at air–tissue interfaces and around objects during functional imaging. Reducing voxel size is one. In the amygdala, for instance, Merboldt and colleagues[21] calculated that voxel sizes of 4 to 8 microliters or less are necessary to recover sufficient signal. Fransson and colleague[22] used a high-resolution acquisition method to receive signal in the hippocampus using coronal acquisitions and in-plane resolution of two square millimeters and slice thickness of one millimeter. For most centers, this approach is impractical, both to a lack of non-standard sequences on clinically oriented machines and because for many systems the associated reduction on field of view (FOV) is not acceptable. However, for patients with a focal lesion in which a small FOV is all that is necessary, small voxel studies may be appropriate. The loss of CNR within small voxels also may prohibit the practical use of this approach.

To some extent, use of alternative pulse sequences can improve, but not wholly overcome these artifacts. Port and colleagues[23] performed a series of imaging studies on titanium screws embedded in gel to determine parameters that would decrease susceptibility artifacts in echo planar (EPI) images. They reported three factors that can reduce artifacts: reducing the echo time (TE), increasing the frequency matrix, and reducing slice thickness. The latter two approaches are identical to those reported by Merboldt and colleagues[21] for imaging at air–tissue boundaries. However, the effect of reducing TE on susceptibility is controversial. Susceptibility artifacts due to signal loss at air–tissue interfaces are greater with longer TEs. One approach to reducing susceptibility artifact is to reduce the TE. Gorno-Tempini and colleagues[24] used a double echo EPI sequence to compare susceptibility artifacts and BOLD signal changes at tissue interfaces, comparing TEs of 27 and 40 milliseconds. They used a face-processing task, which is known to activate the fusiform gyrus in the base of the temporal lobe, an area likely to suffer from susceptibility-induced signal loss. Whereas the lower TE did not reduce their ability to detect BOLD signal in those regions unaffected by susceptibility artifacts, the lower TE was not sufficient to recover the BOLD signal.

Various pulse sequences have differential effects on susceptibility artifacts. One alternative to the commonly used gradient echo EPI scan is the asymmetric spin echo. Both spin echo and gradient echo sequences base their signal on magnetic susceptibility contrast as described above, as well as in the previous chapters. The spin echo sequence, however, refocuses the spin dephasing caused by field inhomogeneity. The consequence is that a spin echo sequence reduces susceptibility artifacts at air–tissue boundaries, but also will result in CNR loss due to reduced BOLD contrast. At high field, this loss may be an acceptable trade-off. Spin echo sequences tend to recover signal from larger, rather than smaller, boundaries, and thus have been thought to affect unwanted susceptibility artifacts preferentially, including effects in larger blood vessels, while preserving signal changes in the capillaries. The asymmetric spin echo sequence shifts the time differential between the image acquisition and readout, allowing the signal to decay; thus, the amount of reversible dephasing that occurs can be varied by adjusting the length of this shift. The longer the asymmetry, the more the spin echo images resemble a gradient echo image. Stables and colleagues[25] have demonstrated that varying these parameters can optimize for a particular perturbation size (i.e., a small or large blood vessel). Several fMRI studies have used a spin echo sequence effectively in high susceptibility areas such as hippocampus and amygdala.[26–28] Figure 5.2 shows examples of a gradient echo and asymmetric spin echo EPI images using otherwise identical parameters in the same subject. The recovery of signal in high susceptibility areas, especially around a lesion, is quite apparent, although not complete.

Other modifications to the EPI sequence may reduce susceptibility artifacts. Cordes and colleagues[29] advocated using a second refocusing gradient in the slice-selection orientation to reduce susceptibility

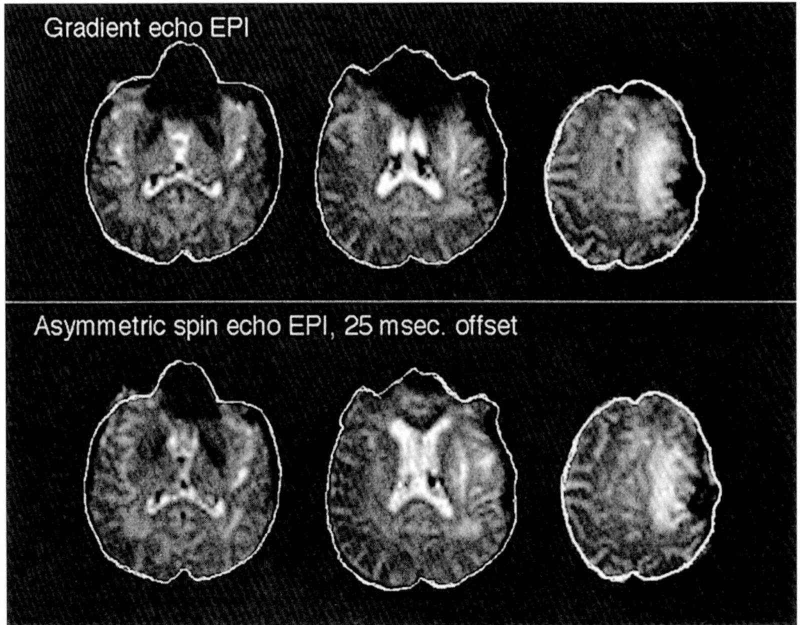


**Figure 5.2.** Gradient echo versus asymmetric spin echo (ASE) EPI. Gradient echo (TR = 2.5, TE = 45, 64 × 64 matrix, FOV = 20, 1 NEX) and asymmetric spin echo (TR = 2.5, TE = 45, offset = 25 msec, 64 × 64 matrix, FOV = 20, 1 NEX) EPI scans in two areas of high susceptibility (left) at air–tissue interfaces in basal temporal and orbitofrontal cortex (right) near the lesion with prior resection. The outlines are derived from a high-resolution spin echo EPI (TR = 4000; TE = 54, 128 × 128 matrix, 20-mm FOV, 5-mm thick, 4 NEX). Note reduced susceptibility in ASE scans in both regions of high susceptibility.

artifacts. A more complicated approach offered by Stenger and colleagues[30] used three-dimensional (3D) tailored radiofrequency (RF) pulses to refocus regions where the susceptibility is greatest, using a modified spiral *k*-space trajectory.

In spiral scanning, *k*-space is traversed in a spiral pattern emanating either from the center to the exterior (spiral-in), the reverse (spiral-out), or in some combination (e.g., dual-echo in-out). Glover and Law[31] reported that a spiral-in trajectory or combinations of in–out trajectories can both increase SNR while reducing susceptibility. Yang and colleagues[32] developed a reverse spiral scanning technique simultaneous with perfusion imaging with arterial spin labeling. Comparisons of susceptibility artifacts between forward and reverse spiral scanning suggested less susceptibility in the reverse sequence, with adequate BOLD signal in high-susceptibility regions. Other techniques to reduce susceptibility artifacts in spiral scans include a sensitivity-encoded (SENSE) sequencing[33] that shortens the readout duration, thus minimizing signal loss. However, the effects of BOLD signal recovery were less dramatic.

### Mapping the Oxy/Deoxyhemoglobin Signal

The choice of mapping signal has become an interesting debate. Although the debate has not yet entered the clinical arena, it deserves brief mention here. Following functional activation, cerebral blood flow (CBF) increases in excess of the cerebral metabolic rate of oxygen ($CMRO_2$), thereby causing a decrease in deoxyhemoglobin (due to an overperfusion of oxyhemoglobin).[34] This functional change in the relative abundance of the different hemoglobin moieties is responsible for the increased BOLD MR signal observed with functional activation. This theory is consistent with several studies that have documented that functional CBF increases exceed that of $CMRO_2$ using multiple modalities, including: positron emission tomography (PET);[35] optical imaging of intrinsic signals (OIS);[5,36] and optical imaging of fluorescent dyes.[37] Recently, an initial decrease in BOLD signal, or initial dip, has been reported that precedes the increased BOLD signal described above. The initial dip is thought to represent an initial burst in oxidative matabolism, which increases local deoxyhemoglobin concentrations before any perfusion changes occur.[37,38] It has been proposed that if this initial negative signal does in fact represent an initial burst in oxidative metabolism, it may be more highly spatially correlated with electrophysiological activity than the later positive BOLD signal.[39] Accordingly, Kim and colleagues[40] was able to use the initial dip signal in cats to map ocular dominance columns in cats using BOLD techniques.

## Study and Task Design

Issues in task design—particularly choice of activation and control tasks, as well as difficulty level—are important considerations in all fMRI studies; however, in the clinical arena, these difficulties take on special significance, as errors in task design can lead to false conclusions that may harm patients. Here, three issues of particular importance in clinical fMRI will be discussed: choice of control conditions, the effect of practice on observed fMRI activations, and the appropriate level of difficulty given the population to be studied.

### Task Selection

Functional MRI activations represent a contrast between two conditions; in the earliest fMRI studies, this contrast was identified by simple subtracting rest or control condition images from those acquired during a task.[41,42] This simple subtraction approach assumes (1) a hierarchical organization of brain function, (2) that the investigator can accurately decompose a complex task, and (3) cognitive activity and brain function are insignificant during rest conditions.

The assumption that an investigator can accurately decompose a task into its components is a challenge in itself. Not all subjects will repeatedly use the same strategy to perform a task, nor can all the cognitive processes that are required to complete a given task function be deduced easily. This challenge is even more difficult in a clinical population in which there may be subclinical or overt cognitive deficits that may alter the strategies used to perform a task. Tasks that are suitable for brain mapping in the general healthy population may not be appropriate in an impaired population. Finally, this approach assumes that cognitive functions linearly summate to produce the observed fMRI signals, and that there is no interaction between cognitive functions that may produce a unique output based on the combination of tasks.

To test the assumptions of linearity of hierarchical structure, Sidtis and colleagues compared activation maps using simple subtraction (maps were generated by subtracting a rest condition from a task condition) and complex subtractions (maps were generated by subtracting two tasks that were presumed to only differ with respect to a single parameter).[43] The three tasks used were syllable repetition, phonation, and lip closure. Syllable repetition was assumed to be a combination of phonation and lip closure for the purposes of this study. Lip closure maps were generated by simple subtraction of the rest condition from the lip closure condition, and complex subtraction maps were generated by subtracting the phonation condition from the syllable repetition condition. The simple and complex subtraction maps were different both with respect to signal intensities and distribution, suggesting that the condition of additivity necessary to decompose complex tasks by subtraction was not present in the data, calling into question subtraction methodology and the assumption that tasks can accurately decompose.

Stark and Squire examined activation patterns associated with rest conditions (used as a baseline) to determine if rest is necessarily an appropriate control or baseline, with particular attention to memory tasks looking at the medial temporal lobe.[44] The authors measured fMRI signals during seven different tasks: novel pictures, familiar pictures, noise detection, odd/even discrimination, arrow discrimination, moving fixation, and rest. The first two tasks were considered memory tasks, whereas the last five were considered to be various controls. Not surprsingly, the authors demonstrated that identifying activity in the medial temporal lobe (including hippocampal and parahippocampal structures) varied depending on the control condition used. In fact, the authors reported that activity within these structures was higher during the rest condition than during other control conditions. Consequently, identifying activity in the ROI intimately depended on the control condition used. This study highlights two important points. First, rest does not mean that the brain is quiescent; the brain is cognitively active even during rest. Second, fMRI activations represent contrasts between two conditions and do not indicate whether a part of the brain was active. Rather, it means there was not a significant enough change in neuronal activity relative to baseline to evoke a functional hemodynamic response. This highlights the need for careful selection of baseline tasks and even more careful interpretation of observed activation patterns.

Gusnard and Raichle[45] reviewed the concept of a physiological baseline, suggesting that in fact the brain has a high level of activity at baseline, and that this must be considered when using rest as a control condition and when interpreting functional activation studies. Importantly, they provided a thorough discussion of task-related decreases in activation and argued that while some of these decreases may represent a task-dependent decrease in cerebral activity, many decreases seem to be task-independent, representing an organized mode of brain function, which is attenuated during various goal-directed behaviors.[45]

### Practice Effects

Paradigm design is not only important with respect to selection of tasks, but also with respect to task timing. Several studies now indicate that practicing a task can significantly alter activation patterns, revealing different maps that may represent alternative strategies for performing the given task, such as automatization.[46–49] Raichle and associates were the first to report that functional activation patterns can be altered by relatively brief periods of practice.[46] Comparing a novel verbal-response selection task with reading visually presented nouns, they found a practice-related decrease in cortical activation of those regions mediating performance at the beginning of the task after only 15 minutes of practice. Moreover, other brain regions increased activity, such that, with practice, the verbal-response task more resembled the reading task. This practice effect was reversed by introducing a novel list of words, allowing the authors to conclude that the activation patterns associated with practice represented an automatization of the task that was reversible. Van Mier and colleagues[48] and Petersen and colleagues[47] reported similar findings of shifts in activation patterns, or changes in functional neuroanatomy, from one part of the brain to another with practice. This is thought to represent an activity-dependent shift in effortful task performance to skilled, automatic task performance.

Similarly, Madden and colleagues[49] reported a decrease in functional activation with practice in the two populations they studied: young adults (20–29 years) and older adults (62–79 years). Using a verbal-recognition memory task, this group characterized activation patterns during encoding, baseline, and retrieval and found that activation patterns were different (both increased magnitude and different spatial distribution) between these populations for each task. Interestingly, despite differences both groups initially demonstrated practice-related effects, showing decreased activation magnitude, although the practice effects were greater in the younger population than in the elderly. The authors concluded that older adults required a more distributive network of brain activation in order to perform the given task and, whereas task performance improved with practice, the smaller practice effect observed in the older group represents a continual recruitment of cognitive processes and attention to support task execution. This is not required in the younger population, who can learn and automate more quickly and effectively.

Not all groups, however, have reported activation of additional areas with practice. Garavan and associates argued that if the core task is unchanged by practice, then practice may cause a decreased magnitude of activation, but will not necessarily recruit additional areas of the brain.[50] Using a visuospatial working memory (VSWM) task, they reported decreased fMRI activations in the four areas of interest with activation, but did not report seeing additional areas of activation with practice. They suggested that their observations are consistent with the fact that the task used continues to tax the VSWM system and could not be automated completely, regardless of amount of practice. This raises an interesting consideration that not all cognitive tasks are equally susceptible to practice effects.

The existence of practice effects and relatively rapidity of onset are important technical considerations in implementing a functional brain-mapping study, especially if one wishes to identify those brain regions that are actively involved in and essential to task performance. Most fMRI studies take approximately one hour to complete, during which time brain-activation patterns may be modified secondary to practice. Therefore, it is critical to plan experiments efficiently and to continually provide novel stimuli and tasks in order to assure that practice-related changes do not taint the results (unless, of course, practice-related effects are under investigation.)

### Task Difficulty

Another important consideration that is intimately related to the concept of practice is task difficulty. It is hypothesized that the changes seen due to practice are largely due to decreases in task difficulty with practice, and therefore automatization of task performance. If a task is too easy, the task may activate brain areas involved with performing automatic activities without taxing the appropriate cognitively critical areas of interest. In contrast, if a task is too difficult, it may recruit additional attentional areas and supplementary areas (areas that a task may not normally activate) to help execute a task.

The paradigm of mapping a paretic or plegic patient offers an excellent means of discussing task difficulty and its effects on fMRI activations. For these patients, the effort and difficulty to complete a motor task is undoubtedly greater than for a healthy volunteer. The source of the paresis (i.e., intracerebral versus spinal) will influence the fMRI activation pattern. In a study of patients with central masses near the motor strip, fMRI activations of primary motor cortex decreased with increasing paresis, independent of the distance of the central mass from the motor strip, although the degree of paresis did not correlate with the magnitude of the observed fMRI signal.[3,10] The observed decrease in primary motor activation cannot be unambiguously attributed do decreased number of functional neurons in the motor strip compression due to mass effect (although the observation was independent of distance of the mass from the central strip), tumor-mediated changes in local cerebral hemodynamics, changes in global perfusion due to the presence of a neoplasm, or a combination of these factors.[3] It is critically important from the perspective of clinical brain mapping to consider if a better primary motor strip mapping signal could have been obtained by changing the level of difficulty of the given motor task. Could a more significant signal be elicited from the primary motor strip if the motor task was made more complex and drove the remaining primary motor neurons harder? What if the motor task was made simpler? Could a simpler task induce greater activation by giving the remaining primary motor neurons a task they are fully capable of executing? These may be important points of consideration in interpreting clinical data.

In the same study, the investigators reported larger secondary motor activations within patients with paresis than without paresis. This is most likely attributable to the difficulty of the task for the paretic patients.[3] Similar to the case of elderly patients recruiting a broader network of neurons than younger controls in order to execute a memory task,[49] the paretic patients may be recruiting additional cortical areas in order to execute a task that is relatively difficult for them given their current medical condition. Krings and colleagues therefore concluded, With increasing task complexity (or with decreasing motor skills), this network must increase its excitatory output, resulting in a higher neuronal activity, more pronounced regional cerebral blood flow changes.[3]

In tasks of higher cognitive functioning, the problem of task difficulty may be even more complex. For example, in our work with patients who have a genetic risk for Alzheimer's disease (AD), older volunteers with normal memory, but who carried the APO-4 allele (which conveys a strong risk of AD), had an increase in the magnitude and spatial extent of brain activation on fMRI in comparison to age- and memory-matched controls.[51] This increase in activation correlated with functional decline after two years. However, among subjects who have mild AD, the same memory paradigms produced the opposite effect; there was a significant decrease in magnitude, spatial extent, and total number of regions showing activation in those subjects who had great difficulty performing the task.

Patients with aphasia due to brain lesions showed similar alterations in brain activity. For instance, Sonty and colleagues[52] showed that patients with primary progressive aphasia had activation like normal patients in primary language areas, but also had additional language activation in regions outside language cortices, suggesting the use of compensatory strategies. Kim and collegues[40] found that the pattern of reorganization within patients with focal lesions varied across individuals and appeared related to whether the lesions were cortical or subcortical. Calvert and colleagues[53] found that patterns of fMRI activation during language tasks in a frontal lobe cerebrovascular accident (CVA) patient depended upon the task; increased right-hemisphere Broca's analog was activated during the most difficult task, whereas the left-hemisphere Broca's was active for a matched control subject.

Together, the existing data suggest that patients with deficits tend to utilize compensatory strategies that engage additional brain regions to accomplish the task. The pattern of fMRI activation during compensation may give a false impression about localization of function; for instance, increased compensatory RH, activation may incorrectly suggest the patient has right-hemisphere speech dominance. Thus, clinical use of fMRI for localization of function must take into account the patient's level of cognitive performance. Impaired performance can easily lead to false conclusions about functional localization, particularly in language tasks.

Ultimately, it is important to consider whether differences in activation patterns across conditions or groups represent differences in brain organization and function or an artifact of differential capability to cope with task difficulty. It is suggested that investigators pay close attention to task difficulty in designing, interpreting, and drawing conclusions from their clinical studies, especially when the general medical condition of one group is significantly different than the comparison group.

## Analysis

Adequate study and task design is not sufficient to be able to draw strong conclusions from a clinical fMRI study. Careful selection of analysis techniques and attention to the particular challenges of analysis limitations is necessary in order to accurately interpret the results of the study. Analysis in the clinical studies differs from other studies most significantly with respect to the type of analysis done: within subject versus group analysis. Attention also must be paid to the technique used to quantify fMRI activations and techniques used to minimize false–positive and false–negative results.

### Within Subject Versus Group Analysis

The vast corpus of data in functional imaging relies almost exclusively on group-averaged data. Early efforts in PET, and later fMRI research, focused on developing superior tools for registering and ultimately warping brains from different subjects into a common space in order to increase SNR through subject averaging. While these efforts have been extremely useful in making it possible to answer broad questions about human cognition, these approaches add little to the clinical utility of these skills. Here, we differentiate between clinical research studies, which have and will continue to use group averaging procedures, from true clinical fMRI, in which a clinician will attempt to make a diagnosis or decision for a single individual based on their fMRI results. First, the broad nature of the question to be answered will be considered.

Why will patients be referred for fMRI? Common current applications are to make a decision relevant to surgical intervention, such as, in what hemisphere is language located? Or where within a hemisphere does a particular functional reside? Future applications may include diagnosis: does a particular pattern of activation indicate a diagnosis of dyslexia, autism, obsessive compulsive disorder, or even malingering, to name a few. The optimal analysis technique will depend upon the question asked. In general, the former category of questions will be answered best by within-subject analysis, and in these cases, there will be a strong emphasis on reliability, reproducibility, and signal magnitude and on accounting for factors that may alter one of these variables. In the latter case, approaches may contrast a particular brain against a databank of brains with and without the disorder in question, calculating the degree of difference for the normative sample and similarity to a diagnostic group probabilistically. While this approach is not currently available, new attempts to find functional landmarks such as the International Consortium for Human Brain Mapping should further such efforts. Here, we will focus on reliability of methods for within-subject analysis in the common current applications.

Given an experimental design that includes at least one activation and *control* condition, several approaches to analysis may reveal active brain regions. Statistical approaches, including correlation coefficients between MR signal and a predicted response curve, *t*-tests comparing activation versus control pixel intensities, on Komogorov–Smirnov tests that show differences not only in mean, but also in variance, all produce a statistical value that the investigator must threshold and display in some way. Current controversies include how to threshold data and whether to use a statistical value or magnitude measure (percent change) or to count volume of activation—that is, the number of pixels exceeding a statistical threshold as a dependent variable. Each technique has its advantages and disadvantages, but few studies have carefully examined the reliability and validity of various approaches.

## Dependent Measures

Functional MRI activations can be quantified broadly into two dimensions: spatial extent and magnitude of activation. Calculating activation size by means of pixel counting has become the most common approach to quantifying fMRI activity, especially in the clinical arena. This approach to activity quantification has several limitations that are discussed below. As an example, the application of pixel counting to studies of language lateralization will be reviewed.

Binder and colleagues[54] compared language lateralization using both fMRI and the intracarotid amobarbital procedure (IAP, the Wada test). For fMRI activations, they studied the contrast between semantic word categorization and a perceptual discrimination task, observing variable amounts of right and left hemisphere activation. The variable activation was quantified using a laterality index (LI), defined as $[V_L - V_R]/[V_L + V_R] \times 100$, where $V_L$ and $V_R$ are activation volumes for the left and right hemispheres, respectively, such that a LI of −100 indicates complete left-sided dominance and a score of +100 would indicate complete right-sided dominance. Volume of activation was defined as the number of pixels exceeding a statistical threshold of correlation with a derived hemodynamic function. A similar index was calculated for errors made during Wada testing using the error rates for each hemisphere injected. Statistical comparisons between the two different measures of laterality, or asymmetry, indicated a strong correlation between the two procedures. This led the authors to suggest a model of relative laterality, which was not completely novel because studies had already indicated by that time that the non-dominant hemisphere had participated in language processing.[54]

These results are striking considering the methodology used. As discussed earlier in this chapter, disruption-based mapping (i.e., Wada testing) and activation-based mapping (i.e., fMRI) may map very different processes. Whereas Wada testing will identify those areas that are essential for language function, fMRI identifies all areas that are involved, essential or not, with language processing. For example, activation paradigms used in fMRI mapping may engage a number of brain systems not specifically related to language, including, including, motor, sensory, and attentional systems that may not be essential and therefore may not cause language disturbance by Wada testing. The high-correlation of the two methods is therefore impressive. The authors proposed that their use of a control paradigm (perceptual discrimination task), in part, controls for these factors, which is probably, in fact, true, but it cannot account for all the methodological differences that seemingly are unimportant in the analysis. They proposed that this be accounted for by the control task.

Beyond differences in methodology between the two techniques, the use of pixel counting to compare relative activity between the two hemispheres may not be valid under all circumstances. Pixel counting has been shown to be remarkably susceptible to noise, and therefore may not be an accurate or precise way of quantifying relative fMRI activation.[55,56] Moreover, this methodology does not account for differences in the magnitude of activation at activated pixels. What if the LI were 0 (indicating equal number of active pixels in both hemispheres), but the average magnitude of activation were three times greater in the left hemisphere? Should one conclude that there is no hemispheric asymmetry? The reliability of language lateralization studies is limited by the preponderance of left-hemisphere–dominant subjects included in the studies and the concomitant lack of right-hemisphere–dominant individual individuals. Therefore, it is not possible to conclude, with confidence, that fMRI using pixels counting is, in fact, a reliable method of identifying hemispheric dominance.

The limitations of using fMRI for language lateralization is demonstrated by Springer and colleagues, who studied 100 normal subjects and 50 epilepsy patients to compare laterality in the two populations.[57] Methods were similar to that of Binder and colleagues[54] except that Wada testing was not used to confirm results. Despite reports in the literature that approximately four percent of the general population is right-hemisphere dominant,[57] the authors did not identify any right-dominant individual in their normal population of 100 (expected number should have been four). Amongst their epilepsy population, four percent demonstrated right-hemisphere dominance, allowing the authors to conclude that laterality is differentially affected in early onset epilepsy patients than in normal populations. The low base rate of right-hemisphere speech makes it very difficult to compare populations accurately. Moreover, without a gold standard against which to validate results, there is no objective means to conclude that the data are valid.

A study by Lehericy and associates, in which they studied 10 patients for temporal surgery, compared fMRI activity with WADA testing, looking at LI in direct lobes using different language tasks: semantic verbal fluency, covert sentence repetition, and story listening.[59] This group also used LI as a measure of fMRI activity, counting pixels that exceeded a statistical threshold. The only statistically significant relationships identified were between the asymmetry of frontal-lobe fMRI activations for semantic verbal fluency and covert sentence repetition and Wada asymmetry indices. Functional MRI asymmetry in the temporal lobes (regardless of language task) did not correlate with Wada asymmetries. Moreover, story listening did not correlate with any Wada asymmetry indices in any lobe. It would be interesting to re-analyze this data to determine if better correlation could be identified across tasks and lobes if signal magnitude where considered instead of only the number of pixels exceeding the statistical threshold. This study highlights that fMRI is not completely reliable for assessing asymmetries and that measures of asymmetry may be task and lobe dependent.

## Conjunction Analysis

Considering the intrinsic noise associated with fMRI data acquisition (both physiological and equipment related), alternative strategies have been devised in order to extract significant mapping signals that are consistent across tasks (see Figure 5.3).[60,61] Conjunction analysis identifies all voxels in the brain that exceed statistical threshold for two or more independent, yet related, tasks. By Bayes theorem, the probability of observing significant pixels by chance on multiple scans is equal to the product of the prior probability of chance activation on each. For example, if two separate tasks are used, using a Pearson's correlation

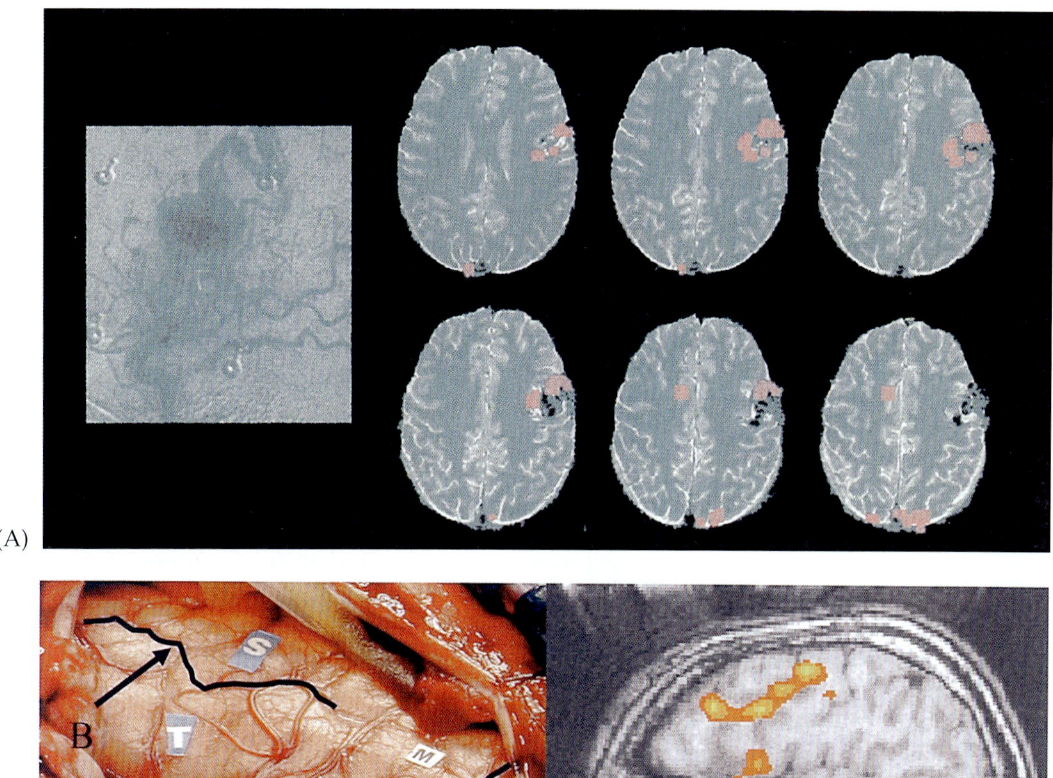


**Figure 5.3.** (A,B) Functional MRI activations adjacent to AVM. Significant fMRI activations are commonly identified adjacent to a left frontal lobe AVM. In this image, fMRI activations of language expression (created by conjunction analysis) are seen adjacent to a frontal AVM, identifying Broca's Area. Note that activations are not identified within the vascular malformation. Functional MRI activations were both qualitatively and quantitatively similar to the intraoperative electrocortical stimulation maps (B). Adapted with permission from Pouratian N, Bookheimer SY, Rex DE, Martin NA, Toga AW. Utility of pre-operative functional magnetic resonance imaging for identifying language cortices in patients with vascular malformations. *J Neurosurg*. 2002(a);97:21–32.

coefficient threshold of 0.2, the probability of correlation by chance for each individual task is 0.063, and the joint probability is less than 0.004. By using a low statistical threshold for each individual scan, conjunction analysis minimizes the probability of eliminating functionally significant voxels due to noise, which effectively reduces false–negative results. However, by requiring that the same voxel must be active across multiple tasks, this analysis minimizes false–positive results by ensuring that only functionally significant voxels are considered in the final analysis.

The power of this technique was recently demonstrated by Pouratian and colleagues in a study comparing language-related fMRI activations with intraoperative electrocortical stimulation map (ESM).[61] The authors created conjunction fMRI maps of expressive language (conjunction of two of three expressive language tasks: visual object naming, word generation, and auditory response naming) and receptive language (conjunction of visual responsive naming and sentence comprehension) and compared these fMRI activations with intraoperative ESM (Figure 5.3A, B). For the population studied, the authors reported sensitivity and specificity values of expression fMRI activations of up to 100% and 66.7%, respectively, in the frontal lobe, and of comprehension fMRI activations of up to 96.2% and 69.8%, respectively, in the parietal/temporal lobes.

Based on the differences between ESM and fMRI methodology, false–positives consistent with an imperfect specificity should be expected. Whereas ESM is a disruption-based technique that will identify only those areas that are essential to language processing, fMRI is an activation-based technique that will identify all regions of the brain that demonstrate activity-related changes, whether those areas are essential or supplementary. Consequently, areas that are negative for language by ESM may still demonstrate fMRI activations, producing false–positives. The use of the conjunction analysis, however, minimizes this false–positive rate by only identifying those areas that are consistently activated across language tasks. Nonetheless, there clearly are still supplementary and non-essential language areas that are not identified by ESM, but that are consistently active across fMRI activations.

## Reproducibility

Reproducibility of fMRI activations, either within subjects or across studies, is rarely addressed. Nonetheless, it is an important consideration, especially now that functional brain mapping is being used increasingly for quantification of brain activity and clinical decision making.[54,61]

Cohen and DuBois reported the most extensive and quantitative study to date of fMRI signal reproducibility, with surprising results with respect to signal stability.[55] Studying both visual and motor cortex, they reported that counting pixels exceeding statistical significance is remarkably unstable, with values varying by 750% across trials. This large degree of variability is attributed to differences in noise levels across trials although the actual activation magnitude is likely the same across trials. (Noise may be composed of a variety of artifacts and physiological factors.) The noise variance propagates through to statistical calculations and produces a widely varying number of pixels that exceed statistical threshold. In contrast, the slope of the regression line, which is essentially the percent signal change, is much more stable across trials and subjects, with less than 20% variability across trials. Monte Carlo simulations support the assertion that even in very poor contrast-to-noise ratio (CNR) conditions, the percent signal change can be determined with relatively good accuracy and precision.[55]

Huetell and McCarthy[56] arrived at a similar conclusion regarding the value of activation size: Group or condition differences may result from differences in voxelwise noise exacerbated by averaging small numbers of trials. By progressively averaging an increasing number of trials to determine activation size, they found that activation size increases exponentially, reaching a plateau at approximately 150 trials averaged a number that is far less than most conventional fMRI studies. This uncertainty in activation size is attributed to noise, highlighting how intrinsic fMRI noise sources can significantly alter activation sizes.

These studies argue strongly for the lack of reliability of activation size as a measure of response magnitude. Instead, measuring the percent signal change or the slope of the regression line is a much more reliable measure of response magnitude. The latter method of measuring percent signal change is also preferable because it can detect changes in response magnitude across tasks in voxels that are already activated in the original task. Investigators should not only be interested in areas of additional activity, but also in changes in response magnitude of already activated regions.[62] Even if pixel counting were a reliable method, it would not be able to account for such differences. Due to the limited reliability of merely counting pixels, we recommend comparing percent signal change within a statistically defined ROI across trials or tasks in order to compare reliable measures.

## Applying fMRI to Clinical Planning

### Significance of Signal Localization

Earlier, the concept that the fMRI activation is intimately related to and depends upon the characteristics of neurovascular coupling was introduced. The uncertainty and imprecision of neurovascular coupling introduces one of the biggest challenges and one of the most significant sources of error in interpreting clinical fMRI studies. It is well accepted that the time courses of electrophysiological and hemodynamic responses are different by orders of magnitude. Most investigators also assume tight spatial coupling between electrophysiologically active cortex and the observed hemodynamic response. This, in fact, is probably not as robust a relationship as most assume, limited by neurovascular mechanisms and fMRI physics.

Depending on the scan sequence used, the BOLD fMRI signals often center in adjacent sulci[39,63,64] and can be up to one centimeter away from electrophysiologically active cortex.[39] The sulcal localization suggests that the positive BOLD fMRI signal may not be a very specific mapping signal. Offering relatively poor spatial colocalization with electrophysiological maps and emphasizing changes occurring in vasculature rather than within the cortex.[34,63–65] Alternative mapping signals have been suggested, like the initial dip that may offer a more precise colocalization with electrophysiologically active cortex.[37,38]

Despite the imprecision of spatial localization, fMRI mapping signals are still useful and have been shown to spatially correlate with electrophysiologically active.[66] However, in most cases, in order to achieve spatial colocalization, a sphere of influence of fMRI activity often is assumed to be approximately 0.5–1.0 centimeters in order to achieve high correlation rates.[61,66–69] Because of the spatial imprecision of fMRI, especially when doing whole head imaging, it is important not to over interpret small differences in spatial extent or lack of difference in spatial extent as representing a clear difference in activation patterns or a lack of difference in activation patterns, respectively.

### Reliability of Signal Adjacent to Pathology

The reliability of fMRI signals has been called into question both with respect to susceptibility artifact induced by intracerebral pathologies and surgical interventions (e.g., atertiovenous malformations, cavernous angiomas, surgical clips), and with respect to the mass effect and possible physiological disturbance induced by the presence of pathology.

With respect to susceptibility artifact, it is clearly impossible to obtain a signal from within a pathology with significant susceptibility artifact. The question remains as to whether reliable signals can be obtained from adjacent to the pathologies. In a study of 14 patients, Schlosser and colleagues reported that fMRI signals within patients with frontal-lobe tumors were comparable to signals in normal controls.[13] Similarly, Righini and colleagues found little difference in motor activations between the affected and unaffected hemispheres in 17 patients with frontoparietal masses.[2] Pouratian and colleagues also recently reported that functional activations, which correlate with intraoperative cortical stimulation mapping, can consistently and reliably be measured adjacent to vascular malformations (i.e., AVMs and cavernous hemangiomas).[61] These reports are consistent with our findings at UCLA, in which we regularly and successfully map motor and language cortices within patients scheduled for neurosurgical intervention near eloquent cortices (see Figure 5.4).

Reports of abnormal fMRI activations adjacent to pathology like represent cases in which the pathology has infiltrated the cortex of interest, and therefore altered normal cortical function, cerebral hemodynamic, or both. Because of the importance of preserving eloquent function, if fMRI maps are being used for neurosurgical guidance, it is imperative to verify preoperative fMRI maps intraoperatively with intraoperative direct cortical stimulation mapping in order to ensure preservation of eloquent function.

## Relationship to Outcomes

Although many studies have investigated the relationship between fMRI and electrophysiological maps,[67–72] very few studies have quantified the sensitivity and specificity of fMRI activations relative to electrophysiological maps or determined the relationship between fMRI

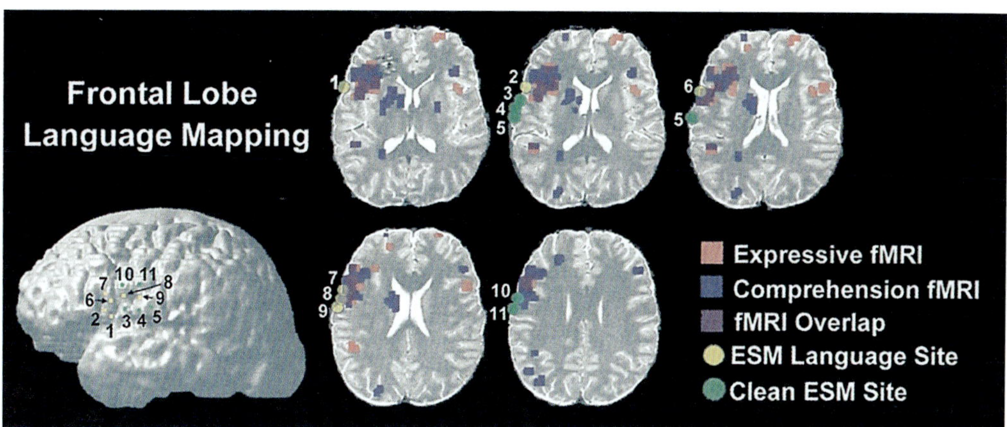


**Figure 5.4.** Frontal lobe language mapping using fMRI with conjunction analysis. Yellow circles are areas essential for language as determined by ESM. Green circle s are areas that, when stimulated, did not disrupt language function. Red activations are conjunction fMRI maps of language expression. Blue activations are conjunction fMRI maps of language comprehension. Electrocortical stimulation map sites are shown with a five-millimeter radius (determined to produce the highest sensitivity with the least cost to specificity) and parietal/temporal. Red (expression) activations tend to overlap with, or are adjacent to, essential (yellow) ESM sites, but avoid non-essential (green) ESM sites. Blue activations in the frontal lobe also appear predictive, but with lower specificity in this subject than the expression fMRI activations. Adapted with permission from Pouratian N, Bookheimer SY, Sex DE, Martin NA, Toga AW. Utility of pre-operative functional magetic resonance imaging for identifying language cortices in patients with vascular malformations. *J Neurosurg*. 2002(a);97:21–32.

maps and clinical outcomes. These are ultimately the most important factors to be determined with respect to the utility of fMRI as a clinical tool. As fMRI analysis techniques are improved, fMRI will surely play an increasing role in identifying clinically relevant motor and language areas, as well as other eloquent cortices.

As long-term outcomes are ultimately the most important variable in clinical neurosurgery, outcomes studies like that of Haglund and colleagues,[73] which characterized clinical outcomes postoperatively relative to distance of resection from essential language sites as defined by ESM, need to be done across different tasks and cortices to determine the best approach to clinical fMRI mapping.

## Conclusions

Functional MRI is a powerful brain-mapping tool whose use has grown exponentially over the last decade. Unfortunately, our understanding of signal etiology, neurovascular coupling, and physiological baselines have not evolved at the same rate. As with most other imaging modalities, fMRI will rapidly enter the clinical arena as a commonly used and accepted modality. Before then, it is important to acknowledge and address many of the limitations that continue to challenge this modality. Moreover, as with any clinical test, it will be important to quantify its sensitivity, specificity, and relationship to outcomes in the future. Different clinical applications, experimental paradigms, analysis approach, and even equipment can produce different results; valid application of fMRI to clinical cases will have to demonstrate reliability and validity for each application separately. The field should move rapidly towards developing uniform approaches to clinical fMRI that are valid, reliable, and replicable across centers. We believe that for most applications, clinical decisions should not rest solely on fMRI results. Rather, fMRI may augment existing clinical tools as validation of the techniques continues.

## References


1. Belliveau JW, Kennedy DN Jr, McKinstry RC, Buchbinder BR, Weisskoff RM, Cohen MS, Vevea JM, Brady TJ. Functional mapping of the human visual cortex by magnetic resonance imaging. *Science.* 1991;254(5032): 716–719.
2. Righini A, de Divitiis O, Prinster A, Spagnoli D, Appollonio I, Bello L, Scifo P, Tomei G, Villani R, Fazio F, Leonardi M. Functional MRI: primary motor cortex localization in patients with brain tumors. *J Comput Assist Tomogr.* 1996;20:702.
3. Krings T, Topper R, Willmes K, Reinges MHT, Gilsbach JM, Thron A. Activation in primary and secondary motor areas in patients with CNS neoplasms and weakness. *Neurology.* 2002(a);58.
4. Mazziotta JC, Huang SC, Phelps ME, Carson RE, MacDonald NS, Mahoney K. A noninvasive positron computed tomography technique using oxygen-15–labeled water for the evaluation of neurobehavioral task batteries. *J Cereb Blood Flow Metab.* 1985;5(1):70–78.
5. Frostig RD, Lieke EE, Ts'o DY, Grinvald A. Cortical functional architecture and local coupling between neuronal activity and the microcirculation revealed by in vivo high-resolution optical imaging of intrinsic signals. *Proc Natl Acad Sci USA.* 1990;87:6082–6086.
6. Villringer A, Planck J, Hock C, Schleinkofer L, Dirnagl U. Near infrared spectroscopy (NIRS): a new tool to study hemodynamic changes during activation of brain function in human adults. *Neurosci Lett.* 1993;154: 101–104.
7. Penfield W, Boldrey E. Somatic motor and sensory representation in the cerebral cortex of man as studied by electrical stimulation. *Brain.* 1937;60: 389–443.
8. Jahanshahi M, Rothwell J. Transcranial magnetic stimulation studies of cognition: an emerging field. *Exp Brain Res.* 2000;131:1–9.
9. Villringer A, Dirnagl U. Coupling of brain activity and cerebral blood flow: basis of functional neuroimaging. *Cerebrovasc Brain Metab Rev.* 1995;7(3): 240–276.
10. Krings T, Reinges MHT, Willmes K, Nuerk HC, Meister IG, Gilsbach JM, Thron A. Factors related to the magnitude of T2* MR signal changes during functional imaging. *Neuroradiology.* 2002(b);44:459–466.
11. Holodny AI, Schulder M, Liu WC, Wolko J, Maldjian JA, Kalnin AJ. The effect of brain tumors on BOLD functional MR imaging activation in the adjacent motor cortex: implications for image-guided neurosurgery. *Am J Neuroradiol.* 2000;21:1415–1422.
12. Schreiber A, Hubbe U, Ziyeh S, Hennig J. The influence of gliomas and nonglial space-occupying lesions on blood-oxygen-level-dependent contrast enhancement. *Am J Neuroradiol.* 2000;21:1055–1063.
13. Schlosser R, Husche S, Gawehn J, Grunert P, Vucurevic G, Geserich T, Kaufmann B, Rossbach W, Stoeter P. Characterization of BOLD-fMRI signal

during a verbal fluency paradigm in patients with intracerebral tumors affecting the frontal lobe. *Magn Reson Imaging.* 2002;20:7–16.
14. Schmitz B, Bettiger BW, Hossmann KA. Brief hypercapnia enhances somatosensory activation of blood flow in rat. *J Cereb Blood Flow Metab.* 1996;16:1307–1311.
15. Bock C, Schmitz B, Kerskens CM, Gyngell ML, Hossmann KA, Hoehn-Berlage M. Functional MRI of somatosensory activation in rat: effect of hypercapnic up-regulation on perfusion and BOLD-imaging. Magn Reson Med. 1998;39:457–461.
16. Bandetti PA, Wong EC. A hypercapnia-based normalization method for improved spatial localization of human brain activation with fMRI. *NMR Biomed.* 1997;10:197–203.
17. Kruger G, Kastrup A, Glover GH. Neuroimaging at 1.5 T and 3.0 T: comparison of oxygenation-sensitive magnetic resonance imaging. *Magn Reson Med.* 2001;45(4):595–604.
18. Ojemann G, Ojemann J, Lettich E, Berger M. Cortical language localization in left, dominant hemisphere. An electrical stimulation mapping investigation in 117 patients. *J Neurosurg.* 1989;71:316–326.
19. Devlin JT, Russell RP, Davis MH, Price CJ, Wilson J, Moss HE, Matthews PM, Tyler LK. Susceptibility-induced loss of signal: Comparing PET and fMRI on a semantic task. *Neuroimage.* 2000;11:589–600.
20. Cohen MS, Weisskoff RM. Ultra-fast imaging. *Magn Reson Imaging.* 1991;9: 1–37.
21. Merboldt KD, Fransson P, Bruhn H, Frahm J. Functional MRI of the human amygdala? *Neuroimage.* 2001;14(2): 253–257.
22. Fransson P, Merboldt KD, Ingvar M, Petersson KM, Frahm J. Functional MRI with reduced susceptibility artifact: high-resolution mapping of episodic memory encoding. *Neuroreport.* 2001;12(7):1415–1420.
23. Port JD, Pomper MG. Quantification and minimization of magnetic susceptibility artifacts on GRE images. *J Comput Assist Tomogr.* 2000;24(6): 958–964.
24. Gorno-Tempini ML, Hutton C, Josephs O, Deichmann R, Price C, Turner R. Echo time dependence of BOLD contrast and susceptibility artifacts. *Neuroimage.* 2002;15(1):136–142.
25. Stables LA, Kennan RP, Gore JC. Asymmetric spin-echo imaging of magnetically inhomogeneous systems: theory, experiment, and numerical studies *Magn Reson Med.* 1998;40(3):432–442.
26. Stern CE, Corkin S, Gonzalez RG, Guimaraes AR, Baker JR, Jennings PJ, Carr CA, Sugiura RM, Vedantham V, Rosen BR. The hippocampal formation participates in novel picture encoding: evidence from functional magnetic resonance imaging. *Proc Natl Acad Sci USA.* 1996;93(16): 8660–8665.
27. Hariri A, Bookheimer SY, Mazziotta J. A neural network for modulating the emotional response to faces. *Neuroreport.* 2000;11(1):43–48.
28. LaBar KS, Gatenby JC, Gore JC, LeDoux JE, Phelps EA. Human amygdala activation during conditioned fear acquisition and extinction: a mixed-trial fMRI study. *Neuron.* 1998;20(5):937–945.
29. Cordes D, Turski PA, Sorenson JA. Compensation of susceptibility-induced signal loss in echo-planar imaging for functional applications. *Magn Reson Imaging.* 2000;18(9): 1055–1068.
30. Stenger VA, Boada FE, Noll DC. Three-dimensional tailored RF pulses for the reduction of susceptibility artifacts in T (*) (2)-weighted functional MRI. *Magn Reson Med.* 2000;44(4):525–531.
31. Glover GH, Law CS. Spiral-in/out BOLD fMRI for increased SNR and reduced susceptibility artifacts. *Magn Reson Med.* 2001;46(3):515–522.

32. Yang Y, Gu H, Zhan W, Xu S, Silbersweig DA, Stern E. Simultaneous perfusion and BOLD imaging using reverse spiral scanning at 3T: characterization of functional contrast and susceptibility artifacts. *Magn Reson Med.* 2002;48(2):278–289.
33. Weiger M, Pruessmann KP, Osterbauer R, Bornert P, Boesiger P, Jezzard P. Sensitivity-encoded single-shot spiral imaging for reduced susceptibility artifacts in BOLD fMRI. *Magn Reson Med.* 2002;48(5):860–866.
34. Cohen MS, Bookheimer SY. Localization of brain function using magnetic resonance imaging. *Trends Neurosci.* 1994;17:268–277.
35. Fox PT, Raichle ME. Focal physiological uncoupling of cerebral blood flow and oxidative metabolism during somatosensory stimulation in human subjects. Proc Nat Acad Sci USA. 1986;83:1140–1144.
36. Malonek D, Grinvald A. Interactions between electrical activity and cortical microcirculation revealed by imaging spectroscopy: implications for functional brain mapping. *Science.* 1996;272:551–554.
37. Vanzetta I, Grinvald A. Increased cortical oxidative metabolism due to sensory stimulation: implications for functional brain imaging. *Science.* 1999;286:1555–1558.
38. Menon RS, Ogawa S, Hu X, Strupp JP, Anderson P, Ugurbil K. BOLD based functional MRI at 4 Tesla includes a capillary bed contribution: echo-planar imaging correlates with previous optical imaging using intrinsic signals. *Magn Reson Med.* 1995;33:453–459.
39. Cannestra AF, Pouratian N, Bookheimer SY, Martin NA, Becker D, Toga AW. Temporal spatial differences observed by functional MRI and human intraoperative optical imaging. Cereb Cortex. 2001;11:773–782.
40. Kim DS, Duong TQ, Kim SG. High-resolution mapping of iso-orientation columns by fMRI [see comments]. *Nat Neurosci.* 2000;3:164–169.
41. Kwong KK, Belliveau JW, Chesler DA, Goldberg IE, Weisskoff RM, Poncelet BP, Kennedy DN, Hoppel BE, Cohen MS, Turner R, et al. Dynamic magnetic resonance imaging of human brain activity during primary sensory stimulation. *Proc Natl Acad Sci USA.* 1992;89:5675–5679.
42. Ogawa S, Tank DW, Menon R, Ellermann JM, Kim SG, Merkle H, Ugurbil K. Intrinsic signal changes accompanying sensory stimulation: functional brain mapping with magnetic resonance imaging. *Proc Natl Acad Sci USA.* 1992;89:5951–5955.
43. Sidtis JJ, Strother SC, Anderson JR, Rottenberg DA. Are brain functions really additive? *Neuroimage.* 1999;9:490–496.
44. Stark CEL, Squire LR. When zero is not zero: The problem of ambiguous baseline conditions in fMRI. *Proc Natl Acad Sci USA.* 2001;98:12760–12765.
45. Gusnard DA, Raichle ME. Searching for a baseline: Functional imaging and the resting human brain. *Nat Rev Neurosci.* 2001;2:685–694.
46. Raichle ME, Fiez JA, Videen TO, MacLeod AK, Pardo JV, Fox PT, Petersen SE. Practice-related changes in human brain functional anatomy during nonmotor learning. *Cereb Cortex.* 1994;4:8–26.
47. Petersen SE, van Mier H, Fiez JA, Raichle ME. The effects of practice on the functional anatomy of task performance. *Proc Natl Acad Sci USA.* 1998; 95:853–860.
48. Van Mier H, Tempel LW, Perlmutter JS, Raichle ME, Petersen SE. Changes in brain activity during motor learning measured with PET: effects of hand of performance and practice. *J Neurophysiol.* 1998;80:2177–2199.
49. Madden DJ, Turkington TG, Provenzale JM, Denny LL, Hawk TC, Gottlob LR, Coleman RE. Adult age differences in the functional neuroanatomy of verbal recognition memory. *Hum Brain Map.* 1999;7:115–135.

50. Garavan H, Kelley D, Rosen A, Rao SR, Stein EA. Practice-related functional activation changes in a working memory task. *Microsc Res Tech.* 2000;51:54–63.
51. Bookheimer SY, Strojwas MH, Cohen MS, Saunders AM, Pericak-Vance MA, Mazziotta JC, Small GW. Patterns of brain activation in people at risk for Alzheimer's disease. *N Engl J Med.* 2000;343(7):450–456.
52. Sonty SP, Mesulam MM, Thompson CK, Johnson NA, Weintraub S, Parrish TB, Gitelman DR. Primary progressive aphasia: PPA and the language network. *Ann Neurol.* 2003;53(1):35–49.
53. Calvert GA, Brammer MJ, Morris RG, Williams SC, King N, Matthews PM. Using fMRI to study recovery from acquired dysphasia. *Brain Lang.* 2000; 71(3):391–399.
54. Binder JR, Swanson SJ, Hammeke TA, Morris GL, Mueller WM, Fischer M. Determination of language dominance using functional MRI: a comparison with the Wada test. *Neurology.* 1996;46:978–984.
55. Cohen MS, DuBois RM. Stability, repeatability, and the expression of signal magnitude in functional magnetic resonance imaging. *J Magn Reson Imaging.* 1999;10:33–40.
56. Huettel SA, McCarthy G. The effects of single-trial averaging upon the spatial extent of fMRI activation. *Neuroreport.* 2001;12:2411–2416.
57. Springer JA, Binder JR, Hammeke TA, Swanson SJ, Frost JA, Bellgowan PSF, Brewer CC, Perry HM, Morris GL, Mueller WM. Language dominance in neurologically normal and epilepsy subject: A functional MRI study. *Brain.* 1999;122:2033–2045.
58. Rasmussen T, Milner B. The role of early left-brain injury in determining lateralization of cerebral speech functions. *Ann NY Acad Sci.* 1977;299: 355–369.
59. Leh Rich S, Cohen L, Bazin B, Samson S, Giacomini E, Rougetet R, Hertz-Pannier L, Le Bihan D, Marsault C, Baulac M. Functional MR evaluation of temporal and frontal language dominance compared with the Wada test. *Neurology.* 2000;54.
60. Bookheimer SY, Zeffiro TA, Blaxton T, Malow BA, Gaillard WD, Sato S, Kufta C, Fedio P, Theodore WH. A direct comparison of PET activation and electrocortical stimulation mapping for language localization. *Neurology.* 1997;48:1056–1065.
61. Pouratian N, Bookheimer SY, Rex DE, Martin NA, Toga AW. Utility of preoperative functional magnetic resonance imaging for identifying language cortices in patients with vascular malformations. *J Neurosurg.* 2002(a); 97:21–32.
62. Price C, Wise R, Ramsay S, Friston K, Howard D, Patterson K, Frackowiak R. Regional response differences within the human auditory cortex when listening to words. *Neurosci Lett.* 1992;146:179–182.
63. Lai S, Hopkins AL, Haacke EM, Li D, Wasserman BA, Buckley P, Friedman L, Meltzer H, Hedera P, Friedland R. Identification of vascular structures as a major source of signal contrast in high resolution 2D and 3D functional activation imaging of the motor cortex at 1.5T: preliminary results. *Magn Reson Med.* 1993;30:387–392.
64. Pouratian N, Bookheimer SY, O'Farrell AM, Sicotte NL, Cannestra AF, Becker D, Toga AW. Optical imaging of bilingual cortical representations: Case report. *J Neurosurg.* 2000;93:686–691.
65. Duong TQ, Kim DS, Ugurbil K, Kim SG. Spatiotemporal dynamics of the BOLD fMRI signals: toward mapping submillimeter cortical columns using the early negative response [in process citation]. *Magn Reson Med.* 2000;44: 231–242.

66. Pouratian N, Sicotte N, Rex D, Martin NA, Becker D, Cannestra AF, Toga AW. Spatial/temporal correlation of BOLD and optical intrinsic signals in humans. *Magn Reson Med.* 2002b;47:766–776.
67. Roux FE, Boulanouar K, Ranjeva JP, Manelfe C, Tremoulet M, Sabatier J, Berry I. Cortical intraoperative stimulation in brain tumors as a tool to evaluate spatial data from motor functional MRI. *Invest Radiol.* 1999a;34: 225–229.
68. Corina DP, Poliakov A, Steury K, Martin R, Mulligan K, Maravilla K, Brinkly JF, Ojemann GA. Correspondences between language cortex identified by cortical stimulation mapping and fMRI. *Neuroimage.* 2000;11:S295.
69. Lurito JT, Lowe MJ, Sartorius C, Mathews VP. Comparison of fMRI and intraoperative direct cortical stimulation in localization of receptive language areas. *J Comput Assist Tomogr.* 2000;24:99–105.
70. Mueller WM, Yetkin FZ, Hammeke TA, Morris GL 3rd, Swanson SJ, Reichert K, Cox R, Haughton VM. Functional magnetic resonance imaging mapping of the motor cortex in patients with cerebral tumors. *Neurosurgery.* 1996;39:515–520; discussion 520–511.
71. Roux FE, Boulanouar K, Ranjeva JP, Tremoulet M, Henry P, Manelfe C, Sabatier J, Berry I. Usefulness of motor functional MRI correlated to cortical mapping in Rolandic low-grade astrocytomas. *Acta Neurochir.* 1999b; 141:71–79.
72. Rutten GJ, van Rijen PC, van Veelen CW, Ramsey NF. Language area localization with three-dimensional functional magnetic resonance imaging matches intrasulcal electrostimulation in Broca's area. *Ann Neurol.* 1999; 46:405–408.
73. Haglund MM, Berger MS, Shamseldin M, Lettich E, Ojemann GA. Cortical localization of temporal lobe language sites in patients with gliomas. *Neurosurgery.* 1994;34:567–576; discussion 576.

# Part II

## Neuroanatomical Atlas

# 6

# Neuroanatomical Atlas

Feroze B. Mohamed and Scott H. Faro

In this chapter we have displayed several important areas of normal-functioning adult brain images generated using fMRI BOLD imaging. The fMRI shown here highlight areas of brain activation arising from simple motor tasks, visual functions, auditory and complex language, and listening paradigms. A somatotopic fMRI mapping of the human motor cortex was created for the foot, knee, trunk, shoulder, wrist, hand, face, tongue, and abdomen. The fMRI experiments in these conditions were carried out by simple box-car type block design experiments. These included a rest condition where no activity was performed, followed by an activation period where the subject was asked to perform a specific task. The representation of visual function, as well as language and auditory areas, were also obtained using a block design.

These pictures represent some of the most important and commonly studied areas of the brain and might serve as a reference or template for users of fMRI for brain mapping. The images shown here are represented in radiological co-ordinates and are presented in three different orientations (axial, coronal, and sagittal). The blue cross hair represents the area of interest, and the region was labeled based on the Talaraich atlas. The color map overlying the images are statistical maps and the graded change in color from yellow to orange represent varying statistical value from low to high statistical significance. A composite display showing the motor homunculus with corresponding fMRI activation maps is shown at the end of the chapter. The post-processing of the fMRI data was performed with SPM'99 software (Statistical Parametric Mapping, Wellcome Department of Cognitive Neurology, University College of London) running under the Matlab (The Mathworks, Inc.) environment. A Pentium-based PC was used to generate all the images shown in this section.

**Axial** **Coronal** **Sagittal**

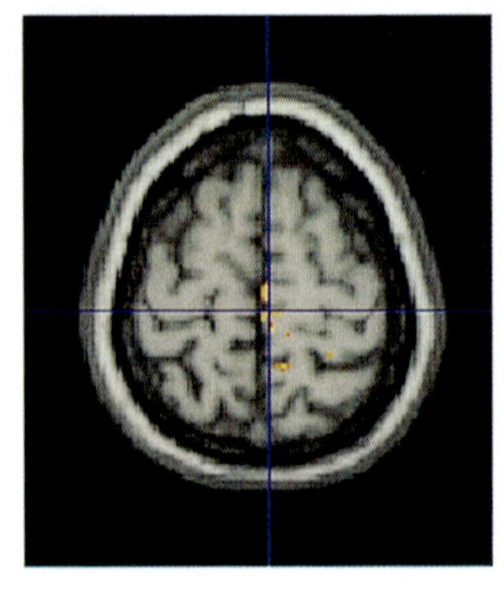
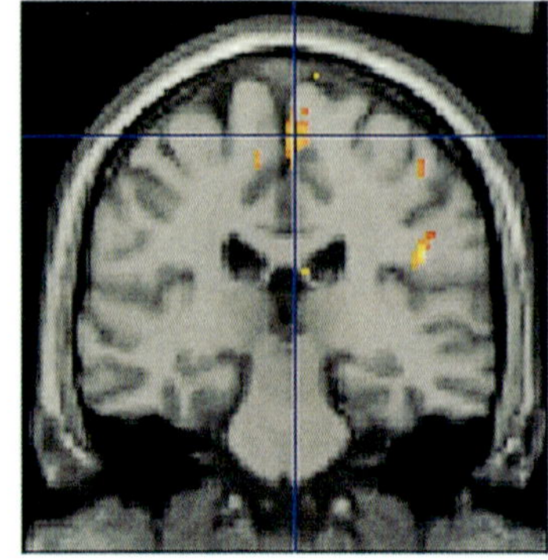
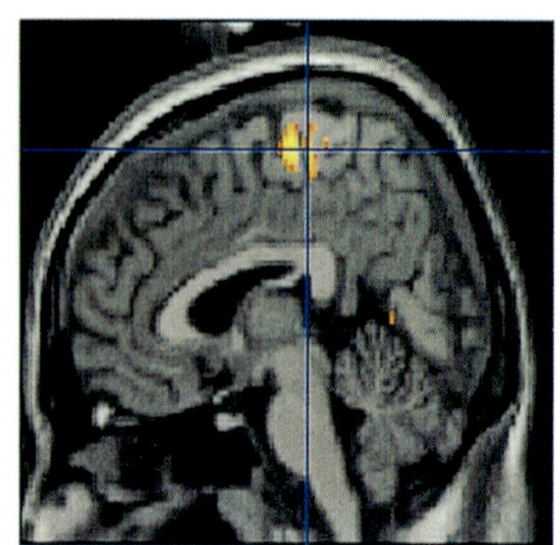

A. Foot representation.

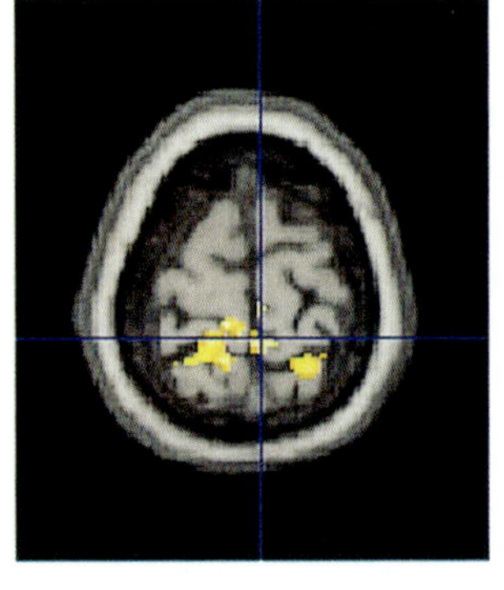
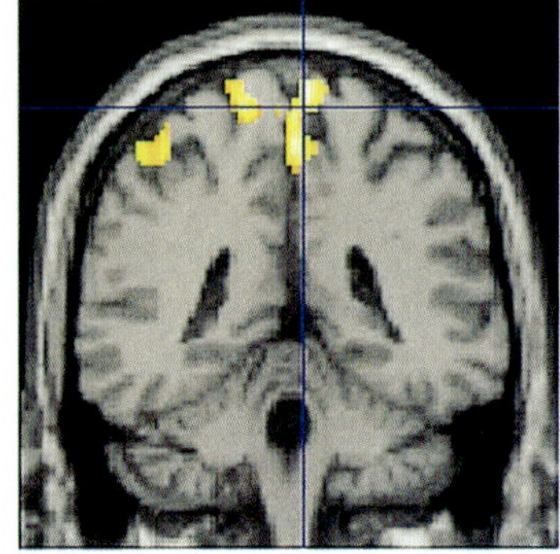
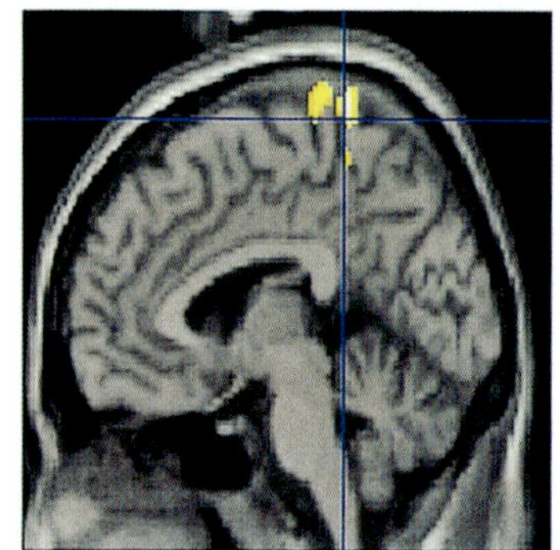

B. Knee representation.

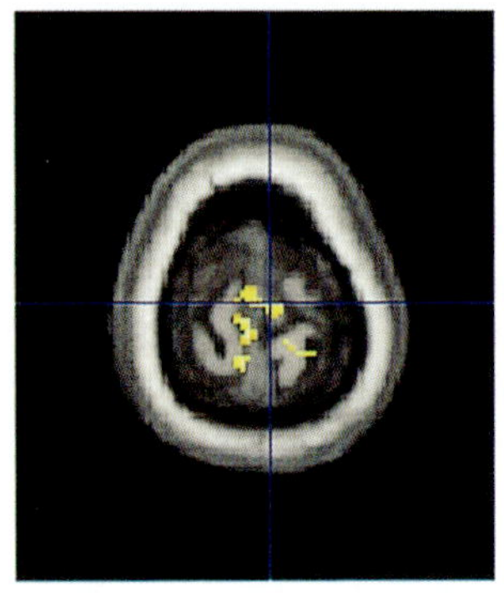
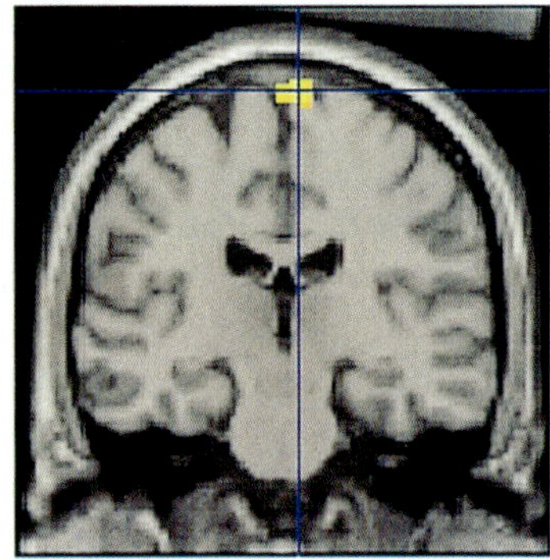
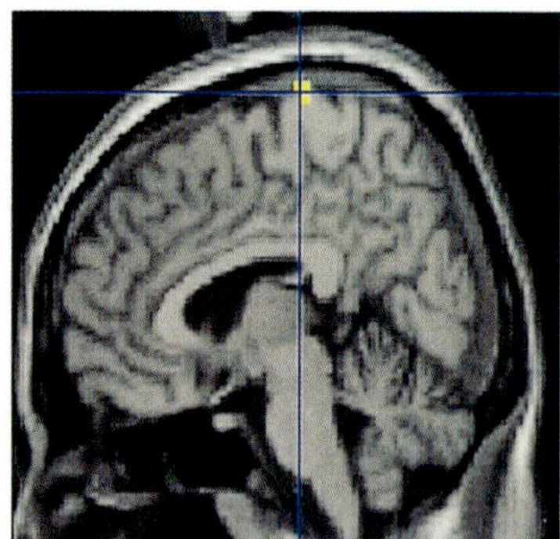

C. Trunk representation.

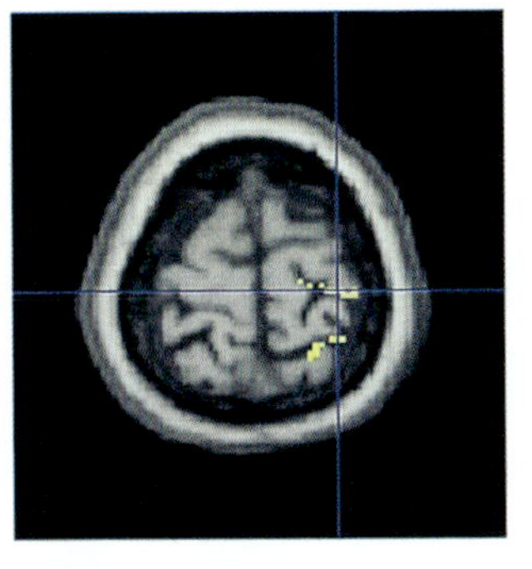
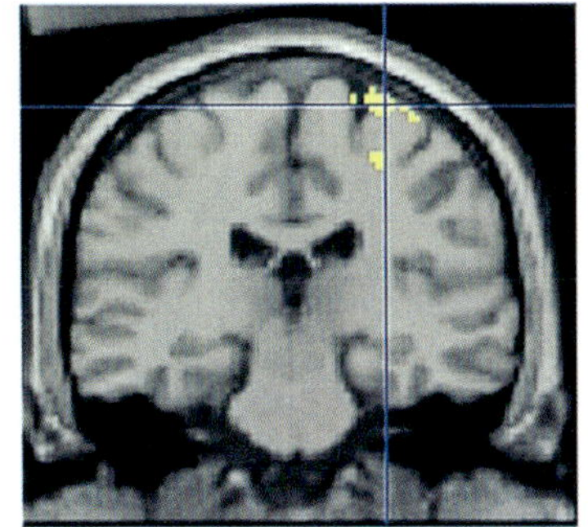
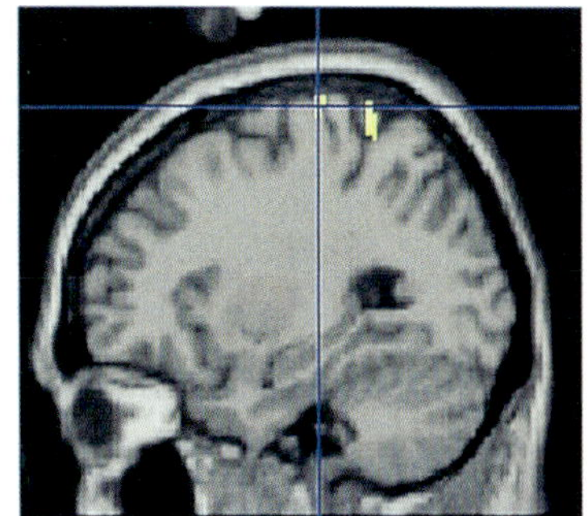

D. Wrist representation.

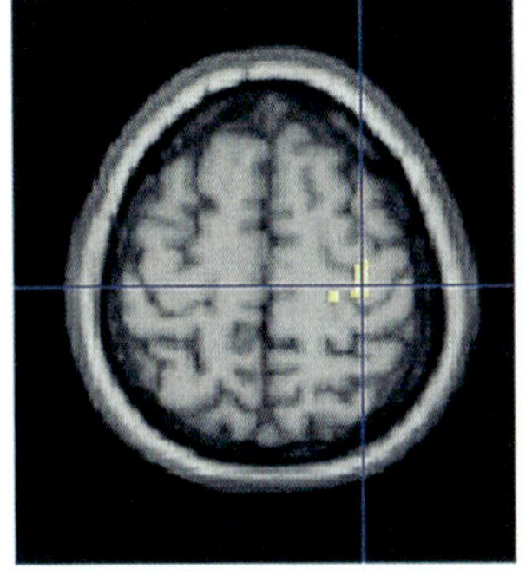
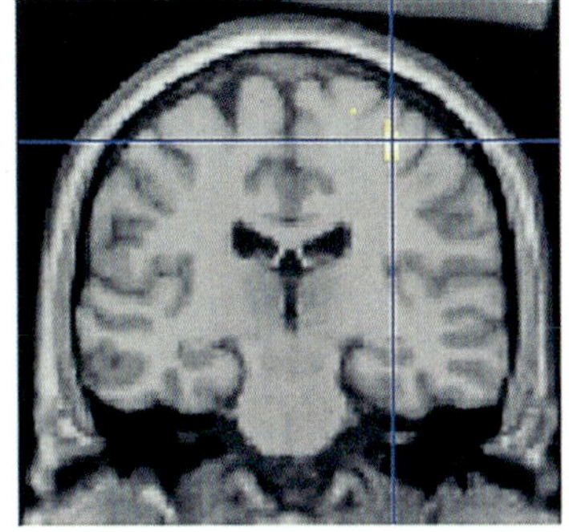
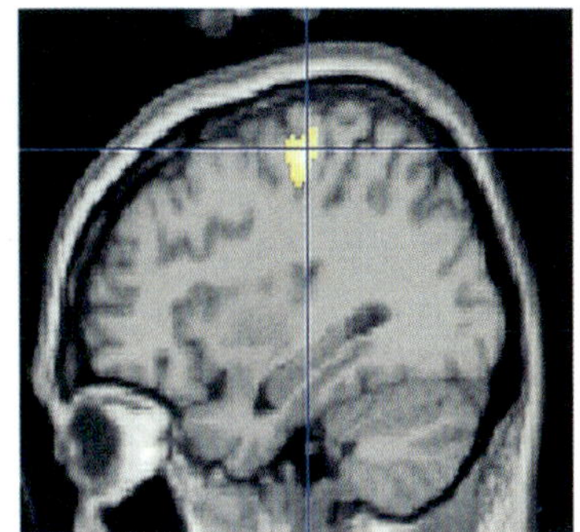

E. Hand representation.

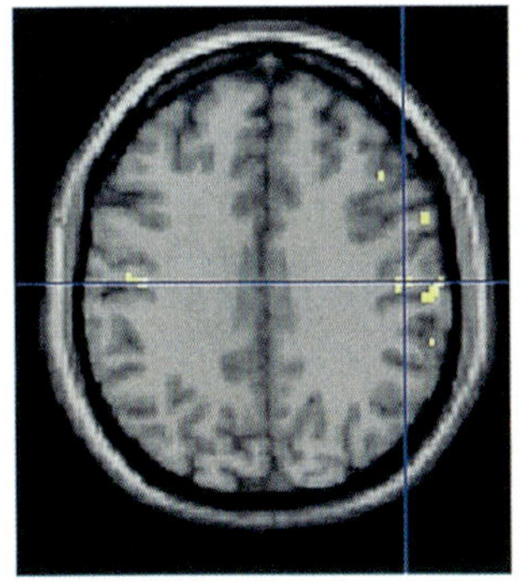
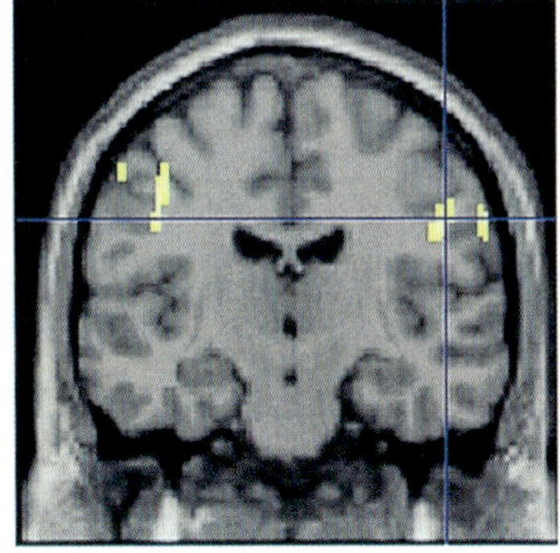
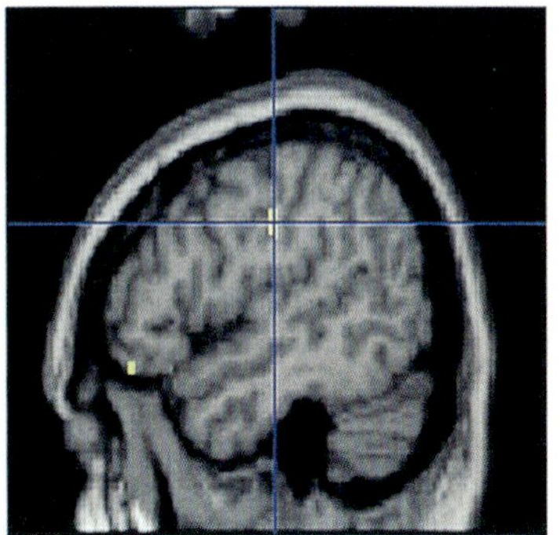

F. Face representation.

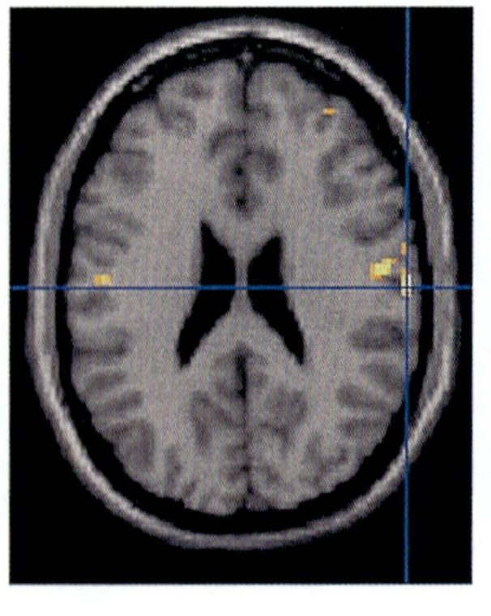
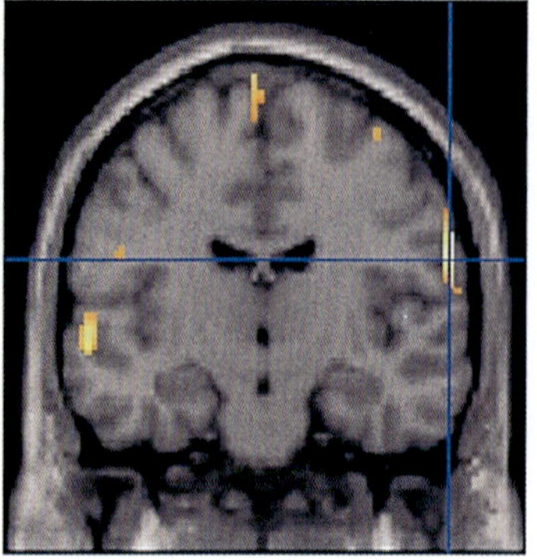
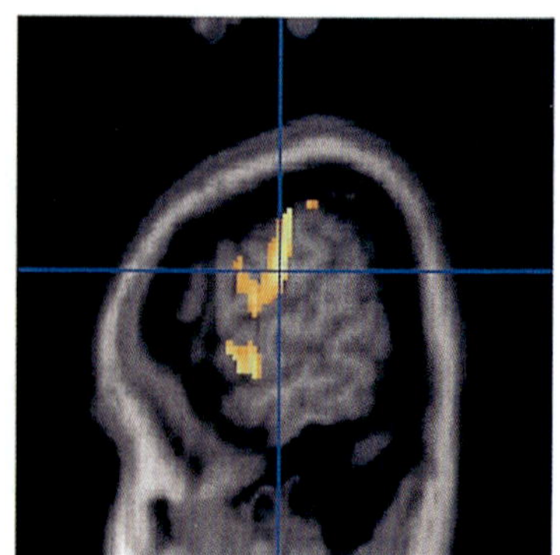

G. Tongue representation.

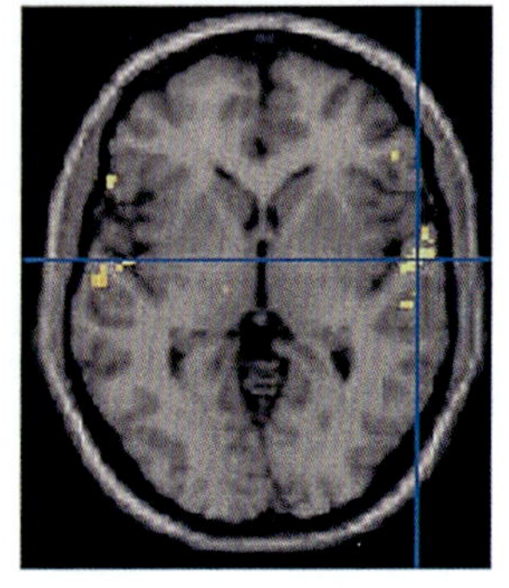
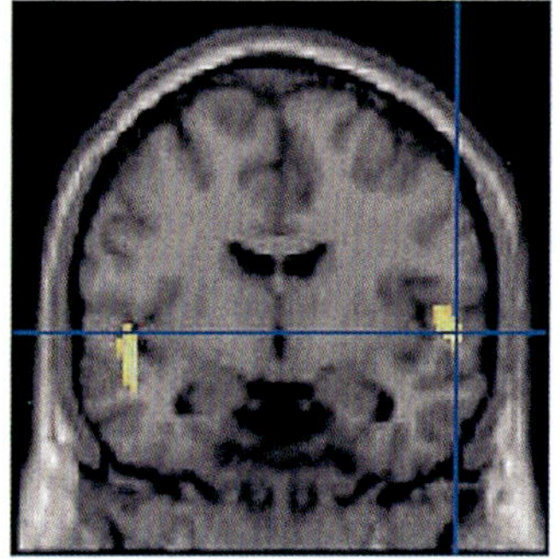
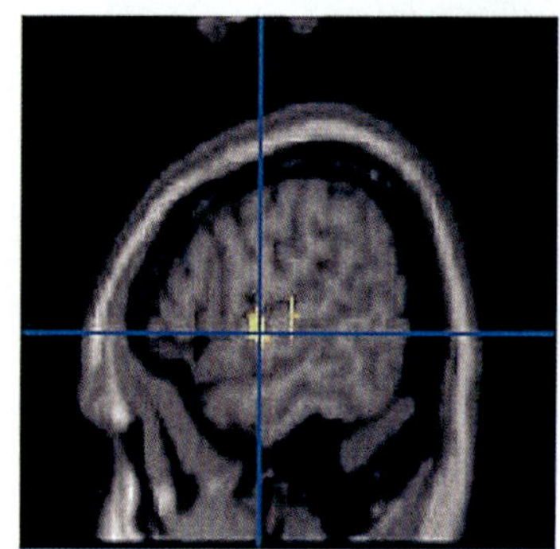

H. Low Auditory Tone (220 Hz)

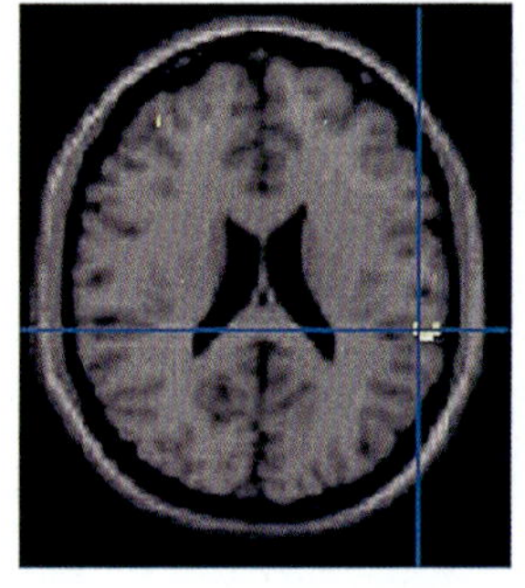
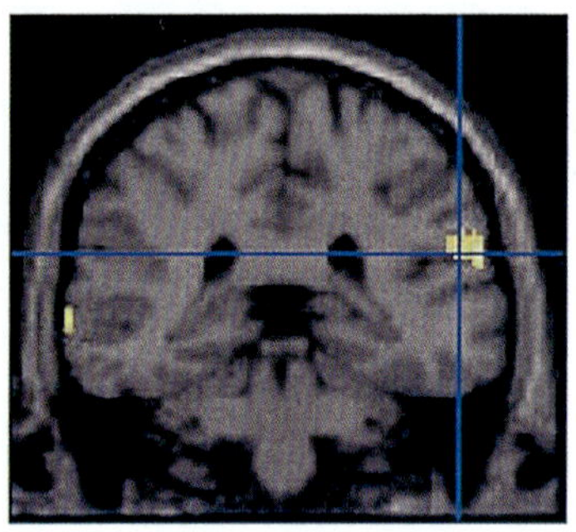
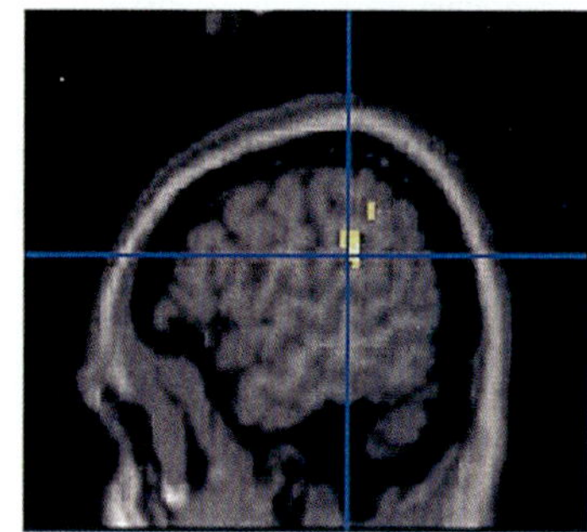

I. High Auditory Tone (1000 Hz)

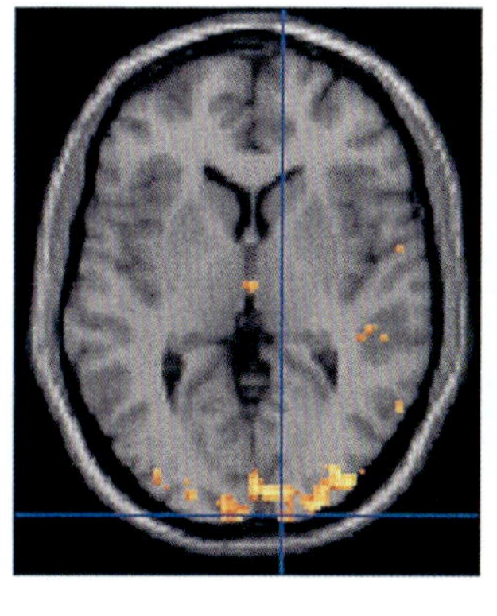
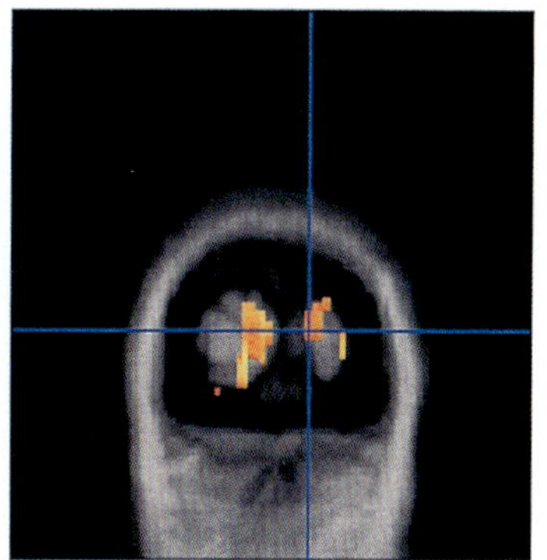
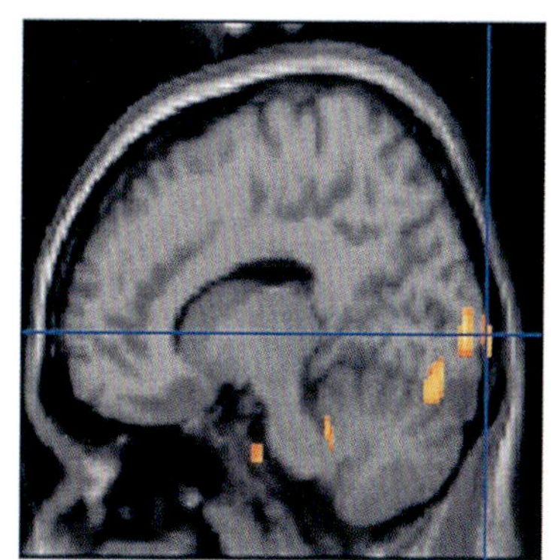

J. Visual Cortex activation

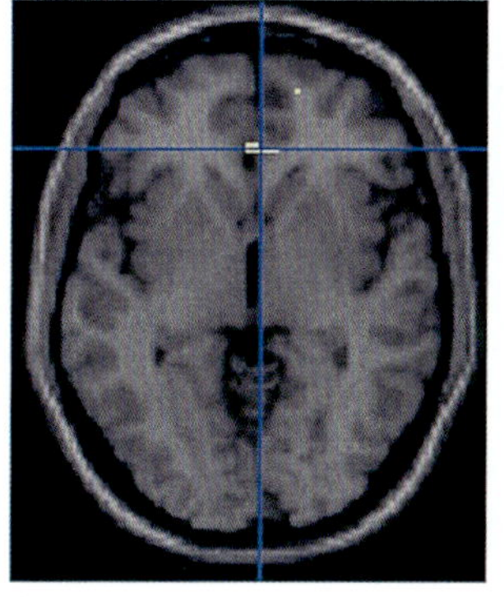
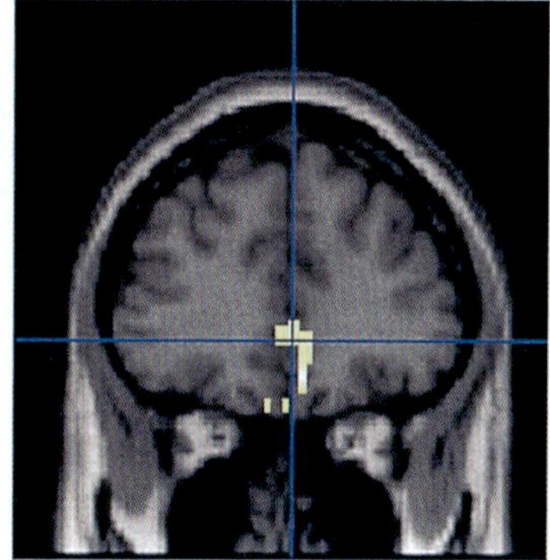
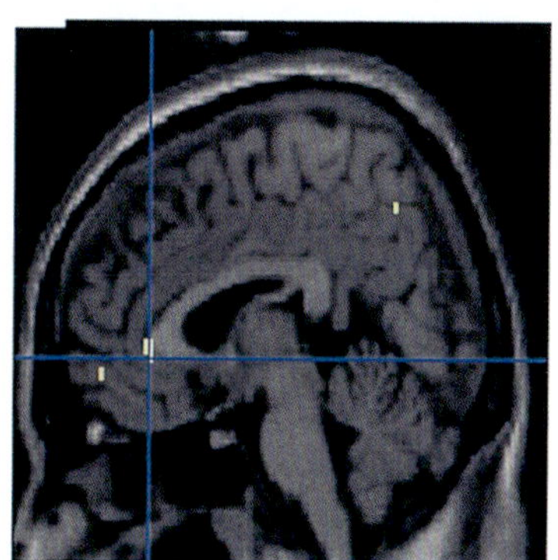

K. Limbic Lobe (Anterior Cingulate)

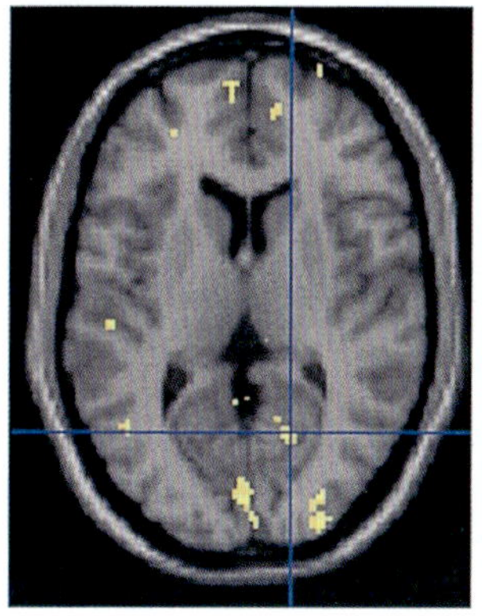
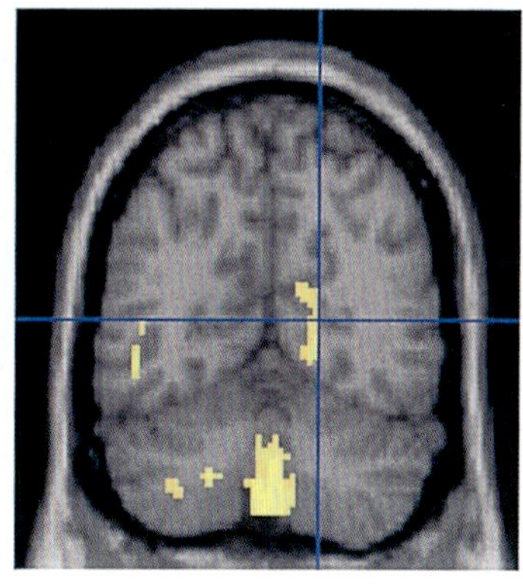
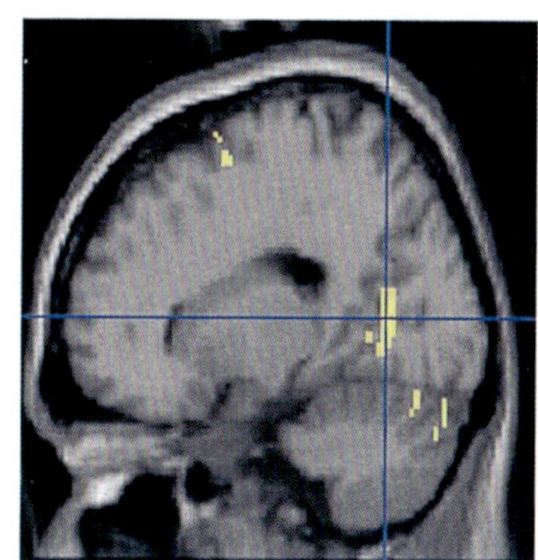

L. Limbic Lobe (Posterior Cingulate)

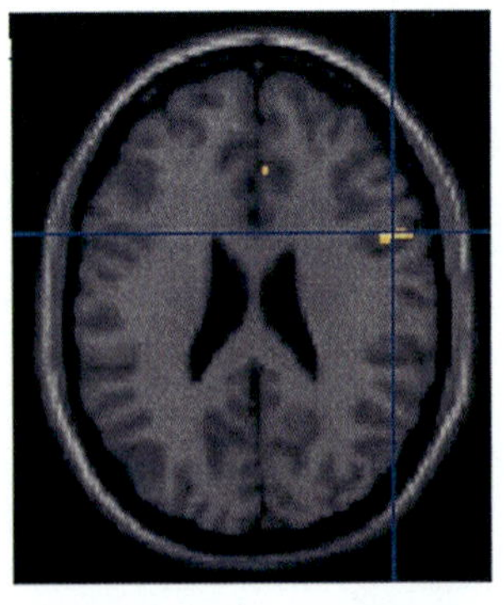
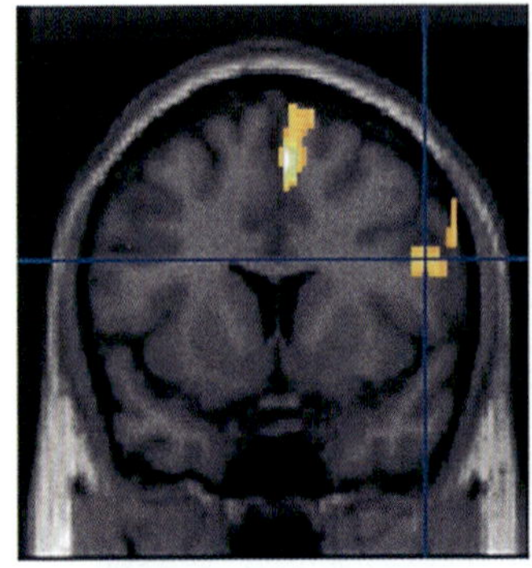
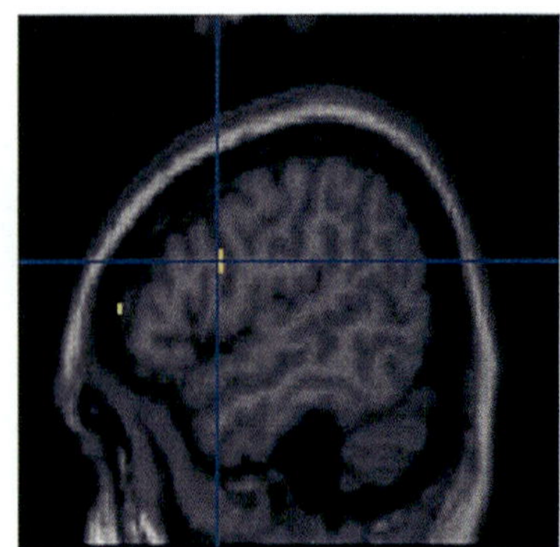

M. Frontal Lobe: Inferior Frontal Gyrus

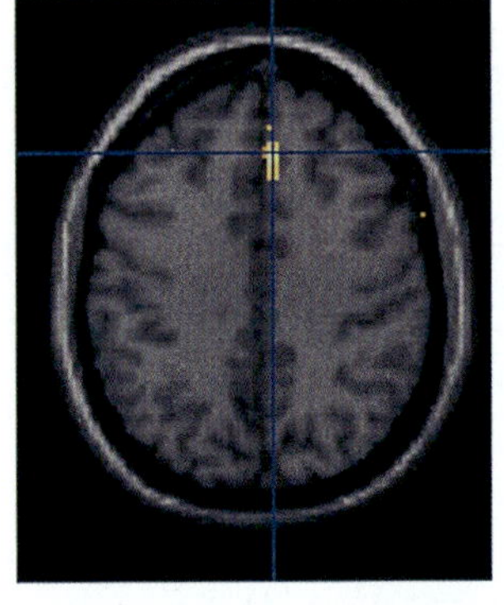
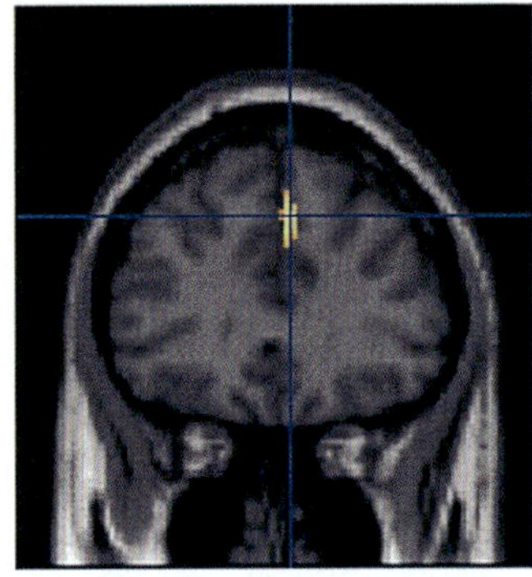
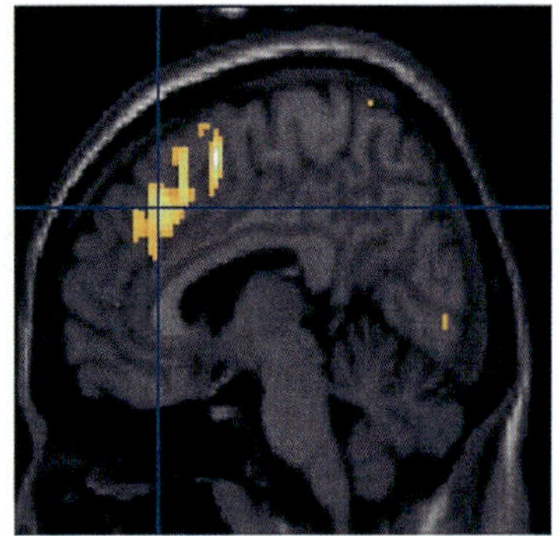

N. Frontal Lobe: Medial Frontal Gyrus

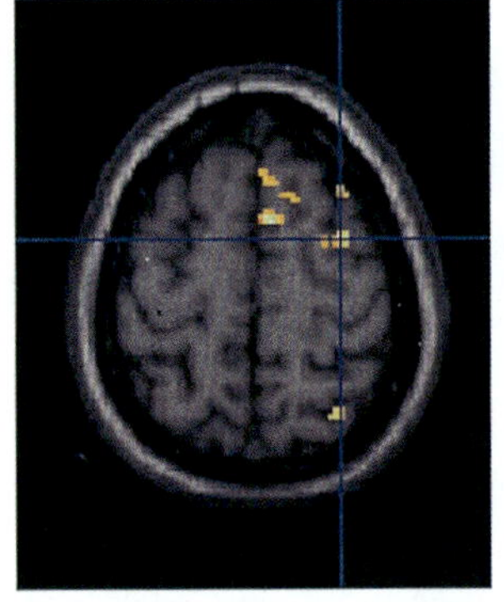
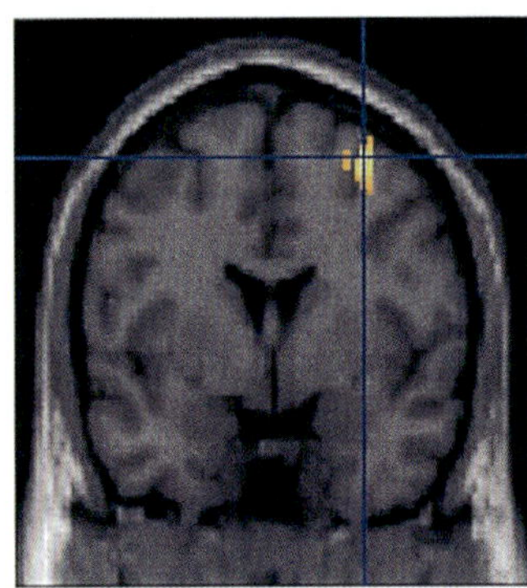
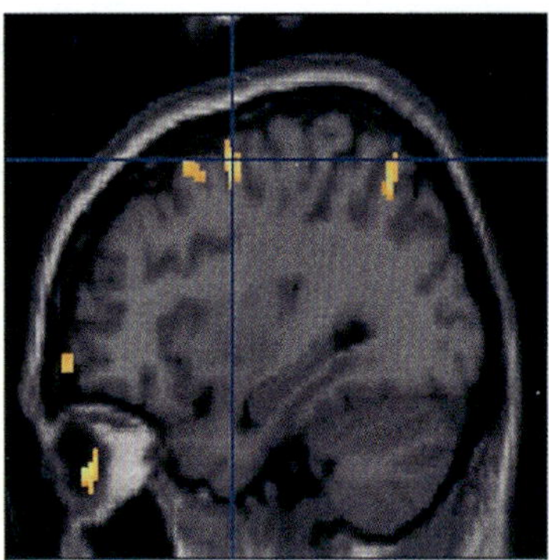

O. Frontal Lobe: Middle Frontal Gyrus

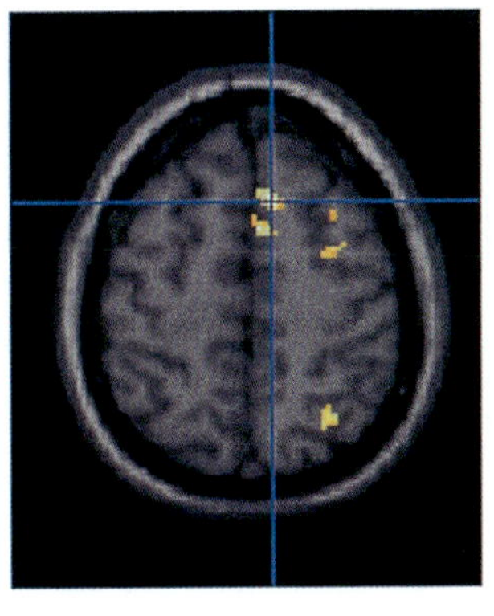
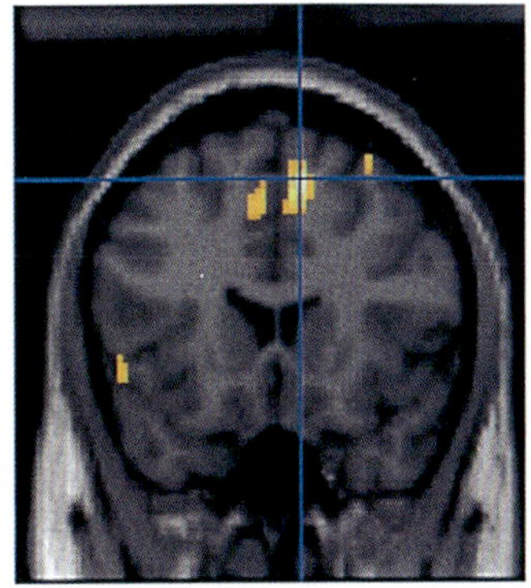
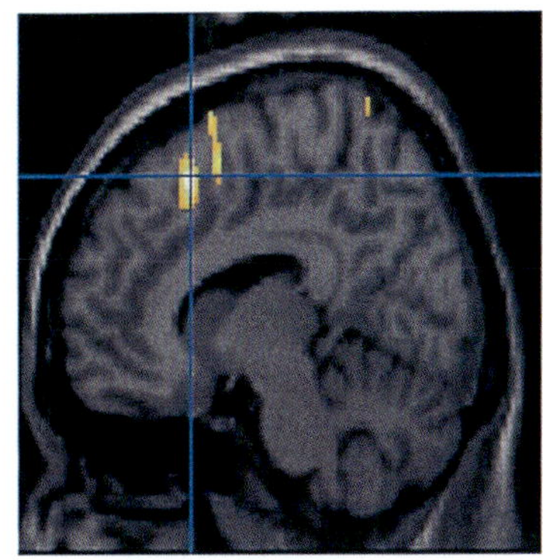

P. Frontal Lobe: Superior Frontal Gyrus

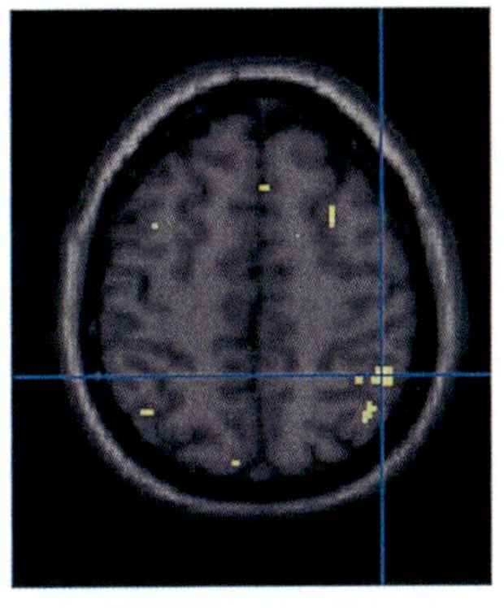
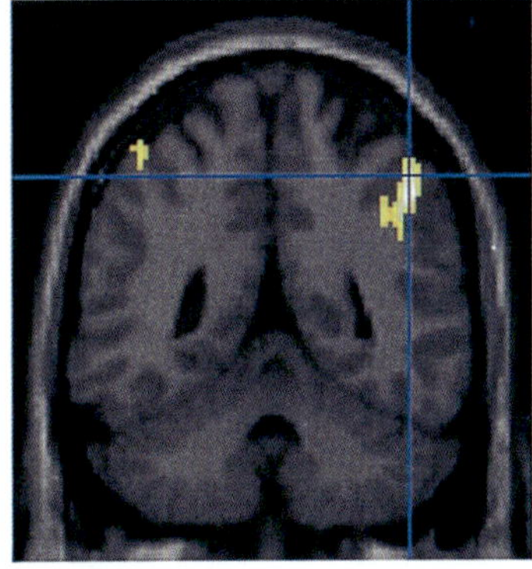
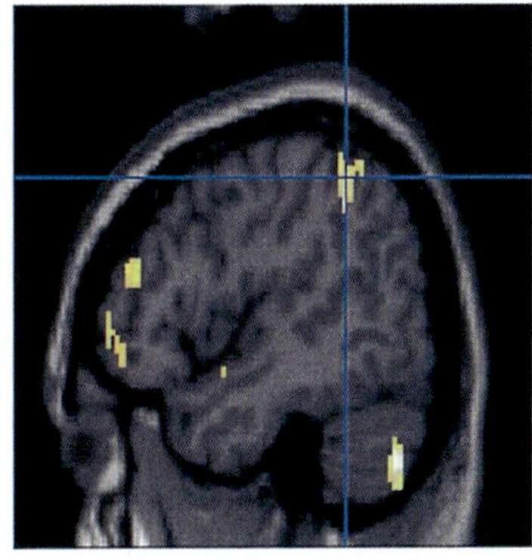

Q. Parietal Lobe: Inferior Parietal Lobule

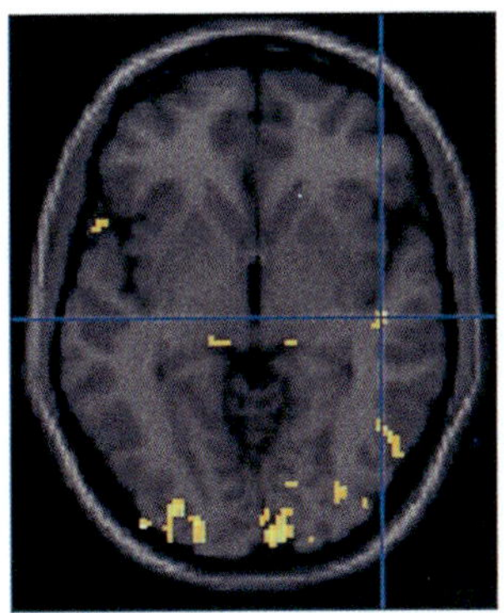
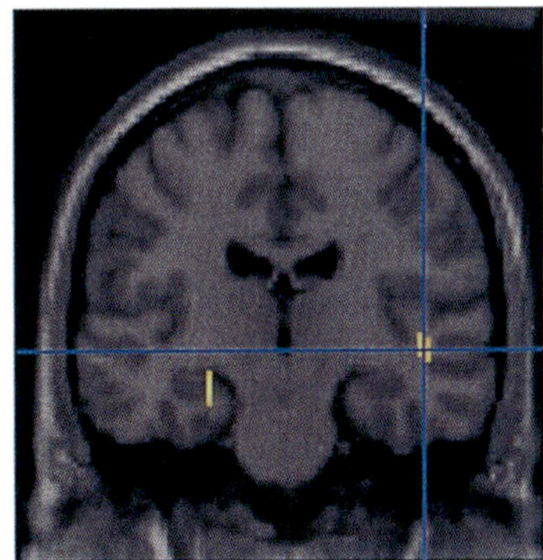
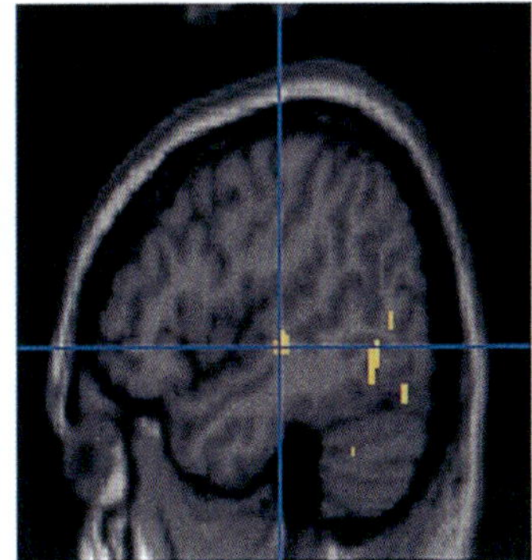

R. Temporal Lobe: Wernicke's Area

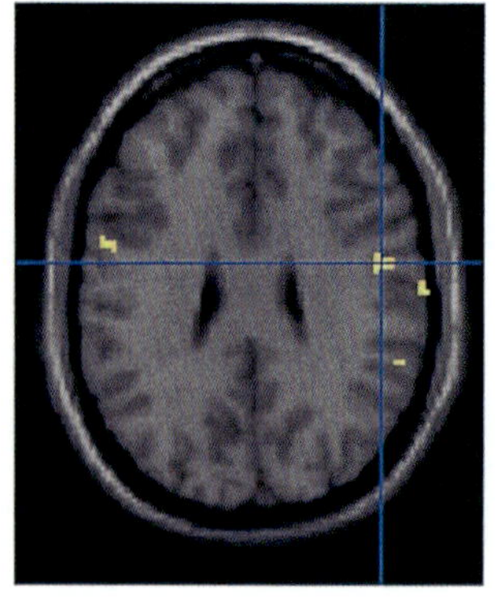
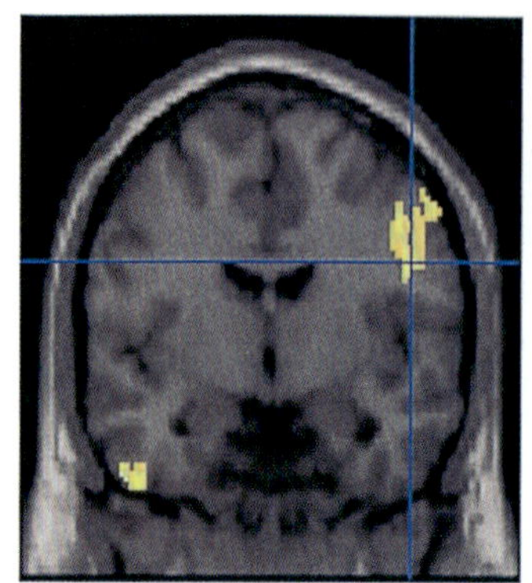
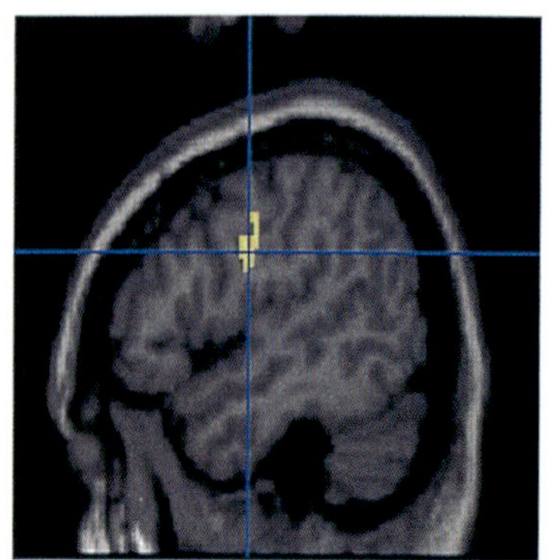

S. Broca's Motor Area

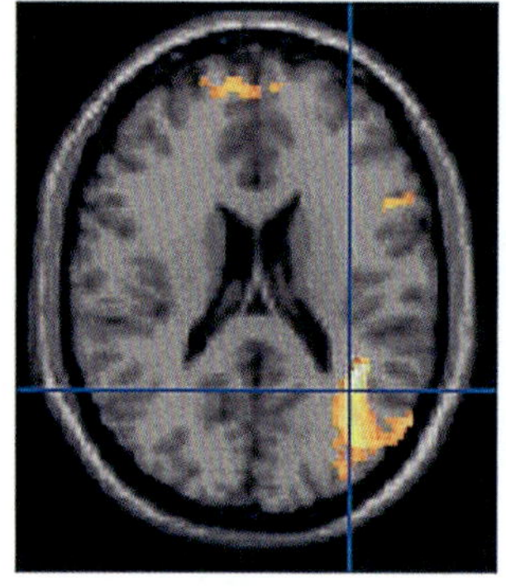
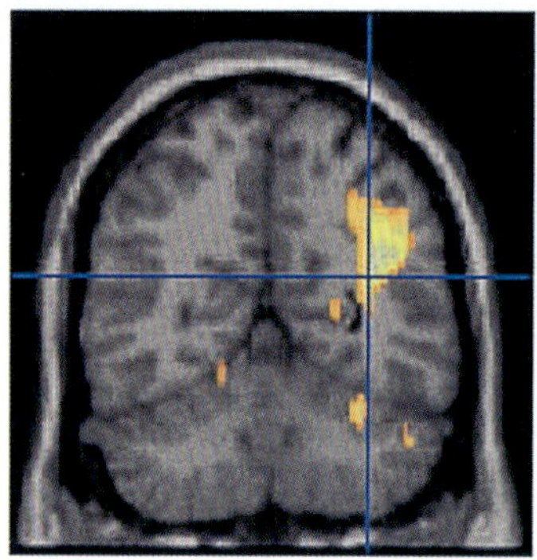
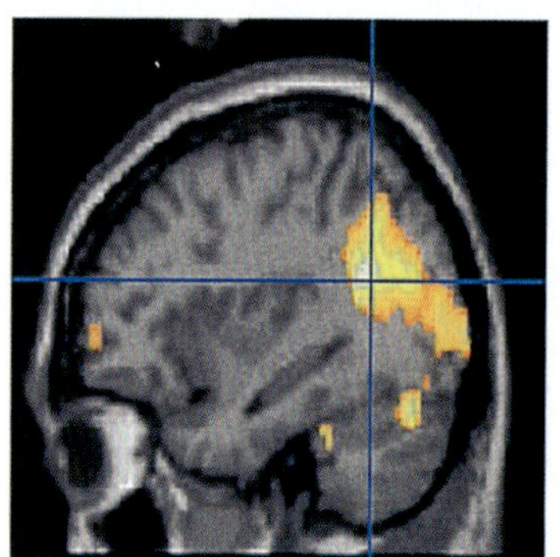

T. Parietal Occipital Lobe: Object Naming Task.

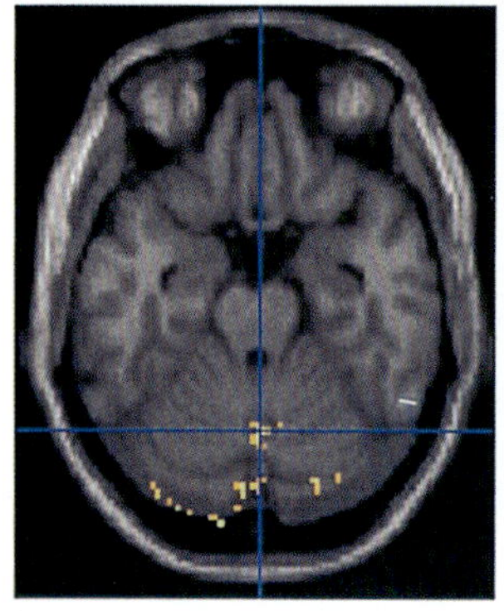
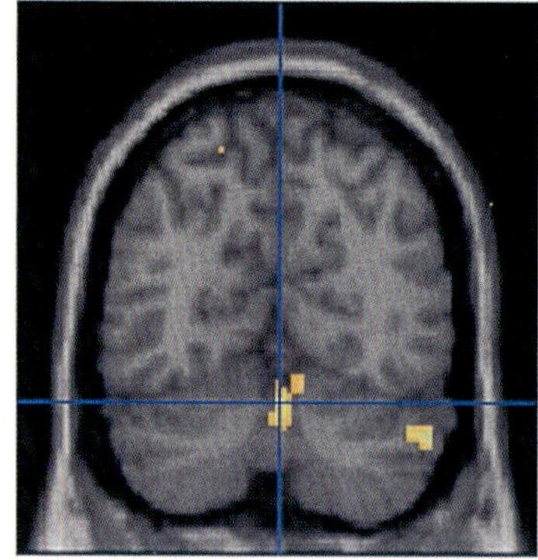
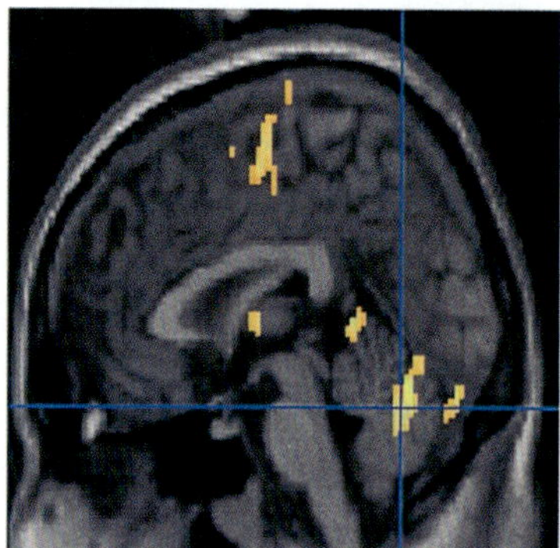

U. Cerebellum: Coordination Motor Task.

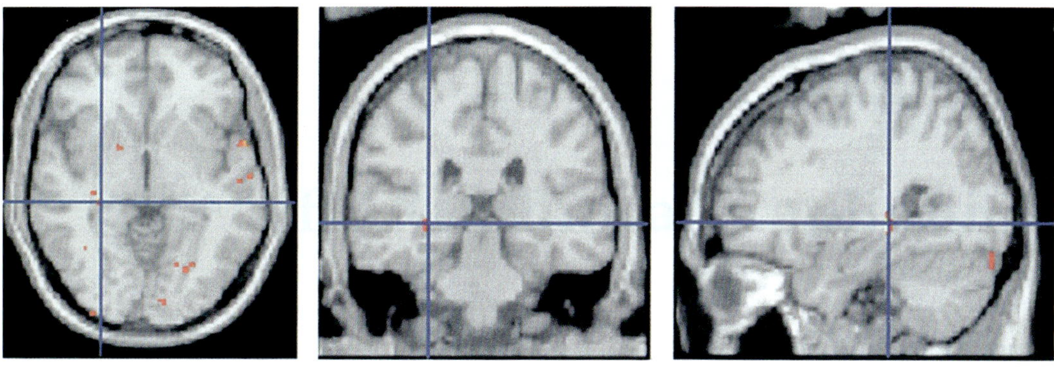

V. Temporal Lobe: Hippocampal Activation

Somatotopic mapping in the human somatosensory motor cortex along with corresponding functional MRI activation patterns.

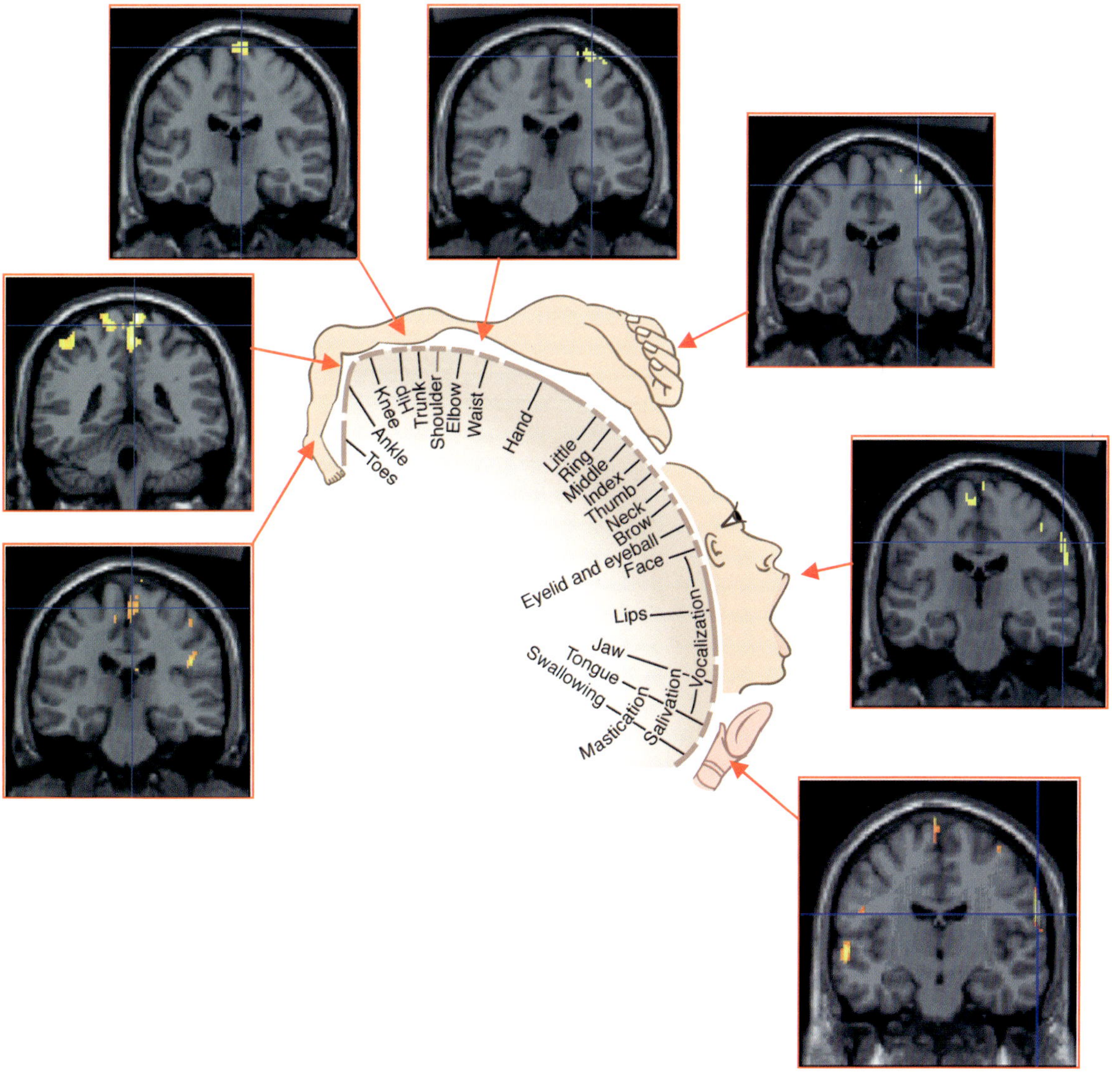

Toes
Ankle
Knee
Hip
Trunk
Shoulder
Elbow
Waist
Hand
Little
Ring
Middle
Index
Thumb
Neck
Brow
Eyelid and eyeball
Face
Lips
Vocalization
Jaw
Tongue
Swallowing
Mastication
Salivation

# 7

# Brain Mapping for Neurosurgery and Cognitive Neuroscience

Joy Hirsch

## Historical Milestones That Enable Imaging of Cortical Processes That Underlie Mental Events Using MRI

One of the primary goals of neural science is to understand the biological underpinnings of cognition. This goal is based on the assumption that cognitive events emerge from brain events and that behavior can be explained in terms of neural processes. Francis Crick referred to this as "the Astonishing Hypothesis."[1] According to this view, the biological principles that underlie cognition link the structure and function of the brain.

> The Astonishing Hypothesis is that "You," your joys and your sorrows, your memories and your ambitions, your sense of personal identity and free will, are in fact no more than the behavior of a vast assembly of nerve cells and their associated molecules. As Lewis Carroll's Alice might have phrased it: "You're nothing but a pack of neurons."† This hypothesis is so alien to the ideas of most people alive today that it can truly be called astonishing.
>
> Francis Crick, 1994, *The Astonishing Hypothesis*, p.3

Using neuroimaging methods, it is possible to observe active cortical areas associated with cognitive processes in healthy human volunteers. This capability has stimulated a renewed focus on the physiological bases of cognition. In particular, the implementation of non-invasive, functional imaging techniques such as functional magnetic resonance imaging (fMRI) offers an unprecedented global view of the complexities of the intact working human brain, including local neural circuits (cortical columns), regions, and large-scale systems of interconnected regions. Functional imaging provides a unique view of the cortical activation patterns associated with specific mental processes such as seeing, hearing, feeling, moving, talking, and thinking. Thus, the potential to realize a neural basis for various aspects of cognition has emerged with the development of neuroimaging.

Conventional definitions of cognition do not directly address the biological components of mental events. For example, *Dorland's Illustrated Medical Dictionary* defines cognition as "operations of the mind by which we become aware of objects of thought or perception; it includes all aspects of perceiving, thinking and remembering."[2] *The American Heritage Dictionary* offers a similar definition for cognition as "the mental process of knowing, including aspects such as awareness, perception, reasoning and judgment, and that which comes to be known, as through perception, reasoning, or intuition, and knowledge."[3] However, in his seminal book, *Cognitive Psychology*, Ulrich Neisser defined cognition as "*all processes* by which the sensory input is transformed, reduced, elaborated, stored, recovered, and used."[4] This definition could be interpreted to encompass biological processes, although none were specifically proposed by Neisser. An essential focus of neuroimaging is to link models of cognition to biological processes.

Medical reports of associations between specific brain injuries and functional deficits provided the initial basis for the assumed linkage between specific brain areas and behavior. As early as 1841, Broca reported language production deficits in patients with specific damage to the left frontal lobe, and in 1874, Wernicke reported deficits in language comprehension and expression in patients following specific damage to the left temporal lobe. Since then, Broca's and Wernicke's Areas have become established as regions of cortex associated with aspects of speech production and comprehension, respectively. Around the same time, Harlow reported profound personality changes following an unfortunate frontal-lobe injury in his now well-known patient, Phineas Gage.[5] Nearly a century later, Penfield pioneered the experimental technique of direct cortical stimulation during neurosurgical procedures. His observations confirmed the functional specializations of the speech-related areas and demonstrated topographical maps associated with sensory and motor functions.[6] Along with the documented associations between lesions and specific functions, Penfield's reports of cortical stimulations that elicited memories, tastes, and other mental events supported the profound link between brain structure and cognitive function widely accepted within the mainstream of clinical neurology and neurosurgery. For example, it had been noted that severing a segment of the optic nerve always resulted in visual field loss (Figure 7.1), and similarly, severing a primary motor projection always resulted in a contralateral plegia.

One of the key principles that links brain function and mental events is the relationship between neural activity and blood flow. In 1881, Angelo Mosso, a physiologist, studied a patient who had survived an injury to the skull. Due to the nature of the injury, it was possible to observe blood-flow–related pulsations to the left frontal lobe that occurred during certain cognitive events. Mosso concluded that blood flow within the brain was coupled to mental events. Roy and Sherrington[7] subsequently proposed a specific mechanism to couple blood flow and neural activity based on direct measurements on dogs. More recently, using $H_2{}^{15}O$ as a tracer of blood flow in the human brain, Raichle and colleagues[8] confirmed this fundamental relationship

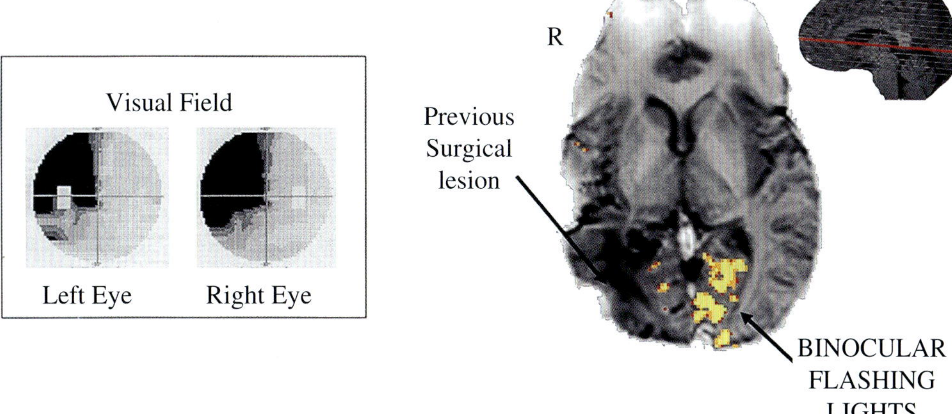


**Figure 7.1.** Static visual fields indicate a homonymous quadrantic field defect in the left superior quadrant that is associated with damage to the visual projection fibers within the right occipital lobe following resection of a lesion within the right hemisphere occipital region. Functional magnetic resonance imaging activation during binocular viewing of flashing lights (8 Hz) demonstrates unilateral cortical responses (left hemisphere only), reflecting the loss of visual responses in this topographically mapped area of the visual field.

between blood flow and local neural activity. This seminal physiology work provided the basis for positron emission tomographic (PET) imaging of active cortical tissue during the execution of a task. The technique was demonstrated by Fox and Raichle[9] with a simple sensory and motor activation paradigm, where hemodynamic variations (as indicated by a radioactive tracer of water molecules) were observed within the pre- and post-central gyri.

Typically, PET activation studies depend upon subtractive comparisons of images acquired during a task and images acquired during a rest or control condition. The logic of this technique is that the difference image represents the neural activity present in the task condition and not in the control; for example, activity associated with viewing a flashing checkerboard minus activity associated with viewing a fixation dot presumably reveals the effect of the flashing checkerboard on specialized neural structures. Unfortunately, the PET camera does not provide a detailed image of brain structure; therefore, computational techniques to register the locations of the gamma ray events to brain anatomy obtained by other higher-resolution techniques such as magnetic resonance imaging (MRI) were developed. These procedures also include algorithms to register the anatomical and PET images of multiple subjects based on a standard human brain atlas. When all subject brains are registered to the same atlas, the difference images of multiple subjects can be averaged to obtain conserved and generalizable results.

These advances in PET techniques enabled the first neuroimaging study of cognitive processes relating to language.[10] The study differntiated cortical patterns of activation associated with four separate word tasks: passively viewing words, listening to words, speaking words, and generating words. These early PET studies firmly established the proof-of-principle that activity associated with cognitive events was observable in the living human brain via hemodynamic variations within locally active neural areas. However, due to risks associated with injections of radioactive tracers, limitations to the number of times a subject can be studied, the relatively coarse resolution, and the relatively few PET facilities available for research, the imaging of cortical activity associated with cognitive processes has advanced most rapidly using a newer, noninvasive, higher-resolution, and more available technique, functional magnetic resonance imaging (fMRI).

## Development of Magnetic Resonance Imaging (MRI) to Visualize Living Brain Structure

Since the invention of the microscope in 1664, imaging technology has guided the mainstream of basic research in biology by revealing structures not visible to the naked eye, including the cell, organelles, molecules, and even atoms. Despite its electronic and computational developments, the microscope is not suited for the imaging of living structures occluded beneath surface tissues such as skin, muscle, and bone. This occlusion problem was solved with the development of MRI, where internal structures within the living body can be resolved at submillmeter scales.

The development of MRI incorporated a long chain of discoveries (Figure 7.2), beginning with the discovery of molecular beam magnetic resonance in 1936 by Isidor Rabi at Columbia University. Shortly thereafter, in 1945, Edward Purcell and Felix Bloch independently discovered nuclear magnetic resonance (NMR) in condensed matter, followed by Erwin Hahn's observations of nuclear magnetic relaxation and the discovery of spin echo in 1949. A pinnacle event in the development of MRI was made in 1971 by Raymond Damadian who discovered that biological tissues have different relaxation rates. A year later, the first magnetic resonance image of a tube phantom was produced by Paul Lauterbur using a magnetic gradient to produce spatial resolution of the image. The first MRI of a human body part (a finger) was published in 1976 by Peter Mansfield and colleagues. Mansfield and colleagues also developed a key enhancement of a high-speed imaging sequence, echo planar imaging, which enabled three-dimensional (3D) acquisitions of body organs (such as the brain) within seconds. A year later, Damadian produced the first magnetic resonance image of a human whole body (cross sectional chest) and in 1980 produced the first human whole body commercial MRI scanner.

## The Development of fMRI

Recent advances in MRI have extended imaging of brain structures to include the identification of active neural tissue in the cortex. The chain of discoveries that led to the generation of MR images of the working brain include Michael Faraday's discovery in 1845 that dried blood has magnetic properties, and Linus Pauling's discovery in 1936

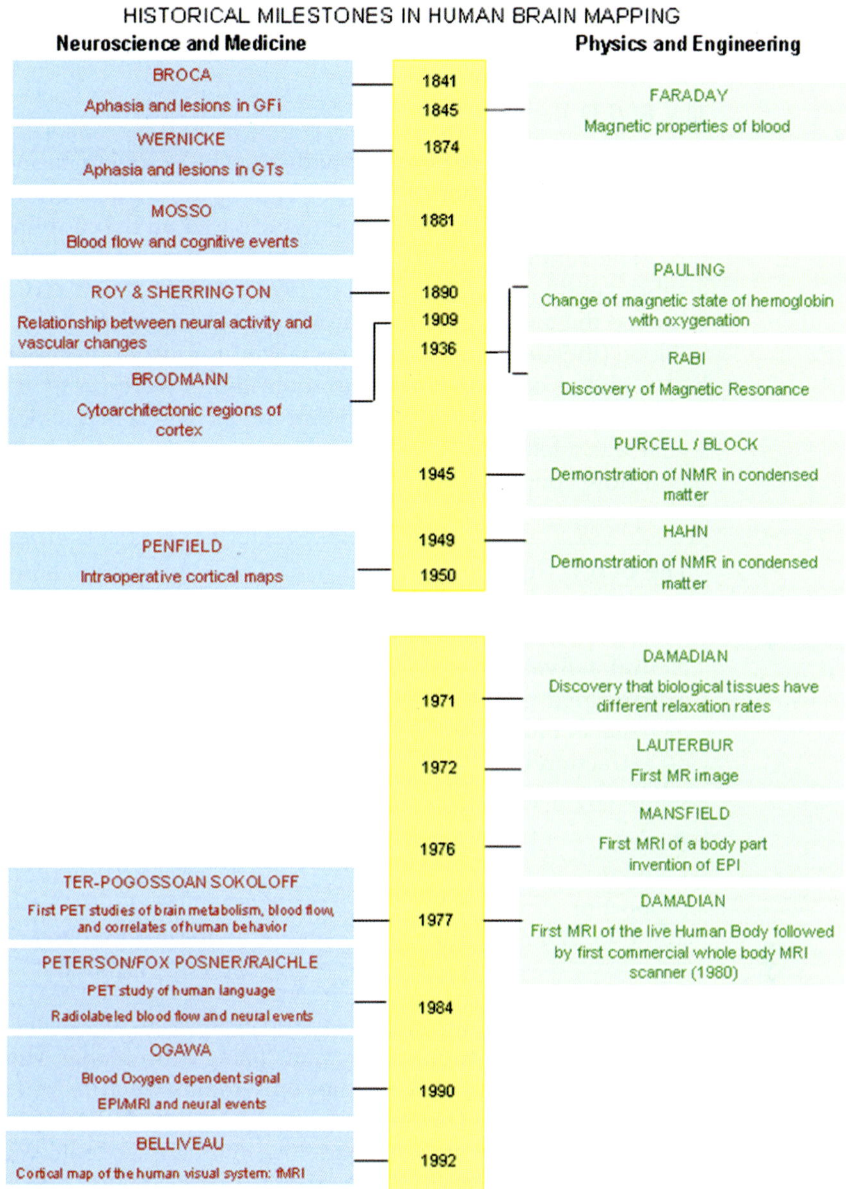


**Figure 7.2.** Historical milestones in human brain mapping. The timeline marks milestones in neuroscience and medicine in parallel with physics and engineering that lead to the development of functional magnetic resonance imaging (fMRI) and the ability to image active human cortical tissue corresponding to specific cognitive function.

that the magnetic properties of hemoglobin change with the state of oxygenation.

### The BOLD Response

These discoveries lay dormant with respect to functional neuroimaging until after the development of high-speed MRI of brain structure and PET imaging of active neural tissue based on the coupling of blood flow. The fundamental breakthrough discovery of the blood oxygen level-dependent (BOLD) signal in 1990 by Seiji Ogawa and colleagues followed the observation that the MR signal originating from the occipital lobe (the area of the brain specialized for visual processing) in rats had a higher contrast when the room lights were on than when the lights were off. Ogawa reasoned that the increased magnetic resonance signal was related to changes in oxygenated hemoglobin resulting from blood flow coupled to neural activity.[11]

**The BOLD Signal**

| **Physiology** | **Physics** |
|---|---|
| **Neural activation** is associated with an increase in blood flow $O_2$ extraction is relatively unchanged | **Deoxy HGB is paramagnetic** and distorts the local magnetic field, causing signal loss |
| **Result:** Reduction in the proportion of deoxy HGB in the local vasculature | **Result:** Less distortion of the magnetic field results in local signal increase |

Within two years, John Belliveau and colleagues replicated Ogawa's visual stimulation studies in humans using echo planar MRI, demonstrating the potential to reveal not only brain structure, but also brain function using MR. This technique, which exploited the fundamental link between the MR signal, blood flow, and neural events, was referred to as functional magnetic resonance imaging (fMRI) (see review by John Gore[12] for a more detailed description of these relationships). Figure 7.3 illustrates a BOLD signal (right) originating from the right hemisphere (R) region of postcentral gyrus (indicated by the arrow and yellow cluster) in response to touch of the left hand. The active region is contralateral to the stimulation and well established as an area functionally specialized for tactile sensation.

## Hypothesis of Functional Specialization

One of the central assumptions that drives research and clinical applications that link cortical structure and function is that specific brain areas are involved in specific aspects of behavior such as action, per-

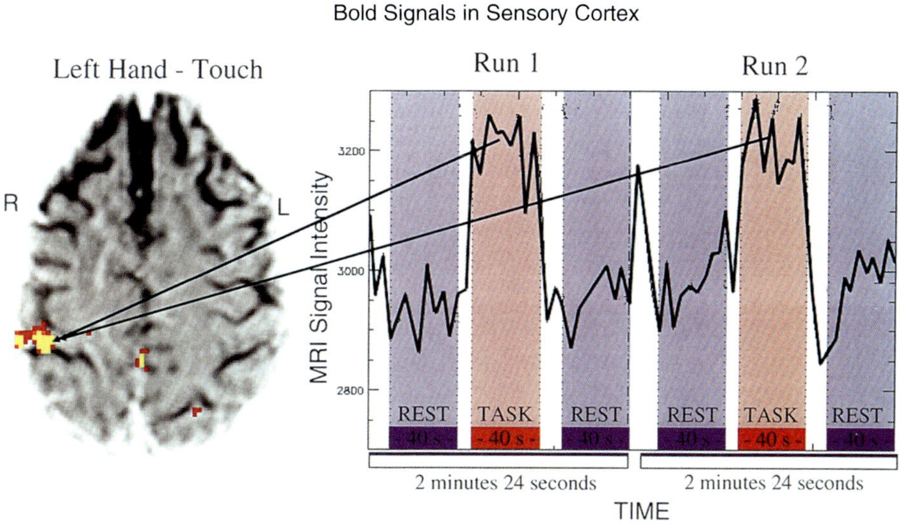

**Figure 7.3.** Cortical activity associated with tactile stimulation of the left hand. Signals illustrate the BOLD changes in MR susceptibility observed in response to passive tactile stimulation of the left hand of a healthy volunteer. Signals originate from a single voxel (1.5 × 1.5 × 4.5 mm) on two separate runs. Each run lasted 2 minutes 24 seconds, during which 36 images were acquired, including 10 images for each of three epochs: initial resting baseline (purple bar), task (left-hand touch) (pink bar), and final resting baseline (purple bar). All voxels in the brain for which the statistical criteria were met (the average amplitude of the signal during the activity epoch was statistically different from the baseline signal) are indicated by either a yellow, or red color superimposed on the T2*-weighted image at the voxel address and signify decreasing levels of statistical confidence. Arrows point to the source voxel, which is centered within a cluster of similar (yellow) voxels and located in the right (R) hemisphere of the brain along the postcentral gyrus. Reprinted with permission from Hirsch J, Ruge MI, Kim KHS, Correa DD, Victor JD, Relkin NR, LaBar DR, Krol G, Bilsky MH, Souweidane MM, DeAngelis LM, Gutin PH. An integrated fMRI procedure for preoperative mapping of cortical areas associated with tactile, motor, language, and visual functions. *Neurosurgery*. 2000;47(3):711–722. Copyright © 2000 Lippincott Williams & Wilkins.

ception, cognition, affect, and consciousness. As discussed above, cognitive deficits in patients with brain damage have led to the conclusion that the brain is functionally specialized at a coarse spatial scale (e.g., at the scale of lobes and hemispheres); for example, visual-related cortex includes occipital lobe, inferior temporal lobe, and posterior parietal lobe; auditory-related cortex includes superior temporal lobe; somatosensory-related cortex includes postcentral gyrus; motor-related cortex includes precentral gyrus; and explicit memory-related cortex includes hippocampus and temporal lobe. It is now widely believed that the brain is also functionally specialized at a finer scale.

In the case of the well-studied visual system, over 30 separate and distinct visual cortical areas are organized into well-defined processing pathways. Visual signals from the retina are transmitted to the lateral geniculate nucleus of the thalamus, and then to primary visual cortex where visual information fans out to the extrastriate visual cortical areas. The extrastriate visual areas serve many different aspects of visual perception and visually guided behavior. Among the dimensions suggested for independent visual analysis are: brightness, texture, color, depth, movement, shape, face recognition, and object recognition. While specializations for these functions are active topics for investigation, Figure 7.4 illustrates the well-known specialization of primary visual cortex for primitive stimuli such as on/off full-field stimulation. Similar specializations exist for language, sensory, motor, and auditory systems, and provide the focus for recent developments in cortical function mapping that protect these systems during invasive neurosurgical procedures.

## Identification and Preservation of Cortical Areas Specialized for Essential Tasks

Functional maps for individual subjects aim to identify functional specializations specific to that particular subject. In the case of functional mapping prior to a surgical procedure, the goal is to identify regions

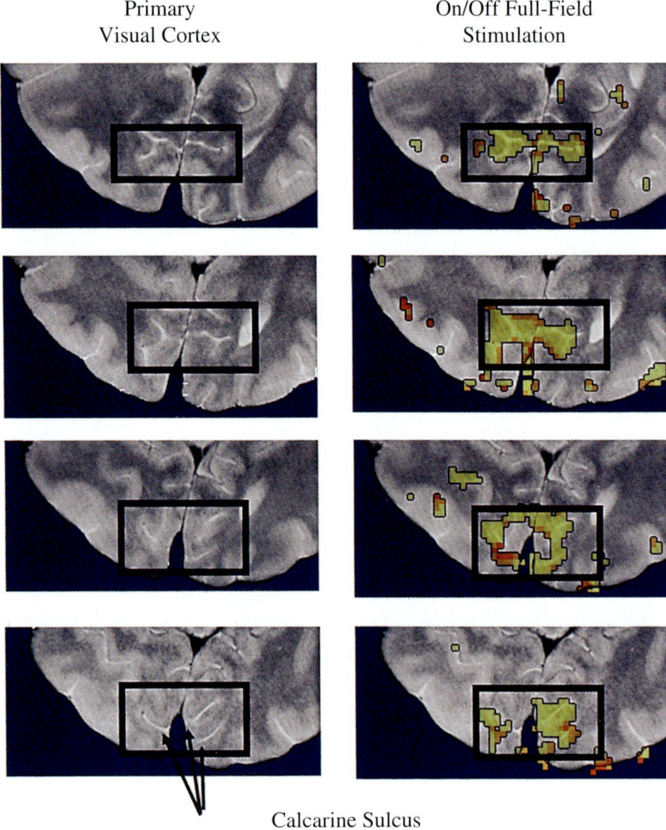


**Figure 7.4.** Boxed areas surround the anatomical calcarine sulcus in contiguous 3-mm-thick axial slices (left column). The right column illustrates cortical activity (fMRI) observed during viewing of full-field 8 Hz on-off stimulation. The proximity of the activity patterns and the calcarine sulcus (primary visual cortex) is consistent with the hypothesis of functional specificity for this simple stimulation.

of the individual patient's brain that are employed for functions (such as motor movements, tactile sensation, language functions, vision, and audition) that might be at risk because of the location of the surgery. The presence of a space-occupying lesion or long-term seizure-genic conditions can modify or shift functional foci, and normal assumptions do not necessarily apply. In these cases, functional images are acquired at the highest-possible resolution and integrated into the appropriate treatment plan. Ideally, individual effects are studied by comparisons that occur before and after a therapeutic intervention where functional changes would be expected.

The preservation of function during a brain tumor resection is an essential goal of neurosurgery, and various intraoperative and preoperative brain mapping techniques are currently employed for this purpose. These techniques aim to identify cortical areas involved in sensory, motor, and language functions and have become standard practice. They include intraoperative electrophysiology with motor and language mapping, preoperative Wada tests, and visual field examinations. However, the added risk, time, and expense of multiple mapping procedures favors a single, noninvasive, preoperative procedure that could prove effective for mapping these functions. Functional MRI, has emerged as such a technique. Functional MRI maps of sensory and motor functions, either alone or in combination with other neuronavigation techniques,[13–15] have been shown effective in directing brain tumor resection procedures away from cortical regions with residual function.[13,16–22]

Tasks employed for functional mapping of sensory and motor-sensitive regions have generally been developed by separate research groups in the service of neurosurgical planning. As a consequence, many task variants have been employed. For example, motor tasks are sometimes accomplished by single finger–thumb tapping,[19] and in other cases by multiple finger–thumb tapping.[17,23,24] Other approaches include self-paced clenching and spreading of the hand,[22,25–27] or sponge squeezing.[18,20] Tactile stimulation has included palm brushing,[18] compressed air puffs to the hand,[20] and scratching the ventral surface of the hand.[19] Similarly, functional mapping of language areas has also been accomplished by a range of tasks and procedures including object naming and verb generation,[28] production of the names of animals starting with a given letter,[17] word generation in alphabetical order,[29] or auditory noun presentations with a required category response.[30] It is not known, however, how these various tasks compare with respect to sensitivity or targeted regions of interest. Assessment of cortical activity associated with visual stimulation has been accomplished with intermittent binocular photic stimulation,[17,24,31] as well as with various projected pattern stimuli.[32] The length of the activity period and the number of epochs in a run are also non-standard. Additional variation is introduced to the literature by different levels of statistical stringency and multiple data-processing procedures. Although all of these tasks for sensory, motor, language, and visual functions may be individually effective, an integrated and standardized battery of tasks could optimize application for neurosurgical planning.

Within a cohesive task battery, it is desirable to maximize reliability by using multiple tasks to target related functions. One such battery of fMRI tasks targets cortical regions associated with tactile, motor, language, and visual-sensitive cortical areas.[33] The task battery targets functions selective for regions frequently considered most critical for surgical decisions. All functions are repeated using both active (volitional) and passive (receptive) modes to assure that it is applicable to patients with a range of symptoms and performance capabilities. Any subset of these tasks may be selected for specific clinical objectives while retaining the advantages of the standardized procedures with validations based on responses of both healthy volunteers and patients.

### A Multifunction Task Battery

The specific tasks selected for this task battery are intended to be nearly universally applicable and employ common stimuli and procedures.[34] The tasks consist of four separate procedures (Figure 7.5) including:

1. Passive tactile stimulation of a hand (either the dominant hand or the hand relevant to the hemisphere of surgical interest) with a mildly abrasive plastic surface that is gently rubbed on the palm and fingers. Simultaneously, the patient views a reversing checkerboard pattern (8 Hz). This visual stimulation also aids in head stabilization of the patient.
2. Active hand movement (finger–thumb tapping) using either the same hand, as in the passive tactile stimulation, or both hands during a repeat of the simultaneous visual stimulation (reversing checkerboard).
3. Picture naming by internal (silent) speech in response to visually displayed, black-and-white, line drawings[35] presented at four-second intervals. These drawings are selected from an appropriate range of the Boston Naming test.

**fMRI Task Battery for Cortical Mapping of Sensory, Motor, Language and Vision-Related Areas**

| | | | |
|---|---|---|---|
| 1. | **SENSORY**<br>**Touch/hand** | + | **VISION**<br>**Reversing Checkerboard** |
| 2. | **MOTOR**<br>**Finger/Thumb tapping** | + | **VISION**<br>**Reversing Checkerboard** |
| 3. | **LANGUAGE/active**<br>**Picture Naming** | + | **VISION**<br>**Pictures** |
| 4. | **LANGUAGE/passive**<br>**Listening to Words** | + | **AUDITION**<br>**Spoken words** |

**Figure 7.5.** A summary of the functions mapped by the four conditions in the fMRI task battery. Reprinted with permission from Hirsch J, Ruge MI, Kim KHS, Correa DD, Victor JD. Relkin NR, LaBar DR, Krol G, Bilsky MH. Souweidane MM, DeAngelis LM, Gutin PH. An integrated fMRI procedure for preoperative mapping of cortical areas associated with tactile, motor, language, and visual functions. *Neurosurgery*. 2000;47(3):711–722. Copyright © 2000 Lippincott Williams & Wilkins.

4. Listening to recordings of spoken words (names of objects) presented through headphones designed to reduce scanner noise. A visual fixation cross helps prevent head movement.

The aims of these four conditions include: 1) localization of sensory and motor cortices, and by inference, location of the central sulcus; 2) localization of language-related activity, and by inference, the locations of Broca's and Wernicke's Areas and the dominant hemisphere for speech; and 3) localization of primary and secondary visual areas.

Each of the targeted functions and structures associated with each task is illustrated in Figure 7.6 for a healthy volunteer. The sensory and motor tasks target post- and precentral gyrus (GPoC and GPrC), respectively, and are illustrated in the left panels. These figures also illustrate the expected overlap along the pre- and postcentral gyrus between activity associated with sensory and motor stimulation. The language tasks target putative Broca's and Wernicke's Areas that are found within inferior frontal gurus (GFi) and superior temporal gyrus (GTs), respectively, on the dominant hemisphere for language (middle panels of Figure 7.6). Both areas are redundantly targeted by expressive (active) and receptive (passive) language tasks, and by both visual

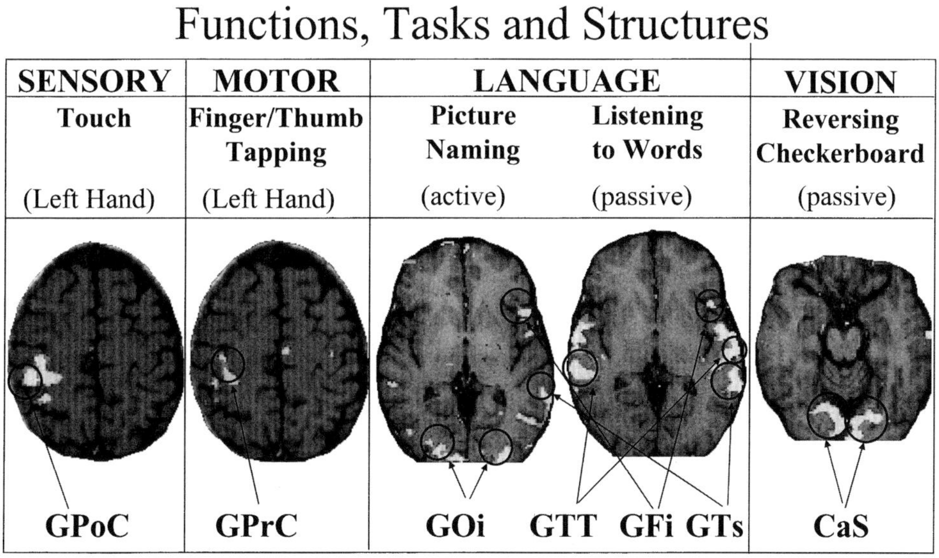

Functions, Tasks and Structures

| SENSORY | MOTOR | LANGUAGE | | VISION |
|---|---|---|---|---|
| Touch | Finger/Thumb Tapping | Picture Naming | Listening to Words | Reversing Checkerboard |
| (Left Hand) | (Left Hand) | (active) | (passive) | (passive) |
| GPoC | GPrC | GOi GTT | GFi GTs | CaS |

**Figure 7.6.** Selected slices for a healthy brain illustrate targeted (circled) structures labeled according to the Talairach and Tournoux Human Brain Atlas[45] for each of the functions and tasks: sensory, passive touch of the hand (left) using a rough plastic surface targets the post-central gyrus (GPoC); motor, active finger–thumb tapping targets the pre-central gyrus (GPrC); language, picture naming (expressive) and listening to spoken words (receptive) target the inferior frontal gyrus (GFi; Broca's Area) and the superior temporal gyrus (GTs; Wernicke's Area) on the dominant hemisphere; and vision, viewing of the reversing checkerboard and picture naming target the calcarine sulcus (CaS) and the inferior occipital gyrus (GOi). Primary auditory activity expected to be associated with the listening task also is observed bilaterally in the transverse temporal gyrus (GTT), middle panel. Reprinted with permission from Hirsh J, Ruge MI, Kim KHS, Correa DD, Victor JD, Relkin NR, LaBar DR, Krol G, Bilsky MH, Souweidane MM, DeAngelis LM, Gutin PH. An integrated fMRI procedure for preoperative mapping of cortical areas associated with tactile, motor, language, and visual functions. *Neurosurgery*. 2000;47(3):711–722. 

and auditory modalities. Visual and auditory systems also are revealed by the activity in inferior occipital gyrus (GOi) and the transverse temporal gyrus (GTT), respectively, left and right language panels. Vision-related activity elicited by the reversing black-and-white checkerboard stimulations also targets primary visual cortex found along the calcarine sulcus (CaS), illustrated in the far-right panel of Figure 7.6. Given the high levels of statistical confidence, ($p$ values from $\leq 0.0001$ to $\leq 0.0005$), it can be assumed that activity not circled also represents true physiological activations that are task-related and distributed outside the targeted regions of interest.

### Healthy Volunteers and Patients

Development of this test battery was based upon a total of 63 healthy volunteers (24 female and 39 male) who participated in the evaluation of the specific set of tasks targeted to identify brain regions most likely to be surgical regions of interest for 1) primary brain tumor, 2) brain metastasis, 3) seizure disorder, or 4) cerebral vascular malformation. A total of 125 patients also participated. These patients were surgical candidates and presented with surgical regions of interest that included sensorimotor ($n = 63$), language ($n = 56$), or visual ($n = 6$) functions.

### Sensitivity of Task Battery: Healthy Volunteers

Each task was associated with the targeted region of interest, and the percentage of cases showing activity in those regions (sensitivity) was determined (Table 7.1A). This task battery provides two opportunities to observe the targeted region; for example, whereas the superior temporal gyrus (GTs) was activated in only 73% of cases during picture naming, it was activated in 100% of healthy volunteers during listening to spoken words (Table 7.1, column 5). Overall, the sensitivity of the entire battery to identify language-related cortex in the superior temporal gyrus is 100% for the population of healthy volunteers, as indicated on the bottom row, Composite Sensitivity. Specifically, the composite sensitivity is the result of a logical operating room (OR) decision rule based on two tasks that target a specific region. Central sulcus and visual cortex were identified in 100% of cases and Broca's Area in 93%.

### Sensitivity of Task Battery: Surgical Population

Following task-sensitivity determinations for healthy volunteers, similar determinations were made for surgical candidates with pathology in the specified cortical regions of interest. This enabled assessment of the fMRI task within the affected pathological cohort. These subgroups served as the basis for evaluation of the respective tasks, although all patients completed all tasks in the battery, regardless of the region of surgical interest. Table 7.1B reports the task sensitivity within each surgical group, thus indicating the sensitivity in the presence of pathology. The tactile stimulation revealed activity in the

**Table 7.1. Evaluation of Task Sensitivity**

| | | A. Healthy Subjects Targeted regions of interest | | | | B. Surgical Patients Surgical regions of interest | | | |
|---|---|---|---|---|---|---|---|---|---|
| Task | Structure | Central Sulcus ($n = 30$) | Broca's Area ($n = 45$) | Wernicke's Area ($n = 45$) | Visual Cortex ($n = 15$) | Central Sulcus ($n = 63$) | Broca's Area ($n = 22$) | Wernicke's Area ($n = 34$) | Visual Cortex ($n = 6$) |
| Touch | GPoC | 100% | | | | 94% | | | |
| Finger-Thumb Tapping | GPrC | 100% | | | | 89% | | | |
| Picture | GFi | | 90% | | | | 72% | | |
| Naming | GTs | | | 73% | | | | 65% | |
| Listening to | GFi | | 93% | | | | 54% | | |
| Spoken Words | GTs | | | 100% | | | | 88% | |
| Checkerboard | CaS | | | | 100% | | | | 100% |
| Pictures | GOi | | | | 100% | | | | 100% |
| Composite Sensitivity (Logical OR) | | 100% | 93% | 100% | 100% | 97% | 77% | 91% | 100% |

Reprinted with permission from Hirsch J, Ruge MI, Kim KHS, Correa DD, Victor JD, Relkin NR, LaBar DR, Krol G, Bilsky MH, Souweidane MM, DeAngelis LM, Gutin PH. An integrated fMRI procedure for preoperative mapping of cortical areas associated with tactile, motor, language, and visual functions. *Neurosurgery*. 2000;47(3):711–722. Copyright © 2000 Lippincott Williams & Wilkins.

well as occasional word-finding difficulties. Preoperative neuropsychological evaluation revealed no language deficits. Magnetic resonance imaging revealed a rounded, partially hemorrhagic lesion, 4.5 centimeters in diameter located in the left posterior temporal lobe. To optimize a therapeutic plan, functional maps were obtained using the multifunction task battery; results are summarized in Figure 7.7. The central sulcus was identified clearly by the sensory and motor tasks (top rows). The language tasks revealed language-related activity on the left hemisphere adjacent to both the posterior margins and the anterior margins of the mass (GTs and GFi; middle rows). The visual stimulation was reliably associated with signals within and along the primary visual areas (CaS). Due to the proximity of the language-related activity to the tumor, an awake craniotomy with electrophysiological mapping of motor and language functions was performed.

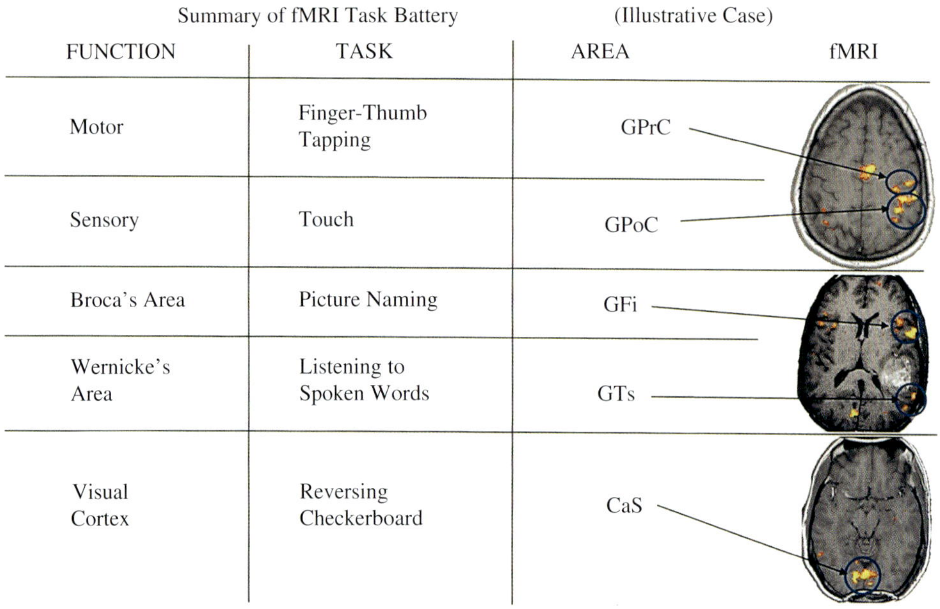

Summary of fMRI Task Battery (Illustrative Case)

| FUNCTION | TASK | AREA | fMRI |
|---|---|---|---|
| Motor | Finger-Thumb Tapping | GPrC | |
| Sensory | Touch | GPoC | |
| Broca's Area | Picture Naming | GFi | |
| Wernicke's Area | Listening to Spoken Words | GTs | |
| Visual Cortex | Reversing Checkerboard | CaS | |

**Figure 7.7.** Selected slices (right) illustrate cortical responses associated with each of the tasks and the targeted regions of interest for case example 1. Sensory and motor tasks elicited activity within pre- and post-central gyri and predicted the location of the central sulcus on multiple contiguous slices. The slice illustrated in the right top row shows a relatively inferior representation. The two language tasks—picture naming and listening to spoken words—elicited activity in the left hemisphere within the inferior frontal gyrus (GFi) and the superior temporal gyrus (GTs; arrows). In this case, the specific locations of the activity within the GFi and GTs were replicated on both tasks and the overlapping regions were taken as the best predictor of Broca's and Wernicke's Areas, respectively. Finally, the reversing checkerboard (bottom row) indicated primary visual cortex, as illustrated by the activity labeled calcarine sulcus (CaS). Similar to the language-related regions, these regions were replicated across the multiple visual tasks and served to increase confidence in these results. Reprinted with permission from Hirsch J, Ruge MI, Kim KHS, Correa DD, Victor JD, Relkin NR, LaBar DR, Krol G, Bilsky MH, Souweidane MM, DeAngelis LM, Gutin PH. An integrated fMRI procedure for preoperative mapping of cortical areas associated with tactile, motor, language, and visual functions. *Neurosurgery*. 2000;47(3):711–722. 

## Integrative Mapping of Sensory and Motor Functions

Recording of SSEPs indicated the location of the central sulcus (Figure 7.8, left columns), which was confirmed by direct cortical stimulation of precentral gyrus (middle columns). Comparison with the location of central sulcus by fMRI (right column) indicates good agreement with both techniques, as illustrated by the arrows.

## Interoperative Mapping of Language Functions

Direct cortical stimulation of the left inferior frontal gyrus with the Ojemann Bipolar stimulator disrupted the patient's ability to count,

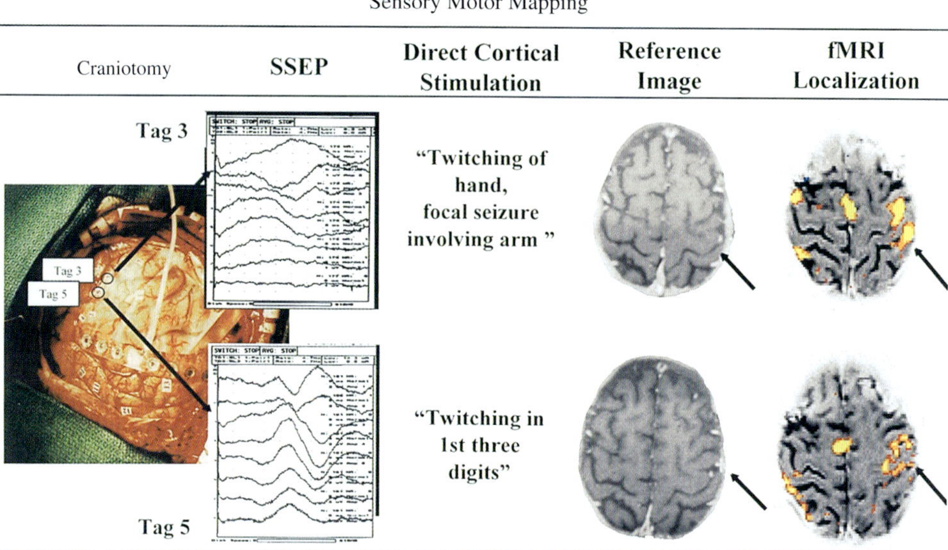


**Figure 7.8.** Needle-recording electrodes were placed at Erb's Point and stimulating electrodes were placed over the left or right median nerve at the wrist. Following craniotomy and exposure of cortex, subdural strip electrodes were placed in the operative field. The median nerve was stimulated to elicit epicortical responses measured with the electrodes. A consistent phase reversal between electrode sites (tags 3 and 5, column 2) was taken as the physiological identification of sensorimotor cortex, and therefore, the central sulcus (indicated by arrows on the reference images in column 4). These recordings of somatosensory-evoked potentials (SSEP) were made with an 8-Channel Viking IV7 and standard filter settings (30 Hz to 3 kHz). Direct cortical stimulation of the exposed cortex directed by the SSEP results was performed using the Ojemann bipolar stimulator (one second trains of one millisecond pulses at 60 Hz) varied from two milliaperes (mA) to 18 mA, peak to peak, resulting in hand twitching and a focal seizure of the right arm (top row) and twitching of the first three digits of the hand (bottom row). Using a frameless-based intraoperative navigation system (BrainLAB GmbH, Munich, Germany), the tagged locations were referenced to anatomical axial MR images localized using a viewing wand and subsequently compared with areas of activation on corresponding fMRI images, as illustrated by comparison of the images in columns 4 and 5 (arrows). The T2* images (right column) and the conventional T1 images (reference image) were not acquired at exactly corresponding plane orientations, accounting for the variation in the two structural images and limiting the precision with which the electrophysiological and fMRI locations can be compared. Reprinted with permission from Hirsch J, Ruge MI, Kim KHS, Correa DD, Victor JD, Relkin NR, LaBar DR, Krol G, Bilsky MH, Souweidane MM, DeAngelis LM, Gutin PH. An integrated fMRI procedure for preoperative mapping of cortical areas associated with tactile, motor, language, and visual functions. *Neurosurgery.* 2000;47(3):711–722. 

and a similar stimulation of the superior temporal gyrus produced language disturbances, including literal paraphasic errors and word-finding difficulties, respectively (Figure 7.9). Sites of observable responses were tagged with numbers, photographically documented, and cross referenced to the fMRI, as illustrated by arrows.

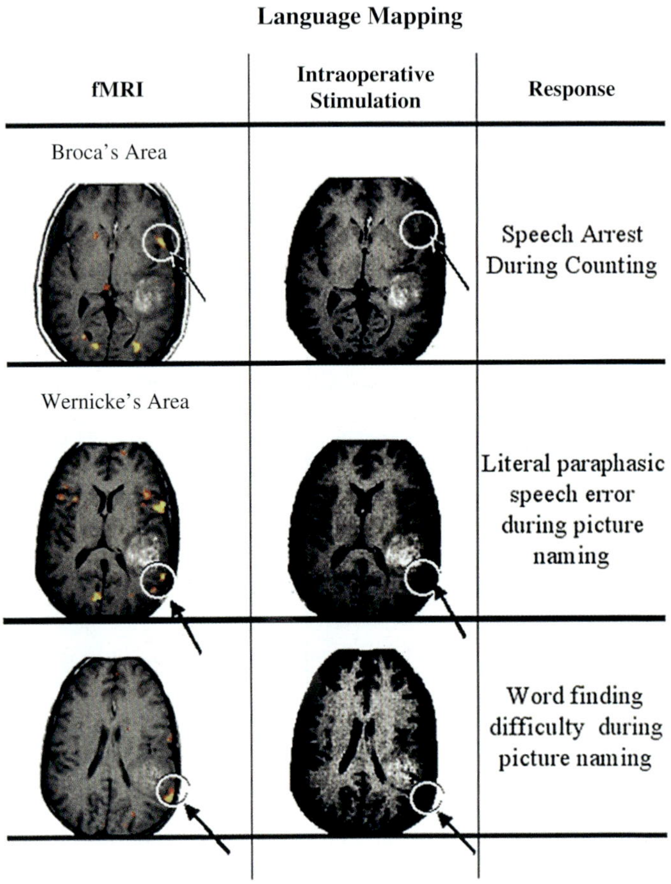

**Language Mapping**

| fMRI | Intraoperative Stimulation | Response |
|---|---|---|
| Broca's Area | | Speech Arrest During Counting |
| Wernicke's Area | | Literal paraphasic speech error during picture naming |
| | | Word finding difficulty during picture naming |

**Figure 7.9.** After craniotomy and recording of SSEPs, the patient was awakened and asked to count forward and backward while the cortex in putative Broca's Area was stimulated. Subsequently, the picture-naming paradigm used in the fMRI battery of tasks was administered and stimulation at the site where fMRI maps indicated the location of Broca's Area resulted in speech disruption (top row). Stimulation was systematically repeated and extended to temporal lobe cortex, and sites of activation revealed by the fMRI maps were specifically targeted as indicated by the circles in the middle and bottom column. These stimulations resulted in paraphasic speech errors and word-finding difficulties as indicated, consistent with disruption of Wernicke's Area-related functions that occurred in the two separate locations as indicated. The corresponding preoperative fMRI maps shown on the left column confirm the correspondence of cortical areas (circles and arrows). Reprinted with permission from Hirsch J, Ruge MI, Kim KHS, Correa DD, Victor JD, Relkin NR, LaBar DR, Krol G, Bilsky MH, Souweidane MM, DeAngelis LM, Gutin PH. An integrated fMRI procedure for preoperative mapping of cortical areas associated with tactile, motor, language, and visual functions. *Neurosurgery*. 2000;47(3):711–722. Copyright © 2000 Lippincott Williams & Wilkins.

### Postsurgical Status

A total resection was achieved that spared these functional regions. The pathology was consistent with an ependymoma. Immediately post-surgery, no impairments in language function were detected. However, the postoperative recovery of the patient was complicated by a temporary mixed aphasia and seizures. Subsequently, within 10 days, the patient's condition was substantially improved, and no further adjuvant treatment was planned. A six-month postsurgical fMRI scan was consistent with previous findings, and neuropsychological evaluation revealed residual, mild word-finding difficulties and occasional literal paraphasic errors.

### Case Example 2: Language Mapping—Late Bilingual Patient

In this case, the patient was a native of Italy who emigrated to the United States as a young adult and then learned English. When she was 44 years old, she began to experience episodes of word-finding difficulty in both Italian and English, as well as slowed speech production. An MRI obtained during a medical evaluation revealed a large tumor in the left inferior posterior frontal region of her brain expected to be associated with speech production (Figure 7.10A). In order to determine the location of her language areas relative to her tumor, a functional MRI was acquired using the task battery described above for each language, which revealed: 1) separate locations for her native (Italian) and second language (English), and 2) that both languages were displaced from the expected locations by the tumor. These displacements were confirmed during surgery and the tumor was resected without damage to either language function. Approximately two years later, she remains tumor free, with excellent English and Italian language function. A follow-up fMRI scan indicated the language areas associated with each language have shifted back to the expected locations within the brain (Figure 7.10B). The separation of the locations active during the native language and the second language within Broca's Area is consistent with previous findings of separation between L1- and L2-sensitive areas, when L2 was acquired during adulthood.[41]

### Case Example 3: Language Mapping—Early Bilingual Patient

A 23-year-old right-handed bilingual woman who works as a waitress in her father's Italian restaurant was seen on an emergency basis following the sudden onset of supplementary motor seizures. An MRI revealed the presence of a left posterior frontal cystic lesion suggestive of cystic astrocytoma. Although the patient was born and educated in the United States, she was raised in a household that spoke Italian and became bilingual during her early language development. Functional MRI of her language areas for both languages revealed over-lapping clusters in putative Broca's Area (left inferior frontal gyrus) as illustrated in Figure 7.11A, which was not changed following surgery (Figure 7.11B), consistent with the absence of postsurgical morbidity.

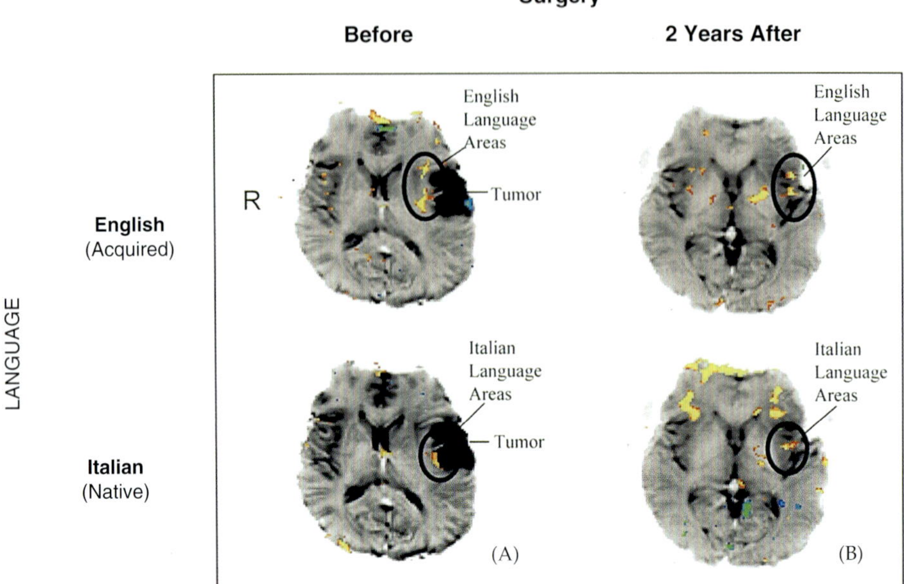


**Figure 7.10.** Language mapping of a late bilingual patient. Object naming was performed in the native language (Italian), and also in the acquired language (English). Typical of Late Bilingual individuals, the languages occupied distinct regions of Broca's Area (A). These distinct regions were preserved following surgery and are consistent with her clinical outcome of no deficits in either language (B).

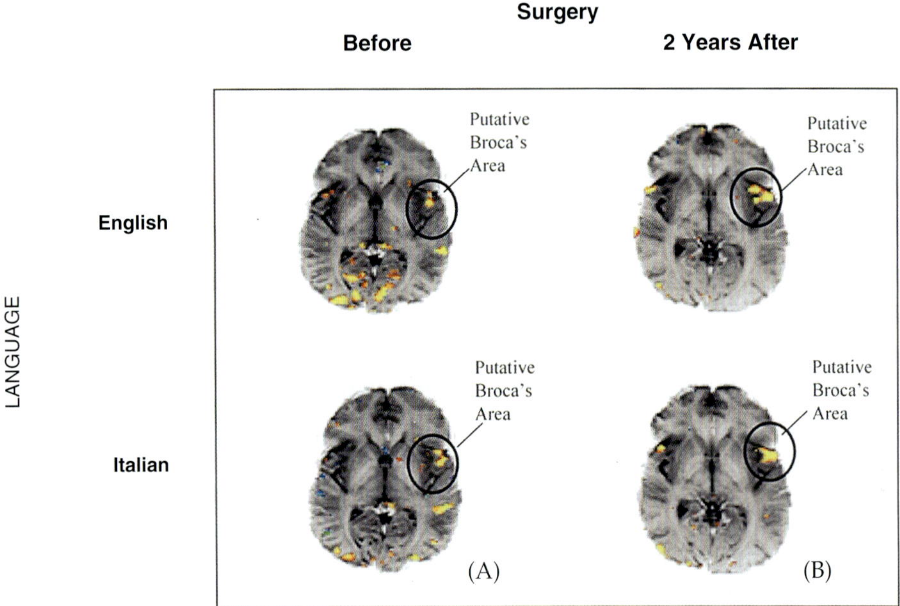


**Figure 7.11.** Language mapping of an early bilingual patient. Object naming as for the Case 2 patient (Figure 7.10) was performed in both languages, Italian and English. Typical of early bilingual individuals, the activity clusters associated with both languages were largely overlapping within Broca's Area (A). This single language area was preserved following resection (B), consistent with the absence of post-surgical morbidity.

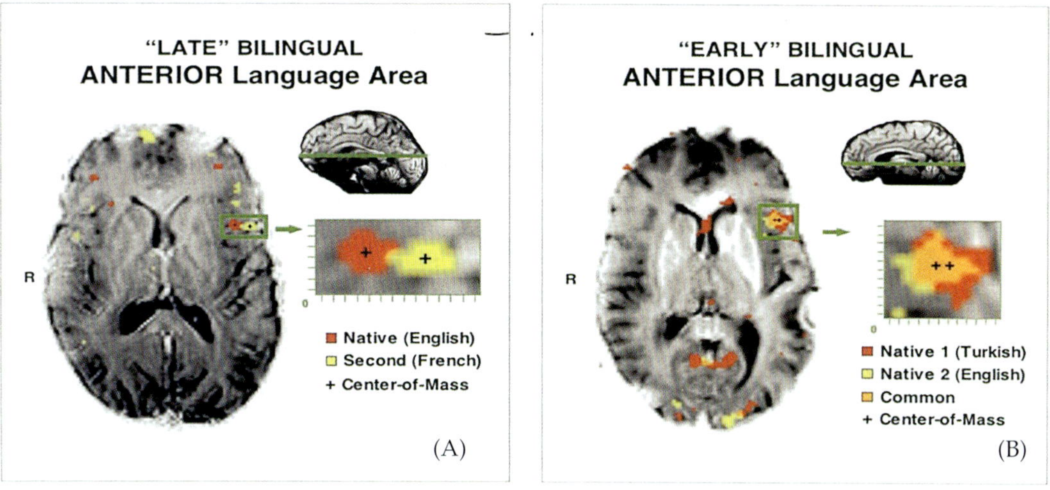


**Figure 7.12.** Examples of main findings based on two samples of healthy volunteers who were either late (A) or early (B) bilinguals. Cluster centroids and variances (spreads) were determined for activity associated with each language. A significant separation between centroids of activity was found for late bilingual subjects and not for the early bilingual subjects in Broca's Area. No differences were observed within Werniche's Area. Reprinted with permission from Kim KHS, Relkin NR, Lee K-M, Hirsch J. Distinct cortical areas associated with native and second languages. *Nature*. 1997;388:171–174.

Cases 2 and 3 illustrate earlier findings that document different cortical organization with respect to early and late acquisition of a second language. Kim and colleagues[41] showed that the average centroid separation in putative Broca's Area during L1 and L2 production in late bilingual subjects was approximately seven millimeters, whereas in early bilingual subjects, the language activations were indistinguishable (Figure 7.12).

## Case Example 4: Motor Mapping

An 11-year-old female with a completely unremarkable medical history presented following the occurrence of a grand mal seizure. Imaging revealed a large mass along the lateral margin of right central sulcus (Figure 7.13A). Due to the risk to sensory and motor functions, a surgical resection was recommended, and recommended treatment consisted of seizure management. Seeking a second opinion, parents sought a medical center with fMRI mapping capability; the functional map revealed that the tumor had displaced eloquent sensory and motor sensitive cortex medially and posteriorly from the expected positions (Figure 7.13B). Based on this information, an anterior surgical route resulted in a complete and total resection of a ganglioglioma without functional deficit. Six months postsurgery she returned for a follow-up map that revealed the expected functional pattern (Figure 7.13C). She had returned to her normal activities, including soccer, dance, and rock climbing.

A novel feature of this battery of integrated fMRI tasks is the redundancy in the measurements; for example, language-sensitive regions are mapped by both active (expressive) and passive (receptive) tasks,

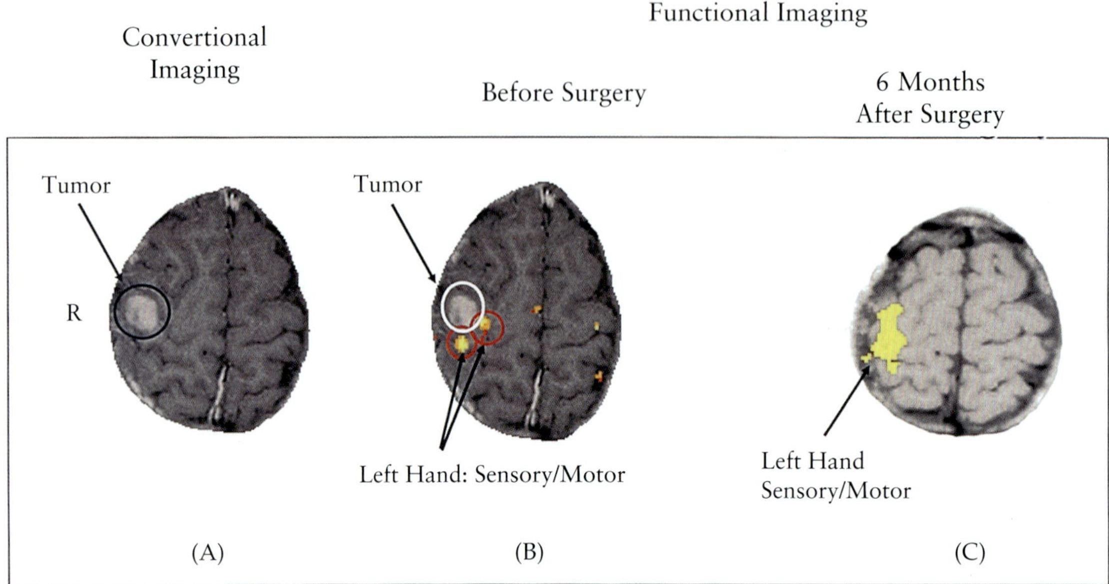


**Figure 7.13.** (A) Conventional T1 image reveals right hemisphere mass located on the margins of the central sulcus. (B) Functional map of tactile and finger–thumb tapping suggests displacement of eloquent cortex. (C) Six months after surgery, the patient is disease-free, without deficits consistent with the sensory and motor activity revealed by fMRI.

as are the regions sensitive to motor (active tapping) and sensory (passive touching) tasks. Visual areas also are assessed by passive viewing of the reversing checkerboard stimulus (no response required) and active viewing of pictures during a naming task in which a response was required. Advantages to employing more than one task associated with a particular function to isolate eloquent cortical areas include improved confidence when replications are observed, and improved sensitivity when the activity is observed during either an active or a passive performance. This feature translates into a greater likelihood of a successful map for patients with neurologic deficits. Together, the task sensitivity and accuracy observed for these fMRI maps suggests that this multifunction task battery yields a reliable estimate of the locations of critical functions potentially at risk during brain surgery, and thus extends the potential of a single preoperative fMRI brain mapping procedure to facilitate optimal outcomes for neurosurgery.

Based on our experience with this fMRI task battery, the images serve both pre- and intraoperative objectives. On the preoperative side, the fMRI maps have contributed to our estimates of the risk–benefit ratio and to the decision whether or not to offer surgery to the patient, although these decisions are based on the entire medical situation taken together, and not on any single factor. Communication between the surgeon and the patient is also facilitated by images that summarize the relevant structure and function issues. On the intraoperative side, as illustrated above, the fMRI results have also served to direct the intraoperative electrophysiology, and thereby have contributed to the efficiency of the intraoperative procedures. However, it has been observed that the information offered by the preoperative fMRI map is often more distributed than that of the intraoperative map, and the question of which active regions are essential to the function is not directly addressed by fMRI.[42] A false–positive interpretation is therefore possible based on these associated patterns of activity, whereas a false–negative finding is also possible due to sensitivity, compliance, and imaging artifacts. The likelihood of both types of errors is reduced with repetitions and checks for internal consistency, as suggested by this integrated task battery. However, advances to resolve these issues may depend upon additional techniques, such as transcranial magnetic stimulation (TMS) to confirm the essential nature of an area identified by fMRI.

Many future enhancements of this initial task battery are possible using methods that determine task sensitivity and clinical validity, as well as improve confidence by reducing the risk of either false–positive or false–negative findings. The battery could be extended to include memory functions, high-level cognitive tasks, and perhaps even emotion and affect, and continued development could improve the tasks to target the sensory/motor and language areas. Techniques employed for the development of this integrated battery of functions could serve as a basis to develop other similar probes, and thus extend the potential role of fMRI in neurosurgical planning to encompass more precision and diversity in structure and function relationships.

## Determination of the Anatomy and Topography of Cortical Areas Specialized for Cognitive Tasks

In contrast to language, sensory/motor, and visual systems, our current understanding of the mechanisms of higher functions is not so closely linked to a specified neurophysiological substrate. This is due, in part, to the fact that many aspects of cognition cannot be studied in animals; therefore, the burden of our understanding falls historically on research in human subjects. The emergence of neuroimaging provides a new opportunity to test hypotheses and map the underlying mechanisms of cognition in healthy individuals without reliance on lesions or disease processes. The neural bases of various aspects of cognition are now observable using imaging techniques. Determinations of the anatomy and topography of cortical areas specialized for cognitive tasks are possible and can contribute to models that integrate multiple functionally specialized areas to perform cognitive tasks. These objectives are discussed below in the context of specific functions, including attention, working memory, executive processes, and consciousness, with an emphasis on the unifying notion that the neurobiological pathways are multiregional with complex covariations.

> While there has been general agreement that operations performed by the sensory and motor systems are localized, there has been much more dispute about higher-level cognitive processes. It is still undetermined whether higher-level processes have defined locations, and if so, where these locations would be.
>
> Posner and Raichle, *Images of Mind*, 1994, p.16

As discussed above, the functional neuroanatomy of cognitive processes is revealed by comparing the BOLD response elicited by various experimental and control tasks and is typically characterized by a voxel-by-voxel statistical comparison of the signal amplitude during the activity epoch, with the average signal amplitude during a baseline resting or control epoch. The basic assumption is that neuronal activity is increased in a functionally specialized area during the execution of a task that employs that specialization. Locations of active areas, cluster sizes, and dynamic properties of the signal can be compared across cognitive conditions. Tasks are designed to either include or exclude the cognitive component of interest and the signals elicited from these tasks are compared.

## Conservation of Effects versus Individual Differences: Generalizing the Results

Investigations of the neural basis for cognitive processes are aimed toward findings generalizable to the population at large. Neuroimaging studies on single subjects can be assumed to include effects that are conserved across all subjects (generalizable), as well as effects that are specific to that individual subject. Results that are present in all or most cases given a sufficiently large sample size can be assumed to reflect a fundamental specialization characteristic of the population, whereas intermittently present results can be assumed to represent other less-conserved (individual) processes. A theoretical basis for inferences to a population based on functional imaging data is currently under development. However, preliminary estimates of a sufficient sample size based on expected levels of variation exceed six subjects.[43] This proposed minimum is consistent with the general practice to employ six to ten subjects per condition in fMRI studies. However, based on other models using a two-tailed test of significance at a criterion level of $p \leq 0.05$ and a power of 80%, Desmond and Glover[44] suggested a sample size of 11 to 12, and most recent analyses of covariation and connectivity may require sample sizes up to 20 subjects.

Inferences to a population based on imaging data generally require registration of individual brains and a standard stereotactic coordinate system. Although registration procedures are an area of active development, the conventional method (originally developed for PET studies) employs the *Co-Planar Stereotaxic Atlas of the Human Brain*.[45] Acquired brain images are registered to that atlas by reference to the anterior–posterior commissure line and active areas are labeled accordingly and assigned an address in $x$, $y$, $z$ stereotactic coordinates. One popular tool for accomplishing this objective is available in Statistical Parametric Mapping (SPM),[46] a software package developed for processing neuroimaging data. Other representations of brain structure and functions include flat maps and inflated brains.

### Method of Cognitive Subtraction

The cognitive subtraction paradigm requires two tasks: an experimental task that engages the cognitive component of interest, and a baseline or control task that engages all of the processes included in the cognitive task except for the cognitive component of interest. The neural correlates of the cognitive task of interest are presumed to be revealed by a subtraction of the baseline activity from the activity observed during the experimental task. Examples of the cognitive subtraction design are found in the early PET studies, where, for example, the effect of viewing a fixation dot was subtracted from the effect of viewing a flashing checkerboard to reveal the neural effect of the checkerboard alone. Although the subtractive approach was employed successfully in those early studies, it is limited by the difficulty of selecting tasks that differ only with respect to the cognition of interest. If differences between the experimental task and the comparison baseline task are due to a combinatorial effect not present with either task alone, then the conclusion could be misguided. These assumptions often are referred to as the assumptions of linear additivity or pure insertion, and depend upon the partitioning of complex cognitive tasks into independent subcomponent processes.

### Method of Cognitive Conjunction

In contrast to the identification of differences between the elicited activity of two cognitive tasks by subtraction, a conjunction analysis reveals the activity common to multiple tasks. For example, in an investigation to identify the neural substrate specialized for object naming, the same task can be performed using multiple sensory systems—that is, objects that are seen, heard, and felt are named during an imaging study. The conjunction of neural activity present in all three naming tasks is assumed to represent the neural activity associated with naming alone, and the processes associated with the sensory-related activity are assumed to be excluded by virtue of the fact that such activity is not common to all tasks (as illustrated in Figure 7.14).

Some of the same assumptions for the subtractive approach described above apply. First, it is assumed that the cognitive processes engaged by each task are performed similarly across the sensory modalities. However, there is considerable evidence for intermingling of modality-specific and domain-general mechanisms in some tasks. For example, mental imagery tasks may draw upon modality-specific subsystems, which would not be observed by this method. Thus, the conjunctive method applied to cross-modal studies identifies a subset

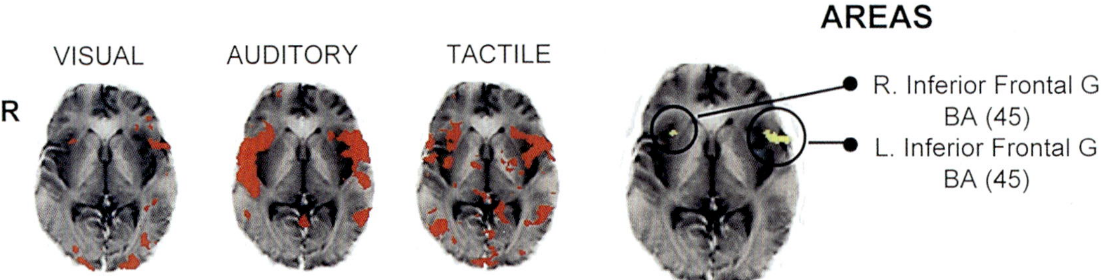


**Figure 7.14.** Conjunction of BOLD responses during object naming across three sensory modalities. Voxels active during visual stimulation (left), auditory stimulation (middle), and tactile stimulation (right) are indicated in orange for one slice of brain. The conjunction image (yellow) illustrates the supramodal activity common to all three modalities of stimulation following a Boolean AND operation. This activity occurs in left and right inferior frontal gyrus (BA 45) and is taken to represent the aspects of object naming not primarily associated with a specific sensory modality for this single subject. Reprinted from Hirsch J, Rodriguez-Moreno D, Kim KHS. Interconnected large-scale systems for three fundamental cognitive tasks revealed by functional MRI *J Cogn Neurosci.* 2001;13(3):1–16. Reprinted with permission from MIT Press Journals.

of domain-general processes, but may fail to recognize all components critical to task performance.

On the other hand, the conjunctive approach, applied to within-modal studies, can serve to enhance confidence in a result by isolating activity that is repeated on multiple runs of the same task. This strategy is based on the assumption that signals originating from noise sources are distinguished from signals originating from real events by the probability of a repeat occurrence at the same location. Voxels that are reliably activated on multiple separate occasions result in a low false–positive rate that can be empirically determined based on images acquired either during resting states or on images acquired on a spherical container of copper sulfate solution that simulates brain (phantom). For this reason, conjunctions often are employed in clinical and neurosurgical applications to enhance confidence in a result by isolating the activity that is elicited on at least two runs of the same task.[34,40,41] However, because repeated stimuli do not usually elicit as robust a response as novel stimuli, all repetitions of a task are optimally performed using equal but different stimuli. Thus, in the case of an object-naming task, all objects would be novel but equated for variables such as familiarity and difficulty, etc., during the multiple runs in order to be optimized for the within-modal conjunction approach.

## Integration of Functionally Specialized Areas Associated with Cognitive Tasks: The Network Approach

Although functional differentiation of single brain areas is a well-established principle of cortical organization, recent approaches to human cognition have focused on the integration of groups of specialized areas into long-range units that may collectively serve as the comprehensive neural substrate for specific cognitive tasks. An early empirical foundation for this emerging view is found in the work of Mishkin and Ungerleider,[47] who described ventral and dorsal pathway segmentation during visual tasks that required either object identification or object localization, respectively. More recently, direct interactions between brain regions that participate in specific functions have been proposed as evidence for this systems model; for example, covariations between BOLD responses in separate cortical areas during complex attention tasks have been examined using a statistical approach called structural equation modeling, which can determine whether the covariances between areas are due to direct or indirect interactions.[48] This analysis technique identifies the groups of areas associated with a task, and also characterizes changes in regional activity and interactions between regions over time. Other approaches to identify function-specific long-range systems associated with language and attention processes are illustrated below.

> A central feature in the organization of the large-scale network is the absence of one-to-one correspondences among anatomical sites, neural computations and complex behaviors. According to this organization, an individual cognitive or behavioral domain is subserved by several interconnected macroscopic sites, each of which subserves multiple computations, leading to a distributed and interactive but also coarse and degenerate (one-to-many and many-to-one) mapping of anatomical substrate onto neural computation and computation onto behavior.
>
> M.—Marsel Mesulam, 1998[49]

### Functional Neuroanatomy of Language Processes: A Large-Scale Network

Models of the neural correlates for elementary language processes often include left hemisphere regions involved in a variety of language functions, including Broca's and Wernicke's Areas, and are generally consistent with a network model. To demonstrate this network, an object naming task using auditory, visual, and tactile stimuli can be employed. A cross-modality conjunction technique (above) isolates effects not dependent upon sensory processes. Results are consistent with the view that the task of naming objects elicits activity from a set of areas within a neurocognitive system specialized for language-related functions (Figure 7.15). The colored circles on the glass brain represent average locations of activity centroids on the standard atlas brain ($x$, $y$, $z$ coordinates) as indicated on the table. There are five regions in this neurocognitive system (all located within the left hemisphere), including putative Broca's Area (inferior frontal gyrus, BA 44 and 45), putative Wernicke's Area (superior temporal gyrus, BA 22),

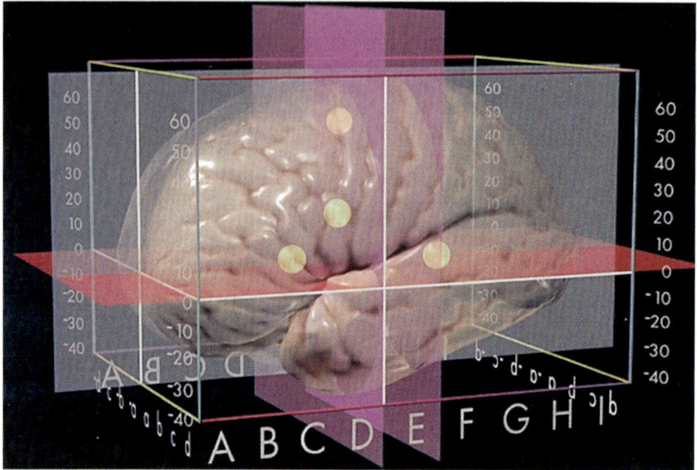


| Anatomical Region | Area | Center of mass x | y | z |
|---|---|---|---|---|
| Medial Frontal Gyrus (GFd) | 6 | 9 | −6 | 53 |
| Superior Temporal Gyrus (GTs) | 22 | 57 | −26 | 9 |
| Inferior Frontal Gyrus (Gfi) | 44 | 49 | 10 | 25 |
| Inferior Frontal Gyrus (Gfi) | 45 | 40 | 25 | 8 |

**Figure 7.15.** A fixed large-scale network for object naming. The network of areas that subserve object naming as determined by conjunction across three sensory modalities consists of medial frontal gyrus (GFd, BA 6), superior temporal gyrus (GTs, BA 22; putative Wernicke's Area), and inferior frontal gyrus (Gfi, BA 44,45; putative Broca's Area) in the left hemisphere. These areas are portrayed as colored circles in a three-dimensional glass brain based upon the Talairach and Tournoux Human Brain Atlas[45] and stereotactic coordinate system. The table appearing below contains the average group coordinates ($x$, $y$, $z$) of the included regions. Reprinted from Hirsch J, Rodriguez-Moreno D, Kim KHS. Interconnected large-scale systems for three fundamental cognitive tasks revealed by functional MRI. *J Cogn Neurosci.* 2001;13(3):1–16. Reprinted with permission from MIT Press Journals.

and medial frontal gyrus (BA 6). Thus, these results are consistent with the view that the functional specialization for this elementary language task involves a system of language-related areas rather than a single area.

## Functional Neuroanatomy of Attention Processes: A Large-Scale Network

Like language, the ability to direct attention is involved in a range of cognitive tasks. Functional imaging studies by Mesulam[49] and others suggest that spatial attention is mediated by a large scale distributed network of interconnected cortical areas within the posterior parietal cortex, the region of frontal eye fields, and the cingulate cortex. Kim and colleagues[50] used a conjunction analysis to compare activity associated with two different types of visuospatial attention shifts: one based on spatial priming and the other based on cues that directed spatial expectancy to test the hypothesis of a fixed area network for both tasks. The activation foci observed for the two tasks were nearly overlapping, indicating that both were subserved by a common network of cortical and subcortical areas. The main findings of this study were consistent with a model of spatial attention that is associated with a fixed large-scale distributed network specialized to coordinate multiple aspects of attention. Alternative hypotheses that predict that task variations are associated with an increase in the number of involved areas can be rejected. However, an observed rightward bias for the spatial priming task suggested that activation within the system showed variations specific to the attributes of the attentional task (Figure 7.16).

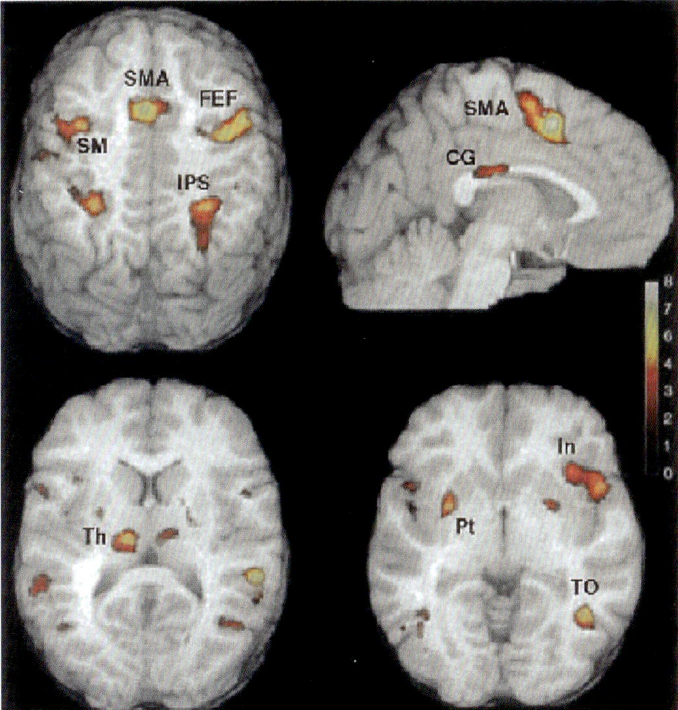


**Figure 7.16.** A fixed large-scale network for spatial attention. The network of areas that subserve visuospatial attention shifts consists of supplementary motor area—anterior cingulate cortex (SMA, BA 6), frontal eye fields (FEF, BA 6), and the banks of the intraparietal sulcus (IPS, BA 7,40). This network was determined by a conjunction analysis of activation related to visuospatial attention tasks based on two different types of information, spatial priming and spatial expectancy. Although the same areas are involved in both tasks, a rightward bias in the intraparietal sulcus (IPS) was observed for the spatial priming task and suggests that, within this network, task-related variations are present. Reprinted from *NeuroImage* Vol. 9. Kim Y-H, Gitelman Dr, Nobre AG, Parrish TB, LaBar KS, Mesulam M-M. The large-scale neural network for spatial attention displays multifunctional overlap but differential asymmetry, 269–277. Copyright © 1999, with permission from Elsevier. (Neurologic coordinates)

## Tests of Cognitive Theory Based on Mapping of Neural Correlates

Advances in our understanding of the biological components of cognition are dependent upon the development of functional tasks that reveal specific cognitive processes; therefore, tasks are selected to target some aspect of cognition that can be varied so that the specific processing requirements are increased or decreased. Current neuroimaging investigations of language, attention, memory, executive processes, and even consciousness generate hypotheses based on theoretical frameworks and behavioral models and develop stimulation paradigms that cause the subject to engage the targeted functions. This section presents a selection of models, hypotheses, cognitive functions, and tasks that have been investigated by neuroimaging techniques. Although more in-depth coverage of many of these topics is presented elsewhere, the objective here is to illustrate the advantages of neuroimaging for understanding the biological components of various cognitive processes rather than to provide a comprehensive survey of each of these cognitive processes.

### Functional Neuroanatomy of Working Memory: A Fixed-or Variable-Area Network

Mechanisms for cognitive functions such as reasoning, problem solving, and language are critically dependent upon working memory processes that briefly maintain a limited amount of information in a mental scratch pad for ongoing processing. To test the hypothesis that a working memory system is subserved by a fixed number of brain areas, Smith and Jonides[51] employed a memory task (*N*-Back) that varied cognitive load. The logic of the experiment follows: If the hypothesis of a fixed number of regions was supported, then increasing the difficulty of the task, and thereby the cognitive load, would increase the amount of activity in each of the component areas. However, if the hypothesis of a variable area network was supported, then increasing the difficulty of the task would activate additional areas.

### The *N* Back Task and a Test of a Cognitive Theory

The *N*-Back task, illustrated in Figure 7.17, was developed as a cognitive tool to vary memory task difficulty (load). The subject views a series of letters separated by fixation points. In the 0-Back condition, the subject responds whenever one of the presented letters matches a standard presented at the beginning of the run. In the 1-Back condition, the subject responds when there is a match to the preceding letter. In the 2-Back condition, the subject responds when there is a match to the letter 2-Back in the series, and similarly for the 3-Back condition.

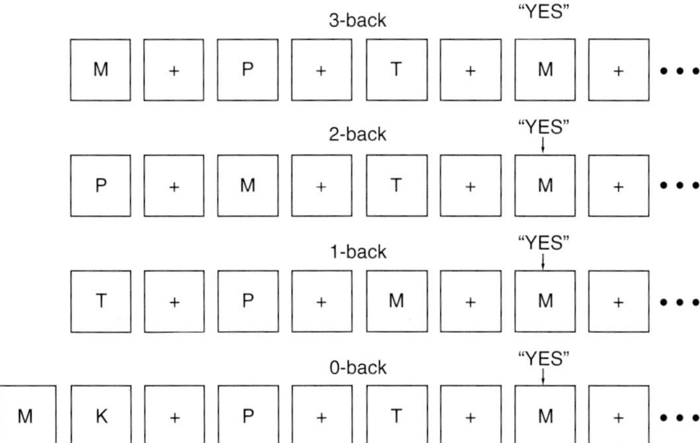


**Figure 7.17.** Variation in working memory load based on the *N*-Back task. The *N*-Back task engages working memory by requiring the subject to remember a previous event and respond if a present stimulus (target) is identical to that previously presented stimulus. Task load can be increased by increasing the distance between the target and its match, e.g., 0-, 1-, 2-, 3-Back. Reprinted from *Cognitive Psychology*, Vol. 33, Smith EE, Jonides J. Working memory: A view from neuroimaging, 5–42. Copyright © 1997, with permission from Elsevier.

Results of this study showed a clear increase in the volume of activity, with the increase in difficulty (load) of the task (Figure 7.18). However, the specific regions involved did not vary with increases in load supporting the fixed-number-of-areas hypothesis for a working memory system.

## Functional Neuroanatomy of Selective Attention: A Neurological Model of Cognitive Interference

The ability to filter task-related stimuli to guide responses is referred to as selective attention. An experimental task that requires the subject to attend to certain stimulus characteristics while ignoring others that elicit a competing response engages a system of selective attention. The Stroop task is a classical cognitive task first developed for use in behavioral studies of cognitive interference and is an ideal task for functional imaging studies that seek to identify the neural substrate associated with selective attention mechanisms.

### *The Stroop Task*

In the classical Stroop task, a subject views a series of words in different colored inks. Each word is the name of a color. The subject is instructed to produce the color of the ink. In the incongruent case, the word and the ink color of the written word are different, resulting in longer reaction times than in the congruent case where the word and ink color match. For example, if the ink color was blue but the word was red (incongruent), the reaction time to report "blue" (the ink color) would be longer than when the word and the ink color were both blue (congruent) (Figure 7.19).

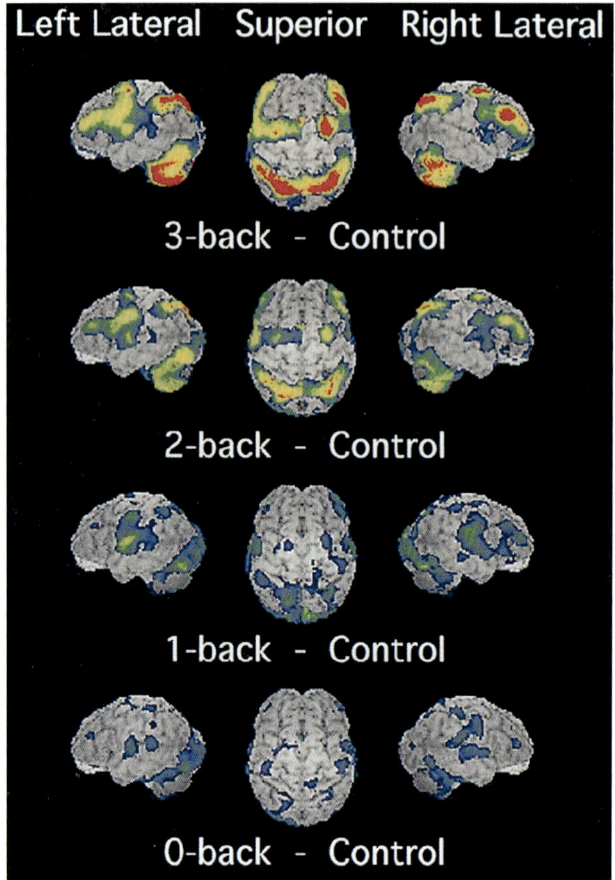


**Figure 7.18.** Cortical responses during the *N*-Back task. Left and right lateral, as well as a superior, views of the average PET images are shown. All images are difference images that reflect the subtraction of a control condition in which subjects responded to every stimulus. The different colors reflect the significance of the activation, with red areas being most significant. Robust responses for the 3-Back condition relative to 0-, 1-, and 2-Back conditions are taken as evidence of increased neural activity associated with increased memory load. Reprinted from *Cognitive Psychology*, Vol. 33, Smith EE, Jonides J. Working memory: A view from neuroimaging, 5–42. Copyright © 1997, with permission from Elsevier.

Cognitive models that account for results obtained by the Stroop task propose that subjects must inhibit the automatic reading response and selectively attend to the color of the letters in order to successfully perform the color-naming task. A neuroimaging study designed to probe the neural basis for this type of cognitive interference, that is, the mechanisms of selective attention,[52] compared BOLD responses to congruent and incongruent conditions in an event-related neuroimaging study (see following section on event-related paradigms). The results are shown in Figure 7.20 for incongruent (A) and congruent conditions (B), respectively. The incongruent condition is associated with robust distributed responses as compared to the congruent condition, sug-

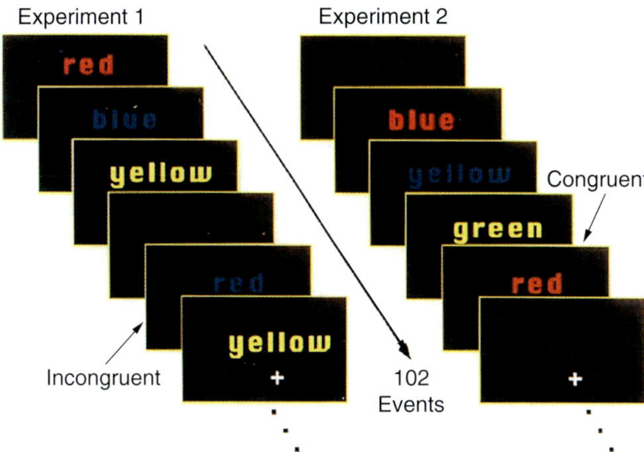


**Figure 7.19.** The classical Stroop color word interference task. In congruent cases, the color of the ink matches the color of the word. In incongruent cases, the color of the ink is different from the color of the word. The words are presented sequentially to subjects who respond by indicating the color of the ink for each word. Reprinted from Leung H-C, Skudlarski P, Gatenby JC, Peterson BS, Gore JC. An event-related functional MRI study of the Stroop color word interference task. *Cereb Cortex*. 2000;10:552–560. Reprinted by permission of Oxford University Press.

gesting that a distributed large-scale neural network is employed during selective attention. The results also suggest a possible correspondence between the selective attention mechanisms engaged in this study and visuospatial attention mechanisms.

## Functional Neuroanatomy of Executive Processes: Separate or Combined Systems

Current models of cognition often include undefined mechanisms (frequently referred to as a black box) to account for executive processes such as the allocation of attentional resources among competing tasks. Functional neuroimaging techniques and experimental paradigms, such as the dual performance task and the Go No-Go task, have been developed to observe the neural correlates of these executive functions and attempt to define the black box in neurophysiological terms.

D'Esposito and colleagues[53] introduced an fMRI task paradigm that required subjects to perform two tasks simultaneously, referred to as a dual performance task (see diagram on page 172). Comparison of the BOLD responses elicited during each task alone and both tasks together enabled tests of hypotheses about the neural system involved in the execution of competing tasks. Specifically, the hypothesis of a modular executive system predicts the recruitment of additional regions during the dual task condition, whereas the fixed-areas hypothesis predicts an increase in volume of the areas activated by a single task.

within that system are modified with development. In both children and adults, the percent change in the amplitude of the BOLD signal responses in the anterior cingulate and the orbital frontal gyri was correlated with the number of false alarms, which also suggests putative within-system processes associated with the emergent response inhibition behavior.

## Integration of Temporal and Spatial Information to Map Executive Processes

A common theme in the aforementioned neuroimaging studies of cognitive functions is the identification of the underlying cortical networks associated with each function and the question of fixed versus variable areas for related functions. In the case of the language, attention, memory, and cognitive control systems illustrated above, the results suggest that a fixed number of areas (rather than the recruitment of new areas) are modulated with increased load. This is an active area of research, and new evidence from studies using techniques such as electrophysiological recordings and event-related fMRI to probe within-system effects may be required to elucidate the modulation of processes both within and across these systems.

### Integration of ERP and fMRI

New investigations that focus on within-system processes and the modulation of a specialized system consisting of a fixed set of distributed areas require probes of the computations performed within neural systems. A new class of multi-technique experiments are currently being developed that elucidate the spatial localization of active regions (fMRI), as well as the temporal co-variations between these cortical or subcortical regions, as reflected in event-related potentials. These techniques may be employed either simultaneously or sequentially and require an adaptation of the blocked fMR experiments (event-related fMRI) and a task specialized for both fMRI and electrophysiological approaches.

### Event-Related fMRI

As in conventional event-related electrophysiology, individual trials (events) are presented separately (rather than in a continuous block), and the signal is selectively averaged across like trials. This acquisition scheme is illustrated in Figure 7.21, where both block and event-related schemes are shown.[56] Event-related fMRI offers an additional class of task designs that expand and elaborate investigations of cognitive processes. Given that the BOLD response tracks neuronal activity with hemodynamic delays on the order of about two to four seconds, it is possible to reliably identify the activity associated with each successive trial.

There are several advantages to event-related fMRI:

1) By detecting signals that are linked to individual trial events rather than to blocks, the observations can parallel other behavioral and evoked response potential studies that are also linked to individual events. Thus, the added value of precise temporal data from other integrated methods in combination with the high-resolution data of fMRI extends the range of questions that can be addressed.

2) An event-related approach is particularly useful when subject response is a factor, as in the case where it is necessary to separate trials in which there was a correct response from trials in which the response was not correct or trials where the stimulus was novel from trials where the stimulus was repeated or to isolate the acquisitions associated with bistable perspectives of ambiguous figures as reported by the subject during the experiment. Thus, the event-related approach allows trials to be categorized post hoc on the basis of the subject's behavior.

3) Some events cannot be presented in a blocked design, as in cases involving a surprise element or the occurrence of an oddball stimulus that is distinguished from the expected context. In those cases, an event-related approach is required.

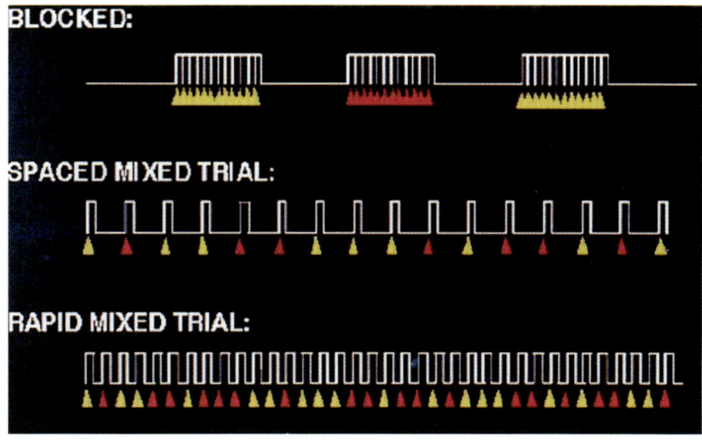


**Figure 7.21.** Blocked-versus event-related fMRI paradigms. Schematic diagrams illustrate the difference between two forms of imaging paradigms: blocked trials and event-related trials. Each schematic shows two trial types indicated by either yellow or red arrows. In blocked trial paradigms (labeled Blocked), the trial types are clustered together in succession so that the same trial type or condition occurs for an extended period of time. Event-related trials, by contrast, intermix different trial types either by spacing them widely apart to allow the hemodynamic response from one trial to decay before the next trial occurs (labeled Spaced Mixed Trial), or by presenting them rapidly (labeled Rapid Mixed Trial). Reprinted from Dale AM, Buckner RL. Selective averaging of rapidly presented individual trials using fMRI. *Hum Brain Mapp.* 1997;5:329-340. Copyright © 1997 Wiley. Reprinted with permission of Wiley-Liss, Inc., a subsidiary of John Wiley & Sons, Inc.

### The Oddball Task

Cortical mechanisms specialized for novelty oddball detection compare incoming information with relevant memories to register a novel event. Opitz and colleagues[57] reported the spatial and temporal properties of cortical mechanisms involved in the detection of novel tones by combining evoked response potential and fMRI measures. The evoked response potential methods lack precision with respect to the spatial source of the signal as detected by scalp electrodes because these sources must be inferred from two-dimensional scalp topography and using dipole fitting algorithms. Temporal resolution of signals, however, is within milliseconds. By combining evoked response potential and fMRI, both temporal and spatial properties of the cortical responses corresponding to novelty can be investigated. Although registration of these separate data domains remains a challenge, results of the Opitz study relate specific evoked response potential responses to bilateral superior temporal gyrus and right pre-frontal cortex, suggesting coordinated activity between areas previously associated with novelty using event-related fMRI techniques.

A similar evoked response potential and fMRI experiment by Kruggel and colleagues[58] employed a visual oddball task using illusory contours that deviated from the prevailing visual stimuli (no illusory contours). Results replicated previous fMRI findings, indicating the activation of extrastriate visual cortex in the appreciation of the illusory contours (perceived between the corner elements of Kanizsa squares) and the lack of this activation during viewing of stimuli in which the corner elements were rotated out of alignment. Additionally, the evoked response potential results confirmed a sequential activation of striate to extra striate visual cortex consistent with hierarchal models of visual processing. Thus, integration of approaches that optimize both spatial and temporal information relating to neural mechanisms and both perceptual and cognitive processes offers new directions and precision to probe the neural basis of mental events.

## The Functional Neuroanatomy of Very High Level Cognitive Processes

Guided by the Astonishing Hypothesis of Francis Crick,[1] it is assumed that the biological components of even very high-level cognitive processes, such as consciousness, are observable. Although still in a nascent stage, the study of consciousness with neuroimaging techniques is a rapidly developing area of research. As in the neuroimaging of related cognitive processes, including language, attention, working memory, and executive control, an investigation of consciousness is largely dependent upon the development of appropriate paradigms and evaluation of relevant theory.

Dehaene and Naccache[59] have developed one theoretical framework for the investigation of consciousness that consists of a global neuronal work space. This framework postulates that, "at any given time, many modular cerebral networks are active in parallel and process information in an unconscious manner." As information becomes conscious, however, the neural population that represents the information is mobilized by top-down attentional amplification into a state of coherent activity that involves many neurons distributed throughout the brain. The long-distance connectivity of these workspace neurons can, when they are active for a minimal duration, make the information available to a variety of processes, including perceptual categorization, long-term memorization, evaluation, and intentional action. According to this theoretical framework, the global availability of information throughout the workspace is what is subjectively experienced as a conscious state.

> The fact that consciousness is a private, first-person phenomenon makes it more difficult to study than other cognitive phenomena that, although being equally private, also have characteristic behavioural signatures. Nonetheless, by combining cognitive and neurobiological methods, it is possible to approach consciousness, to describe its cognitive nature, its behavioral correlates, its possible evolutionary origin and functional role; last but not least, it is possible to investigate its neuroanatomical and neurophysiological underpinnings.
>
> Antonio R. Damasio, 1998[60]

A major obstacle to applying neuroimaging techniques to the investigation of consciousness is the inability to establish a task that varies the state of consciousness; that is, consciousness is not started and stopped in synchrony with a particular task, as is assumed in many cognitive tasks. The global workspace hypothesis suggests a distributed neural system or workspace with long-distance connectivity that interconnects multiple specialized brain areas in a coordinated, although variable, manner.[61] This framework challenges current neuroimaging paradigms based on conventional experimental paradigms and views of functional specialization.

One approach to circumvent this obstacle is based on the specific hypothesis that conscious humans are engaged continuously during resting states in "adaptive cognitive processes that involve semantic knowledge retrieval, representation in awareness and directed manipulation of represented knowledge for organization, problem solving and planning." Thus, comparison of resting activation and task activations during a neuroimaging study might reveal neural processes associated with consciousness. Binder and colleagues[62] used fMRI to measure brain activity during rest and during several contrasting activation paradigms, including a perceptual task (tone-monitoring) designed to interfere with ongoing thought processes and a semantic retrieval task (noun categorization) designed to engage on-going thought processes similar to those hypothesized to occur during rest. Higher signal values were observed during the resting state than during the tone-monitoring task in a network of left hemisphere cortical regions. These areas were equally active during the semantic task.

This finding is consistent with the hypothesis that perceptual tasks interrupt specific ongoing processes during rest that are associated with many of the same brain areas engaged during semantic retrieval. Thus, neuroimaging observations suggest that on-going processing during a conscious resting state involves an underlying neural substrate similar to that employed in cognitive tasks such as semantic processing.

Another paradigm that employs masked (too brief for cognitive awareness) presentations of emotional facial expressions has been found to modulate BOLD and PET-related hemodynamic responses originating in the amygdala.[63,64] In these studies, the amygdala was involved in 1) nonconscious responses that reflected the emotional valence of stimuli, and 2) was spatially differentiated depending upon level of awareness. Both findings confirm a neural substrate that is active and responsive without awareness.

The resting-state and masking paradigms, as well as other ongoing neuroimaging investigations of related aspects of consciousness, including perceptual awareness, awareness during varying levels of anesthesia, and awareness in patients in vegetative and minimally conscious states, can be expected to contribute to an emerging understanding of the neural basis of consciousness and the neural basis for related events that occur without awareness. Imaging paradigms that are established to investigate the neural underpinnings of cognition also provide foundations for emerging investigations of the neural underpinnings of consciousness and bring neural science closer to the goal of understanding the biological underpinnings of the mind.

## Acknowledgments

This chapter was written in collaboration with Sarah Callahan, a psycholinguistic student in my laboratory, who not only researched and provided essential original sources, but also was a partner in the development of the ideas and conceptual organization. Without her critical contributions, this chapter would not have emerged in print.

## References

1. Crick F. *The Astonishing Hypothesis: The Scientific Search for the Soul.* New York: Charles Scribner's Sons; 1994.
2. *Dorland's Illustrated Medical Dictionary.* 27th ed. Philadelphia, PA: W.B. Saunders Co. (Harcourt Brace Jovanovich Inc.); 1988.
3. *The American Heritage Dictionary of the English Language.* 4th ed. Boston, MA: Houghton Mifflin Co.; 2000.
4. Neisser U. *Cognitive Psychology.* New York; Appleton: 1967.
5. Damasio H, Grabowski T, Frank R, Galaburda AM, Damasio AR. The return of Phineas Gage: Clues about the brain from the skull of a famous patient. *Science.* 1994;264:1102–1105.

6. Penfield W. *The Mystery of the Mind.* Princeton, NJ; Princeton University Press: 1975.
7. Sherrington R. *J Physiol.* 1890;11:85.
8. Raichle ME, Martin WRW, Herscovitch P, Mintun MA, Markham J. Brain blood flow measured with intravenous H215O. II. Implementation and validation. *J Nucl Med.* 1983;24:790–798.
9. Fox PT, Raichle ME. Stimulus rate dependence of regional cerebral blood flow in human striate cortex demonstrated by positron emission tomography. *J Neurophysiol.* 1984;51:1109–1120.
10. Peterson SE, Fox PT, Posner MI, Mintun M, Raichle ME. Postiron emission tomographic studies of the processing of single words. *J Cogn Neurosci.* 1989;1(2):153–170.
11. Ogawa S, Lee T-M, Nayak AS, Glynn P. Oxygenation-sensitive contrast in magnetic resonance image of rodent brain at high magnetic fields. *Magn Reson Med.* 1990;14:68–78.
12. Gore JC, Principles and practice of functional MRI of the human brain. *J Clin Invest.* 2003;112:4–9.
13. George JS, Aine CJ, Mosher JC, Schmidt MD, Ranken DM, Schlitt HA, Wood CC, Lewine JD, Sanders JA, Belliveau JW. Mapping function in the human brain with magneto encephalography, anatomical magnetic resonance imaging, and functional magnetic resonance imaging. *J Clin Neurophysiol.* 1995;12:406–429.
14. Nimsky C, Ganslandt O, Kober H, Moller M, Ulmer S, Tomandl B, Fahlbusch R. Integration of functional magnetic resonance imaging supported by magnetoencephalography in functional neuronavigation. *Neurosurgery.* 1999;44(6):1249–1255.
15. Stapleton SR, Kiriakopoulos E, Mikulis D, Drake LM, Hoffman HJ, Humphreys R, Hwang P, Otsubo H, Holowka S, Logan W, Rutka JT. Combined utility of functional MRI, cortical mapping, and frameless stereotaxy in the resection of lesions in eloquent areas of brain in children. *Pediatr Neurosurg.* 1997;26:68–82.
16. Atlas SW, Howard RS, Maldjian J, Alsop D, Detre JA, Listerud J, D'Esposito M, Judy KD, Zager E, Stecker M. Functional magnetic resonance imaging of regional brain activity in patients with intracerebral gliomas: findings and implications for clinical management. *Neurosurgery.* 1996;38(2):329–338.
17. Latchaw RE, Xiaoping HU, Ugurbil K, Hall WA, Madison MT, Heros RC. Functional magnetic resonance imaging as a management tool for cerebral arteriovenous malformations. *Neurosurgery.* 1995;37(4):619–625.
18. Lee CC, Jack CR Jr, Riederer SJ. Mapping of the central sulcus with functional MR: Active versus passive activation tasks. *Neuroradiology.* 1998; 19:847–852.
19. Mueller WM, Yetkin FZ, Hammeke TA, Morris GL III, Swanson SJ, Reichert K, Cox, Haughton VM. Functional magnetic resonance imaging mapping of the motor cortex in patients with cerebral tumors. *Neurosurgery.* 1996;39(3):515–521.
20. Puce A, Constable T, Luby ML, Eng M, McCarthy G, Nobre AC, Spencer DD, Gore JC, Allison T. Functional magnetic resonance imaging of sensory and motor cortex: comparison with electrophysiological localization. *J Neurosurg.* 1995;83:262–270.
21. Schulder M, Maldijian JA, Liu WC, Holodny AI, Kalnin AT, Mun IK, Carmel PW. Functional image-guided surgery of intracranial tumors located in or near the sensorimotor cortex. *Neurosurgery.* 1998;89:412–418.
22. Yousry TA, Schmid UD, Jassoy AG, Schmidt D, Eisener WE, Reulen HJ, Reiser MF, Lissner J. Topography of the cortical motor hand area: prospec-

tive study with functional MR imaging and direct motor mapping at surgery. *Radiology.* 1995;195:23–29.
23. Debus J, Essig M, Schad LR, Wenz F, Baudendistel K, Knopp MV, Engenhart R, Lorenz WJ. Functional magnetic imaging in a stereotactic setup. *Magn Reson Imaging.* 1996;14(9):1007–1012.
24. Fried I, Nenov VI, Ojemann SG, Woods RP. Functional MR and PET imaging of rolandic and visual cortices for neurosurgical planning. *J Neurosurg.* 1995;83:854–861.
25. Chapman PH, Buchbinder BR, Cosgrove GR, Jiang HJ. Functional magnetic resonance imaging for cortical mapping in pediatric neurosurgery. *Pediatr Neurosurg.* 1995;23:122–126.
26. Fandino J, Kollias S, Wieser G, Valavanis A, Yonekawa Y. Intraoperative validation of functional magnetic resonance imaging and cortical reorganization patters in patients with brain tumors involving the primary motor cortex. *J Neurosurg.* 1999;91:238–250.
27. Pujol J, Conesa G, Deus J, Lopez-Obarrio L, Isamat F, Capdevila A. Clinical application of functional magnetic resonance imaging in presurgical identification of the central sulcus. *J Neurosurg.* 1998;88:863–869.
28. Herholz K, Reulen H, von Stockhausen H, Thiel A, Ilmberger J, Kessler J, Eisner W, Yousry TA, Heiss W. Preoperative activation and intraoperative stimulation of language-related areas in patients with glioma. *Neurosurgery.* 1997;41(6):1253–1262.
29. Hinke RM, Hu X, Stillman AE, Kim SG, Merkle H, Salmi R, Ugurbil K. Functional magnetic resonance imaging of Broca's area during internal speech. *NeuroReport.* 1993;4:675–678.
30. Binder JR, Frost JA, Hammeke TA, Bellgowan PSF, Rao SM, Cox RW. Conceptual processing during the conscious resting state: A functional MRI study. *J Cogn Neurosci.* 1999;11(1):80–93.
31. Kollias SS, Landau K, Khan N, Golay X, Bernays R, Yonekawa Y, Valavanis A. Functional evaluation using magnetic resonance imaging of the visual cortex in patients with retrochiasmatic lesions. *Neurosurgery.* 1998;89:780–790.
32. Tootell RB, Reppas JB, Kwong KK, Malach R, Born RT, Brady TJ, Rosen BR, Belliveau JW. Functional analysis of human MT and related visual cortical areas using magnetic resonance imaging. *J Neurosci.* 1995;15:3215–3230.
33. Hirsch J, Rodriguez-Moreno D, Kim KHS. Interconnected large-scale systems for three fundamental cognitive tasks revealed by functional MRI. *J Cogn Neurosci.* 2001;13(3):1–16.
34. Hirsch J, Ruge MI, Kim KHS, Correa DD, Victor JD, Relkin NR, Labar DR, Krol G, Bilsky MH, Souweidane MM, DeAngelis LM, Gutin PH. An integrated fMRI procedure for preoperative mapping of cortical areas associated with tactile, motor, language, and visual functions. *Neurosurgery.* 2000;47(3):711–722.
35. Kaplan EF, Goodglass H, Weintraub S. The Boston naming test. 2nd ed. Philadelphia, PA: Lea & Febiger: 1983.
36. Dinner DS, Luders H, Lesser RP, Morris HH. Cortical generators of somatosensory evoked potentials to median nerve stimulation. *Neurology.* 1987;37:1141–1145.
37. Cedzich C, Taniguchi M, Schafer S, Schramm J. Somatosensory evoked potential phase reversal and direct motor cortex stimulation during surgery in and around the central region. *Neurosurgery.* 1996;38:962–970.
38. Puce A. Comparative assessment of sensorimotor function using functional magnetic resonance imaging and electrophysiological methods. *J Clin Neurophysiol.* 1995;12:450–459.

39. Wada J, Rasmussen T. Intracarotid injection of sodium amytal for the lateralization of cerebral speech dominance. *J Neurosurg.* 1960;17:266–282.
40. Ruge MI, Victor JD, Hosain S, Correa DD, Relkin NR, Tabar V, Brennan C, Gutin PH, Hirsch J. Concordance between functional magnetic resonance imaging and intraoperative language mapping. *J Stereotact Funct Neurosurg.* 1999;72:95–102.
41. Kim KHS, Relkin NR, Lee K-M, Hirsch J. Distinct cortical areas associated with native and second languages. *Nature.* 1997;388:171–174.
42. Ojemann G, Ojemann J, Lettich E, Berger M. Cortical language localization in left, dominant hemisphere. *J Neurosurg.* 1989;71:316–326.
43. Friston KJ, Holmes AP, Price CJ, Büchel C, Worsley KJ. Multisubject fMRI studies and conjunction analysis. *Neuroimage.* 1999;10:385–396.
44. Desmond JE, Glover GH. Estimating sample size in functional MRI (fMRI) neuroimaging studies: statistical power analyses. *J Neurosci Methods.* 2002;118:115–128.
45. Talairach J, Tournoux P. *Co-Planar Stereotaxic Atlas of the Human Brain.* New York; Thieme: 1988.
46. Friston KJ, et al. *Human Brain Mapping.* 1995;2:189.
47. Mishkin M, Ungerleider LG. Contribution of striate inputs to the visuospatial functions of parieto-preoccipital cortex in monkeys. *Behav Brain Res.* 1982;6(1):57–77.
48. Buchel C, Friston KJ. Modulation of connectivity in visual pathways by attention: Cortical interactions evaluated with structural equation modelling and fMRI. *Cerebral Cortex.* 1997;7(8):768–778.
49. Mesulam M-M. From sensation to cognition. *Brain.* 1998;121:1013–1052.
50. Kim Y-H, Gitelman DR, Nobre AC, Parrish TB, LaBar KS, Mesulam M-M. The large-scale neural network for spatial attention displays multifunctional overlap but differential asymmetry. *NeuroImage.* 1999;9:269–277.
51. Smith EE, Jonides J. Working memory: A view from neuroimaging. *Cogn Psychol.* 1997;33:5–42.
52. Leung H-C, Skudlarski P, Gatenby JC, Peterson BS, Gore JC. An event-related functional MRI study of the Stroop color word interference task. *Cereb Cortex.* 2000;10:552–560.
53. D'Esposito M, Detre JA, Alsop DC, Shin RK, Atlas S, Grossman M. The neural basis of the central executive system of working memory. *Nature.* 1995;378:279–281.
54. Adcock RA, Constable RT, Gore JC, Goldman-Rakic PS. Functional neuroanatomy of executive processes involved in dual-task performance. *Proc Natl Acad Sci USA.* 2000;97(7):3567–3572.
55. Casey BJ, Trainor RJ, Orendi JL, Schubert AB, Nystrom LE, Giedd JN, Castellanos FX, Haxby JV, Noll DC, Cohen JD, Forman SD, Dahl RE, Rapoport JL. A developmental functional MRI study of prefrontal activation during performance of a Go-No-Go task. *J Cogn Neurosci.* 1997; 9(6):835–847.
56. Rosen BR, Buckner RL, Dale AM. Event-related functional MRI: Past, present, and future. *Proc Natl Acad Sci USA.* 1998;95:773–780.
57. Opitz B, Mecklinger A, Friederici AD, von Cramon DY. The functional neuroanatomy of novelty processing: Integrating ERP and fMRI results. *Cerebr Cortex.* 1999;9(4):379–391.
58. Kruggel F, Herrmann CS, Wiggins CJ, von Cramon DY. Hemodynamic and electroencephalographic responses to illusory figures: Recording of the evoked potentials during functional MRI. *Neuroimage.* 2001;14:1327–1336.
59. Dehaene S, Naccache L. Towards a cognitive neuroscience of consciousness: Basic evidence and a workspace framework. *Cognition.* 2001;79:1–37.

60. Damasio AR. Investigating the biology of consciousness. *Phil Trans R Soc Lond B Biol Sci.* 1998;353:1879–1882.
61. Dehaene S, Kerszberg M, Changeux JP. A neuronal model of a global workspace in effortful cognitive tasks. *Proc Natl Acad Sci USA.* 1998; 95(24):14529–14534, November 24.
62. Binder JR, Price CJ. Functional imaging of language. In: Cabeza R, Kingstone A, eds. *Handbook of Functional Neuroimaging of Cognition.* Cambridge, MA: MIT Press. pp. 187–251.
63. Whalen PJ, Rauch SL, Etcoff NL, McInerney SC, Lee MB, Jenike MA. Masked presentations of emotional facial expressions modulate amygdala activity without explicit knowledge. *J Cogn Neurosci.* 1998;18(1):411–418.
64. Morris JS, Ohman A, Dolan RJ. Conscious and unconscious emotional learning in the human amygdala. *Nature.* 1998;393:467–470.

# 8

# Applications of fMRI to Psychiatry

Deborah A. Yurgelun-Todd, Perry F. Renshaw, and Lisa A. Femia

## Introduction

The application of functional neuroimaging to characterize cortical dysfunction in patients with psychiatric disorders provides one of the most exciting in vivo techniques for the identification of both pathophysiologic factors and treatment effects. In recent years, the number of functional techniques that fall into this category has continued to increase. However, functional magnetic resonance imaging (fMRI) refers to a non-invasive method to assess cortical activation by measuring changes in oxidation and regional blood flow. The most frequently used fMRI paradigms involve primary sensory stimulation, including visual stimulation and motor sequencing.

Functional brain imaging studies have historically been limited both by the need to use radioactive tracers and by poor temporal resolution. Developments in the area of MR imaging may largely surmount these limitations. First, the development of high-speed, echo planar imaging devices has greatly enhanced the temporal resolution of MRI. With echo planar imaging, single image planes can be acquired in 50 to 100 milliseconds or multiple image planes can be acquired each second. Functional MRI studies, which may be performed with or without a high-speed MR scanner, selectively detect image parameters that are proportional to cerebral blood flow (CBF) or cerebral blood volume (CBV). This strategy capitalizes on the fact that, in general, focal changes in neuronal activity are coupled closely to changes in CBF and CBV.

Functional MRI studies generally are divided into two separate classes. The first includes studies that make use of endogenous physiologic factors to detect changes in cerebral activation, often referred to as the non-contrast techniques.[1] The second group of studies requires the intravenous administration of a paramagnetic agent and comprises the contrast techniques.[2] Non-contrast techniques make use of either T1-weighted pulse sequences to detect changes in blood flow or, more commonly, T2-weighted pulse sequences to detect changes in the local concentration of paramagnetic deoxyhemoglobin. The latter method has been referred to as blood oxygen level-dependent (BOLD) imaging.

In a BOLD experiment, regional brain activation is associated with changes in both blood flow and blood volume, generally leading to a washout of paramagnetic deoxyhemoglobin, which results in an increase in local signal intensity.

Blood oxygenation level-dependent studies have several limitations from the perspective of performing clinical research studies. At 1.5 Tesla (T), the magnitude of the observed signal intensity changes is relatively small. For instance, photic stimulation, which induces a substantial increase in occipital cortical blood flow, produces only a two to four percent MR signal intensity increase. The application of functional imaging techniques during complex cognitive functions may result in even smaller changes in signal intensity. One reason is that higher-order functions, such as attentional processing, are subserved by widely distributed networks. Furthermore, studies of more medial cortical regions, such as the cingulate cortex, have been difficult to carry out because of the limited signal available in functional activation and MRI experiments completed with standard imaging hardware.[3] These factors reduce the likelihood of finding unique anatomical correlates for higher cognitive functions and may contribute to the relatively small cortical activation observed during cognitive tasks compared with primary sensory activation.

Previous investigations also have suggested that the magnitude of BOLD signal intensity changes may vary with subject age and gender. To investigate the effects of age and sex on cortical activation, Ross and colleagues[4] measured signal intensity changes during photic stimulation in a group of young adults and in a group of elderly subjects. The older study subjects produced significantly less signal change in response to photic stimulation compared with younger subjects. An examination of the younger group revealed that women demonstrated significantly less signal change in response to photic stimulation as compared with men, and men produced greater activation in the right occipital lobe. This study suggests that both age and sex are important covariates in analyzing fMRI data.

Furthermore, a number of medications directly alter vascular tone and modify BOLD signal changes, presenting an important confound for studies of subjects with psychiatric illness. Finally, the uncoupling of CBF and CBV, which occurs acutely after cerebral activation and produces the BOLD effect, appears to resolve with prolonged stimulation. In response to these problems, many research groups are developing noncontrast fMRI methods, which have a greater sensitivity to changes in cerebral flow.

The contrast method is a tracer kinetic technique using a bolus injection of a paramagnetic contrast agent to produce changes in tissue magnetic susceptibility and MR image intensity. During the first pass of the contrast agent, MR signal intensity may decrease by as much as 20 to 40%. This method may be used to map the distribution of CBV at rest or to measure changes in response to cerebral activation. Resting CBV maps have been shown to correlate well with positron emission tomography (PET) images of fluorodeoxyglucose uptake and with hexamethyl propyleneamine oxime (HMPAO) single-photon emission computed tomography (SPECT) images of CBF. Additionally, the development of a multiple bolus method for performing dynamic susceptibility contrast (DSC-MRI) studies may facilitate the measurement of drug effects on cerebral hemodynamics.

Magnetic resonance brain imaging technologies offer exceptional promise for greater clarification and understanding of psychopathology. Neuroimaging techniques may one day make or confirm psychiatric diagnoses, and neuroimaging profiles may even be incorporated into the diagnostic criteria for certain psychiatric disorders. Moreover, the potential clinical applications extend beyond diagnosis. Ultimately, neuroimaging data may be valuable for predicting natural course of illness, as well as for monitoring treatment response. Currently, the clinical utility of fMRI to patients has thus far been limited, as no findings have been shown to be diagnostically specific for any psychiatric illness or treatment. Although many hospitals and research facilities complete MRI on psychiatric patients, this information cannot, as yet, be used reliably to generate a psychiatric diagnosis; however, scans often are used to rule out the presence of a neurological illness. This chapter highlights the promise that fMRI studies hold for the evaluation of patients with mental illness by briefly reviewing applications of fMRI to the study of schizophrenia, major depression, bipolar disorder, substance abuse, autism spectrum disorders, and obsessive–compulsive disorder (OCD).

## Functional MRI in Psychiatry

### Developmental Disorders

Autism spectrum disorders (ASD) are classified in the DSM-IV as developmental disabilities with behavioral deficits existing in each of the three main domains of functioning: social interactions, communication, and interests or activities.[5] Within the last decade, research related to clinical diagnoses of autistic disorder and Asperger's disorder, both found under the ASD umbrella, has increased tremendously, specifically with a focus on utilizing neuroimaging techniques.[6] While these disorders have been shown to be devastating life-long debilitating symptoms in many individuals, no well-defined physiological marker or indicator of ASD exists. Currently, the application of modern medical technology to clinical populations is used to rule out more general medical conditions. The clinical diagnosis of ASD relies solely on behaviorally oriented diagnostic tools designed to identify deficits in children through observation, clinical testing, and parental reports.[7] While these diagnostic tools have shown better reliability and validity in identifying an overall population of children with ASD, overall scores have been inadequate in distinguishing between the vast combinations of symptoms and symptomology degrees seen in these children.[8,9] The importance of distinguishing subsets of autism sharing common symptoms and symptom degrees may play an essential role in clinical diagnosis, etiology, and treatment planning.

Whereas the use of neuroimaging technologies has the ability to provide important new insight into the nature of autism, to date, the majority of empirical research focusing on morphometric analysis has produced inconsistent and contradictory results in the identification of regional brain abnormalities. A critical review highlights the heterogeneous nature of these disorders, suggesting that inconsistencies in results, possibly due to the use of heterogeneous subject pools, would have been more representative of the complexity of this disorder if both group and individual statistical analysis of functional brain activity were employed (see Table 8.1).[10] Based on neuroanatomic research, which reports a significant difference in amygdalar volume of autistic individuals as compared to normal control subjects, researchers have begun to explore the functional role of the amygdala and other regions associated with affect processing during facial affect tasks in individuals with autism.[11–14] Functional MRI research on autism, although limited, has illustrated that individuals diagnosed with autistic disorder demonstrate an alternate method of facial processing when compared to normal healthy control subjects.[15–17] Pierce and colleagues showed normal control subjects to have a consistent pattern of activation within the fusiform face (fusiform gyrus) and amygdala during facial affect tasks.[17] A stringently defined group of autistic patients were presented with the same facial affect task and showed activation sites differing from subject to subject. All autistic subjects showed significantly decreased activation sites in the left amygdala and fusiform face area.[17] The consistent increased activation of the amygdala in control subjects, but not in autistic individuals, also can be seen during implicit facial tasks and theory of mind facial tasks. In contrast to control subjects, when autistic individuals were asked to respond with a button press to determine the emotion of a facial photograph, they again showed no activation in the left amygdalahippocampal region and left cerebellum.[16] During a facial task utilizing photographs of eyes, autistic individuals again demonstrated decreased rates of activation in the left amygdala, left inferior frontal gyrus, and right insula when compared to control subjects.[15] A follow up study by Schultz and colleagues[18] has also shown autistic patients demonstrate activation decreases or no activation in the fusiform gyrus and activation decreases in the amygdala, inferior occipital gyrus, and superior temporal sulcus during viewing of neutral faces. These findings suggest a consistent alternative method of facial processing in individuals diagnosed with autism as compared to normal healthy individuals. The identification of various alternative activation areas during similar tasks for each autistic patient illustrates a physiological variation within the broader diagnosis of autism, which may or may not be identified behaviorally. This variation further supports the importance of identifying additional markers in understanding and treatment of these disorders (Figure 8.1).[15–17]

## Substance Abuse and Dependence

Drug abuse and addiction remain critical public health problems in the United States, associated with serious adverse behavioral, health, and social consequences for individuals, their families, and society. Recent data indicate that 13.6 million Americans 12 years of age and older

Table 8.1. Summary of fMRI Research in Autistic Spectrum Disorders Population

| Authors | Subjects | fMRI paradigm | Results |
|---|---|---|---|
| Pierce et al., 2001[17] | 7 male autistic patients; 8 sex- and age-matched healthy controls | Facial perception task | Autistic patients showed a significant decrease in activation in the fusiform gyrus and left amygdala when compared to controls. |
| Schultz et al., 2000[18] | 14 male autistic or Asperger's Disorder patients; 28 healthy controls | Objects or faces were visually presented. Subjects pressed a button to indicate similarity or dissimilarity | Overall results show patients to have decreased or no activation in fusiform gyrus and also decreased activation in the inferior occipital gyrus, superior temporal sulcus and amygdala when compared to controls. |
| Critchley et al., 2000[16] | 9 high-functioning male autistic patients; 8 healthy males | Two experiments presenting alternating facial stimuli high with emotion and neutral: 1) subject indicates emotion with button press, 2) indicates gender with button press | Overall, patients had increased activation versus controls in left superior temporal gryus and left peristriate visual cortex. Task 1, controls, but not patients, exhibited activation in left cerebellum and left amygdalahippocampal region. Task 2, controls had activation in the left middle temporal gyrus, patients did not. |
| Baron-Cohen et al., 1999[15] | 6 autistic or Asperger's Disorder patients; 12 matched controls | Two tasks using visual viewing of photographs with eyes: 1) subject indicates gender with button press, 2) indicates mental state with button press | Task 2, patients showed increased activations in superior temporal gyrus bilaterally, whereas controls showed an increase in left inferior frontal gyrus, right insula, and left amygdala. |

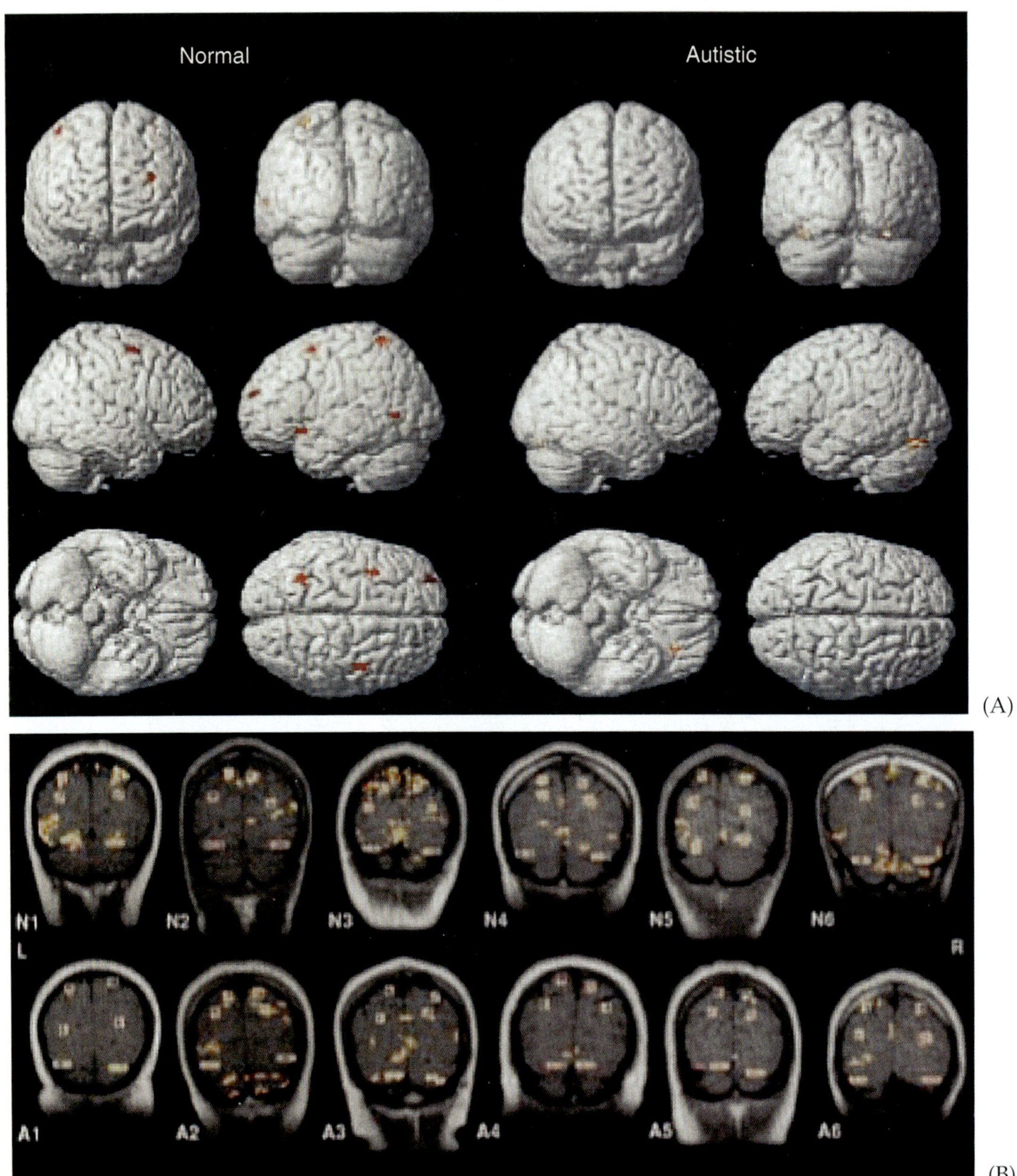


**Figure 8.1.** (A) Surface views for normal (left) and autistic (right) subjects (Belmonte and Yurgelun Todd, 2003). (B) Single slice projections of functional regions of interest during task-versus-fixation in normal (top) and autistic (bottom) subjects. Reprinted from *Cognitive Brain Research*, Vol. 17, No. 3, 2003, pp 651–664, Belmonte M and Yurgelun-Todd DA. Functional anatomy of impaired selective attention and compensatory processing in autism. Copyright © 2003, with permission from Elsevier.

were current users of illegal drugs in 1998. The American Psychiatric Association considers the abuse of alcohol, amphetamines, caffeine, cannabis, cocaine, hallucinogens, inhalants, nicotine, opioids, phencyclidine, and sedatives to be diagnosable disorders. Despite aggressive intervention efforts during the last decade, the overall prevalence of drug use has remained relatively constant. Ominously, drug use among youths has increased significantly over this same time period. Medically, drug-induced deaths have increased over the last decade, reaching a total of 15,973 in 1997, and the Drug Abuse Warning Network has noted consistent increases in hospital emergency room mentions of marijuana-, heroin-, and cocaine-related episodes. Economically, illegal drug use accounted for an estimated 110 billion dollars in expenses and lost revenue in the United States in 1995.

It has been reported that the reinforcing effects of abused drugs may be related to their effects on specific neural circuits, and neuroimaging methods provide an important set of techniques for the identification of pathways that mediate the cognitive changes and reinforcing effects of drugs. Magnetic resonance techniques are particularly well suited for identifying withdrawal and treatment effects. While fMRI has yet to be applied clinically to drug abuse, research has begun to exemplify this importance of functional brain activity on understanding both the phenomenon of craving and the neurophysiological effects of narcotics, such as cocaine (see Table 8.2A).

Although the role of craving in subsequent drug taking continues to be debated, the elucidation of the neurochemical mechanisms that lead to craving may provide new therapeutic opportunities for the treatment of cocaine dependence. Functional MRI methods may provide a means to characterize more fully brain regions that produces the euphoria associated with cocaine.[18] These investigators noted increases in signal intensity in the ventral tegmentum, the pons, the basal forebrain, the caudate, the cingulate, and most regions of the lateral prefrontal cortex, which were temporally concordant with self-reports of a post drug rush. Reviews of fMRI studies related to cocaine abuse highlight the consistent finding of altered activation of the prefrontal cortex, indicating therapeutic inventions may benefit from functional neuroimaging of this region.[19,20] During the presentation of audiovisual stimuli containing alternating levels of neutral and drug-related scenes, male subjects with a history of crack cocaine use showed significant activation in the anterior cingulate and left dorsolateral prefrontal cortex as compared to control subjects. Self-reported levels of craving for drug users correlated to regional activation, whereas it did not in control subjects.[21] Additionally, it also has been demonstrated that, as compared to control subjects, individuals addicted to cocaine demonstrated increased activation of the anterior cingluate and decreased frontal lobe activation during videotapes designed to elicit the desire to use cocaine.[22] Functional MRI BOLD imaging also has been used to investigate the neural circuits affect by the use of cocaine. Cocaine-related reduction of cortical activation in the primary visual cortex and primary motor cortex has been shown in long-term cocaine users.[23]

Table 8.2A. Summary of fMRI Research in Cocaine Users

| Authors | Subjects | fMRI paradigm | Results |
|---|---|---|---|
| Wexler et al., 2001[22] | Cocaine addicts; healthy controls | Viewing of videotapes designed to elicit happy and sad feelings and the desire to use cocaine. | Addicts viewing cocaine tapes showed decreased activation in the anterior cingulate (not present in sad, happy, or in any tapes for controls) and decrease activation in the frontal lobe. |
| Li et al., 2000[23] | Long-term cocaine users | Three test conditions: Rest, after saline injection, and after cocaine injection. | Decreased activation in the primary visual cortex and primary motor cortex after cocaine administration. |
| Maas et al., 1998[21] | Males with history of crack cocaine; 6 male controls | Viewing of drug-related and neutral scenes. | Increased activation in the anterior cingulate and left dorsolateral prefrontal cortex in cocaine-using group during drug-related scenes. Correlation between self-reported levels of craving and activation found. |
| Breiter et al., 1997[18] | Cocaine-dependent patients | Cocaine and saline infusions, imaged 5 minutes pre and 13 minutes post infusion. Simultaneous ratings were attained for rush, high, low, and craving. | Increase in, but short, signal intensity in the ventral tegmentum, the pons, the basal forebrain, the caudate, the cingulated, and most regions of the prefrontal cortex, which correlated to ratings of rush. Increased, but sustained, in Nac/SCC, right parahippocampal gyrus, and some regions of the lateral prefrontal cortex that correlated to ratings of craving. Sustained decrease in amygdala also correlated with craving ratings. |

Table 8.2B. Summary of fMRI Research in Marijuana Users

| Authors | Subjects | fMRI paradigm | Results |
|---|---|---|---|
| Yurgelun-Todd et al., 1998[24] | Chronic marijuana smokers at two time points of abstinence; healthy control subjects | Two tasks: A right-hand and left-hand psychomotor task and visual working memory task | Smokers with 24 hour and 28 day abstinence showed decreased activation in the dorsolateral prefrontal cortex and an increased activation in the cingulate when compared to controls. |

Dynamic susceptibility contrast MRI is an alternative technique to BOLD imaging. Compared to BOLD, DSC-MR imaging allows data to be collected over the 5- to 10-second first pass of paramagnetic contrast agent through the cerebral vasculature; therefore, data is much less sensitive to motion artifact. Within each voxel, the signal intensity change may be on the order of 10%, and the resulting images may have spatial resolution on the order of 0.02 cubic centimeters. On a 1.5-T MR scanner, DSC-MRI experiments may be repeated every two minutes. The principal limitations to the DSC-MRI method are the requirement for an intravenous catheter and the fact that the data are presented in terms of change in relative CBV, as opposed to a direct measurement of blood flow. One study applying DSC-MRI to study the effects of cocaine included 23 healthy and neurologically normal men who underwent DSC-MRI measurements of global CBV at baseline and 10 minutes after intravenous, double-blind placebo or cocaine administration.[24] Both cocaine doses induced global CBV decreases that were statistically significant, and the magnitude of the CBV decrease was consistent with reports of cocaine-induced reductions in absolute global blood flow in SPECT studies. For those subjects receiving cocaine, strong correlations were detected between drug-induced CBV change and self-reported ratings of high and euphoria. Thus, greater high and euphoria ratings were associated with smaller decrements in CBV. Additional DSC-MRI studies have been performed to identify sex-based differences in cerebral vasoconstriction.[25] Nine healthy, neurologically normal women with a history of occasional cocaine use underwent DSC-MRI scans after both phases of their menstrual cycle. On each occasion, global CBV was determined before and after the single-blind administration of cocaine. A greater CBV reduction in the luteal phase was noted in eight of nine subjects studied in both the follicular and the luteal menstrual cycle phases. Independent of the mechanism, these results highlight the importance of evaluating the cerebrovascular effects of cocaine in separate cohorts of both men and women.

Studies of marijuana users have reported deficits in cognitive functioning, particularly in the executive and attentional systems. Functional MRI techniques have been applied in order to gain a better understanding of the extent to which these functions may recover with dry substances and the specific time course of recovery (see Table 8.2B). Chronic marijuana smokers have been examined with fMRI at two time points during a 28-day supervised abstinence period.[26] Subjects completed two tasks: a right-hand and left-hand psychomotor task and a visual working memory task. Whereas control subjects produced significant activation in the dorsolateral prefrontal cortex during the challenge paradigm, marijuana smokers demonstrated diminished activation in this region after 24 hours of abstinence. This effect remained after 28 days of abstinence, although some increase in the dorsolateral prefrontal cortex activation was noted. In contrast, smokers produced increased activation in the cingulate cortex at both time points, whereas control subjects did not. These results indicate that even after extended abstinence periods, specific differential patterns of cortical activation exist in subjects with a history of heavy marijuana use (Figure 8.2).

### Schizophrenia

Schizophrenia often is considered the most serious psychiatric disorder, with classic symptoms of auditory hallucinations and bizarre delusions. Affecting approximately one percent of the population in late adolescence or early adulthood, the illness is lifelong, with significant morbidity and disability. Because of its severity, fMRI research directed at psychiatric illnesses has dedicated more time to schizophrenia than any other illness. Despite these exhaustive efforts, the clinical applications of fMRI in schizophrenia are still preliminary (see Table 8.3A–8.3F).

Early investigations of altered functional brain activation in schizophrenic patients utilizing fMRI began with sensory paradigms and simple motor tasks (see Table 8.3A). It has been demonstrated that the mean signal intensity change in the primary visual cortex was significantly greater in patients with schizophrenia than in comparison subjects when presented with alternating blocks of flash photic stimulation and darkness.[27] Other groups have supported this hypothesis of cortical dysfunction in schizophrenic patients and reported a decrease in activation of both sensorimotor cortices and the supplementary motor area during a finger-to-thumb opposition task (Figure 8.3).[28] More recent and complex motor paradigms have investigated the effects of medication on patients with schizophrenia, illustrating the possible use of fMRI as a method to investigate treatment response. Schizophrenic patients have been examined before and after four treatments with olanzapine using a simple finger-tapping task.[29] Data from this study indicates that significant changes in right cerebellar activation with patients following treatment demonstrates a pattern of activity more similar to control subjects than at baseline. During a unilateral self-pace finger-tapping task, untreated schizophrenic patients have been found to demonstrate a greater increase in activation in the ipsilateral cerebellum and the contralateral basal ganglia as compared to control subjects or medicated schizophrenic patients.[30] Given the differential activation seen within subgroups of schizophrenic patients, additional research has been aimed at examining altered cortical activation in schizophrenic patients who rely heavily on pharmacological treatment. During a self-generated left-handed finger opposition task, unmedicated schizophrenic patients and patients treated with typical neuroleptics showed the same patterns of activation in the high-order sensorimotor areas, whereas patients treated with typical or atypical antipsychotic showed decreased activation.[31] Patients treated with a stable pharmacological regime with typical neuroleptics showed reduced activation in sensorimotor cortices (contra- and ipsilateral) as compared to patients on antipsychotics. These findings support prior research identifying now-significant differences in activation patterns during motor tasks between control subjects and schizophrenic patients, suggesting the motor cortex has no role in the identification of schizophrenia.[32,33]

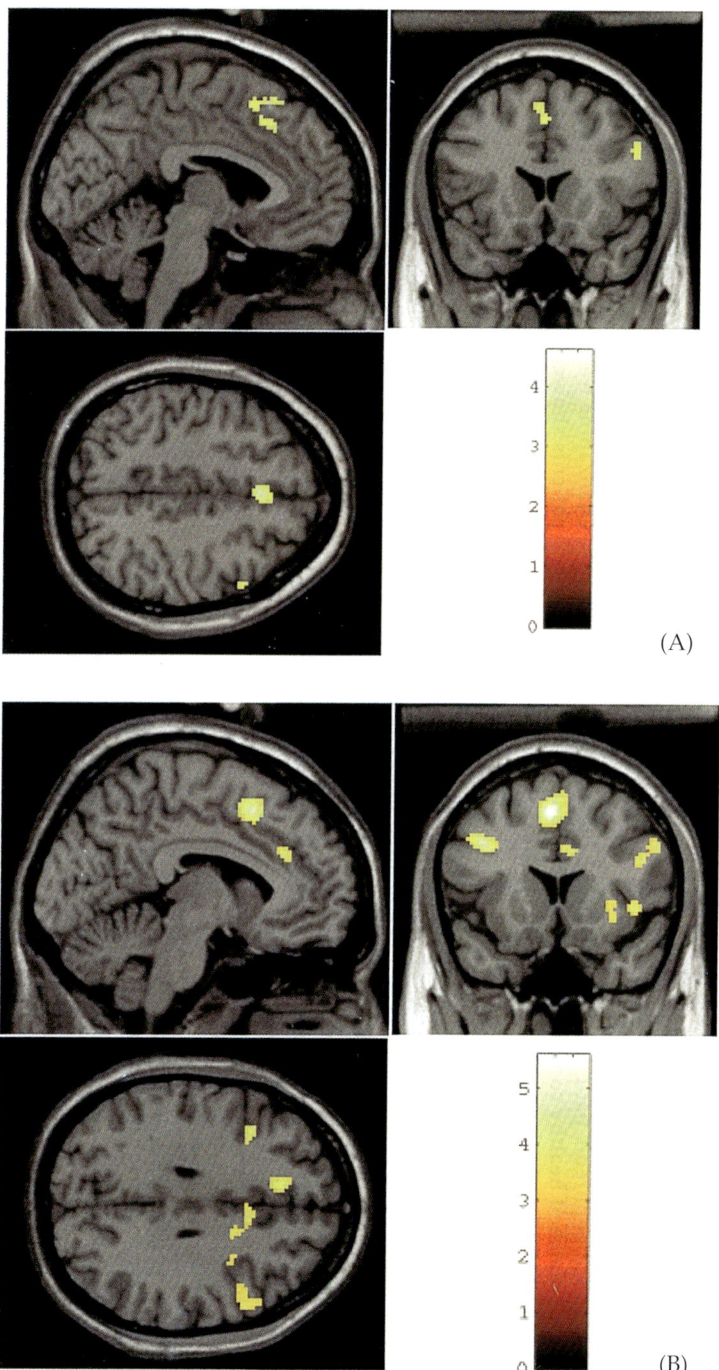


**Figure 8.2.** Illustration of brain activation during a working memory task in heavy cannabis users after 1–24 hrs discontinuation and control subjects. (A) Control subjects. (B) Heavy cannabis users. (Neurologic coordinates)

Table 8.3C. Summary of fMRI Research Pertaining to Schizophrenia Using Working Memory Task Paradigms

| Authors | Subjects | fMRI paradigm | Results |
| --- | --- | --- | --- |
| Ramsey et al., 2002[42] | Medicated schizophrenic patients; medication-naïve schizophrenic patients; healthy controls | XT-Task—Executive function task requiring logical reasoning alongside a closely matched control task | After correction for performance, deductive-reasoning brain activity (Brodmann's Areas) did not differ between controls and medicated schizophrenics, but did remain different between controls and medication-naïve schizophrenics. |
| Manoach et al., 2001[41] | Schizophrenic patients; normal controls | Scanned twice during a working memory task | Overall, no group activations or performance differences were found between the two scans. In schizophrenics, however, individual differences in activation were significant from first scan to the next. |
| Manoach et al., 2000[40] | Schizophrenic patients; normal controls | Working memory task (Modified Sternberg Item Recognition Task) | Before and after correction for performance, schizophrenics showed activation in the basal ganglia and thalamus, whereas controls did not. Schizophrenics showed decreased working memory performance and differential dorsolateral prefrontal cortex activation. |
| Callicott et al., 2000[39] | Schizophrenic patients; healthy controls | Working memory task | Exaggerated and inefficient cortical activity in the dorsolateral prefrontal cortex. |
| Manoach et al., 1999[38] | Schizophrenic patients; normal controls | Reward performance on working memory task (Modified Sternberg Item Recognition Task) | Schizophrenics had increased activation in the left dorsolateral prefrontal cortex, which was inversely correlated with task performance (measured by errors). |

Table 8.3D. Summary of fMRI Research Pertaining to Schizophrenia Using Cognitive Challenge Paradigms

| Authors | Subjects | fMRI paradigm | Results |
|---|---|---|---|
| Riehemann et al., 2001[44] | Neuroleptic-naïve schizophrenic patients; matched controls | Wisconsin Card Sorting Task | Schizophrenics showed decreased activation in right frontal and left temporal lobe, and the cerebellum. |
| Carter et al., 2001[4] | Medicated Schizophrenic patients; healthy controls | Continuous Performance Task | Controls, unlike schizophrenics, showed error-related activity in the anterior cingulate cortex. |
| Volz et al., 1999[45] | Schizophrenic patients on stable neuroleptics; healthy controls | The Continuous Performance Task | Schizophrenics showed decreased activation in the right mesial prefrontal cortex, the right cingulate, and the left thalamus. |
| Volz et al., 1997[43] | Chronic schizophrenic patients on stable neuroleptics; healthy controls | Wisconsin Card Sorting Task | Schizophrenics showed decreased activation in the right prefrontal cortex and a trend of increased left temporal activity. |

Table 8.3E. Summary of fMRI Research Pertaining to Schizophrenia Using Emotional Processing Paradigms

| Authors | Subjects | fMRI paradigm | Results |
|---|---|---|---|
| Phillips et al., 1999[46] | Right-handed schizophrenic patients (half paranoid and half non paranoid); healthy controls | Three 5-minute experiment: Black-and-white facial photographs of happiness alternated with black-and-white facial photographs of fear, anger, or disgust | As a whole, schizophrenics showed less activation and poorer performance. Non-paranoid patients did not activate neural regions associated with perception of stimuli. Paranoid patients showed increased activation when compared to non-paranoids. |
| Schneider et al., 1998[47] | Medicated male schizophrenic patients; matched controls | Happy and sad mood induction | In contrast to controls, schizophrenics showed no amygdala activation during sadness induction. |

Table 8.3F. Summary of fMRI Research Pertaining to Hallucinatory Symptoms in Schizophrenia

| Authors | Subjects | fMRI paradigm | Results |
|---|---|---|---|
| Lawrie et al., 2002[49] | Schizophrenic patients; healthy controls | Visually presented sentences with last word missing; patient was instructed to think of last word | Correlation coefficients between the left temporal cortex and left dorsolateral prefrontal cortex were inversely correlated with severity of auditory hallucinations in patients. |
| Lennox et al., 2000[50] | Medicated schizophrenic patients | Scanned while having hallucinations in scanner | During hallucinations, all subjects showed activation in the temporal cortex and prefrontal cortex. |
| Woodruff et al., 1997[48] | Male schizophrenics patients with a history of auditory hallucinations but were not actively hallucinating; male schizophrenic patients with no history of auditory hallucinations; non-psychiatric males | Auditory perception of externally presented speech | Patients (both with and without hallucinations) showed a decrease in left temporal lobe activation, and as a combined group also showed an increase in right temporal activation when compared to controls. |

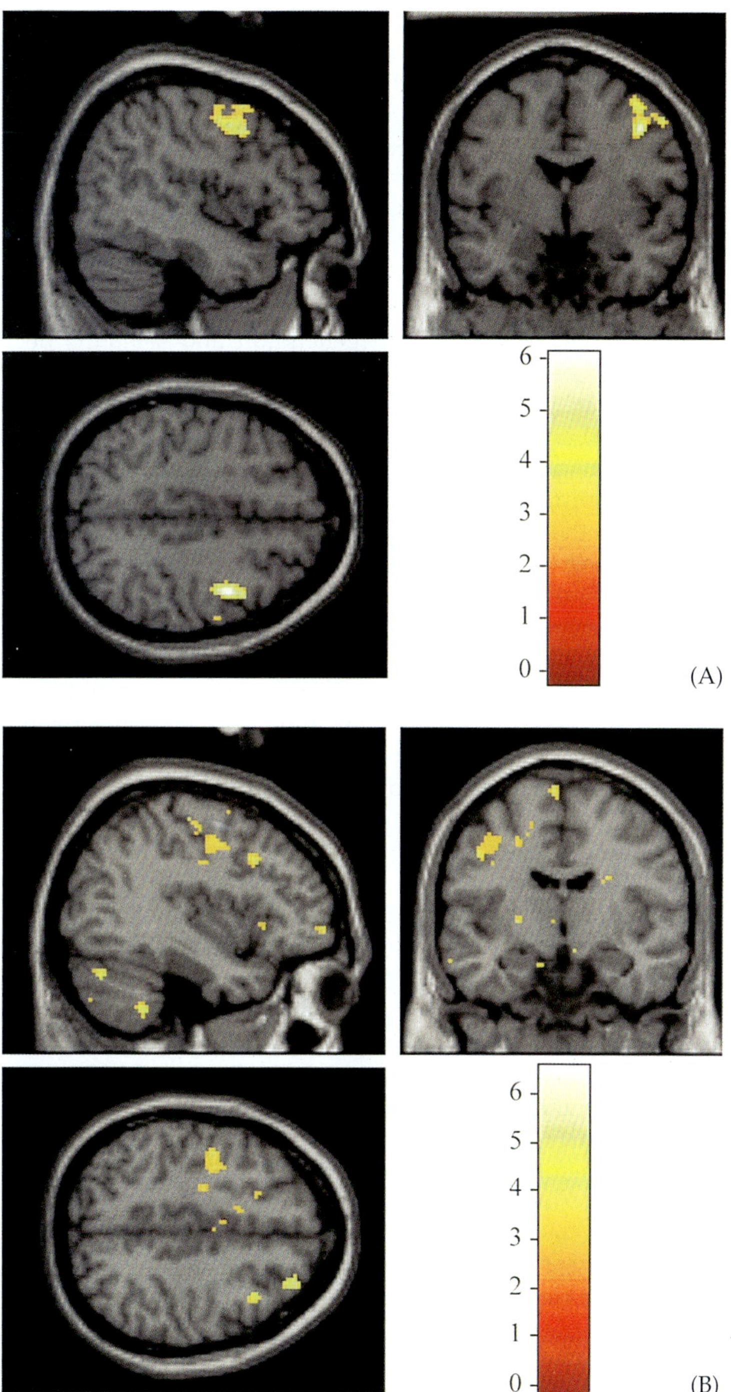


**Figure 8.3.** Illustrating activation from a schizophrenic patient during (A) left and (B) right finger tapping. Images are based on SPM analysis of data. (Neurologic coordinates)

A number of investigations have used paradigms directed at assessing neural activation during cognitive verbal and memory tasks as a method of determining altered neural processing between schizophrenic patients and control subjects (see Table 8.3B). Abnormal language functions, including difficulties with word-association tasks and verbal fluency, have been noted in schizophrenic patients. Schizophrenic patients and normal control subjects have been investigated with fMRI using a verbal cognitive challenge paradigm.[34] Normal control subjects produced higher mean differences for frontal lobe activation and lower mean temporal lobe activation as compared to schizophrenic patients. During a verb generation and semantic decision task, language processing has been shown to be less lateralized in schizophrenic patients than in control subjects.[35] Schizophrenic patients showed an increased activation in the right hemisphere and a decreased language lateralization associated with more severe hallucinations. Schizophrenic patients also demonstrated reversed laterality of activation in the superior temporal cortex when asked to engage in a task involving word retrieval during continuous speech while looking at an inkblot.[36] Further differences seen in schizophrenic patients during verbal cognitive tasks report that patients with schizophrenia have less activation in the superior and inferior posterior temporal regions during a silent reading task.[37] In this same study, acutely psychotic patients with schizophrenia, more so than non-actively psychotic patients, were shown to have significant activation decreases in posterior (occipito-temporal) and increases in anterior (frontal, insular, and striatal) brain areas when compared to control subjects (Figure 8.4).

Schizophrenic patients have shown both a decrease in performance and altered activation patterns in the dorsolateral prefrontal cortex during working memory tasks (Table 8.3C). Using the Modified Sternberg Item Recognition Paradigm, it has been demonstrated that schizophrenic patients' performance were inversely correlated with a greater activation in the left dorsolateral prefrontal cortex.[38] Similarly, using a working memory paradigm in schizophrenic patients, an increase in cortical activity has been shown in the dorsal prefrontal cortex.[39] During the same working memory task, fMRI has demonstrated schizophrenic patients to have activation in the basal gangalia and thalamus before and after correction for performance, whereas control subjects showed no activation in these regions.[40] A recent study investigating the test–retest reliability of fMRI using working memory paradigms showed no significant difference in group activations or performance for two scans done on separate occasions; however significant individual differences within the schizophrenic patient group across two scans were noted.[41] The effects of medication and performance in schizophrenic patients in relation to previous findings of hypofrontality also have been investigated, specifically within the dorsolateral prefrontal cortex during executive functioning.[42] Functional MRI activation differences have been shown in medication-naïve schizophrenic patients, medicated schizophrenic patients, and control subjects during a deductive reasoning protocol (modified XT-task).[42] Decreases in task performance were found in both patients groups and

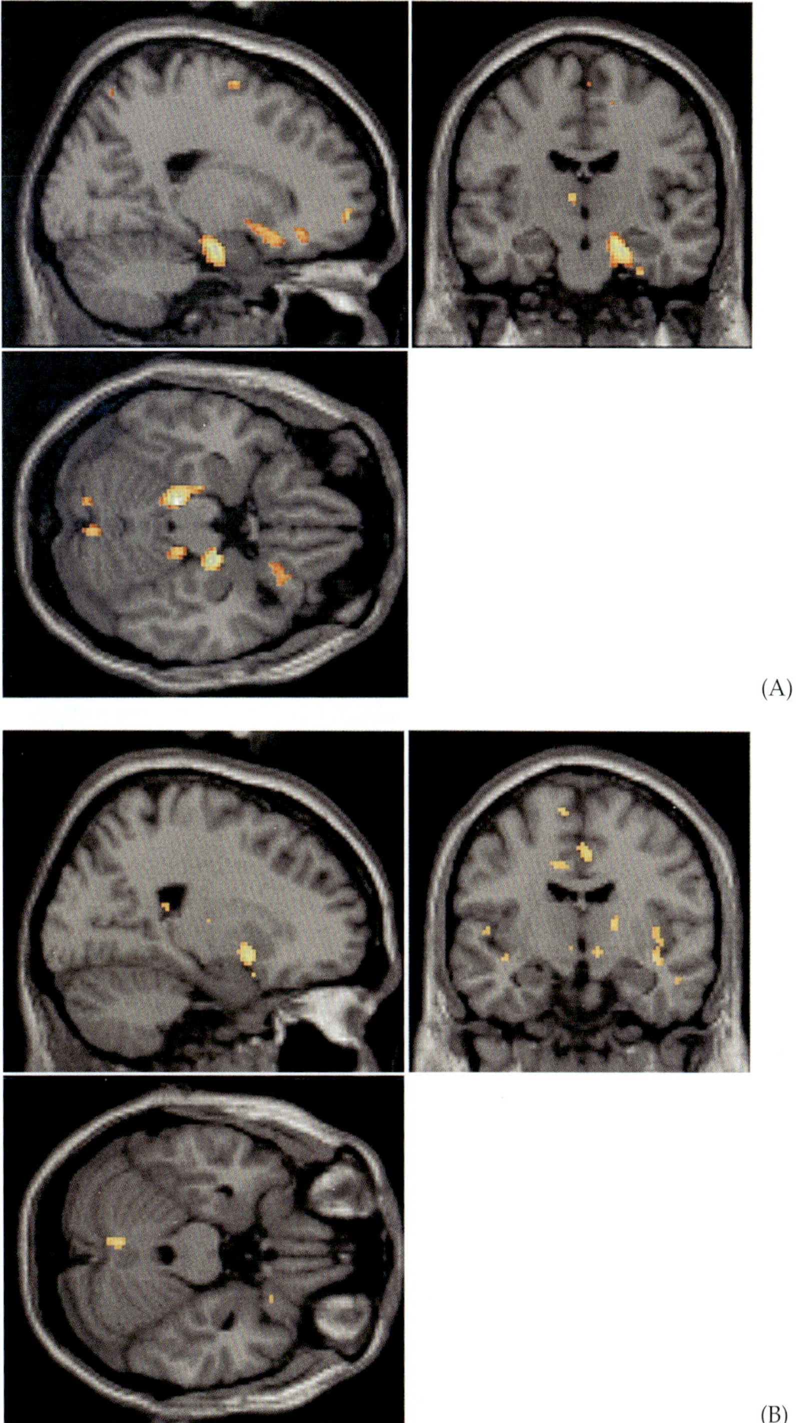


**Figure 8.4.** Illustration of contrast of activation between schizophrenic and control subjects during a Semantic Priming Task. (A) Shows increased activation in patients with schizophrenia during an indirect priming task with an ISI of 50 ms. (B) Shows increased activation in schizophrenics during an indirect priming task with an ISI of 750 ms. (Neurologic coordinates)

brain activity associated with logical reasoning, as defined by combined voxel counts for 11 volume of interests per hemisphere following the division of Brodmann areas, showed a positive correlation in all groups. After correction for performance, logical reasoning brain activity differences were not maintained between control subjects and medicated schizophrenic patients, whereas differences between medication-naïve schizophrenic patients and these groups were maintained. As a whole, these studies demonstrate the importance of controlling for individual sources of variation, performance, and medication status when utilizing fMRI procedures.

Altered frontal activation in patients with schizophrenia also has been examined using other challenge paradigms in combination with BOLD fMRI methods (see Table 8.3D). Previous neuroimaging studies of schizophrenic patients performing the Wisconsin Card Sorting Test (WCST) have reported decreased prefrontal activation as compared with nonpsychiatric populations. Functional MRI techniques have been applied to neuroleptic-stable chronic schizophrenic patients and control subjects while performing the WCST.[43] The control subjects demonstrated right lateralized frontal activation; in contrast, the schizophrenic patients demonstrated a lack of activation in the right prefrontal cortex and a trend toward increased left temporal lobe activation. Performance for the two groups was essentially equivalent, indicating that altered activation patterns could not be accounted for by poor performance. Using a similar paradigm, neuroleptic-naïve schizophrenic patients demonstrated reduced activation in the cerebellum, right frontal lobe, and left temporal lobe during the WCST.[44] Paradigms using the Continuous Performance Task (CPT) also have suggested hypofrontality in schizophrenic patients. Volz and colleagues scanned schizophrenic patients maintained on a stable regime of neuroleptics and healthy control subjects during the CPT.[45] Schizophrenic patients showed decreased activation in the right mesial prefrontal cortex, the right cingulate, and the left thalamus relative to control subjects. A similar paradigm using a CPT reported that only control subjects demonstrated error-related activity in the anterior cingulate cortex; schizophrenic patients did not show this effect, arguing against efficient processing in this region.[4]

Investigations on altered emotional processing have been an integral part of psychiatric research and have begun to play a role in the study of schizophrenia (see Table 8.3E). Schizophrenic patients divided into paranoid and nonparanoid subtypes, and control subjects during the viewing of facial expressions of fear, anger, disgust, and mild happiness have been examined with fMRI (Figure 8.5).[46] Overall, schizophrenic patients showed less cortical activation and poorer performance. Nonparanoid patients did not activate neural regions that are normally linked with perception of the prefrontal cortex, the right cingulate, and the left thalamus. In a prior experiment, medicated male schizophrenic patients and matched control subjects were scanned during a paradigm that induced happiness or sadness.[47] Schizophrenic patients, unlike control subjects, showed no activation in the amygdala during the induction of sadness.

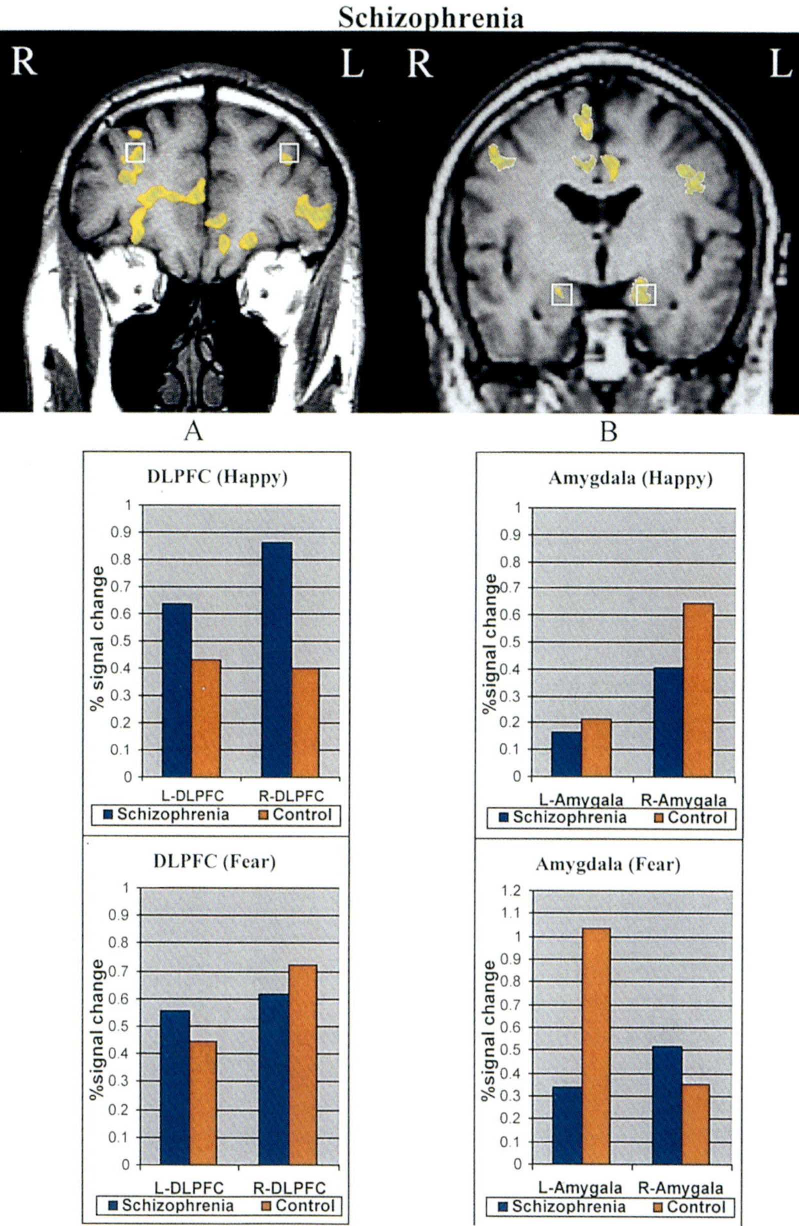


**Figure 8.5.** Location of regions of interest (ROIs) selected for study, shown on a coronal section of a control subject as an example. Image A was obtained while the subject was viewing a happy face; image B was obtained while the subject was viewing a fearful face. (A) Squares indicate right and left dorsolateral prefrontal cortex. (B) Squares indicate right and left amygdala. Average overall percent signal change in the left and right amygdala, and dorsolateral prefrontal cortex (DLPFC) in response to happy affect ("Happy") and fearful affect ("Fear") in schizophrenic and control subjects.

Limited studies have begun to look at the structural correlates of hallucinations (see Table 8.3E). It has been investigated whether schizophrenic patients with a history of hallucinations would exhibit a less left-lateralized response to auditory perception of externally presented speech than both nonpsychiatric subjects and schizophrenic patients without hallucinations.[48] Their study samples included male schizophrenic patients with a history of auditory hallucinations who were not actively hallucinating, male schizophrenic patients who had never experienced auditory hallucinations, and nonpsychiatric control subjects. Schizophrenic subjects—with and without hallucinations—exhibited a decrease in left temporal lobe activation in response to external auditory stimulations as compared to control subjects. The combined group, however, also demonstrated an increase in right temporal activation compared with control subjects. While investigating the activation patterns of schizophrenic patients and control subjects during a task requiring the completion of 128 visually presented sentences, the correlation coefficients between left temporal cortex and left dorsolateral prefrontal cortex were found to be negatively correlated with the severity of auditory hallucinations of schizophrenic patients.[49] Using a 3 Tesla MRI, it has been reported that medicated schizophrenic patients showed activation in the temporal and prefrontal cortices during episodes of hallucinations.[50]

Research directed at identifying cortical dysfunction during cognitive challenges in schizophrenic patients versus other psychiatric illnesses, illustrates the possible future utility of fMRI as a tool for differential diagnosis. A comparison of schizophrenic and bipolar patients on cognitive challenge paradigms, such as the Stroop Color Word test, illustrates significant differences between the groups within specific regions of interest. A recent investigation that utilized fMRI techniques reported that during the color naming task, a highly significant difference was detected between a group of schizophrenic and bipolar patients, demonstrating nearly opposite patterns of activation within the VOA subdivision of the anterior cingulate cortex.[51] Although the schizophrenic patients showed a reduction of signal change on both the left and right sides of the VOA, bipolar patients exhibited a bilateral increase during the color naming task, a similar pattern as control subjects (see Figure 8.6).

Within a second region of interest, the dorsal lateral prefrontal cortex (DLPFC), differences between the groups also emerged. Although the groups demonstrated similar patterns of signal intensity change during the color naming task, bipolar patients showed a much higher magnitude of signal change on both left and right sides, which trended towards significance on the right side as compared to the schizophrenic patients (see Figure 8.7).

Each of the subject groups was able to perform the conditions of the Stroop task within the magnet environment reasonably well, and the two patient groups did not differ significantly from each other on any of the conditions. These findings suggest that all subjects were engaged actively in the tasks, and that no generalized deficit in task performance was present for either diagnostic group. These data

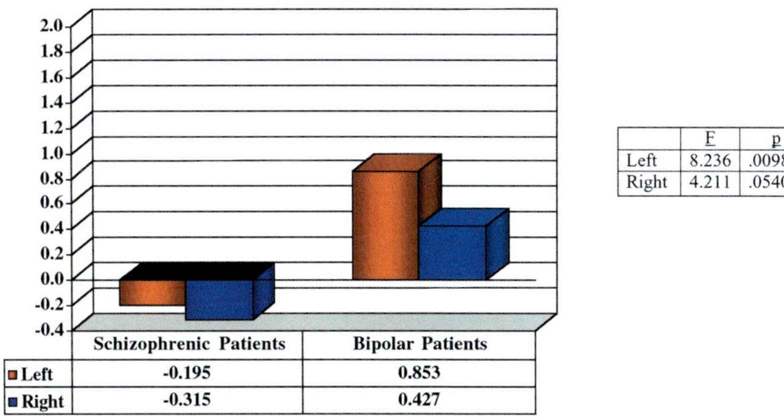


**Figure 8.6.** VOA subdivision: Color naming. Graph demonstrates activation intensities within the VOA subdivision of the anterior cingulate cortex for schizophrenic versus bipolar patients during a modified version of the color-naming task. (From Gruber S, Rogowska R, Yurgelun-Todd DA. Differential activation of anterior cingulated and prefrontal cortex in schizophrenic and bipolar patients: an fMRI study [abstract]. Colorado Springs, CO; International Congress on Schizophrenic Research, 2003.)

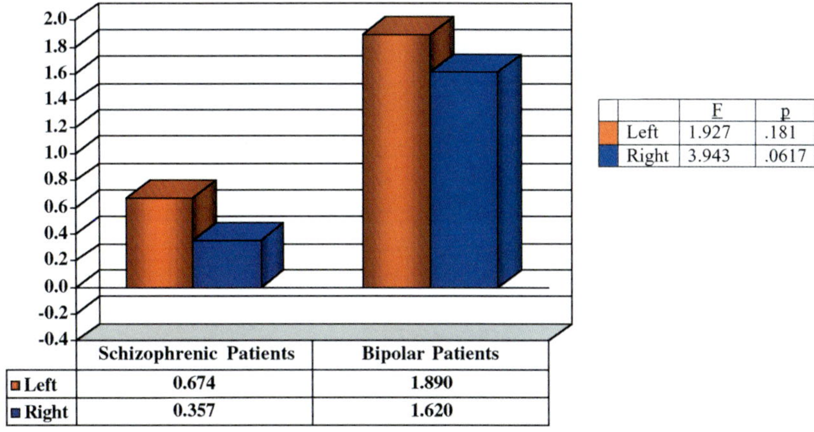


**Figure 8.7.** Dorsolateral prefrontal cortex subdivision: Color naming. Graph demonstrates activation intensities within the DLPFC for schizophrenic versus bipolar patients during a modified version of the color-naming task. From Gruber S, Rogowska R, Yurgelun-Todd DA. Differential activation of anterior cingulated and prefrontal cortex in schizophrenic and bipolar patients: an fMRI study [abstract]. Colorado Springs, CO; International Congress on Schizophrenic Research, 2003.

support the theory of altered frontal function in patients with schizophrenia and bipolar disorder, which also has been reported in work using verbal fluency and semantic decision-making tasks.[52] The continual identification of group differences during cognitive tasks and others, such as Loeber and colleagues' identification of cerebellar blood volume to be highest in schizophrenic patients and lowest in bipolar patients when compared to control subjects using DSC fMRI, indicate that fMRI techniques are perhaps well suited for examining between-group differences that may not be evident on standard behavioral measures.[53]

## Mood Disorders

The two most severe affective illnesses are major depression and bipolar disorder. Major depression is characterized by persistent feelings of deep despair accompanied by at least four of the following symptoms: sleep disturbances, disruption of appetite, apathy, lethargy, feelings of hopelessness or worthlessness, difficulty concentrating, or suicidal thoughts. The World Health Organization (WHO) has concluded that by the year 2020, major depression will be the second most debilitating disease to affect mankind, following only ischemic heart disease. Bipolar disorder is associated with episodes of mania and depression. It affects approximately one percent of the population. Chronic treatment with mood stabilizers, antipsychotics, and/or anticonvulsants, is generally required, and suicide occurs in 10 to 15% of all patients.

While fMRI research investigating major depression and bipolar disorder compared to nonpsychiatric populations shows consistent regional activation differences, empirical studies remain limited, causing a restraint on its ability to be used as a clinical tool (see Table 8.4). Emotional paradigms utilizing film clips or facial photographs to induce feelings of sadness, happiness, or fear have shown significant differences in prefrontal, cingulate gyrus, and amygdala activation between depressed, bipolar, and normal control subjects (Figure 8.8). It has been reported that patients with major depression had greater activation in the medial prefrontal cortex and in the right cingulate gyrus during the passive viewing of a film clip inducing sadness when compared to normal control subjects.[54] While viewing positive and negatively valenced stimuli, it has been shown that depressed patients, unlike control subjects, displayed no activation to positive stimuli at baseline.[55] Following treatment with venlafaxine, depressed patients showed a significant increase in activation to the same positive stimuli. Likewise, depressed patients initially showed an increased activation in the left amygdala compared to control subjects when viewing masked emotional faces. Post treatment, depressed patients exhibited a decreased activation in the left amygdala, whereas activation in control subjects for baseline and follow-up scans did not differ.[56] Using negatively and positively valenced words as stimuli, an increased amygdalar activation has been demonstrated to negative words in depressed patients that extended significantly longer when compared to control subjects.[57] Similarly, bipolar patients showed increased amygdala activity during the viewing of fearful facial affect when compared to normal control subjects (Figure 8.9). Activation of the dorsal lateral prefrontal cortex in bipolar patients, however, was reduced when compared to control subjects.[58]

Table 8.4. Summary of fMRI Research in Patients with Mood Disorders

| Authors | Subjects | fMRI paradigm | Results |
|---|---|---|---|
| Siegle et al., 2002 | Depressed patients; never-depressed controls | Alternating emotional (valence identification) and non-emotional processing (Sternberg memory) | Patients had longer-lasting amygdalar activation to negative words in valence identification than did controls. |
| Sheline et al., 2001 | Major Depression Disorder (MDD) patients; matched controls | Viewing of masked emotional faces before and after antidepressant treatment | MDD patients had increased left amygdala activation to all faces (greatest for fearful) compared to controls. Post-treatment MDD had bilateral decreased amygdala activation to all faces. |
| Yurgelun-Todd et al., 2000 | Bipolar affective disorder patients; healthy controls | Viewing of facial photographs depicting fearful or happy affect | Bipolar patients had increased amygdala activity and decreased dorsolateral prefrontal cortex activity during fearful facial affect when compared to controls. |
| Beauregard et al., 1998 | Unipolar depressed patients; healthy controls | Emotional activation (sadness and neutral) | Patients had increased activation in left medial prefrontal cortex and right cingulated gyrus during sadness. |
| Kalin et al., 1997 | Healthy controls; Major Depression Disorder (MDD) patients; MDD patients treated with venalafaxine after baseline scans. | Viewing of positive and negatively valence stimuli | Controls showed activation to both positive stimuli pre and post. MDD patients showed no activation in prescan to positive stimuli, but activation to positive stimuli in postscan. |

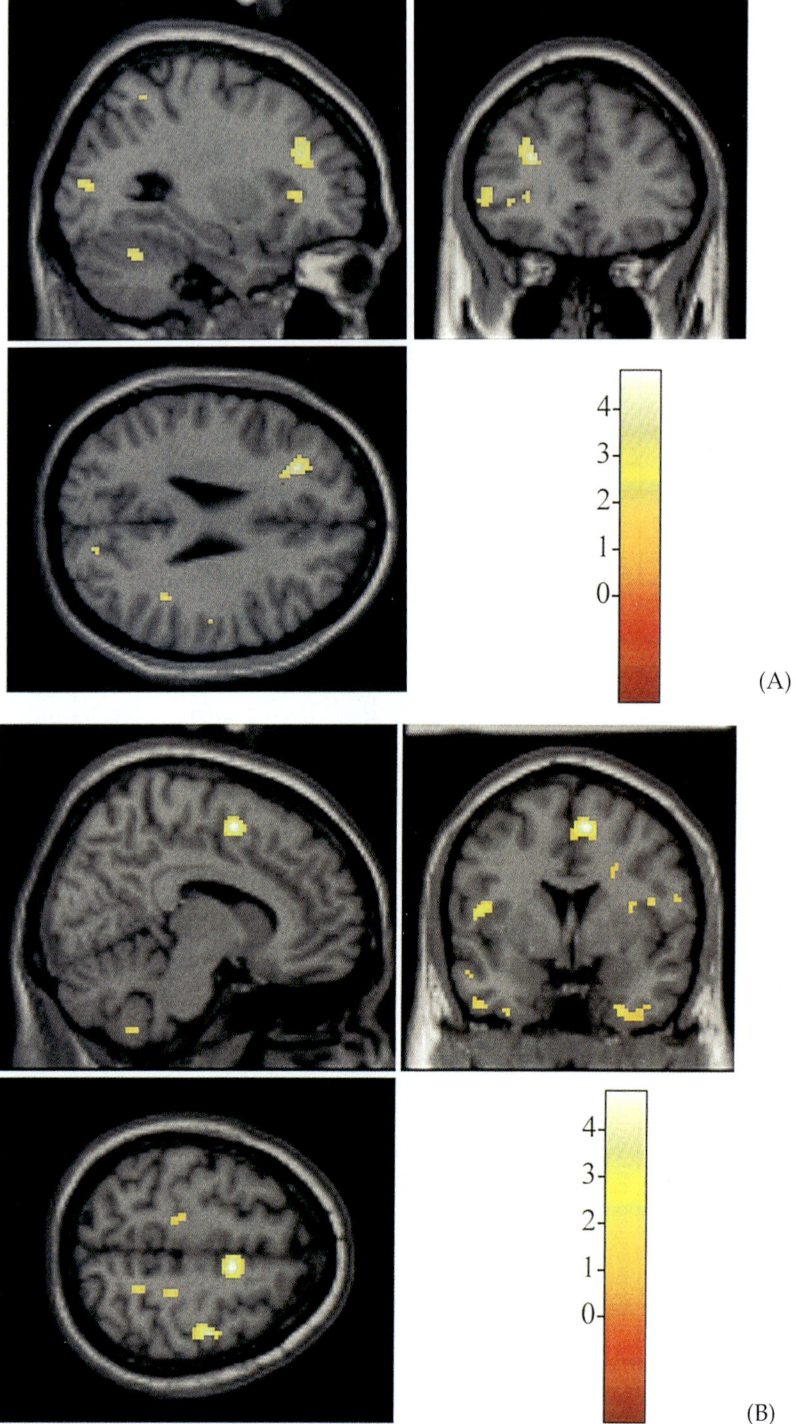


**Figure 8.8.** (A) Illustrating increased frontal activation in control subjects compared with depressed subjects during the viewing of fearful faces. (B) Comparison of activation in depressed adolescents and healthy comparison adolescents during the viewing of happy facial affect. Nonpsychiatric subjects produced significantly greater cingulate activation than depressed subjects during this task. (Neurologic coordinates)

### Obsessive–Compulsive Disorder (OCD)

Obsessive–compulsive disorder is an anxiety disorder in which patients experience recurrent obsessions and compulsions that cause significant distress and occupy a significant portion of the affected person's life. Lifetime prevalence of this disorder is two to three percent. Blood oxygenation level-dependent fMRI studies have afforded much insight into the brain–behavior relationships in patients with OCD (see Table 8.5). Functional MRI techniques have been used to examine the neuroanatomic correlates of OCD in patients and control subjects using symptom provocation.[59] Medicated patients with OCD exhibited increased activation in the medial orbitofrontal, lateral frontal, anterior temporal, anterior cingulated, and insular cortex, as well as caudate, lenticulate, and amygdalar regions in association with OCD symptoms. In contrast, normal subjects did not exhibit activation of any of these regions after provocation. These same findings have been replicated using unmedicated patients with OCD.[60] A study targeted at investigating the differential neural response between two specific symptoms of OCD patients, washing and checking, showed patients predominately concerned with washing to have similar neural activations during the viewing of disgusting pictures and washer-relevant pictures. Patients predominately concerned with checking instead showed activations in the fronto-striatal regions, seen to be associated with the urge to ritualize in OCD during the viewing of washer-relevant pictures.[61] The importance in the identification of differential neural responses associated with varying symptomatology and symptom degrees, as seen in Levine and colleagues' identification of a negative correlation between clinical ratings of OCD symptomatology and the activation of the dorsolateral prefrontal cortex during verbal fluency, has great implications for the future use of fMRI as a tool for treatment development and evaluation.[62]

## Review of Affective Behavior

Affective behavior can be divided into at least four distinct, yet interrelated, processes, which include the perception, experience, expression, and modulation of affect. Research on affect and emotions has often been inconsistent because there has been considerable disagreement as to the best method for defining a subjective state of emotion.[63] Most researchers, however, have accepted that there are basic emotions that are essentially invariant and universally recognized across cultures.[64–69] One aspect of affective perception that recently has received considerable attention is the ability of individuals to identify facial cues of emotion.[70,71]

Recent neuroimaging studies of adults have demonstrated that the amygdala is involved in the perception of emotion, especially fear, displayed in facial expressions.[72–80] The amygdala, a small almond-shaped structure located deep within the medial aspect of each temporal lobe, has been shown to be particularly important for affective conditioning of fear and avoidance responses.[81–85] A number of human

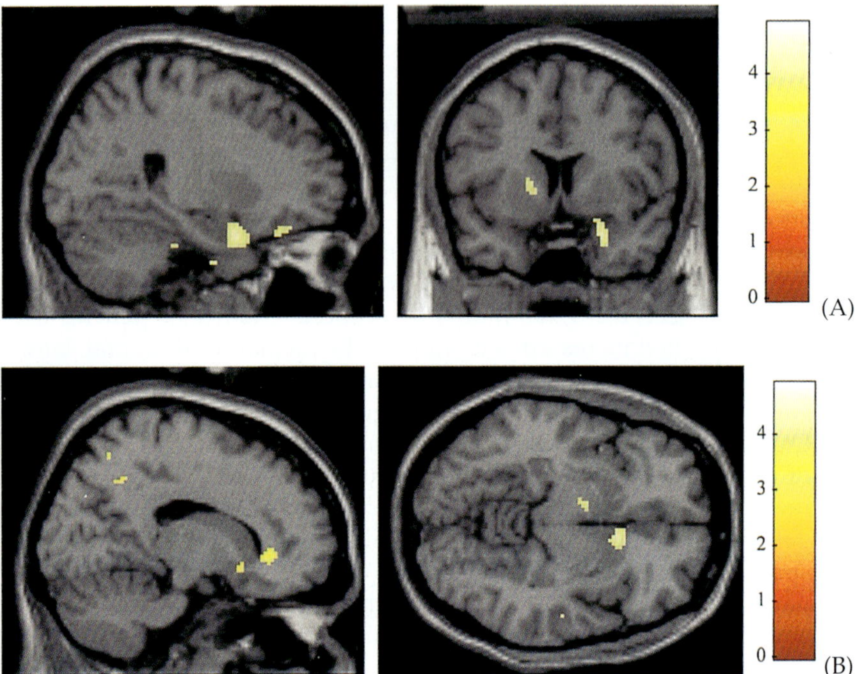


**Figure 8.9.** (A) Illustration of increased parahippocampal activation in patients with bipolar disorder compared with controls during the viewing of fearful faces. (B) Illustration of increased cingulate activation in patients with bipolar disorder compared with controls during the viewing of fearful faces. (Neurologic coordinates)

lesion studies have shown that individuals with bilateral damage to the amygdala show significant deficits in the ability to discriminate threat-related cues in facial expressions; for example, patients with amygdala damage have difficulty discriminating between photographs of threatening and nonthreatening individuals,[86] and are severely deficient in the ability to process facial expressions of fear.[87–89] The prefrontal cortex activation acts in concert with many other distributed neural systems to influence affective experience and perception; for instance, subcortical limbic structures, such as the amygdala, also play a critical role in emotional processing,[90] and may interact directly with the prefrontal cortex to influence affective experience (Figure 8.10).[91]

Recent models have suggested that emotional processing may be modulated by the prefrontal cortex via its influence over the activity of the amygdala.[92] This prefrontal cortex modulation allows for enhancement or attenuation of emotional responses through cognitive processes. The following is an example of an fMRI paradigm aimed at investigating activation differences between healthy adults and adolescents in the perception of fear using facial cues.

## Fearful Face Activation Paradigm

Affective face stimuli consisted of six faces expressing the emotion of fear. The faces were gray-scale black-and-white photographs from the

Table 8.5. Summary of fMRI Research in Patients with Obsessive Compulsive Disorder

| Authors | Subjects | fMRI paradigm | Results |
|---|---|---|---|
| Adler et al, 2000[60] | Medication-free out patients with OCD | Provocative and innocuous stimuli individually created for each patient was presented. Self-ratings of OCD symptoms also were done before and after each exposure to stimuli | Significant activations in the orbitofrontal, superior frontal, dorsolateral prefrontal, anterior, medial, and lateral temporal cortex and the right anterior cingulate. Inverse correlations where found between right superior frontal activation to baseline compulsion symptomatology and left orbitofrontal cortical activation to OCD self-ratings after provocative stimuli. |
| Phillips et al., 2000[76] | Patients with OCD (half with need for washing symptoms and half with need for checking symptoms); age-matched normal controls | Two 5-minute experiments; 1) alternating blocks of disgusting and neutral pictures, 2) alternating blocks of washer-relevant and neutral pictures | Patients with symptoms of washing showed similar activations during both viewing of washer-relevant and disgusting pictures. Patient with symptoms of checking instead showed activations in the frontostriatal regions during viewing of washer-relevant pictures. |
| Levine et al., 1998[62] | Schizophrenic patients with varying degrees of OCD symptoms | Verbal-fluency task and rating of OCD symptoms on the Yale–Brown Obsessive Compulsive Scale and the NIMH scale | As a whole group, no significant relationship between rating scores and activation, however, significant association for a subgroup. For subgroup, a negative relationship between OCD ratings and activation of the left dorsolateral prefrontal cortex was found. |
| Breiter et al., 1996[72] | Medicated patients with OCD; normal controls | Symptom provocation | Patients showed activation in the medial orbitofrontal, lateral frontal, anterior temporal, anterior cingulate, insular cortex, caudate, lenticulate, and amygdalar regions. Controls did not exhibit activation in any of these regions after provocation. |

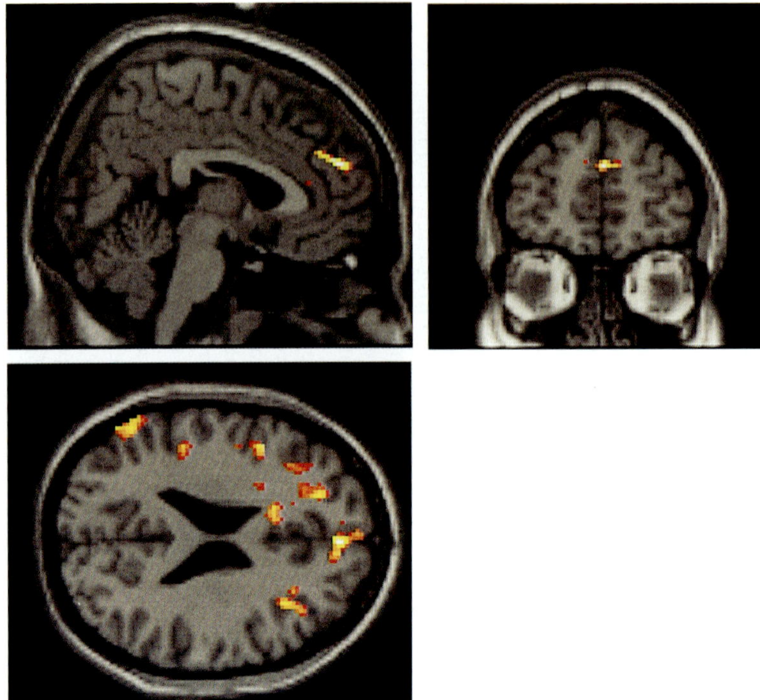

**Figure 8.10.** Illustrating increased activation in subjects with panic disorder compared with activation in healthy controls. All subjects were completing interference subtest of the Stroop test.

Ekman series (photos # 12, 13, 14, 15, 16, 17) and included both male and female posers[93] (see Figure 8.11). Stimuli were generated from a Macintosh computer and back projected from a magnetically shielded LCD video projector onto a translucent screen placed at the end of the scanning table. Stimuli were viewed from a mirror mounted to the head coil. The scanning sequence lasted for 150 seconds, consisting of five alternating 30-second stimulus/rest periods. During baseline and rest periods, subjects maintained visual fixation on a small white circle located in the center of the screen. Three different face photographs were presented during each of the two stimulation periods for a total of six stimulus expressions. Each facial expression was presented for 9.5 seconds with a 0.5-second interstimulus interval. To ensure that subjects maintained fixation during the task, they were asked to report the affect of the faces following the conclusion of the scan. In addition to the fearful face perception condition, subjects also participated in several other cognitive fMRI tasks, the order of which was randomized across subjects. These other tasks included a modified version of the Stroop color–word naming task, and either an angry face or happy face affect perception condition.

The findings of this study converge with other neuroimaging and neurophysiological data to suggest that cerebral development from childhood into early adulthood involves nonlinear transitions in the

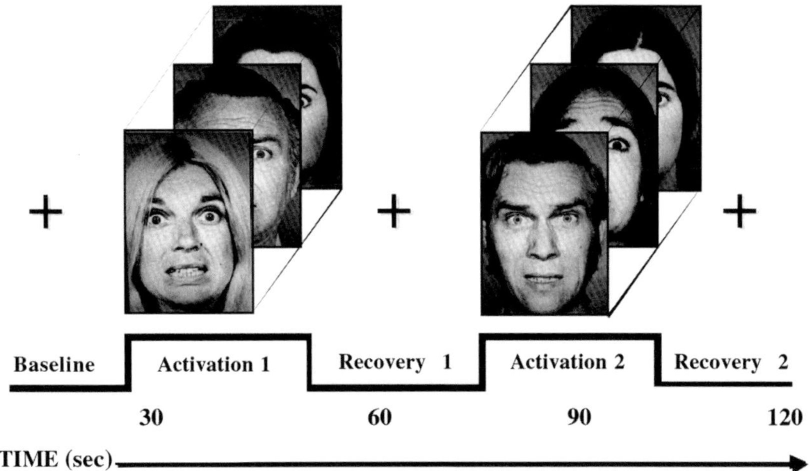


**Figure 8.11.** Emotional processing fMRI paradigm. Faces, taken from the Ekman series (photos # 12, 13, 15, 14, 16, 17),[93] were presented to both adolescents and adult controls in a 1.5T scanner. The scanning sequence lasted for 150 seconds, consisting of five alternating 30-second stimulus/rest periods. During baseline and rest periods, subjects maintained visual fixation on a small white circle located in the center of the screen. Three different face photographs were presented during each of the two stimulation periods for a total of six stimulus expressions. Each facial expression was presented for 9.5 seconds with a 0.5-second interstimulus interval. Printed with permission from Paul Ekman and Associates LLC.

ratio of subcortical to cortical contributions to affective processing and in the lateralization of these affect systems (see Figure 8.12). It has been proposed that a key element of cerebral maturation is the progressive reallocation of cognitive and emotional regulatory systems from lower subcortical regions to the prefrontal cortex.[94] Others also have explored this hypothesis in recent years.[58,73,92]

## Future Implications

There is little question that fMRI methods are considered to play a critical role in psychiatric research. The ability to monitor brain function noninvasively using fMRI techniques in individuals with brain disorders is compelling, especially considering that the months of work often can be summarized in a single image on the cover of a scientific journal. These tools are even more important in psychiatry, as opposed to other medical disciplines, in the context of limited existing knowledge with respect to the pathophysiology of mental illnesses and an absence of valid or compelling animal models of disease. However, research studies conducted to date have not yet identified a role for fMRI as a diagnostic imaging method in psychiatric practice. While it is likely that future fMRI research will provide new insights into psychiatric brain dysfunction, there are obstacles that stand in the way of clinical method development.

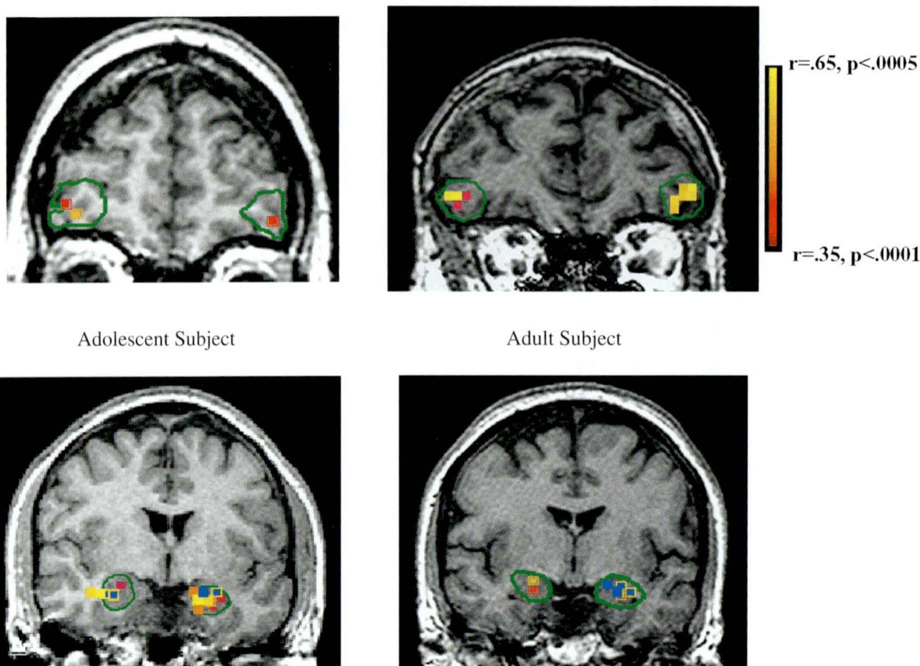


**Figure 8.12.** Activation sites found in adolescents versus adults during viewing of fearful face paradigm seen in Illustration 8.1.

The majority of ongoing psychiatric neuroimaging research is focused on studies of brain activity occurring in groups of subjects with specific disorders. Indeed, National Institutes of Health-funded investigations increasingly involve the use of methods such as single-event fMRI, where averaging across subjects is essential for statistically significant results to be obtained. In a parallel vein, cognitive neuroscience studies often make use of complex paradigms that may not be performed well in persons with psychotic or affective illness. Deconvolving the effects of changes in brain activity with differences in task performance remains a challenging problem. Moreover, there exists a relatively limited understanding of the effects of psychotropic agents—many of which have vasoactive properties—on fMRI parameters.

At the present time, the future use of fMRI in psychiatry is uncertain and progress toward this end has been limited; for example, little effort is being devoted to the identification of relatively simple challenges that can be presented in a block design and that provide distinct patterns of brain activation in single subjects with a specific psychiatric illness. The elucidation of fMRI methods that provide task-independent assessments of cerebral activity, such as DSCI may help to clarify this area of study. Research along these lines would be facilitated greatly if it were to be driven by the vendors of MRI devices. Given the substantial prevalence of psychiatric disorders, these vendors would benefit greatly from the development of psychiatrically relevant fMRI strategies as a means to address a substantial new market.

## References

1. Kwong K, Belliveau J, Chesler D, et al. Dynamic magnetic resonance imaging of human brain activity during primary sensory stimulation. *Proc Natl Acad Sci USA.* 1992;89:5675–5679.
2. Belliveau JW, Rosen BR, Kantor HL, et al. Functional cerebral imaging by susceptibility-contrast NMR. *Magn Reson Med.* 1990;14:538–546.
3. Yurgelun-Todd DA, Renshaw PF. Applications of functional MR imaging to research in psychiatry. *Neuroimaging Clin N Am.* 1999;9:295–308.
4. Carter CS, MacDonald AW 3rd, Ross LL, Stenger VA. Anterior cingulate cortex activity and impaired self-monitoring of performance in patients with schizophrenia: an event-related fMRI study. *Am J Psychiatry.* 2001; 158:1423–1428.
5. American Psychiatric Association. *Diagnostic and Statistical Manual of Mental Disorders.* Washington, DC: American Psychiatric Press; 1994.
6. Filipek PA, Accardo PJ, Baranek GT, Cook EH Jr, Dawson G, Gordon B, et al. The screening and diagnosis of autistic spectrum disorders. *J Autism Dev Disord.* 1999;29:439–484.
7. Filipek PA, Accardo PJ, Ashwal S, Baranek GT, Cook EH Jr. Dawson G, et al. Practice parameter: screening and diagnosis of autism: report of the Quality Standards Subcommittee of the American Academy of Neurology and the Child Neurology Society. *Neurology.* 2000;55:468–479.
8. Hill A, Bolte S, Petrova G, Beltcheva D, Tacheva S, Poustka F. Stability and interpersonal agreement of the interview-based diagnosis of autism. *Psychopathology.* 2001;34:187–191.
9. Lord C, Risi S, Lambrecht L, Cook EH Jr, Leventhal BL, DiLavore PC, et al. The autism diagnostic observation schedule-generic: a standard measure of social and communication deficits associated with the spectrum of autism. *J Autism Dev Disord.* 2000;30:205–223.
10. Femia LA, Yurgelun-Todd DA. Application of MR and its relation to behavioral symptoms in autistic patients.
11. Abell F, Krams M, Ashburner J, Passingham R, Friston K, Frackowiak R, et al. The neuroanatomy of autism: a voxel-based whole brain analysis of structural scans. *Neuroreport.* 1999;10:1647–1651.
12. Aylward EH, Minshew NJ, Goldstein G, Honeycutt NA, Augustine AM, Yates KO, et al. MRI volumes of amygdala and hippocampus in non-mentally retarded autistic adolescents and adults. *Neurology.* 1999;53: 2145–2150.
13. Howard MA, Cowell PE, Boucher J, Broks P, Mayes A, Farrant A, et al. Convergent neuroanatomical and behavioural evidence of an amygdala hypothesis of autism. *Neuroreport.* 2000;11:2931–2935.
14. Sparks B, Friedman SD, Shaw DWW, Aylward E, Echelard D, Artu AA, Maravilla KR, Giedd JN, Munson J, Dawson G, Dager SR. Brain stuctural abnormalities in young children with autism specturm disorder. *Neurology.* 2002;59:184–192.
15. Baron-Cohen S, Ring HA, Wheelwright S, Bullmore ET, Brammer MJ, Simmons A, et al. Social intelligence in the normal and autistic brain: an fMRI study. *Eur J Neurosci.* 1999;11:1891–1898.
16. Critchley HD, Daly EM, Bullmore ET, Williams SC, Van Amelsvoort T, Robertson DM, et al. The functional neuroanatomy of social behaviour: changes in cerebral blood flow when people with autistic disorder process facial expressions. *Brain.* 2000;123:2203–2212.

17. Pierce K, Muller RA, Ambrose J, Allen G, Courchesne E. Face processing occurs outside the fusiform "face area" in autism: evidence from functional MRI. *Brain.* 2001;124:2059–2073.
18. Breiter HC, Gollub RL, Weisskoff RM, Kennedy DN, Makris N, Berke JD, et al. Acute effects of cocaine on human brain activity and emotion. *Neuron.* 1997;19:591–611.
18. Schultz RT, Klin E, Levitan T, Cantey P, Skdlarski P, Gore F, Volkmar R, Cohen DJ. An fMRI study of face recognition, facial expression detection and social judgement in autism spectrum disorders. Paper presented at: International Meeting For Autism Research; 2001; San Diego, CA.
19. Hommer DW. Functional imaging of craving. *Alcohol Res Health.* 1999; 23:187–196.
20. London ED, Bonson KR, Ernst M, Grant S. Brain imaging studies of cocaine abuse: implications for medication development. *Crit Rev Neurobiol.* 1999; 13:227–242.
21. Maas LC, Lukas SE, Kaufman MJ, Weiss RD, Daniels SL, Rogers VW, et al. Functional magnetic resonance imaging of human brain activation during cue-induced cocaine craving. *Am J Psychiatry.* 1998;155:124–126.
22. Wexler BE, Gottschalk CH, Fulbright RK, Prohovnik I, Lacadie CM, Rounsaville BJ, et al. Functional magnetic resonance imaging of cocaine craving. *Am J Psychiatry.* 2001;158:86–95.
23. Li SJ, Biswal B, Li Z, Risinger R, Rainey C, Cho JK, et al. Cocaine administration decreases functional connectivity in human primary visual and motor cortex as detected by functional *MRI. Magn Reson Med.* 2000;43: 45–51.
24. Kaufman MJ, Levin JM, Maas LC, Rose SL, Lukas SE, Mendelson JH, et al. Cocaine decreases relative cerebral blood volume in humans: a dynamic susceptibility contrast magnetic resonance imaging study. *Psychopharmacology (Berl).* 1998b;138:76–81.
25. Kaufman M, Levin J, Mass L. Cocaine-induced cerebral blood volume reduction in women is a function of menstural cycle phase. In: College on Problems of Drug Dependence, Sixtieth Annual Scientific Meeting. Scottsdale, Arizona; 1998.
26. Yurgelun-Todd D, Gruber S, Hanson R, et al. Residual effects of marijuana use: An fMRI study [abstract]. In: College on Problems of Drug Dependence, Sixtieth Annual Scientific Meeting; 1998; Scottsdale, Arizona.
27. Renshaw PF, Yurgelun-Todd DA, Cohen BM. Greater hemodynamic response to photic stimulation in schizophrenic patients: an echo planar MRI study. *Am J Psychiatry.* 1994;151:1493–1495.
28. Schroder J, Wenz F, Schad LR, Baudendistel K, Knopp MV. Sensorimotor cortex and supplementary motor area changes in schizophrenia. A study with functional magnetic resonance imaging. *Br J Psychiatry.* 1995;167: 197–201.
29. Stephan KE, Magnotta VA, White T, Arndt S, Flaum M, O'Leary DS, et al. Effects of olanzapine on cerebellar functional connectivity in schizophrenia measured by fMRI during a simple motor task. *Psychol Med.* 2001; 31:1065–1078.
30. Muller JL, Roder CH, Schuierer G, Klein H. Motor-induced brain activation in cortical, subcortical and cerebellar regions in schizophrenic inpatients. A whole brain fMRI fingertapping study. *Prog Neuropsychopharmacol Biol Psychiatry.* 2002;26:421–426.
31. Braus DF, Ende G, Weber-Fahr W, Sartorius A, Krier A, Hubrich-Ungureanu P, et al. Antipsychotic drug effects on motor activation mea-

sured by functional magnetic resonance imaging in schizophrenic patients. *Schizophr Res.* 1999;39:19–29.

32. Braus DF, Ende G, Hubrich-Ungureanu P, Henn FA. Cortical response to motor stimulation in neuroleptic-naive first episode schizophrenics. *Psychiatry Res.* 2000;98:145–154.
33. Buckley PF, Friedman L, Wu D, Lai S, Meltzer HY, Haacke EM, et al. Functional magnetic resonance imaging in schizophrenia: initial methodology and evaluation of the motor cortex. *Psychiatry Res.* 1997;74:13–23.
34. Yurgelun-Todd DA, Waternaux CM, Cohen BM, Gruber SA, English CD, Renshaw PF. Functional magnetic resonance imaging of schizophrenic patients and comparison subjects during word production. *Am J Psychiatry.* 1996;153:200–205.
35. Sommer IE, Ramsey NF, Kahn RS. Language lateralization in schizophrenia, an fMRI study. *Schizophr Res.* 2001;52:57–67.
36. Kircher TT, Liddle PF, Brammer MJ, Williams SC, Murray RM, McGuire PK. Reversed lateralization of temporal activation during speech production in thought disordered patients with schizophrenia. *Psychol Med.* 2002; 32:439–449.
37. Surguladze SA, Calvert GA, Brammer MJ, Campbell R, Bullmore ET, Giampietro V, et al. Audio-visual speech perception in schizophrenia: an fMRI study. *Psychiatry Res.* 2001;106:1–14.
38. Manoach DS, Press DZ, Thangaraj V, Searl MM, Goff DC, Halpern E, et al. Schizophrenic subjects activate dorsolateral prefrontal cortex during a working memory task, as measured by fMRI. *Biol Psychiatry.* 1999;45: 1128–1137.
39. Callicott JH, Bertolino A, Mattay VS, Langheim FJ, Duyn J, Coppola R, et al. Physiological dysfunction of the dorsolateral prefrontal cortex in schizophrenia revisited. *Cereb Cortex.* 2000;10:1078–1092.
40. Manoach DS, Gollub RL, Benson ES, Searl MM, Goff DC, Halpern E, et al. Schizophrenic subjects show aberrant fMRI activation of dorsolateral prefrontal cortex and basal ganglia during working memory performance. *Biol Psychiatry.* 2000;48:99–109.
41. Manoach DS, Halpern EF, Kramer TS, Chang Y, Goff DC, Rauch SL, et al. Test–retest reliability of a functional MRI working memory paradigm in normal and schizophrenic subjects. *Am J Psychiatry.* 2001;158:955–958.
42. Ramsey NF, Koning HA, Welles P, Cahn W, Van Der Linden JA, Kahn RS. Excessive recruitment of neural systems subserving logical reasoning in schizophrenia. *Brain.* 2002;125:1793–1807.
43. Volz HP, Gaser C, Hager F, Rzanny R, Mentzel HJ, Kreitschmann-Andermahr I, et al. Brain activation during cognitive stimulation with the Wisconsin card sorting test—a functional MRI study on healthy volunteers and schizophrenics. *Psychiatry Res.* 1997;75:145–157.
44. Riehemann S, Volz HP, Stutzer P, Smesny S, Gaser C, Sauer H. Hypofrontality in neuroleptic-naive schizophrenic patients during the Wisconsin Card Sorting Test—a fMRI study. *Eur Arch Psychiatry Clin Neurosci.* 2001;251: 66–71.
45. Volz H, Gaser C, Hager F, Rzanny R, Ponisch J, Mentzel H, et al. Decreased frontal activation in schizophrenics during stimulation with the continuous performance test—a functional magnetic resonance imaging study. *Eur Psychiatry.* 1999;14:17–24.
46. Phillips ML, Williams L, Senior C, Bullmore ET, Brammer MJ, Andrew C, et al. A differential neural response to threatening and non-threatening negative facial expressions in paranoid and non-paranoid schizophrenics. *Psychiatry Res.* 1999;92:11–31.

47. Schneider F, Weiss U, Kessler C, Salloum JB, Posse S, Grodd W, et al. Differential amygdala activation in schizophrenia during sadness. *Schizophr Res.* 1998;34:133–142.
48. Woodruff PW, Wright IC, Bullmore ET, Brammer M, Howard RJ, Williams SC, et al. Auditory hallucinations and the temporal cortical response to speech in schizophrenia: a functional magnetic resonance imaging study. *Am J Psychiatry.* 1997;154:1676–1682.
49. Lawrie SM, Buechel C, Whalley HC, Frith CD, Friston KJ, Johnstone EC. Reduced frontotemporal functional connectivity in schizophrenia associated with auditory hallucinations. *Biol Psychiatry.* 2002;51:1008–1011.
50. Lennox BR, Park SB, Medley I, Morris PG, Jones PB. The functional anatomy of auditory hallucinations in schizophrenia. *Psychiatry Res.* 2000;100:13–20.
51. Gruber S, Rogowska R, Yurgelun-Todd DA. Differential activation of anterior cingulate and prefrontal cortex in schizophrenic and bipolar patients: an fMRI study [abstract]. Colorado Springs, CO; International Congress on Schizophrenic Research: 2003.
52. Curtis VA, Dixon TA, Morris RG, Bullmore ET, Brammer MJ, Williams SC, et al. Differential frontal activation in schizophrenia and bipolar illness during verbal fluency. *J Affect Disord.* 2001;66:111–121.
53. Loeber RT, Sherwood AR, Renshaw PF, Cohen BM, Yurgelun-Todd DA. Differences in cerebellar blood volume in schizophrenia and bipolar disorder. *Schizophr Res.* 1999;37:81–89.
54. Beauregard M, Leroux JM, Bergman S, Arzoumanian Y, Beaudoin G, Bourgouin P, et al. The functional neuroanatomy of major depression: an fMRI study using an emotional activation paradigm. *Neuroreport.* 1998;9: 3253–3258.
55. Kalin NH, Davidson RJ, Irwin W, Warner G, Orendi JL, Sutton SK, et al. Functional magnetic resonance imaging studies of emotional processing in normal and depressed patients: effects of venlafaxine. *J Clin Psychiatry.* 1997;58:32–39.
56. Sheline YI, Barch DM, Donnelly JM, Ollinger JM, Snyder AZ, Mintun MA. Increased amygdala response to masked emotional faces in depressed subjects resolves with antidepressant treatment: an fMRI study. *Biol Psychiatry.* 2001;50:651–658.
57. Siegle GJ, Steinhauer SR, Thase ME, Stenger VA, Carter CS. *Biol Psychiatry.* 2002;51:693–707.
58. Yurgelun-Todd DA, Gruber SA, Kanayama G, Killgore WD, Baird AA, Young AD. fMRI during affect discrimination in bipolar affective disorder. *Bipolar Disord.* 2000;2:237–248.
59. Breiter HC, Rauch SL, Kwong KK, Baker JR, Weisskoff RM, Kennedy DN, et al. Functional magnetic resonance imaging of symptom provocation in obsessive-compulsive disorder. *Arch Gen Psychiatry.* 1996;53:595–606.
60. Adler CM, McDonough-Ryan P, Sax KW, Holland SK, Arndt S, Strakowski SM. fMRI of neuronal activation with symptom provocation in unmedicated patients with obsessive compulsive disorder. *J Psychiatr Res.* 2000; 34:317–324.
61. Phillips ML, Marks IM, Senior C, Lythgoe D, O'Dwyer AM, Meehan O, et al. A differential neural response in obsessive-compulsive disorder patients with washing compared with checking symptoms to disgust. *Psychol Med.* 2000;30:1037–1050.
62. Levine JB, Gruber SA, Baird AA, Yurgelun-Todd D. Obsessive-compulsive disorder among schizophrenic patients: an exploratory study using functional magnetic resonance imaging data. *Compr Psychiatry.* 1998;39:308–311.

63. Kleinginna PR, Kleinginna AM. A categorized list of emtion definitions with suggestions for a consensual definition. *Motiv Emot.* 1981;5:345–379.
64. Camras LA, Oster H, Campos JJ, Miyake K, Bradshaw D. Japanese and American infant's responses to arm restraint. *Dev Psychol.* 1992;28:578–583.
65. Ekman P. Are there basic emotions? *Psychol Rev.* 1992;99:550–553.
66. Ekman P. Strong evidence for universal in facial expressions: a reply to Russell's mistaken critique. *Psychol Bull.* 1994;115:268–287.
67. Ekman P, Davidson RJ, Friesen WV. The Duchenne smile: emotional expression and brain physiology II. *J Pers Soc Psychol.* 1990;58:342–353.
68. Frank MG, Ekman P, Friesen WV. Behavioral markers and recognizability of the smile of enjoyment. *J Pers Soc Psychol.* 1993;64:83–93.
69. Izard CE. Innate and universal facial expressions: evidence from developmental and cross-cultural research. *Psychol Bull.* 1994;115:288–299.
70. Adolphs R, Damasio H, Tranel D, Damasio AR. Cortical systems for the recognition of emotion in facial expressions. *J Neurosci.* 1996;16:7678–7687.
71. Hamann SB, Stefanacci L, Squire LR, Adolphs R, Tranel D, Damasio H, Damasio A. Recognizing facial emotions. *Nature.* 1996;379:497.
72. Breiter HC, Rauch SL, Kwong KK, Baker JR, Weisskoff RM, Kennedy DN, et al. Functional magnetic resonance imaging of symptom provocation in obsessive-compulsive disorder. *Arch Gen Psychiatry.* 1996;53:595–606.
73. Killgore WD, Yurgelun-Todd DA. Sex differences in amygdala activation during the perception of facial affect. *Neuroreport.* 2001;12:2543–2547.
74. Morris JS, Frith CD, Perrett DI, Rowland D, Young AW, Calder AJ, et al. A differential neural response in the human amygdala to fearful and happy facial expressions: Gender differences in mood and cardiovascular responses to socially stressful stimuli. *Nature.* 1996;383:812–815.
75. Morris TL, Masia CL, Bauer TW. Psychometric evaluation of the social phobia and anxiety inventory for children: concurrent validity and normative data. The consequences of a major bile duct injury during laparoscopic cholecystectomy. *J Clin Child Psychol.* 1998;27:452–458.
76. Phillips MD, Phillips ML. Time courses of left and right amygdalar responses to fearful facial expressions. *J Am Board Fam Pract.* 2001;14: 123–130.
77. Phillips EL, Pratt HD. *Indian J Pediatr.* 1998;65:487–494.
78. Phillips ML, Young AW, Senior C, Brammer M, Andrew C, Calder AJ, et al. A specific neural substrate for perceiving facial expressions of disgust. *Am J Clin Hypn.* 1997;40:118–129.
79. Vuilleumier P, Armony JL, Driver J, Dolan RJ. Effects of attention and emotion on face processing in the human brain: an event-related fMRI study. *Neuron.* 2001;30:829–841.
80. Whalen PJ, Rauch SL, Etcoff NL, McInerney SC, Lee MB, Jenike MA. Masked presentations of emotional facial expressions modulate amygdala activity without explicit knowledge. *J Neurosci.* 1998;18:411–418.
81. Aggleton P. Young people, HIV/AIDS and social research. *AIDS Care.* 1992;4:243–244.
82. Davis M. Neurobiology of fear responses: the role of the amygdala. *J Neuropsychiatry Clin Neurosci.* 1997;9:382–402.
83. Davis M, WHalen PJ. The amygdala: vigilance and emotion. *Mol Psychiatry.* 2001;6:12–34.
84. LaBar KS, Gatenby JC, LeDoux JE, Phelps EA. Human amygdala activation during conditioned fear acquisition and extinction: a mixed-trial fMRI study. *Neuron.* 1998;20:937–945.
85. LeDoux G. Fear and the brain: where have we been and where are we going? *Biol Psychiatry.* 1998;44:533–545.

86. Adolphs R, Tranel D, Damasio AR. The human amygdala in social judgement. *Nature.* 1998;393:470–474.
87. Adolphs R. Impaired recognition of emotion in facial expressions following bilateral damage to the human amygdala [see comments]. *J Neuropsychiatry Clin Neurosci.* 1997;9:382–402.
88. Adolphs R. Recognition of facial emotion in nine individuals with bilateral amygdala damage. *Neuropsychologia.* 1999;37:1135–1141.
89. Adolphs R, Tranel D, Damasio H, Damasio AR. Fear and the human amygdala. *J Neurosci.* 1995;15:5879–5891.
90. LeDoux J. Emotional networks and motor control: a fearful view. *Prog Brain Res.* 1996;107:437–446.
91. Garcia RV, RM, Baudry M, Thompson RF. The amygdala modulates prefrontal cortex activity relative to conditioned fear. *Nature.* 1999;402:294–296.
92. Hariri AR, Bookheimer SY, Mazziotta JC. Modulating emotional responses: effects of a neocortical network on the limbic system. *Neuroreport.* 2000;11: 43–48.
93. Ekman P. *Pictures of Facial Affect.* Palo Alto, CA: Consulting Psychologists; 1976.
94. Rubia K, Overmeyer S, Taylor E, Brammer M, Williams SC, Simmons A, et al. Functional frontalisation with age: mapping neurodevelopmental trajectories with fMRI. *Neurosci Biobehav Rev.* 2000;24:13–19.

# 9

# fMRI of Memory in Aging and Dementia

Andrew J. Saykin and Heather A. Wishart

In the human brain, functionally and anatomically defined systems exist for actively encoding, consolidating, and retrieving memories of experiences (episodic memory); accumulating and accessing factual information in a body of knowledge (semantic memory); and processing and manipulating information (working memory). These three declarative memory systems can be distinguished from other nondeclarative memory systems such as procedural learning and priming.[1–4] Brain-behavior studies using a variety of approaches, from lesion-based research to functional magnetic resonance imaging (fMRI), demonstrate distinct, though interrelated, neural circuitry for working, episodic, and semantic memory.[4,5] Each of these three memory systems is affected somewhat differently by aging and dementia. In this chapter, the episodic, semantic, and working memory systems will be considered in turn, with special attention to changes associated with aging and with memory disorders such as Alzheimer's disease and Mild Cognitive Impairment.

## Episodic Memory

Episodic memory refers to memory for events or information encoded with respect to a particular temporal or spatial context.[1] Originally defined to encompass memory for specific information presented, for example, during a testing session, the concept has been reformulated over the years to have at its core the conscious recollection of previous experiences. The emphasis is on memory for experience itself, not knowledge about the world derived from experience.[6] Important distinctions pertaining to episodic memory include the processes or operations that are performed (e.g., novelty versus familiarity discrimination; encoding, consolidation, retrieval); the success with which these processes are performed (i.e., whether they result in the formation of an accurate, inaccurate, or no memory trace); the sensory modality in which the information is received (e.g., auditory, visual); and the nature of the material (e.g., verbal, spatial, pictorial). There are a variety of episodic memory fMRI probes, many of which are designed specifically to address or manipulate certain of these aspects of episodic memory processing; a sample task is shown in Table 9.1.

In general, episodic memory is thought to be subserved by a broad network of brain regions, primarily involving prefrontal and medial temporal circuitry, including the hippocampal formation (dentate gyrus; CA1, CA2, and CA3 fields; and subiculum), entorhinal cortex, perirhinal cortex, parahippocampal complex, and the amygdala.[7–10] Several models of the neural basis of specific episodic memory processes have been proposed. For example, the hippocampal encoding/retrieval (HIPER) model proposes a rostrocaudal gradient of hippocampal activity during encoding and retrieval from episodic memory,[11] although additional data suggest a more complex set of findings regarding hippocampal organization for episodic memory processes.[12,13] According to the hemispheric encoding and retrieval asymmetry (HERA) model, which pertains to the role of prefrontal cortex in memory, left prefrontal regions are involved primarily in retrieval from semantic memory and encoding into episodic memory, and right prefrontal are regions involved in retrieval of information from episodic memory.[9,14,15] This asymmetry is superimposed on a historical, lesion-based, material-specificity model[16] that proposes a left medial temporal specialization for verbal memory and a right medial temporal specialization for nonverbal material that is not readily verbally coded. Early brain insults appear to moderate this model.[17–19] A number of current functional imaging studies focus on the precise roles of medial temporal, frontal and associated parietal, cingulate, thalamic and other areas in specific attentional, learning and memory processes, such as the initiation of retrieval processes, and the evaluation of recovered information.[20–23] For more detail on episodic memory circuitry, the reader is referred to several recent review articles.[9,12,24,25]

## Age Related Changes in Episodic Memory

A large body of literature suggests that episodic memory processes, particularly encoding and retrieval, decline with age.[26–31] Whether this is related to "normal aging" of the brain or to an accumulation of age-related diseases remains a topic of some debate.[32–34] There is some evidence to suggest selective age-related atrophy of prefrontal cortical areas involved in episodic memory circuitry,[35] with relative preservation of medial temporal lobe structures,[35–37] although this too is debatable.[38–40] Furthermore, regenerative processes and reorganization in the adult human brain may help allay development of cognitive problems despite structural brain changes.[41,42] Therefore, significant questions remain as to the neural and cognitive basis of episodic memory decline in aging.

A number of functional neuroimaging, electrophysiological, and behavioral studies suggest that the typical prefrontal functional asymmetries for memory processes in younger adults are diminished or absent in older adults. In other words, research suggests that the HERA

Table 9.1. Sample fMRI Task Characteristics for Episodic, Semantic, and Working Memory

| Study | Memory domain | Cognitive process | Modality | Design | Stimuli[a] | Control condition | Performance monitoring |
|---|---|---|---|---|---|---|---|
| Logan et al., 2002[46] | Episodic memory | Intentional & incidental encoding | Visual | Blocked | Words and faces | Fixation stimulus | Ss completed a recognition test immediately after presentation of the stimuli |
| Saykin et al., 1999[91] | Semantic memory | Category-matching | Auditory | Blocked | Word pairs: category–exemplar pairs (e.g., beverage–milk; vehicle–carrot) and category–function pairs (e.g., beverage–sip, beverage–debate) | Separate phonological task using nonword-matching (e.g., temla–temla; yodb–rea) | Ss pressed a pneumatic bulb in scanner to indicate whether the word pairs matched or not |
| Rypma & D'Esposito, 2000[104] | Working memory | Delayed response | Visual | Event-related | A series of memory sets containing either 2 or 6 stimuli (letters, or objects and locations) were encoded and retained over an unfilled interval | | Ss indicated in scanner whether a single item was or was not part of the memory set just presented |

[a] In all three cases, the different types of stimuli were presented in different runs, e.g., words on one run, faces on another.

model does not hold in normal aging. This concept has been articulated in the Hemispheric Asymmetry Reduction in Old Adults (HAROLD) model.[43] Increased bilateral representation of cognitive functions in older adults may reflect a form of compensatory brain reorganization that helps support normal cognitive function. This would parallel findings on brain functional reorganization following acquired brain damage. For example, in the case of unilateral focal acquired brain damage, recovery of function can be associated with bihemispheric representation (among other types of reorganization) for functions such as language and movement.[44,45] On the other hand, bihemispheric representation simply may reflect diminished selectivity or de-differentiation of the neural substrate of cognition in older adults,[46,47] which may or may not be partly consistent with an interpretation based on compensation, depending on investigators' use of these terms.

A small number of recent fMRI studies speak to the HAROLD model and address issues of compensation versus de-differentiation of the neural substrate of episodic memory in aging. For example, Morcom and colleagues[48] observed overall activation of inferior prefrontal cortex and the hippocampal formation for successful recognition of previously presented words. Activation was relatively left-lateralized in the younger adults, and more bilaterally represented in the older group (Figure 9.1).

Logan and colleagues[46] investigated the brain basis of episodic memory in two fMRI experiments in younger and older adults. Older adults showed less hemispheric asymmetry for intentional encoding of both verbal and nonverbal material, with greater right prefrontal (Brodmann areas 6/44) activation for words, and greater left prefrontal (BA 6/44) activation for face encoding compared to young adults. In

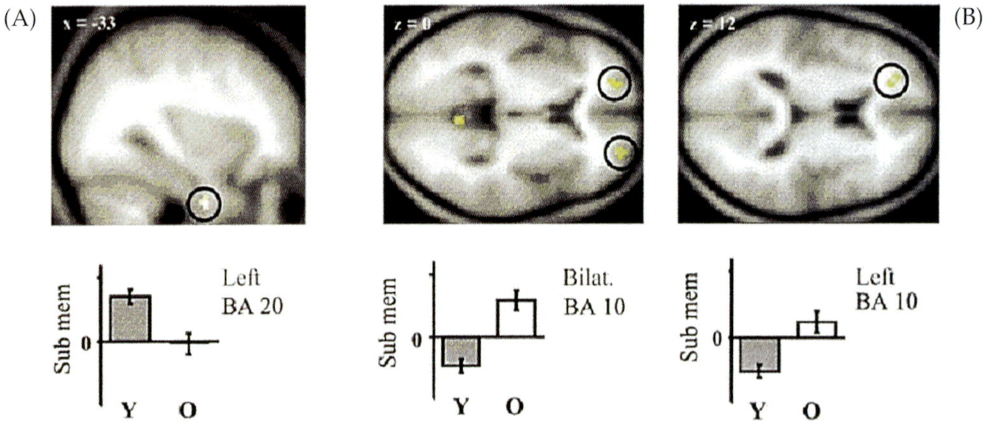


**Figure 9.1.** Brain regions showing age-related differences in activity during successful recognition of previously presented verbal information. Young adults showed greater activation than older adults in left anterior inferior temporal cortex (BA 20) (A). Older adults showed greater activation than young adults in bilateral anterior prefrontal cortex among other regions (B). Reprinted from Morcom AM, Good CD, Frackowiak RS, et al. Age effects on the neural correlates of successful memory encoding. *Brain*. 2003;126(Pt 1):213–229, by permission of Oxford University Press. (Neurologic coordinates)

this study, failure to recruit normal task-related areas did not always occur in conjunction with recruitment of additional brain regions, suggesting that these two types of alteration in brain activity may occur independently in aging. Furthermore, this study provided preliminary evidence that strategy use could overcome the age-related changes in brain activity. During intentional encoding of words, older adults failed to activate a left prefrontal (BA 45/47) region recruited by young adults (Figure 9.2A,B); this is an area thought to be associated with semantic elaboration and successful verbal encoding. However, when supported in the use of deep encoding strategies, activation of this region in older adults approximated that of controls (Figure 9.2C,D). These findings suggest that the regional deficit in activation in older adults during encoding is related to inefficient recruitment of available brain resources, rather than an irreversible loss of the underlying tissue due to cell death or dysfunction.

In a related study, Daselaar and colleagues[49] found that healthy older adults activated mainly left frontotemporal and cingulate areas during deep relative to shallow classification, similar to young adults. However, the older adults showed under-recruitment of left anterior hippocampus relative to the young adults. The authors interpreted this as possible evidence that, despite the capacity to engage brain regions associated with semantic elaboration, age-related impairment of medial temporal system functioning may nonetheless hinder episodic encoding in older adults.

Krause and colleagues[4] reported greater prefrontal connectivity during episodic encoding and retrieval in older adults compared to younger adults on structural equation modeling of fMRI and position emission tomography (PET) data, which lends some further support to the HAROLD model.[50] Furthermore, Krause and colleagues found stronger connectivity involving inferior parietal cortex and less for the hippocampal formation in older compared to younger subjects, consistent with an age-related change in the neural circuitry underlying episodic memory.

Whereas many studies of cognitive aging have used auditory–verbal or spatial stimuli, memory for which generally declines with age, Iidaka and colleagues examined brain activation patterns associated with pictorial memory using fMRI.[51] Based on prior findings that memory for pictures is generally better than memory for words and is relatively preserved in normal aging (especially memory for concrete and meaningful pictorial information), Iidaka and colleagues compared brain activity associated with encoding pairs of concrete-related, concrete-unrelated, and abstract pictures. The concrete-related task made relatively simple cognitive demands (e.g., learning to associate a picture of a cigarette with a picture of an ashtray) and yielded little significant signal change relative to the control condition. The main findings involved the unrelated and abstract pictures. Briefly, both the younger and older participants showed activation of left dorsal prefrontal cortex during encoding of the concrete-unrelated pictures and the abstract pictures. However, compared to the young group, the older adults showed reduced activation in some regions, including right

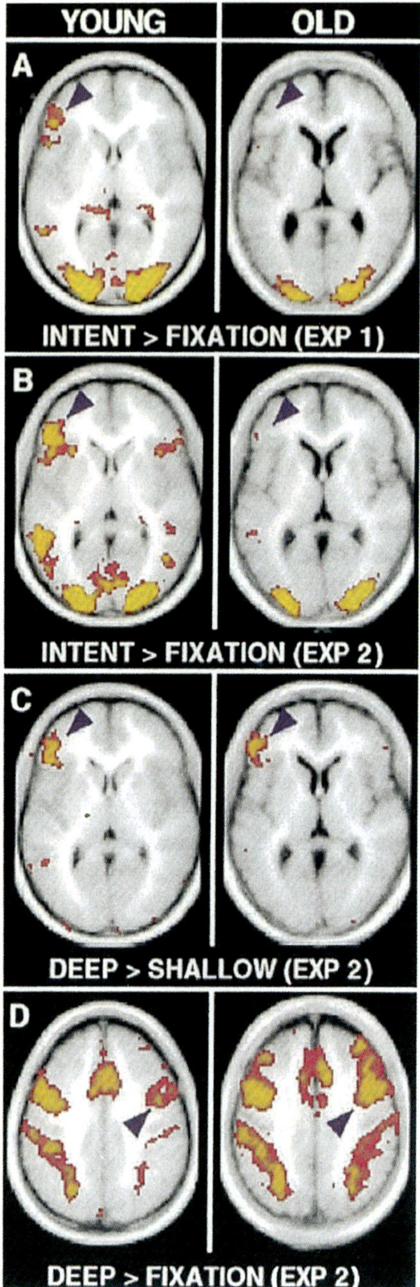


**Figure 9.2.** Brain regions showing age-related differences in activation during encoding of verbal material. Images are presented in neurologic coordinates (left side of brain shown on left side of image), with arrows marking the regions being highlighted. In Experiment 1, young adults showed activation of left BA 45/47 during intentional encoding of words, whereas older adults showed under-recruitment of this region (A). In Experiment 2, this pattern was replicated (B). When older adults were supported in the use of semantic elaboration, under-recruitment of BA 45/47 was reversed (C), but non-selective activation of right BA 6/44 remained (D). Reprinted from Neuron, Vol. 33, Logan JM, Sanders AL, Snyder AZ et al. Under-recruitment and non-selective recruitment: dissociable neural mechanisms associated with aging, 827–840, Copyright © 2002, with permission from Elsevier.

temporo-occipital cortex in the concrete-unrelated condition and bilateral parieto-temporo-occipital areas during abstract picture encoding. There were no regions in which older adults showed greater signal change than controls, providing no evidence of compensatory processing or de-differentiation in the older group, possibly related to the relatively preserved figural recall performance of the older adults on baseline cognitive testing.

In an fMRI study of remote memory in older adults, Haist and colleagues[52] suggested a preferential role for the entorhinal cortex in consolidation of memory over decades. They presented eight older adults with pictures of famous faces from each decade from the 1940s to the 1990s and compared the brain activity to activation patterns for nonfamous faces from the present and the past. While the hippocampus was activated during recognition of the more recent famous faces, parahippocampal activity was present for famous faces from several of the recent and past decades, and right entorhinal activation appeared to be associated with memory for faces extending up to two decades back in time. Although the finding was preliminary, the authors interpreted it as consistent with evidence that damage to the CA1 hippocampal subfield results in a retrograde amnesia of a few years, whereas more-extensive temporal lobe involvement causes a longer period of retrograde amnesia. It is noteworthy that lesion studies typically have reported widespread temporal lobe damage in cases of pronounced retrograde amnesia.[53,54]

In a study of real autobiographical event memories acquired over decades, Maguire and Frith[55] found that younger and older adults activated a similar broad network of regions with one key difference—whereas the younger participants activated the left hippocampus during retrieval, older participants activated the hippocampus bilaterally. This additional hippocampal recruitment was evident despite preserved performance in both groups and was specific to the autobiographical event memories. The authors discuss possible explanations for the finding, including possible increased salience of the spatial context for the memories in the older adults, the fact that older adults have accrued more memories that need to be distinguished, and the possibility that the right hippocampus activated as a compensatory mechanism.

Small and colleagues have used a blood oxygenation level-dependent (BOLD) fMRI signal obtained at rest to estimate regional basal metabolism and examine the integrity of hippocampal subregions in healthy controls and individuals with dementia.[56,57] This method rests on the assumption that basal deoxyhemoglobin levels reflect hemodynamic variables, such as oxygen extraction, that are related to basal metabolism. Using this method, Small examined hippocampal circuitry in 70 individuals ranging in age from 20 to 88 years. In two hippocampal subregions, the subiculum and the dentate gyrus, decline in resting BOLD fMRI signal appeared to occur as a linear function of age. However, decline in the entorhinal cortex was more variable, present only in a subset of older adults. This was interpreted as

relative to age-matched controls. Within the patient group, interindividual variations in frontal activity were related to hippocampal volume. Patients with greater preservation of the hippocampus showed greater activity in bilateral prefrontal regions. This is consistent with the notion that medial temporal and frontal regions form an integrated circuitry subserving episodic memory, and that damage in one part of the circuitry may be reflected in altered activation of other regions. Corkin[73] also found that frontal activation during retrieval was related to the success with which older adults, regardless of whether or not they had AD, recognized previously presented pictures. Position emission tomography (PET) studies provide related data; for example, in one study, patients with mild AD showed reduced functional connectivity of frontal, hippocampal, and other regions during a face-recognition memory task.[77]

Evidence is emerging that functional neuroimaging is sensitive to the earliest stages of dementia before the clinical symptoms of AD or MCI are evident.[78] Bookheimer and colleagues[79] examined cognitively intact, middle-aged to older individuals who were at risk for AD by virtue of their genetic [apolipoprotein E (ApoE) ε4] status. Although not a valid clinical predictor at the individual level, there is a clear correlation between presence of the ε4 allele and likelihood of developing AD.[80] Bookheimer and colleagues found increased intensity and spatial extent of activation in temporal, parietal, and prefrontal regions during episodic encoding and retrieval in individuals who were ε4 positive compared to those without the ε4 allele (Figure 9.4). Baseline activation patterns predicted memory decline over the next two years. The fact that these individuals were recruiting broader areas of brain tissue to accomplish the episodic memory task suggests that changes in activation may occur very early during the course of memory disorders such as AD. These changes may play a compensatory role and may represent an early marker for subsequent cognitive decline. Some of the same researchers reported no differences between ε4 positive and negative groups in fMRI brain activation patterns on an attention/working memory task.[81] This was interpreted as evidence that compensatory brain activation in ε4 carriers is specific to the episodic memory system.

Daselaar and colleagues[82] examined activation patterns associated with successful recognition of incidentally encoded words in healthy adult males. Young adults with normal memory were compared with two older groups, one cognitively intact and the other with mildly impaired memory. During successful encoding, the younger group showed significantly more left anterior medial temporal lobe activation than the older adults with reduced memory, but did not significantly differ from the older adults with normal memory.

Grön and colleagues[83] examined fMRI patterns of brain activity in older adults presenting for first-time medical evaluation of subjective memory complaints. After comprehensive assessment, twelve individuals were diagnosed with probable AD and twelve with major depression. These participants were compared to twelve healthy older adults without cognitive complaints. In general, those participants who were

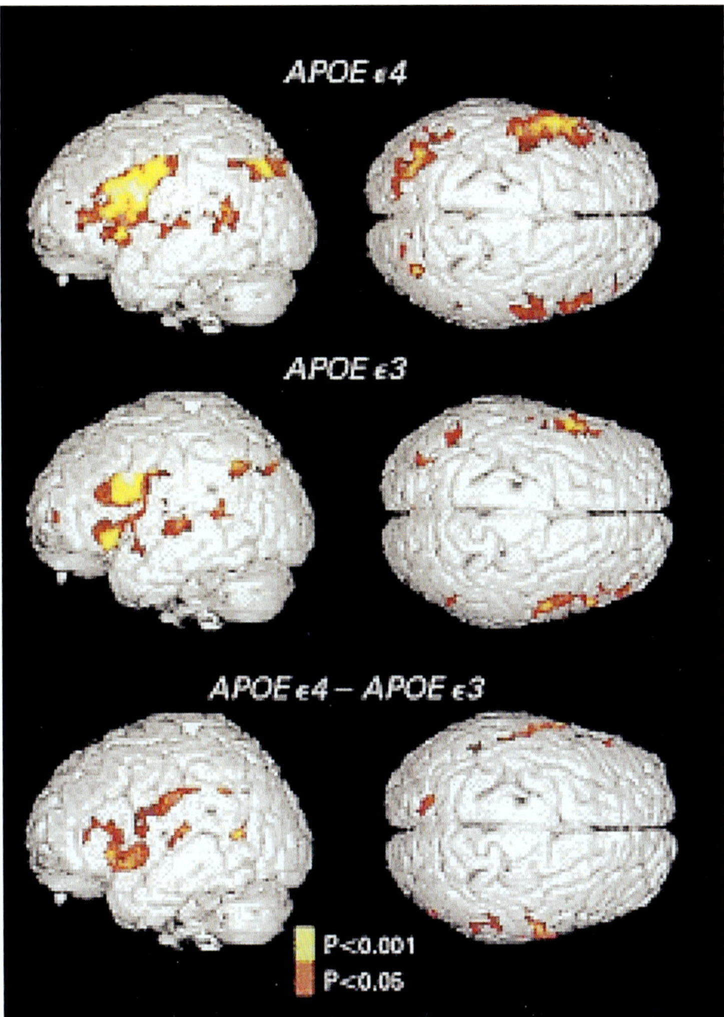


**Figure 9.4.** Brain activation patterns associated with learning and recall in individuals with increased genetic risk for AD (ApoE ε4 carriers) compared to ApoE ε3 carriers. Both groups showed increased activation in left inferior frontal cortex, right prefrontal cortex, transverse temporal gyri bilaterally, left posterior temporal, and inferior parietal regions during learning or recall compared to rest, as shown in the top two panels. However, the intensity and spatial extent of activation was greater in those with the ε4 allele (bottom panel). Reprinted with permission from Bookheimer SY, Strojwas MH, Cohen MS, et al. Patterns of brain activation in people at risk for Alzheimer's disease. *N Engl J Med*. 2000;343(7):450–456. Copyright © 2000 Massachusetts Medical Society. All rights reserved.

diagnosed with AD showed reduced hippocampal activation during episodic memory processing relative to either of the other groups. Increased bilateral prefrontal activity also was seen in the AD patients, consistent with possible attempted compensatory recruitment or de-differentiation.

In a preliminary study of seven patients with mild AD, Rombouts and colleagues recently investigated the effects of rivastigmine, a cholinesterase inhibitor, on brain activity patterns during episodic memory performance (and working memory, as described below).[84] A single dose of the medication led to a bilateral increase in activation in the fusiform gyrus during face encoding. This suggests that rivastigmine affects activity in regions associated with cholingeric circuitry, and that fMRI may be useful in monitoring treatment effects in AD, MCI, and other disorders.

Together, these studies suggest that fMRI is sensitive to preclinical and very early clinical stages of AD and may be useful in early diagnosis, prognosis, and treatment monitoring. Functional MRI may be able to assist in determining whether a drug is effective and the mechanisms by which its effects occur.

## Semantic Memory

Semantic memory is broadly defined as knowledge about the world and includes the set of ideas, words, and symbols that generally are shared by individuals within a culture. Unlike episodic memories, semantic memories are not context dependent. For example, remembering the movie you saw last week depends on episodic memory, but remembering the meaning of the word "movie" depends on semantic memory. As might be expected given the rich associative and inferential processes that can be invoked for the recollection of even simple factual information and words, studies of semantic memory suggest a broad-based neural circuitry, including prominent involvement of several left-hemisphere regions.[9,85] A sample fMRI measure of semantic memory is presented in Table 9.1.

### Semantic Memory in Aging and Dementia

The core component of semantic memory, as reflected by knowledge (crystallized intellect), is thought to be preserved and possibly enhanced during aging, at least under favorable conditions of aging.[34,86] However, the efficiency and accuracy with which information is retrieved from semantic memory can be affected.[87–89] Very little fMRI research on semantic memory in aging and dementia has been conducted to date. Johnson and colleagues[90] examined the relation between age-related whole brain atrophy and brain activation patterns on category-matching fMRI tasks. Across the entire sample, the semantic task activated mainly left superior temporal and bilateral inferior frontal regions, left more than right, likely related to both the semantic and the auditory demands of the task. There were only small group differences in brain activity, with slightly but not significantly greater precentral activation in the younger compared to older adults. The older adults showed global brain atrophy relative to the younger adults, but degree of atrophy was unrelated to BOLD signal on the semantic task. These findings suggest that cognitively intact younger and older adults activate similar brain regions when performing semantic memory operations despite the presence of age-related brain atrophy.

Like episodic memory, semantic memory is affected in AD, although the more profound changes typically occur later in the disease course. Eventually profound deficits in identification and knowledge can emerge.[32] Using fMRI, Saykin and colleagues[91] demonstrated that two semantic category-matching tasks activated left lateral prefrontal and temporal regions, whereas a phonologic control task activated only temporal areas. In patients with mild AD, the spatial extent of left frontal activation on the semantic task was greater than in elderly controls, although accuracy was lower in the patient group. Figure 9.5 shows a surface render of brain activation during semantic decision making for category–function pairs (e.g., match: beverage–sip; mismatch: vehicle–sip). Furthermore, the expanded spatial extent of frontal activation within the patient group was correlated directly with the extent of atrophy in that frontal region.[92] This finding offered preliminary fMRI-based support for the compensatory recruitment hypothesis in semantic memory in AD, suggesting that increased brain activation may help offset disease-related structural changes in the brain, although other reasons for the alterations in brain activation also are possible.

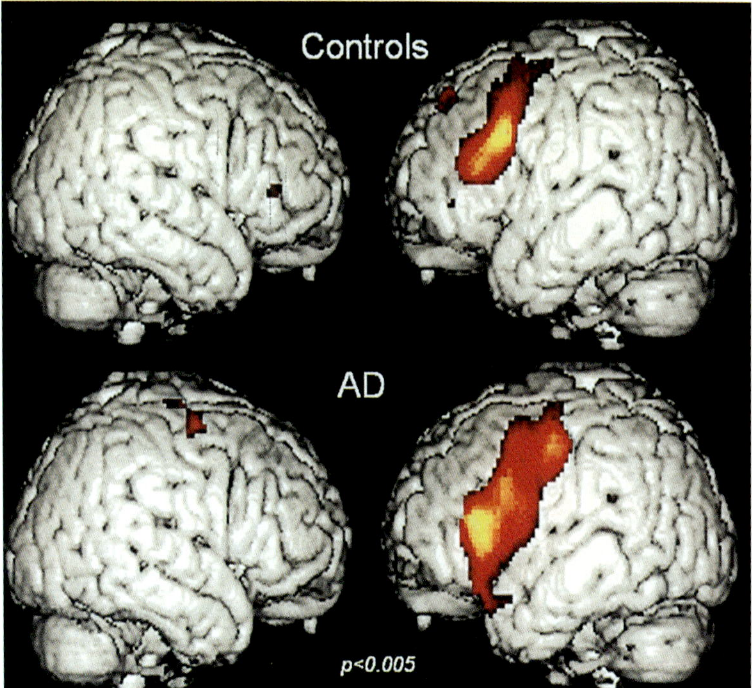


**Figure 9.5.** Surface render of fMRI brain activation during semantic decision making (match versus mismatch) for category–function pairs (e.g., beverage–sip, vehicle–sip). Upper panel is activation for the healthy elderly control group; bottom panel is mild Alzheimer's disease group. Note the expanded spatial extent of activation in the patient group in the left frontal region. Based on further analysis of data published in Saykin AJ, Flashman LA, Frutiger S, et al. Neuroanatomic substrates of semantic memory impairment in Alzheimer's Disease: Patterns of functional MRI activation. *J Int Neurophyschol Soc*. 1999;5:377–392.

Smith and colleagues[93] reported reduced brain activation in inferotemporal regions bilaterally during language tasks in individuals at risk for AD by virtue of their family history and ApoE status. The reduction was present despite the fact that these individuals were cognitively intact at the time of the study, suggesting that subclinical changes are evident in the brain before the onset of symptoms of AD. It is interesting to compare the Smith finding of reduced activation during language tasks in an at-risk sample to the Bookheimer[79] at-risk study, which found an increase in extent of activation during episodic memory. Despite the variability across early studies, the combination of genetic, family history, neuroimaging, and other test data may enhance prediction of risk for AD, and thereby increase the potential to target early intervention appropriately.

## Working Memory

Working memory can be defined as the means by which small amounts of information are maintained in active stores while other cognitive operations are performed. These other operations may include language comprehension, problem solving, and memory encoding, and the ability to hold information in working memory is fundamental to executing these other cognitive processes efficiently and accurately.[2,3,94] According to Baddeley and colleagues, the working memory system has a central executive that, together with an episodic buffer, allocates limited attentional resources to separate subsystems for verbal and nonverbal information.[2,3,95] For a review of models of working memory, see Becker[96] and Baddeley.[3]

Working memory is subserved by a broad network of brain areas, including prefrontal and parietal regions, with greater left lateralization for processing of verbal information and right lateralization for spatial information.[9,97] It has been proposed that there are also separate although overlapping neural representations for visual working memory processes associated with spatial (where) information versus object (what) information. This is analogous to the dissociation in the visual system between dorsal occipitoparietal pathways thought to be involved in the processing of spatial locations and relations among objects and the ventral occipitotemporal pathways that are involved in the processing of the perceptual characteristics that are important for recognition of objects.[98,99] Other conceptualizations hold that it is the type of processing rather than type of information that is related to a dorsal/ventral division of activity during working memory.[97] Various working memory fMRI probes contrast or emphasize different processing demands; a sample task is presented in Table 9.1.

### Working Memory in Aging and Dementia

Behavioral studies indicate age-related changes in working memory,[100,101] and additional changes are seen in AD,[102] although as yet there is a relatively small body of research in this area. There are age-associated structural changes in prefrontal cortex,[35] and AD is associated with diffuse cortical atrophy by later stages of the disease. In the context of these behavioral and structural changes involving working memory circuitry, a small number of studies have used PET[103] and fMRI to examine brain activity associated with working memory in older adults with and without dementia.

Rypma and D'Esposito[104] examined working memory-related brain activity in younger and older adults in three experiments using a delayed-response paradigm. An age-related difference in brain activity was found in a dorsolateral but not ventrolateral prefrontal region of interest, with greater activity in the dorsolateral region during retrieval in younger adults. In addition, speed of processing was related differentially to dorsolateral prefrontal cortical activity in the two age groups. Younger subjects with rapid responding showed less dorsolateral prefrontal cortical activity than younger subjects with slow responses. That pattern was reversed in the older group. Overall, these findings suggest a role for dorsolateral prefrontal cortex in age-related changes in working memory. A subsequent study by Rypma and colleagues using a similar paradigm also showed age-related differences in activity of dorsal, but not ventral, prefrontal cortex.[105] In addition, greater rostral prefrontal cortex activation was evident in the older adults. In a preliminary study, Wishart, Saykin, and colleagues also observed decreased activity in dorsolateral prefrontal cortex in healthy older adults relative to younger controls on a working memory fMRI task, suggesting a different pattern of activity as a function of age.[106] Increased activity was seen in posterior frontal and cerebellar regions. These alterations in activation were related directly to extent of gray matter loss on voxel-based morphometry.[106]

Age-related differences in activity of working memory circuitry may underlie the fact that sentence comprehension declines with age.[107] Using a sentence-comprehension task, Grossman and colleagues demonstrated that older participants showed less left parietal activity than younger adults. However, the older group also showed increases in activity in right inferior parietal, right posterolateral temporal, and left premotor cortex, as well as dorsal portions of left inferior frontal cortex. These findings were interpreted as evidence of upregulation of working memory circuitry in the older adults in order to achieve a level of sentence comprehension that was equivalent to that of the younger adults.[107]

Motivated by findings that estrogen may positively affect brain structure and function, Shawitz and colleagues[108] used fMRI to examine effects of estrogen treatment on brain activity during verbal and nonverbal working memory in a randomized, double-blind, placebo-controlled, cross-over study involving 46 women (aged 33 to 61 years). Treatment with estrogen did not improve the women's performance on working memory tasks, but did lead to alterations in brain activity, some of which were interpreted as consistent with a sharpening of the HERA effect; that is, greater left hemispheric activity was seen during encoding and greater right hemispheric activity was seen during retrieval when the women were on active treatment compared to placebo. In a subsequent study by members of this team, the data from the treatment phase were analyzed further to examine age and performance effects.[94] Using a partial least-squares approach, age-related declines in brain activity were noted in anterior frontal cortex for all three working memory processes studied (encoding, rehearsal, and retrieval). Age-related deficiencies in hippocampal activation also have been demonstrated for feature binding in working memory, the process whereby individual elements of experience are bound together.[109]

In a study comparing patients with AD to individuals with early frontotemporal dementia (FTD) on a working memory task, both groups showed activation of frontal, parietal, and thalamic regions.[110] However, patients with FTD showed less frontal and parietal activation and greater cerebellar activation than those with AD. The authors suggested that fMRI may be useful for differentiating AD and FTD early in the disease course, even when the structural MRI is normal.

Rombouts and colleagues[84] recently examined the effect of cholinergic enhancement on brain activity during working memory in a preliminary sample of patients with mild AD. After a single dose of rivastigmine, activity in prefrontal cortex was enhanced during the basic working memory condition. When the working memory demands were increased, both increases and decreases in activation in different regions were seen. As described above in the *Episodic Memory* section of this chapter, these investigators also found increased brain activity with medication on an episodic memory task. In the first controlled study of its kind (to our knowledge), our group also observed increased prefrontal activity during a working memory task in patients with MCI after short-term treatment with donepezil, another cholinesterase inhibitor.[111]

Overall, the findings point to age-related changes in activity of working memory circuitry, largely characterized by declines in prefrontal and hippocampal regions. However, there is also initial fMRI evidence that upregulation of working memory circuitry may help maximize cognitive function in normal aging,[107] as well as evidence from PET that patients with AD show increased activity in frontal regions relative to controls that could reflect compensatory processing.[103] The Rombouts[112] and Saykin[111] studies indicate the relevance of fMRI for determining the brain regions in which a medication exerts its effects. In addition to clarifying the mechanism of action of psychoactive medications, fMRI may be useful when employed before and after drug treatment to monitor efficacy.

## Methodological Issues in the Use of fMRI in Aging and Dementia Research

A number of methodological considerations must be addressed when conducting and interpreting fMRI research in aging and dementia. For example, there is evidence to suggest that normal aging affects some aspects of the coupling of the hemodynamic response with neural activity. Using a simple reaction time task (one known to evoke similar electrical potentials in young and old adults), D'Esposito and colleagues found in excess of four times more activated voxels in sensorimotor cortex in young than older participants.[113] Other aspects of the hemodynamic response, such as the shape of the curve and the within-group variance, did not significantly differ as a function of age. In contrast, Huettel and colleagues found age differences in the shape of the hemodynamic response, its within-group variability, and the number of activated voxels on a visual task.[114] The younger adults showed a later time to peak, less variability, and twice as many activated voxels as the older adults, although both groups activated similar regions of visual cortex.[114] Age-related prolongation of the time lag in signal change on fMRI also has been reported.[115] Other groups have observed smaller areas[116,117] or larger areas[118] of activation in older adults compared to younger individuals, or no significant differences between groups.[90] Buckner and colleagues observed similar summation of the hemodynamic response across brain regions examined with their sensorimotor task and suggested that even if absolute measurement differences exist between age groups, there should be preservation of relative task-related changes in activation.[119] These issues indicate the need for sophisticated experimental design, post processing, and interpretation of fMRI data in aging research to ensure that reported findings are not spurious effects of basic physiological or artifactual signal differences between young and older groups.

Further technical and scientific issues are encountered when using fMRI to study patients with dementia. Currently, the conditions and importance of alterations in brain activity in individuals with AD are not well understood. For example, does increased activation in patients relative to controls reflect compensation, de-differentiation, or both? If patients perform abnormally on an activation task, how should the resulting activation maps be compared to those of controls? How should atrophy and lesions be taken into account when analyzing and interpreting fMRI data? Approaches that integrate structural neuroimaging, carefully designed activation tasks, and close monitoring of in-scanner mentation and task performance will likely help address such questions.[68] When studying memory, issues related to signal dropout in memory-relevant regions also must be considered.[13]

## Conclusion

Of the three memory systems examined in this chapter, episodic memory has been the most studied using fMRI to date. Although limited largely to cross-sectional data, fMRI research indicates age-related changes in episodic memory circuitry. Reduced prefrontal asymmetry, greater prefrontal connectivity, and altered frontotemporal interaction are observed during episodic memory processing in older adults compared to younger adults. These changes may be a direct effect of structural changes in the aging brain and also may reflect age-related differences in cognitive strategy or approach to the tasks. In individuals with AD, further reductions are seen in hippocampal activity during episodic encoding and in prefrontal cortex activity during episodic retrieval.

Functional MRI research on working memory suggests age-related declines in prefrontal and hippocampal activity. However, there is also evidence to suggest that increased activity of regions within working memory circuitry may occur and help support normal to near-normal functioning in older age despite the presence of structural changes in the brain. Very little fMRI research has been done on semantic memory, which is relatively preserved in aging and in the earliest stages of AD. Two studies by the authors' group suggest that during semantic memory processing, (a) younger and older adults activate similar circuitry, and (b) mild AD patients show an expanded recruitment and/or shifted activation pattern. However, there are as yet too few studies in AD or at-risk groups to make any definitive statements regarding semantic memory-related activation.

Despite significant technical challenges, research using fMRI and other neuroimaging techniques is advancing knowledge of the different effects of aging and dementia on memory systems in the brain. These techniques have major potential implications for early detection of dementia and treatment monitoring, especially if used in combination with genetic testing and emerging PET-based methods for in vivo detection of the neurofibrillary tangles and amyloid plaques of AD.[120–122] Early detection and treatment monitoring are especially important at this time because medications that slow the progression of cognitive decline are available and other treatments, including vaccines, are under development.[120]

## Acknowledgments

The authors wish to thank Heather S. Pixley, Jennifer S. Randolph, Tara McHugh, and Alex Dominguez for their assistance.

## References

1. Tulving E, Donaldson W. *The Organization of Memory.* New York: Academic Press; 1972.
2. Baddeley A. Working Memory. In: Gazzaniga MS, editor. *The Cognitive Neurosciences.* Cambridge, MA: MIT Press; 1995.
3. Baddeley A. Recent developments in working memory. *Curr Opin Neurobiol.* 1998;8(2):234–238.
4. Krause JB, Taylor JG, Schmidt D, et al. Imaging and neural modeling in episodic and working memory processes. *Neural Netw.* 2000;13(8–9): 847–859.
5. Nyberg L, Marklund P, Persson J, et al. Common prefrontal activations during working memory, episodic memory, and semantic memory. *Neuropsychologia.* 2003;41:371–377.
6. Tulving E, Markowitsch HJ. Episodic and declarative memory: role of the hippocampus. *Hippocampus.* 1998;8(3):198–204.
7. Braak H, Braak E, Yilmazer D, et al. Functional anatomy of human hippocampal formation and related structures. *J Child Neurol.* 1996;11(4): 265–275.
8. Van Hoesen GW. Anatomy of the medial temporal lobe. *Magn Reson Imaging.* 1995;13(8):1047–1055.

9. Cabeza R, Nyberg L. Imaging cognition II: An empirical review of 275 PET and fMRI studies. *J Cogn Neurosci.* 2000;12(1):1–47.
10. Desgranges B, Baron JC, Eustache F. The functional neuroanatomy of episodic memory: The role of the frontal lobes, the hippocampal formation, and other areas. *Neuroimage.* 1998;8:198–213.
11. Lepage M, Habib R, Tulving E. Hippocampal PET activations of memory encoding and retrieval: The HIPER model. *Hippocampus.* 1998;8:313–322.
12. Schacter DL, Wagner AD. Medial temporal lobe activations in fMRI and PET studies of episodic encoding and retrieval. *Hippocampus.* 1999;9(1): 7–24.
13. Greicius MD, Krasnow B, Boyett-Anderson JM, et al. Regional analysis of hippocampal activation during memory encoding and retrieval: fMRI study. *Hippocampus.* 2003;13:164–174.
14. Tulving E, Kapur S, Craik FI, et al. Hemispheric encoding/retrieval asymmetry in episodic *memory*: Positron emission tomography findings. *Proc Natl Acad Sci USA.* 1994;91(6):2016–2020.
15. Nyberg L, Cabeza R, Tulving E. PET studies of encoding and retrieval: The HERA Model. *Psychol Bull Rev.* 1996;3:135–148.
16. Milner B. Psychological aspects of focal epilepsy and its neurosurgical management. *Adv Neurol* 1975;8:299–321.
17. Saykin AJ, Gur RC, Sussman NM, et al. Memory deficits before and after temporal lobectomy: Effect of laterality and age of onset. *Brain Cogn.* 1989;9:191–200.
18. Saykin AJ, Robinson LJ, Stafiniak P, et al. Neuropsychological effects of temporal lobectomy: Acute changes in memory, language, and music. In: Bennett T, editor. *Neuropsychology of Epilepsy.* New York: Plenum Press; 1992.
19. Hermann BP, Seidenberg M, Haltiner A, et al. Relationship of age at onset, chronologic age, and adequacy of preoperative performance to verbal memory change after anterior temporal lobectomy. *Epilepsia.* 1995;36(2): 137–145.
20. Cabeza R, Dolcos F, Prince SE, et al. Attention-related activity during episodic memory retrieval: a cross-function fMRI study. *Neuropsychologia.* 2003;41:390–399.
21. Dobbins IG, Rice HJ, Wagner AD, et al. Memory orientation and success: separable neurocognitive components underlying episodic recognition. *Neuropsychologia.* 2003;41(3):318–333.
22. Rugg MD, Henson RN, Robb WG. Neural correlates of retrieval processing in the prefrontal cortex during recognition and exclusion tasks. *Neuropsychologia.* 2003;41(1):40–52.
23. Ranganath C, Johnson MK, D'Esposito M. Prefontal activity associated with working memory and episodic long-term memory. *Neuropsychologia.* 2003;41:378–389.
24. Wagner AD, Koutstaal W, Schacter DL. When encoding yields remembering: insights from event-related neuroimaging. *Philos Trans R Soc London B Biol Sci.* 1999;354(1387):1307–1324.
25. Fletcher PC, Frith CD, Rugg MD. The functional neuroanatomy of episodic memory. *Trends Neurosci.* 1997;20(5):213–218.
26. Nyberg L, Backman L, Erngrund K, et al. Age differences in episodic memory, semantic memory, and priming: relationships to demographic, intellectual, and biological factors. *J Gerontol B Psychol Sci Soc Sci.* 1996; 51(4):234–240.
27. Park DC, Smith AD, Lautenschlager G, et al. Mediators of long-term memory performance across the lifespan. *Psychol Aging.* 1996;11:621–637.

28. Anderson ND, Craik FIM. Memory in the aging brain. In: Tulving E, Craik FIM, editors. *The Oxford Handbook of Memory.* New York: Oxford; 2000:411–425.
29. Balota DA, Dolan PO, Duchek JM. Memory changes in healthy older adults. In: Tulving E, Craik FIM, editors. *The Oxford Handbook of Memory.* New York: Oxford; 2000:395–409.
30. Grady C, Craik FI. Changes in memory processing with age. *Curr Opin Neurobiol.* 2000;10:224–231.
31. Zacks RT, Hasher L, Li KZH. Human memory. In: Craik FIM, Salthouse TA, editors. *The Handbook of Aging and Cognition.* Mahwah, NJ: Erlbaum; 1999:200–230.
32. Flashman LA, Wishart HA, Saykin AJ. Boundaries between normal aging and dementia: Perspectives from neuropsychological and neuroimaging investigations. In: Emory VOB, Oxman TE, editors. *Dementia: Presentations, Differential Diagnosis and Nosology.* 2nd ed. Baltimore, MD: Johns Hopkins University Press; 2003:3–30.
33. Schroots JJF, Birren JE. Theoretical issues and basic questions in the planning of longitudinal studies of health and aging. In: Schroots JJF, editor. *Aging, Health and Competence: The Next Generation of Longitudinal Studies.* Amsterdam: Elsevier; 1993:4–34.
34. Baltes PB. The aging mind: potential and limits. *Gerontologist.* 1993;33(5): 580–594.
35. Raz N, Gunning FM, Head D, et al. Selective aging of the human cerebral cortex observed in vivo: Differential vulnerability of the prefrontal gray matter. *Cereb Cortex.* 1997;7(3):268–282.
36. Bigler ED, Blatter DD, Anderson CV, et al. Hippocampal volume in normal aging and traumatic brain injury. *AJNR Am J Neuroradiol.* 1997; 18(1):11–23.
37. DeCarli C, Murphy DG, Gillette JA, et al. Lack of age-related differences in temporal lobe volume of very healthy adults. *AJNR Am J Neuroradiol.* 1994;15(4):689–696.
38. Greenwood PM. The frontal aging hypothesis evaluated. *J Int Neuropsychol Soc.* 2000;6:705–726.
39. West R. In defense of the frontal lobe hypothesis of cognitive aging. *J Int Neuropsychol Soc.* 2000;6:727–729.
40. Greenwood PM. Reply to West. *J Int Neuropsychol. Soc.* 2000;6:730.
41. Kempermann G, Gage FH. New nerve cells for the adult brain. *Sci Am.* 1999;280:48–53.
42. Reuter-Lorenz PA, Stanczak L, Miller AC. Neural recruitment and cognitive aging: Two hemispheres are better than one, especially as you age. *Psychol Sci.* 1999;10(6):494–500.
43. Cabeza R. Hemispheric asymmetry reduction in old adults: The HAROLD model. *Psychol Aging.* 2002;17:85–100.
44. Muller RA, Rothermel RD, Behen ME, et al. Differential patterns of language and motor reorganization following early left hemisphere lesion: a PET study. *Arch Neurol.* 1998;55(8):1113–1119.
45. Fawcett JW, Rosser AE, Dunnett SB. *Brain Damage, Brain Repair.* New York: Oxford U.P; 2001.
46. Logan JM, Sanders AL, Snyder AZ, et al. Under-recruitment and nonselective recruitment: dissociable neural mechanisms associated with aging. *Neuron.* 2002;33(5):827–840.
47. Cabeza R, Anderson ND, Locantore JK, et al. Aging gracefully: Compensatory brain activity in high-performing older adults. *Neuroimage.* 2002; 17:1394–1402.

48. Morcom AM, Good CD, Frackowiak RS, et al. Age effects on the neural correlates of successful memory encoding. *Brain.* 2003;126(Pt 1):213–229.
49. Daselaar SM, Veltman DJ, Rombouts SARB, Raaijmakers JG, Jonker C. Deep processing activated the medial temporal lobe in young but not old adults. *Neurobiol Aging.* 2003;24(7):1005–1011.
50. Cabeza R, Grady CL, Nyberg L, et al. Age-related differences in neural activity during memory encoding and retrieval: A positron emission tomography study. *J Neurosci.* 1997;17(1):391–400.
51. Iidaka T, Sadato N, Yamada H, et al. An fMRI study of the functional neuroanatomy of picture encoding in younger and older adults. *Cogn Brain Res.* 2001;11(1):1–11.
52. Haist F, Bowden Gore J, Mao H. Consolidation of human memory over decades revealed by functional magnetic resonance imaging. *Nature Neurosci.* 2001;4(11):1139–1145.
53. Kapur N. Focal retrograde amnesia in neurological disease: a critical review. *Cortex.* 1993;29(2):217–234.
54. Kapur N, Ellison D, Smith MP, et al. Focal retrograde amnesia following bilateral temporal lobe pathology. A neuropsychological and magnetic resonance study. *Brain.* 1992;115(Pt 1):73–85.
55. Maguire EA, Frith C. Aging affects the engagement of the hippocampus during autobiographical memory retrieval. *Brain.* 2003;126:1511–1523.
56. Small SA, Tsai WY, DeLaPaz R, et al. Imaging hippocampal function across the human life span: is memory decline normal or not? *Ann Neurol.* 2002;51(3):290–295.
57. Small SA, Wu EX, Bartsch D, et al. Imaging physiologic dysfunction of individual hippocampal subregions in humans and genetically modified mice. *Neuron.* 2000;28(3):653–664.
58. American Psychiatric Association. *Diagnostic and Statistical Manual of Mental Disorders.* (IV ed.). Washington DC: American Psychiatric Press; 1994.
59. Braak H, Braak E, Bohl J. Staging of Alzheimer-related cortical destruction. *Eur Neurol.* 1993;33(6):403–408.
60. de Leon MJ, Convit A, DeSanti S, et al. The hippocampus in aging and Alzheimer's disease. *Neuroimaging Clin N Am.* 1995;5(1):1–17.
61. de Leon MJ, Convit A, George AE, et al. In vivo structural studies of the hippocampus in normal aging and in incipient Alzheimer's disease. *Ann N Y Acad Sci.* 1996;777:1–13.
62. Jack CR, Jr., Petersen RC, O' Brien PC, et al. MR-based hippocampal volumetry in the diagnosis of Alzheimer's disease. *Neurology.* 1992;42(1):183–188.
63. Petersen RC, Doody R, Kurz A, et al. Current concepts in Mild Cognitive Impairment. *Arch Neurol.* 2001;58(12):1985–1992.
64. Petersen RC. Aging, mild cognitive impairment, and Alzheimer's disease. *Neurol Clin.* 2000;18(4):789–806.
65. Petersen RC, Stevens JC, Ganguli M, et al. Practice parameter: Early detection of dementia: Mild cognitive impairment (an evidence-based review). Report of the Quality Standards Subcommittee of the American Academy of Neurology. *Neurology.* 2001;56:1133–1142.
66. Chetelat G, Desgranges B, de la Sayette V, et al. Mapping gray matter loss with voxel-based morphometry in mild cognitive impairment. *Neuroreport.* 2002;13:1939–1943.
67. Saykin A, Wishart H, Flashman L, et al. Gray matter reduction in MCI and in older adults with cognitive complaints [abstract]. *J Int Neuropsychol Soc.* 2003:174.

68. Saykin AJ, Wishart HA. Mild cognitive impairment: Conceptual issues and structural and functional brain correlates. *Sem Clin Neuropsychiatry.* 2003;8:12–30.
69. Small SA, Perera GM, DeLaPaz R, et al. Differential regional dysfunction of the hippocampal formation among elderly with memory decline and Alzheimer's disease. *Ann Neurol.* 1999;45(4):466–472.
70. Rombouts SA, Barkhof F, Veltman DJ, et al. Functional MR imaging in Alzheimer's disease during memory encoding. *AJNR Am J Neuroradiol.* 2000;21(10):1869–1875.
71. Kato T, Knopman D, Liu H. Dissociation of regional activation in mild AD during visual encoding: A functional MRI study. *Neurology.* 2001;57: 812–816.
72. Saykin AJ, Riordan HJ, Burr RB, et al. Functional Magnetic Resonance Imaging: Studies of Memory. In: Bigler ED, editor. *Neuroimaging II: Clinical Applications.* New York: Plenum Press; 1996.
73. Corkin S. Functional MRI for studying episodic memory in aging and Alzheimer's disease. *Geriatrics.* 1998;53(Suppl 1):S13–15.
74. Sperling RA, Bates JF, Chua EF, et al. FMRI studies of associative encoding in young and elderly controls and mild Alzheimer's disease. *J Neurol Neurosurg Psychiatry.* 2003;74(1):44–50.
75. Sperling R, Greve D, Dale A, et al. Functional MRI detection of pharmacologically induced memory impairment. *Proc Nat Acad Sci USA.* 2002; 99(1):455–460.
76. Saykin AJ, Flashman LA, Johnson S, et al. Frontal and hippocampal memory circuitry in early Alzheimer's disease: Relation of structural and functional MRI changes. *Neuroimage.* 2000;11(5):S123.
77. Grady CL, Furey ML, Pietrini P, et al. Altered brain functional connectivity and impaired short-term memory in Alzheimer's disease. *Brain.* 2001;124(Pt 4):739–756.
78. Wagner AD. Early detection of Alzheimer's disease: An fMRI marker for people at risk? *Nature Neurosci.* 2000;3(10):973–974.
79. Bookheimer SY, Strojwas MH, Cohen MS, et al. Patterns of brain activation in people at risk for Alzheimer's disease. *N Engl J Med.* 2000;343(7):450–456.
80. Smith JD. Apolipoproteins and aging: emerging mechanisms. *Ageing Res Rev.* 2002;1(3):345–365.
81. Burggren AC, Small GW, Sabb FW, et al. Specificity of brain activation patterns in people at genetic risk for Alzheimer disease. *Am J Geriatr Psychiatry.* 2002;10(1):44–51.
82. Daselaar SM, Veltman DJ, Rombouts SA, et al. Neuroanatomical correlates of episodic encoding and retrieval in young and elderly subjects. *Brain.* 2003;126(Pt 1):43–56.
83. Gron G, Bittner D, Schmitz B, et al. Subjective memory complaints: objective neural markers in patients with Alzheimer's disease and major depressive disorder. *Ann Neurol.* 2002;51(4):491–498.
84. Rombouts SA, Barkhof F, Van Meel CS, et al. Alterations in brain activation during cholinergic enhancement with rivastigmine in Alzheimer's disease. *J Neurol Neurosurg Psychiatry.* 2002;73(6):665–671.
85. Martin A. Functional neuroimaging of semantic memory. In: Cabeza R, Kingstone A, editors. *Handbook of Functional Neuroimaging of Cognition.* Cambridge, MA: Bradford; 2001:153–186.
86. Salthouse TA. Speed and knowledge as determinants of adult age differences in verbal tasks. *J Gerontol.* 1993;48(1):29–36.
87. Albert MS, Heller HS, Milberg W. Changes in naming ability with age. *Psychol Aging.* 1988;3(2):173–178.

88. Au R, Joung P, Nicholas M, et al. Naming ability across the adult life span. *Aging Cogn.* 1995;2(4):300–311.
89. Rich JB, Park NW, Dopkins S, et al. What do Alzheimer's disease patients know about animals? It depends on task structure and presentation format. *J Int Neuropsychol Soc.* 2002;8(1):83–94.
90. Johnson SC, Saykin AJ, Flashman LA, et al. Similarities and differences in semantic and phonological processing with age: Patterns of functional MRI activation. *Aging Neuropsychol Cogn.* 2001;8(4):307–320.
91. Saykin AJ, Flashman LA, Frutiger S, et al. Neuroanatomic substrates of semantic memory impairment in Alzheimer's Disease: Patterns of functional MRI activation. *J Int Neuropsychol Soc.* 1999;5:377–392.
92. Johnson SC, Saykin AJ, Baxter LC, et al. The relationship between fMRI activation and cerebral atrophy: Comparison of normal aging and Alzheimer disease. *Neuroimage.* 2000;11(3):179–187.
93. Smith CD, Andersen AH, Kryscio RJ, et al. Altered brain activation in cognitively intact individuals at high risk for Alzheimer's disease. *Neurology.* 1999;53:1391–1396.
94. Mencl WE, Pugh KR, Shaywitz SE, et al. Network analysis of brain activations in working memory: behavior and age relationships. *Microsc Res Tech.* 2000;51(1):64–74.
95. Baddeley AD. Is working memory still working? *Am Psychol.* 2001; 56(11):851–864.
96. Becker JT, Morris RG. Working memory(s). *Brain Cogn.* 1999;41:1–8.
97. D'Esposito M, Aguirre GK, Zarahn D, et al. Functional MRI studies of spatial and nonspatial working memory. *Cogn Brain Res.* 1998;7:1–13.
98. Sala JB, Rama P, Courtney SM. Functional topography of a distributed neural system for spatial and nonspatial information maintenance in working memory. *Neuropsychologia.* 2003;41:341–356.
99. Levy R, Goldman-Rakic PS. Segregation of working memory functions within the dorsolateral prefrontal cortex. *Exp Brain Res.* 2000;133(1):23–32.
100. Van der Linden M, Bredart S, Beerten A. Age-related differences in updating working memory. *Br J Psychol.* 1994;85(Pt 1):145–152.
101. Anders TR, Fozard JL, Lillyquist TD. Effects of age upon retrieval from short-term memory. *Dev Psychol.* 1972;6:214–217.
102. Baddeley AD, Baddeley HA, Bucks RS, et al. Attentional control in Alzheimer's disease. *Brain.* 2001;124:1492–1508.
103. Woodard J, Grafton S, Votaw J, et al. Compensatory recruitment of neural resources during overt rehearsal of word lists in Alzheimer's disease. *Neuropsychology.* 1998;12:491–504.
104. Rypma B, D'Esposito M. Isolating the neural mechanisms of age-related changes in human working memory. *Nature Neurosci.* 2000;3(5):509–515.
105. Rypma B, Prabhakaran V, Desmond JE, et al. Age differences in prefrontal cortical activity in working memory. *Psychol Aging.* 2001;16(3):371–384.
106. Wishart HA, Saykin AJ, McDonald BC, et al. Gray matter volume predicts age-related alterations in brain fMRI activation pattern during working memory [abstract]. *J Neuropsychiatry Clin Neurosci.* 2003;15(2):233.
107. Grossman M, Cooke A, DeVita C, et al. Age-related changes in working memory during sentence comprehension: an fMRI study. *Neuroimage.* 2002;15(2):302–317.
108. Shaywitz SE, Shaywitz BA, Pugh KR, et al. Effect of estrogen on brain activation patterns in postmenopausal women during working memory tasks. *JAMA.* 1999;281(13):1197–1202.

109. Mitchell KJ, Johnson MK, Raye CL, et al. fMRI evidence of age-related hippocampal dysfunction in feature binding in working memory. *Cogn Brain Res.* 2000;10(1–2):197–206.
110. Rombouts SARB, van Swieten JC, Pijenburg YAL, et al. Loss of frontal fMRI actiation in early frontotemporal dementia compared to early AD. *Neurology.* 2003;60:1904–1908.
111. Saykin AJ, Wishart HA, Rabin LA, et al. Cholinergic enhancement of frontal lobe activity in mild cognitive impairment. *Brain* 2004;127(pt 7): 1574–1583.
112. Rombouts SA, Barkhof F, Van Meel CS, et al. Alterations in brain activation during cholinergic enhancement with rivastigmine in Alzheimer's disease. *J Neurol Neurosurg Psychiatry.* 2002;73(6):665–671.
113. D'Esposito M, Zarahn E, Aguirre GK, et al. The effect of normal aging on the coupling of neural activity to the BOLD hemodynamic response. *Neuroimage.* 1999;10:6–14.
114. Huettel SA, Singerman JD, McCarthy G. The effects of aging upon the hemodynamic response measured by functional MRI. *Neuroimage.* 2001;13(1):161–175.
115. Taoka T, Iwasaki S, Uchida H, et al. Age correlation of the time lag in signal change on EPI-fMRI. *J Comput Assist Tomogr.* 1998;22(4):514–517.
116. Mehagnoul-Schipper DJ, van der Kallen BF, Colier WN, et al. Simultaneous measurements of cerebral oxygenation changes during brain activation by near-infrared spectroscopy and functional magnetic resonance imaging in healthy young and elderly subjects. *Hum Brain Mapp.* 2002;16(1):14–23.
117. Ross MH, Yurgelun-Todd DA, Renshaw PF, et al. Age-related reduction in functional MRI response to photic stimulation. *Neurology.* 1997;48(1): 173–176.
118. Ward NS, Frackowiak RSJ. Age-related changes in the neural correlates of motor performance. *Brain.* 2003;126:873–888.
119. Buckner RL, Snyder AZ, Sanders AL, et al. Functional brain imaging of young, nondemented, and demented older adults. *J Cogn Neurosci.* 2000; 12(Suppl 2):24–34.
120. Burggren AC, Bookheimer SY. Structural and functional neuroimaging in Alzheimer's disease: an update. *Curr Top Med Chem.* 2002;2(4):385–393.
121. Shoghi-Jadid K, Small GW, Agdeppa ED, et al. Localization of neurofibrillary tangles and beta-amyloid plaques in the brains of living patients with Alzheimer disease. *Am J Geriatr Psychiatry.* 2002;10(1):24–35.
122. Bondi MW. Genetic and brain imaging contributions to neuropsychological functioning in preclinical dementia. *J Int Neuropsychol Soc.* 2002;8: 915–917.

# 10

# fMRI of Language Systems: Methods and Applications

Jeffrey R. Binder

Language functions were among the first to be ascribed a specific location in the human brain[1] and have been the subject of intense research for over a century. Many researchers across the globe—working in disciplines as varied as linguistics, psychology, neurology, anthropology, and philosophy—have devoted their careers to understanding language processes and their biological bases.

Language research has not been merely an incremental, trivial extension of the classical Wernicke–Broca neuroanatomical model of language. In fact, there is now a wealth of empirical evidence and modeling results that were unavailable to theorists a century ago. These have led to ever more detailed accounts of how language happens in terms of both psychological and physiological processes. It is easy to see, given the difficulty of assimilating this knowledge base, how forays into language mapping based on nineteenth century brain models might easily go astray, producing rather uninteresting and uninterpretable results. This chapter will offer a common vocabulary and an exposure to some of the main issues in language imaging, so that functional imagers might be able to communicate more effectively with language scientists in jointly designing and interpreting fMRI studies.

## Some Proposed Clinical Applications of fMRI Language Mapping

Some current techniques used for language mapping include the intracarotid amobarbital, or Wada, test,[2] subdural grid stimulation mapping,[3] intraoperative cortical stimulation mapping (ICSM),[4] positron emission tomography (PET),[5] and magnetic source imaging (MEG).[6] These methods, while extremely useful, are generally invasive (Wada, subdural grids, ICSM), lacking in spatial precision (Wada), costly, or not widely available (PET, MEG).

Several characteristics of functional magnetic resonance imaging (fMRI) make it a potentially very useful tool for language mapping.

First, the relatively small size of fMRI voxels (typically two to four millimeters on an edge) produces favorable image quality and spatial localization capability. Second, functional data can be registered easily with very high-resolution standard MRI images acquired at the same brain location, enhancing the ability to associate functional foci with specific anatomic structures. Third, activation procedures can be performed repeatedly in the same subject within and across scanning sessions, providing improved statistical power, measures of test–retest reliability, the ability to monitor changes in activation serially over time, and the potential for exploring a range of cognitive processes. Fourth, fMRI can be implemented on the MRI scanners already in place at many medical facilities, with the addition of relatively inexpensive fast acquisition pulse sequences, ancillary coil hardware, and specialized stimulus delivery and response recording systems.

### Presurgical Applications

The primary application for language mapping with fMRI is identifying critically important language areas prior to brain tumor removal or epilepsy surgery. Optimal presurgical evaluation includes estimation and minimization of the surgical risks. Functional brain mapping techniques can contribute to this process in several ways. By determining the location of important brain functions, mapping techniques might help predict the risk of postoperative language deficits. During the surgical procedure itself, functional maps might be used to minimize such deficits by avoiding important functional areas.

A large number of fMRI studies and reviews pertaining to this application have been published.[7–39] One hotly debated issue that can only be touched on briefly in this chapter is whether fMRI will ever be able to completely replace more-invasive procedures such as the Wada test. For further review of this topic, refer to chapter 11. Whether or not this goal ever comes to pass, however, it seems almost certain that fMRI language studies will one day provide valuable adjunctive information concerning lateralization and localization of language. At the least, this information will be useful for identifying patients who require more-invasive mapping, such as ICSM or subdural grids, because of planned surgery in potentially sensitive regions.

### Prediction of Outcome in Aphasia

Functional MRI language activation measures might be useful in predicting long-term outcome in the acute or subacute phase of acquired aphasia. Long-term outcome is known to be predictable from lesion size, severity of the initial deficit, and regional patterns of resting glucose metabolism.[40–47] Functional MRI might conceivably offer independent predictive value by detecting residual functional capacity in perilesional or contralateral homologous brain regions. Aside from the intrinsic value of prognostic information for patients and caregivers, such information also might be useful for cost-effective allocation of resources in the rehabilitation setting. No studies of this potential application have as yet been published, although several fMRI studies have investigated the neurophysiological basis of recovery from aphasia.[48–51]

### Diagnosis

Functional MRI might prove useful for diagnosis of brain illnesses that perturb language processing, but do not cause gross structural changes, such as developmental dyslexia and aphasia, milder forms of autism, schizophrenia, and early dementia. The neurobiological basis for many of these disorders is still not known, and in many cases, it remains unclear whether the disease represents a single entity or many subtypes. With careful study, it may be possible to define signature activation patterns that are highly characteristic of particular illnesses or illness subtypes.[52–54] This information could lead to an improved understanding of such illnesses and how they disrupt normal language processes. These patterns also could be followed over time as an additional indicator of disease progression or stability.

### Monitoring Treatment Effects

A small number of studies have shown changes in language-related activation patterns after remediation or rehabilitation therapy for language disorders.[55] While the primary measure of treatment efficacy will always be improvement in behavioral performance, such physiological measures may offer new insights into the mechanisms by which behavioral performance improves, possibly enabling selection of more specific and effective therapeutic strategies.

## Some Theoretical Principles

Attempts to detect brain activity related to language processing are best preceded by a consideration of two general theoretical questions: What processes are linguistic? If linguistic processes can be carried out autonomously (internally or covertly), when can it be said that these processes are not occurring?

Language processes are those that enable communication. This definition is overly inclusive, however, in that many bodily functions (e.g., cardiac, pulmonary, general arousal, and sustained attention functions) are necessary for communication to occur but are not linguistic in nature. Many linguistic and non-linguistic tasks require neural systems that process auditory or visual sensory information, hold such information in a short-term store, direct attention to specific features or aspects of the information, perform comparative and other operations on the information, select a response based on such operations, and carry out the response. The extent to which any of these systems is specialized for language-related functions (as in, for example, specialized perceptual or working memory systems) is still a matter of debate. Careful consideration of these general-purpose functions is especially relevant for interpreting and designing language studies, which often employ relatively complex tasks involving motor, sensory, attentional, memory, and central executive functions in addition to language. Should these other components be considered part of the language system because they are so necessary for adequate task performance, or should they be delineated from language processes per se? In choosing a control task against which a language task is to be contrasted, investigators tacitly establish which components of the task are not, by their definition, part of the language process in which they are interested. These implicit definitions can vary even among investigators purportedly studying the same language process, leading to apparently conflicting results.[56–58]

Clinicians working with aphasic patients historically have focused on the distinction between expressive and receptive language functions, but a more useful taxonomy of language processes is available from the field of linguistics. These processes include: (1) phonetics, the processes governing production and perception of speech sounds; (2) phonology, the processes by which speech sounds are represented and manipulated in abstract form; (3) orthography, the processes by which written characters are represented and manipulated in abstract form; (4) semantics, the processing of word meanings, names, and other declarative knowledge about the world; and (5) syntax, the processes by which words are combined to make sentences and sentences analyzed to reveal underlying relationships between words. A basic assumption of language mapping is that activation tasks can be designed to make varying demands on these processing subsystems. For example, a task requiring careful listening to word-like nonwords (often called pseudowords, e.g., *pemid*) would make great demands on phonetic perception (and on prephonetic auditory processing and attention), but very little demand on semantic or syntactic processing, given that the stimuli have no (or very little) meaning. In contrast, a task requiring semantic categorization of printed words (e.g., Is it an animal or not?) would make great demands on orthographic and semantic processing, but relatively little on phonetic, phonological, or syntactic processing.

On the other hand, the processing subcomponents of language often act together. The extent to which each component can be examined in isolation remains a major methodological issue, as it is not yet clear to what extent the systems responsible for these processes become active automatically when presented with linguistic stimuli.[59] One familiar example of this is the Stroop effect, in which orthographic and phonological processing of printed words occurs, even when subjects are instructed to attend to the color of the print, and even when this processing interferes with task performance.[60] Other familiar examples include semantic priming effects during word recognition, picture–word interference effects, lexical effects on phonetic perception, orthographic effects on letter perception, and semantic–syntactic interactions during sentence comprehension.[61–69] If linguistic stimuli such as words and pictures evoke obligatory automatic language processing, these effects need to be considered in the design and interpretation of language activation experiments. Use of such stimuli in a baseline condition could result in undesirable subtraction (or partial subtraction) of language-related activation. Because investigators frequently try to match stimuli in control and language tasks very closely, such inadvertent subtraction is relatively commonplace in functional imaging studies of language processing. One example is the widely employed word-generation task, which frequently is paired with a control task involving repetition or reading of words.[56,70,71] In most of these studies, which were aimed at detecting activation related to semantic processing, there has been relatively little activation in temporal and temporoparietal structures that are known, on the basis of lesion studies, to be involved in semantic processing. In contrast, subtractions involving control tasks that use non-linguistic stimuli generally reveal a much more extensive network of left hemisphere temporal, parietal, and frontal language-processing areas.[58,72–75]

A final theoretical issue is the extent to which language processes occur during resting states or states with minimal task requirements (e.g., visual fixation or passive stimulation). Language involves interactive systems for manipulating internally stored knowledge about words and word meanings. In examining these systems, we typically use familiar stimuli or cues to engage processing, yet it seems likely that activity in these systems could occur independently of external stimulation and task demands. The idea that the conscious mind can be internally active independent of external events has a long history in psychology and neuroscience.[76–79] When asked, subjects in experimental studies frequently report experiencing seemingly unprovoked thoughts (including words and recognizeable images) that are unrelated to the task at hand.[79–81] The precise extent to which such thinking engages linguistic knowledge remains unclear,[82,83] but many researchers have demonstrated close parallels between behavior and language content, suggesting that at least some internal thought processes make use of verbally encoded semantic knowledge and other linguistic representations.[82,84,85] Some authors have argued that rest and similar conditions are actually active states in which subjects frequently are engaged in processing linguistic and other information.[86–92] Thus, the use of such states as control conditions for language imaging studies may obscure similar processes that occur during the language task of interest. This is a particularly difficult problem for language studies because the internal processes in question cannot be directly measured or precisely controlled.

## Survey of Language Activation Protocols

This section describes some of the experimental designs that have been used in language activation studies and the results that can be expected. It may be helpful to identify from the outset a few myths about language activation studies that are, in the author's view, somewhat prevalent.

**Myth 1**

Language-related brain activation is difficult to detect and not as robust as motor and primary sensory activation.

In fact, activation magnitude is primarily determined by the type of contrast being performed, that is, how similar or different are the conditions being contrasted. Very robust signals in heteromodal cognitive areas can be readily detected, even in individual brains, given an appropriate task contrast.

**Myth 2**

The pattern of language-related brain activation observed by fMRI depends mainly on the type of language task employed.

In fact, the control task is equally important in determining the pattern of activation. Extremely different patterns can result from the same language task when contrasted with different control or baseline conditions. Conversely, very similar patterns can result from very different language tasks when these are contrasted with different control conditions.

**Myth 3**

An effective language mapping protocol should detect all critical language areas.

It is very unlikely that any single protocol could detect all critical language areas. This is because language is not a single homogeneous process, but rather the product of many interacting neural systems that are engaged to varying degrees depending on task requirements.

**Myth 4**

The main language zones in the brain are Broca's Area (left posterior inferior frontal gyrus) and Wernicke's Area (left posterior superior temporal gyrus).

In fact, these brain areas appear to have very specific rather than general language functions. As such, they are engaged during some language tasks but not others, and their damage results in specific deficits that are often relatively minor. Both traditional lesion studies and language imaging studies have identified a host of other, larger, more general language zones in the prefrontal, lateral temporal, ventral temporal, and posterior parietal cortex of the dominant hemisphere (see References 59, 93, 94 for reviews). The approximate location of some of these zones is shown in Figure 10.1.

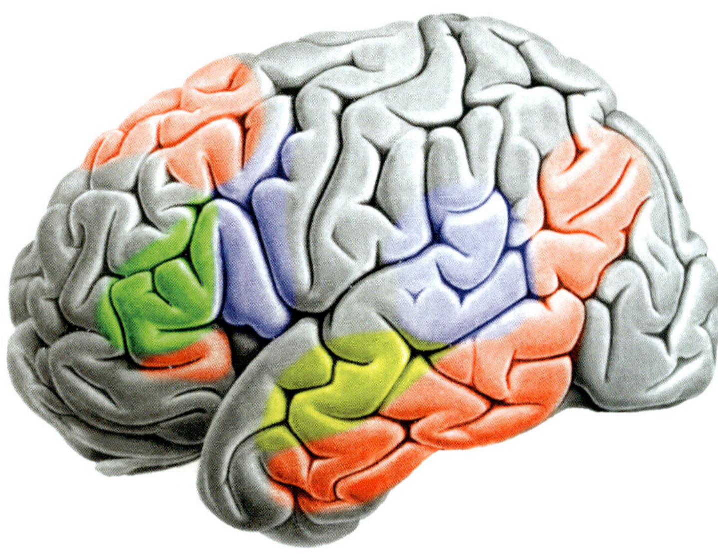

**Figure 10.1.** Schematic drawing of some putative language areas in the dominant hemisphere. Yellow = phoneme and auditory word form perception area. Red = semantic storage and retrieval systems. Blue = phonological access and phonological output systems. Green = general verbal retrieval, selection, and working memory functions.

The variety of possible stimuli and tasks that could be used to induce language processing is vast, and a coherent, concise discussion is difficult. Table 10.1 lists some of the broad categories of stimuli that have been used and some of the brain systems they tend to engage. Auditory nonspeech refers to noises or tones that are not perceived as speech. Such stimuli can be variably complex in their temporal or spectral features and possess to varying degrees the acoustic properties of speech (see References 95–97). They activate early (primary and association) auditory cortex to varying degrees depending on their precise acoustic characteristics. Auditory phonemes are speech sounds that do not comprise words in the listener's language; these may be simple consonant–vowel monosyllables or longer sequences. In addition to early auditory cortex, speech phonemes activate auditory wordform systems that are relatively specialized for the perception of speech

**Table 10.1. Effects of Stimuli on Sensory and Linguistic Processing Systems**

| Stimuli | Early sensory | Auditory wordform | Visual wordform | Object recognition | syntax |
|---|---|---|---|---|---|
| Auditory Nonspeech | Aud | – | – | – | – |
| Auditory Phonemes | Aud | + | – | – | – |
| Auditory Words | Aud | + | – | – | – |
| Auditory Sentences | Aud | + | – | – | + |
| Visual Nonletters | Vis | – | – | – | – |
| Visual Letterstrings | Vis | – | +/– | – | – |
| Visual Pseudowords | Vis | – | + | – | – |
| Visual Words | Vis | – | + | – | – |
| Visual Sentences | Vis | – | + | – | + |
| Visual Objects | Vis | – | – | + | – |

sounds, whether presented in the form of nonwords, words, or sentences.[95–98]

Visual nonletter here refers to any visual stimulus not recognized by the subject. Examples include characters from unfamiliar alphabets, nonsense signs, and false font. Such stimuli can be variably complex and possess to varying degrees the visual properties of familiar letters. They activate early (primary and association) visual cortex depending, to varying degrees, on their visual characteristics. Visual letterstrings are random strings of letters that do not form familiar or easily pronounceable letter combinations (e.g., FCJVB). Visual pseudowords are letterstrings that are not words, but possess the orthographic and phonological characteristics of real words (e.g., SNADE). Letterstrings are claimed to activate a visual wordform area located in the left mid-fusiform gyrus; this area responds more strongly to pseudowords and words than to random letterstrings.[99]

The degree to which these stimuli engage the processes listed in Table 10.1 may depend partly on the task that the subject is asked to perform, although the processes in Table 10.1 seem to be activated relatively automatically, even when subjects are given no explicit task. This is less true for the processing systems listed in Table 10.2, which seem to be strongly task-dependent. The semantic system appears to be partly active even during rest or when stimuli are presented passively to the subject.[87–91] Other tasks seem to suppress semantic processing by requiring a focusing of attention on perceptual, orthographic, or phonological properties of stimuli. Examples include Sensory Discrimination tasks (e.g., intensity, size, color, frequency, or more complex feature-based discriminations), Phonetic Decision tasks in which the subject must detect a target phoneme or phonemes, Phonological Decision tasks requiring a decision based on the phonological structure of a stimulus (e.g., detection of rhymes, judgment of syllable number), and Orthographic Decision tasks requiring a decision based on the letters in the stimulus (e.g., case matching, letter identification). Other tasks, such as reading and repeating, make no overt demands on semantic systems, but probably elicit automatic semantic processing. The extent to which this occurs may depend on how

**Table 10.2. Effects of Task States on Some Linguistic Processing Systems**

| Tasks | Semantics | Output phonology | Speech articulation | Working memory | Other language |
|---|---|---|---|---|---|
| Rest or Passive | + | – | – | – | – |
| Sensory Discrimination | – | – | – | +/– | – |
| Read or Repeat Covert | + | + | – | +/– | – |
| Read or Repeat Overt | + | + | + | +/– | – |
| Phonetic Decision | – | + | – | + | – |
| Phonological Decision | – | + | – | + | – |
| Orthographic Decision | – | +/– | – | – | – |
| Semantic Decision | + | +/– | – | + | Semantic search |
| Word Generation Covert | + | + | – | + | Lexical search |
| Word Generation Overt | + | + | + | + | Lexical search |
| Naming Covert | + | + | – | – | Lexical search |
| Naming Overt | + | + | + | – | Lexical search |

meaningful the stimulus is: sentences likely elicit more semantic processing than isolated words, which in turn elicit more than pseudowords. Finally, many tasks make overt demands on retrieval and use of semantic knowledge. These include Semantic Decision tasks requiring a decision based on the meaning of the stimulus (e.g., "Is it living or non-living?"), Word Generation tasks requiring retrieval of a word or series of words related in meaning to a cue word, and Naming tasks requiring retrieval of a verbal label for an object or object description.

Output Phonology refers to the processes engaged in retrieving a phonological (sound based) representation of a word. These processes are required for both overt and covert reading, repeating, naming, and word generation. In addition, any task that engages reading, such as an orthographic or semantic decision on printed words or pseudowords, will automatically engage output phonological processes to some degree.[60,67,73] In contrast, Speech Articulation processes are engaged fully only when an overt spoken response is produced.[100] Verbal Working Memory is required whenever a written or spoken stimulus must be held in memory. This applies to repetition tasks if the stimulus to be repeated is relatively long, to auditory decision tasks if the auditory stimulus must be remembered while the decision is being made, and to most word-generation tasks, because the cue must be maintained in memory while the response is retrieved. Finally, semantic decision, word-generation, and naming tasks make strong demands on frontal mechanisms involved in searching for and retrieving information associated with a stimulus.

With these somewhat over-simplified stimulus and task characterizations, it is possible to make some general predictions about the processing systems in which the level of activation will differ when two task conditions are contrasted, and thus the likely pattern of brain activation that will be observed in a subtraction analysis. Some commonly encountered examples are listed below and in Table 10.3.

### Language Task: Passively Listening to Words or Sentences

*Control Task: Rest*

As shown in Table 10.1, auditory words activate early auditory cortices and auditory wordform areas. Because both rest and passive stimulation are accompanied by spontaneous semantic processes and make no other overt cognitive demands, no other language systems should appear in the contrast. These predictions are confirmed by many studies employing this contrast, which results primarily in activation of the superior temporal gyrus auditory cortex bilaterally (Figure 10.2A).[57,95,101,102] The activation is relatively symmetrical and bears no relationship to language dominance, as measured by Wada testing.[16]

### Language Task: Passively Listening to Words

*Control Task: Passively Listening to Nonspeech*

Because there are no differences in task requirements in this contrast, and because semantic processing occurs in all passive conditions, the

Table 10.3. Some Task Contrasts Used for Language Mapping and the Regions in which Robust Activations are Typically Observed

| | Ventrolateral prefrontal | Dorsal prefrontal | Superior temporal | Ventrolateral temporal | Ventral occipital | Angular gyrus |
|---|---|---|---|---|---|---|
| Hearing Words vs. Rest | | | B | | | |
| Hearing Words vs. Nonspeech Sounds | | | L > R | | | |
| Word Generation vs. Rest | L > R | | | L > R | B | |
| Word Generation vs. Reading | L | | | | | |
| Object Naming vs. Rest | B | | | L > R | B | |
| Semantic Decision vs. Sensory Discrimination | L | L | L > R | L | | L |
| Semantic Decision vs. Phonological Decision | | L | | L | | L |
| Reading Sentences vs. Letterstrings | L > R | | L > R | L > R | | |

L = left hemisphere, R = right hemisphere, B = bilateral.

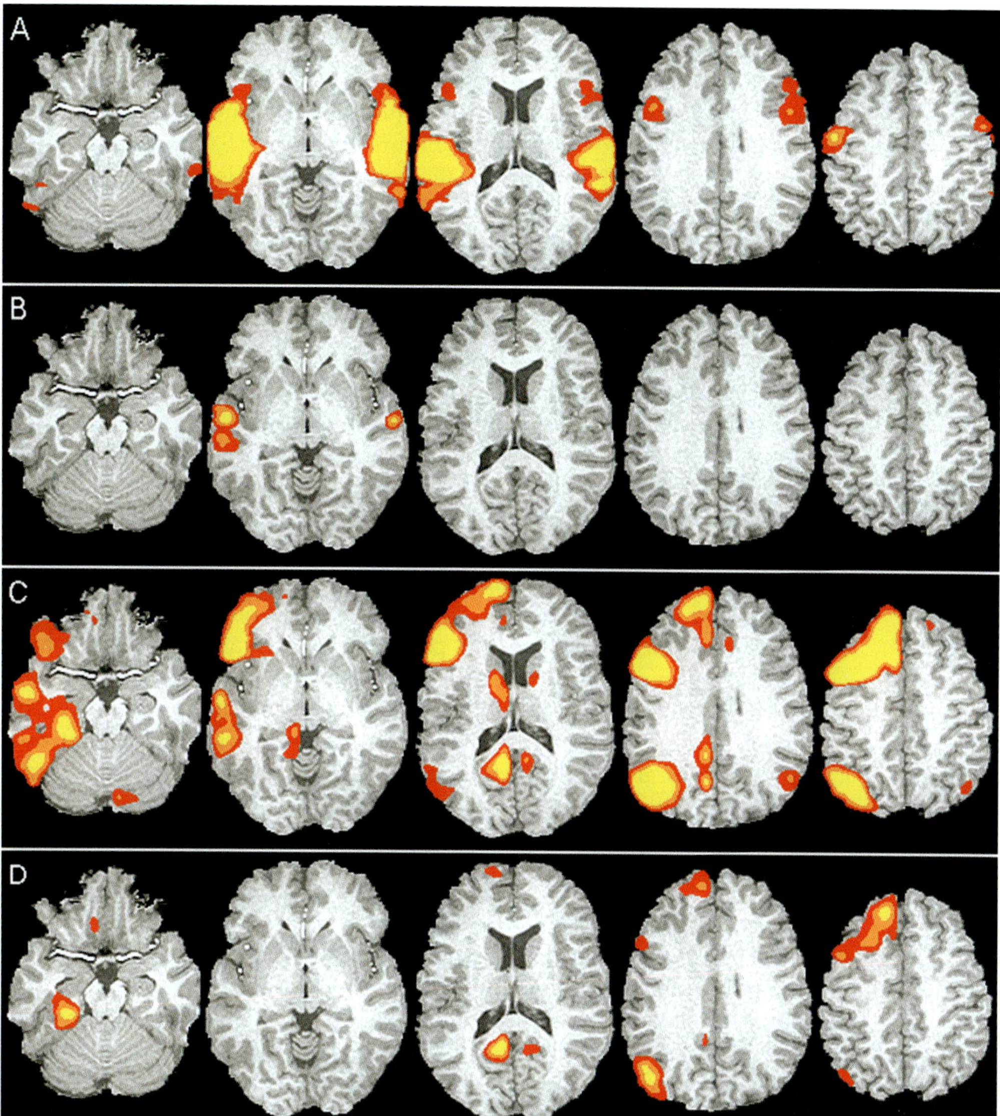


**Figure 10.2.** Group average fMRI activation patterns in neurologically normal, right-handed volunteers during four language paradigms. (A) Passive listening to spoken words contrasted with resting (28 subjects). Superior temporal activation occurs bilaterally. (B) Passive listening to spoken words contrasted with passive listening to tones (same 28 subjects as in (A)). Superior temporal sulcus activation occurs bilaterally, more prominent on the left. (C) Semantic decision on auditory words contrasted with a tone monitoring control task (30 subjects). Activation is strongly left-lateralized in prefrontal, lateral and ventral temporal, angular, and cingulate cortices. (D) Semantic decision on auditory words contrasted with a phonological task using pseudowords (same 30 subjects as in (C)). Activation is strongly left-lateralized in dorsal prefrontal, angular, and posterior cingulate cortices. There is no activation of Broca's or Wernicke's area. The images are serial axial sections spaced at 15-mm intervals through stereotaxic space, starting at $z = -15$. The left hemisphere is on the reader's left. (Neurologic coordinates)

activation pattern depends mainly on acoustic and phonetic differences between the speech and nonspeech stimuli. Studies employing such contrasts reliably show stronger activation by words in the middle and anterior superior temporal sulcus, with some leftward lateralization and little or no activation elsewhere (Figure 10.2B).[95,96,103–105] Similar patterns are observed whether the language stimuli are words or pseudowords.[95]

### Language Task: Word Generation

#### *Control Task: Rest*

Because the rest state includes no control for sensory processing, early auditory or visual cortices may be activated bilaterally depending on the sensory modality of the cue stimulus (Table 10.1) and the rate of cue presentation.[106] In some protocols, a single cue (e.g., a letter or a semantic category) is provided only at the beginning of an activation period; in others, a different cue is provided every few seconds. Unlike rest, word generation makes demands on output phonology, verbal working memory, and lexical search systems (Table 10.2). Speech articulation systems also will be activated if an overt spoken response is required. These predictions are confirmed by many studies employing this contrast, which results primarily in activation of the left inferior frontal gyrus and left > right premotor cortex, systems thought to be involved in phonological production, verbal working memory, and lexical search.[13,14,16,18,57,107–110] There may be weak activation of left posterior temporal or ventral temporal regions, possibly due to engagement of auditory or visual wordform systems.

### Language Task: Word Generation

#### *Control Task: Reading or Repeating*

These tasks can be given in either the visual or auditory modality; it will be assumed here that the same modality is used for both tasks. The stimuli in both cases are single words; thus, no difference in activation of sensory or wordform systems is expected. Both tasks are accompanied by semantic processing (automatic semantic access in the case of the control task, effortful semantic retrieval in the case of word generation) and output phonology processes. The word-generation task makes greater demands on lexical search and on working memory; consequently, greater activation is expected in left inferior frontal areas associated with these processes. These predictions match findings in many studies using this contrast.[56,70,108,111]

### Language Task: Visual Object Naming

#### *Control Task: Rest*

Compared to rest, visual objects activate early visual sensory cortices and object recognition systems bilaterally (Table 10.1).[112–114] There may be additional left-lateralized activation in semantic systems of the ventrolateral posterior temporal lobe.[72,115–118] Unlike rest, naming requires output phonology and lexical search, and, when overt, speech articulation (Table 10.2). These predictions match findings in several studies using this contrast that show extensive bilateral visual system activation and modest left-lateralized inferior frontal activation.[14,116,118,119]

### Language Task: Semantic Decision

#### *Control Task: Sensory Discrimination*

Again, it will be assumed that the same stimulus modality is used for both tasks. If the stimuli used for the sensory discrimination task are non-linguistic (e.g., tones or nonsense shapes), then the semantic decision task will produce relatively greater activation in auditory or visual wordform systems, depending on the sensory modality. In addition, there will be greater activation of output phonology systems, semantic systems, and semantic search mechanisms in the semantic decision task. Working memory systems may or may not be activated, depending on whether or not the sensory task also has a working memory demand. These predictions match findings in studies using this contrast, which show left-lateralized activation of auditory (middle and anterior superior temporal sulcus) or visual (mid-fusiform gyrus) wordform regions, and extensive activation of left prefrontal, lateral and ventral left temporal, and left posterior parietal systems believed to be involved in semantic retrieval (Figure 10.2C).[38,58,75,120,121]

### Language Task: Semantic Decision

#### *Control Task: Phonological Decision*

These tasks also can be given in either the visual or auditory modality; it will be assumed that the same modality is used for both tasks. The stimuli used for phonological decision are either words or pseudowords. Thus, there are no stimulus-related differences between the stimuli, and no difference in activation of sensory or wordform systems is expected. There will be greater activation of semantic systems and semantic search mechanisms in the semantic decision task. These predictions match findings in many studies using this contrast, which show activation of left prefrontal, lateral and ventral left temporal, and left posterior parietal systems believed to be involved in semantic retrieval (Figure 10.2D).[58,88,122–125]

### Language Task: Sentence or Word Reading

#### *Control Task: Passively Viewing Letterstrings*

Compared to letterstrings, sentences enage visual wordform, syntactic, and output phonology systems, and probably working memory if the words are presented one at a time. Both reading and passive viewing probably involve semantic processing. There should be relative left-lateralized activation of the fusiform gyrus (visual wordform), posterior superior temporal gyrus and STS (output phonology), and inferior frontal gyrus (phonology, working memory, syntax). These predictions are consistent with several studies using this contrast.[73,126–129]

These examples cover but a small sample of the possible language activation protocols. There are also numerous published studies employing designs that do not fit neatly into the schema provided here. Many of these represent attempts to further define or fractionate a particular language process, or to define further the functional role of a specific brain region. The reader should appreciate that the review given here is merely a coarse outline of some of the most commonly used types of stimuli and tasks. Above all, it is important to note that activations in a particular part of the language system are seldom all or none, but vary in a graded way depending on the particular stimuli and tasks used.

## Reliability, Validation, and Outcome Prediction Studies

As with any clinical test, the applicability of language mapping techniques to clinical problems depends on the reliability and validity of the test results. It goes without saying that any imaging protocol applied to patients should first be applied in a sample of normal subjects. The initial aims of gathering normative data in this case are: (i) to verify the feasibility of the procedure and estimate the likelihood of obtaining uninterpretable results (i.e., test failures); (ii) to verify that activation occurs in the expected brain regions and is lateralized to the left hemisphere in a random sample of right-handed subjects; (iii) to estimate the range of inter-subject variability that occurs in the normal population; and (iv) to determine the expected test–retest reproducibility of the results. If significant variability in results is observed, a secondary aim is to determine some of the factors (e.g., age, sex, handedness) associated with this variability.

### Normative Studies

Several language mapping protocols have been carried out in relatively large samples of normal subjects.[130–135] All of these protocols produced left-lateralized activation patterns in right-handed subjects. Lateralization has been quantified in most of these studies using some type of left–right difference score. One commonly used version is based on the left–right difference in the number of activated voxels (activation volume), normalized by the total number of activated voxels (i.e., [L – R]/[L + R]). This index varies from –1 (all activated voxels in the right hemisphere) to +1 (all activated voxels in the left hemisphere). This type of index depends on the statistical threshold used to identify voxels as active and tends to increase with increasingly stringent thresholds due to the elimination of false-positive voxels in both hemispheres.[20,31] Others have advocated measures based on magnitude rather than volume of activation.[14,18] Lateralization indices (LI) can be computed for the entire hemisphere or for homologous regions of interest (ROIs). Focusing on language-related ROIs avoids the problem of nonspecific or non-language activation in bilateral sensory, motor, and executive systems that is characteristic of some task contrasts.[31]

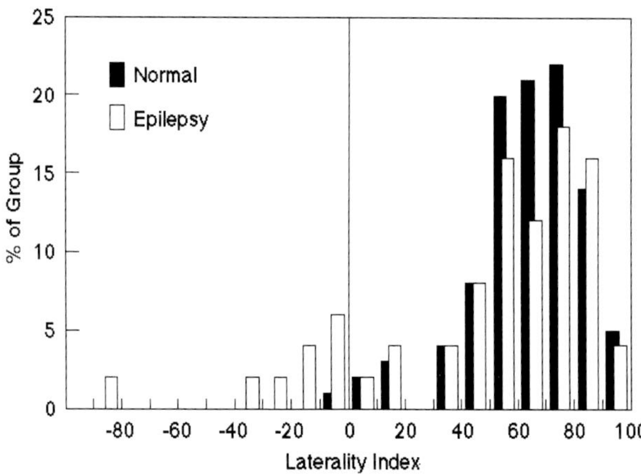


**Figure 10.3.** Frequency distributions of language LI in normal right-handed subjects. Reprinted from Springer JA, Binder JR, Hammeke TA, Swanson SJ, Frost JA, Bellgowan PSF et al. Language dominance in neurologically normal and epilepsy subjects: a functional MRI study. *Brain*. 1999:122:2033–2045. Reprinted by permission of Oxford University Press.

Figure 10.3 shows the range of variability observed for one such LI. The subjects were 100 right-handed healthy adults; they were scanned during a block-design fMRI protocol contrasting an auditory word semantic decision task with an auditory nonspeech sensory discrimination task.[131] Lateralization indices in this group ranged from strong left dominance (LI = 0.97) to roughly symmetrical representation (LI = –0.05), with a group median LI of 0.66. Using a dominance classification scheme based on a cut-off LI value of ±0.20, 94% of subjects were classified as left dominant, 6% were symmetrical, and none had right dominance. Thus, although LI values ranged widely, the vast majority of subjects were left-hemisphere dominant. Similar variability in lateralization among normal, right-handed subjects was observed in two other large studies.[132,136]

Several studies have attempted to identify subject variables associated with language lateralization. One group of investigators, using fMRI to contrast visual pseudoword phonological decision with visual letterstring orthographic decision (a contrast likely to activate visual wordform, phonological output, and working memory systems), found significant effects of gender on lateralization, particularly in the frontal lobe, with women showing relative symmetry of activation and men showing leftward lateralization.[130,137] Other PET,[71,138] fMRI,[132,134,139] and functional transcranial Doppler[136] studies, together involving over 600 normal subjects, have failed to find differences between men and women in terms of lateralization of language functions. Several large series have documented a relative rightward shift of language functions in left-handed and ambidextrous subject samples compared to right-handed subjects.[132,134,140] It is important to note, however, that this difference reflects a group tendency only due to the fact that a larger minority (20–25%) of the non-right-handed subjects are symmetrical or

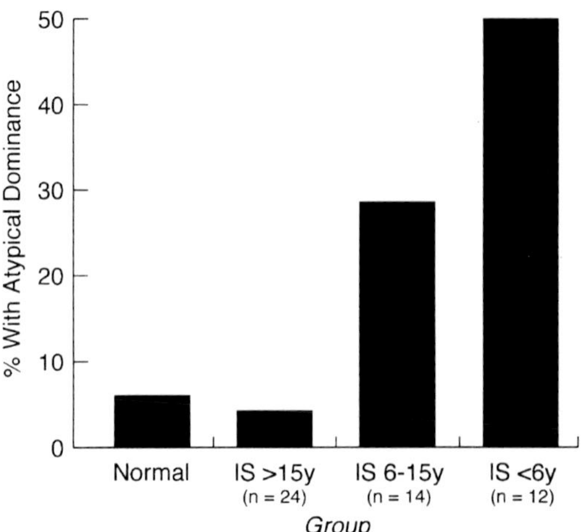


**Figure 10.4.** Frequency of atypical language dominance in normal right-handed subjects (left-most bar) and in epilepsy patients with onset of intractable seizures (IS) after age 15 (IS > 15y), between age 6 and 15 (IS 6–15y), or before age 6 (IS < 6y). Atypical (right or symmetric) language representation is strongly associated with earlier age of seizure onset. Reprinted from Springer JA, Binder JR, Hammeke TA, Swanson SJ, Frost JA, Bellgowan PSF et al. Language dominance in neurologically normal and epilepsy subjects: a functional MRI study. *Brain*. 1999;122:2033–2045. Reprinted by permission of Oxford University Press.

right dominant. Most left-handed and ambidextrous subjects are, like right-handers, left-dominant for language. These estimates of language dominance and handedness effects in normal subjects agree very well with earlier Wada language studies in patients with late-onset seizures.[131,141,142]

Two studies have reported age effects on language dominance, manifested as a decline in the LI (greater symmetry of language processing) with increasing age.[131,134] Similar declines in hemispheric specialization have been observed for other cognitive domains,[143,144] and may reflect recruitment of homologous functional regions as compensation for age-related declines in neural functional capacity. Level of education had no effect on LI in the one study in which it was assessed.[131]

Two fMRI studies directly compared LIs from a sample of normal subjects with those from patients with epilepsy.[20,131] Both studies included only right-handed individuals to avoid confounding effects of handedness. Patients with epilepsy had a higher incidence of atypical (symmetric or right-lateralized) language dominance; this was particularly true for patients with left-sided seizure foci.[20] In one study, there was a clear relationship between LI and age of onset of seizures ($r = 0.50$, $p < 0.001$), with language tending to shift more toward the right hemisphere with earlier onset (Figure 10.4).[131] These effects are in agreement with Wada studies showing effects of side of seizure focus and age at onset on language lateralization.[141,142,145,146]

## Test–Retest Reliability

Test–retest reliability of language activation procedures has not been sufficiently studied. There are two clinical issues to consider, the first being the reliability of activation of specific voxels across different testing sessions, which is an obvious concern if the goal is to identify specific brain regions that are potentially critical for language. Several authors mention good test–retest reproducibility in a few subjects, although without quantitative analyses.[14,132,147] In one of the first quantitative studies of this issue, Rutten and colleagues measured the overlap of activated voxels across two test sessions as the proportion activated in both sessions relative to the minimum number activated in either the first or second session.[31] Functional data from the two sessions were registered to a common anatomical image and apparently were not spatially smoothed. The results were somewhat disappointing: the best overlap, achieved by combining data from three different activation paradigms and thereby maximizing statistical power, was only 40%. This implies that, for any given activated voxel, there is less than a 50% chance that the same voxel will be activated on retesting with the same protocol. A very similar result (approximately 45% overlap between sessions) was reported in another study using very similar methods.[39]

There are, however, several reasons why these estimates may be overly pessimistic. First, accurate measurement of reproducibility at the single-voxel level requires exquisitely precise spatial registration of voxels across sessions, as well as identical placement of the voxel grid relative to brain tissue across sessions in order to achieve identical partial-volume averaging effects; neither of these goals seems practically possible. Therefore, a more realistic measure of reproducibility might be based on spatially smoothed versions of the activation maps or on activation in anatomically defined regions of interest. Second, it is clear that reproducibility depends on how accurately the level of activation is estimated within each session, that is, on the statistical power, which is determined largely by the number of image volumes acquired.[148] The data of Rutten and colleagues show this effect clearly: when data from any one of the three activation paradigms was analyzed alone, thereby reducing by two-thirds the number of image volumes included in the activation analysis for each session, reproducibility dropped to 25% or less. Thus, it seems reasonable to expect that test–retest reproducibility (i.e., reliability of the activation map) can be optimized simply by increasing the number of image volumes acquired at each session. This increase in reliability will, however, be a decelerating exponential function of image volume number; thus, there will be a point at which significant improvement in reliability cannot be attained without exceeding the practical limits on image acquisition in a single session. These limitations have yet to be worked out for any fMRI language protocols.

The second clinical issue concerns the reliability of language lateralization measurements. Two large studies (with 54 patients[149] and 34 patients[39]) examined this question from the point of view of reliability within a testing session. Both studies involved epilepsy patients performing a Semantic Decision versus Sensory Discrimination paradigm; both examined the correlation between a language LI based on data from the first half of the imaging session and LI based on the second half of the session (intrasession reliability). Results were remarkably similar, showing correlations of 0.89[149] and 0.90.[39] Other investigators measured reliability of the language LI across sessions.[20,31,39] Rutten and colleagues found a correlation of approximately 0.80 across sessions in nine normal subjects using the combined data from three activation tasks. Interestingly, the correlation did not change across different activation thresholds. This means that, although the LI in any given session is affected by the stringency of the activation threshold, that LI relative to the LIs of other subjects will not change as long as the same threshold is applied to all subjects. Adcock and colleagues found a correlation of 0.65 between LIs[95] from two different sessions in 31 subjects (a mix of normals and epilepsy patients). This value seems somewhat low, although the authors state that "in all cases the categorical definitions of laterality on the first and second examinations were in agreement." Finally, Fernández and colleagues observed a correlation of 0.82 in a sample of 12 epilepsy patients scanned in two different sessions on the same day.[39] Collectively, these results suggest a relatively high degree of reproducibility of language LIs derived by fMRI.

## Wada Comparisons

Demonstration that a language mapping procedure produces left-lateralized activation, and that this functional lateralization varies in the expected direction with handedness and seizure focus, provides good preliminary validation that the activated regions are truly related to language. Further evidence is available from at least three sources: (i) comparison of fMRI results with Wada language lateralization testing in the same patients; (ii) comparison of fMRI results with cortical stimulation mapping of language in the same patients; and (iii) correlation with language outcomes after brain surgery. Other potential sources of validation, which will not be discussed further here, include comparisons with putative language lateralization and localization measures derived from PET,[150] magnetoencephalography,[6] EEG,[151] transcranial magnetic stimulation,[152] functional transcranial Doppler,[153] dichotic listening,[135] and MRI structural morphometry.[154]

Preliminary results suggest a high level of agreement between fMRI and Wada tests on measures of language lateralization (see chapter 11, Table 11.1, 286–287).[7–10,13,14,16,19–22,38] Most of these studies involved relatively small sample sizes (7–20 patients) and relatively few crossed-dominant individuals. A variety of task contrasts have been employed, including Semantic Decision versus Sensory Discrimination,[7,19,38] Semantic Decision versus Orthographic Decision,[8] Word Generation versus Rest,[9–11,13,14,16,20–22] Object Naming,[14,22] and Word or Sentence Reading.[14,22] In the largest of these early studies, an fMRI language laterality index based on a Semantic Decision versus Sensory Discrimination contrast was compared to an analogous index based on the Wada test in 22 epilepsy patients.[7] The two indices were highly correlated ($r = 0.96$), and there were no disagreements in dominance classification. In a subsequent analysis using the same methods, dominance classification by Wada and fMRI was concordant in 48 of 49 (98%) consecutive patients with valid exams.[149]

While semantic decision and word-generation paradigms generally produce high (90–100%) concordance rates (although see Reference 11), results obtained with Sentence Listening versus Rest,[16] Object Naming versus Rest,[14] and Object Naming versus Sensory Discrimination[22] protocols were not correlated with Wada results. This lack of concordance probably stems from the fact that these contrasts produce strong activation in auditory and visual sensory systems that are not strongly lateralized and only weak activation in prefrontal language areas. Word-generation tasks, on the other hand, produce strong frontal activation, but relatively weak temporal and parietal activation. The most concordant results obtained with these tasks are thus based on activation in a frontal ROI. This characteristic of the word-generation task is potentially problematic for clinical applications in patients with temporal lobe pathology, for several reasons. First, it is possible that language lateralization in such cases could differ for the frontal and temporal lobes, and it would be preferable to know the dominance pattern in the region in which surgery is to be undertaken. Second, if the goal is not simply to determine language dominance, but rather to detect language-related cortex with optimal sensitivity for surgical planning, then lack of dominant temporal or parietal lobe activation represents a clear failure of the task paradigm. Another major limitation of the word-generation task is that it requires spoken responses, which are somewhat problematic for fMRI studies. As a result, all of the cited studies have used covert responding in which subjects are asked simply to think of words. The absence of behavioral confirmation of task performance is not a problem if the goal is simply to calculate a lateralization index in the setting of at least some measurable activation. If, on the other hand, there is little or no activation, or the goal is to localize activation with optimal sensitivity, it can never be known whether lack of activation implies lack of cortical function or is simply an artifact of poor task compliance.

## Comparisons with Cortical Stimulation Mapping

A number of studies have compared fMRI language maps with language maps obtained using cortical stimulation mapping.[14,23–30,38] These studies are of great potential interest because they permit a test of whether fMRI activation foci represent critical language areas. Some regions activated during language tasks may play a minor supportive role rather than a critical role, and resection of these active foci may not necessarily produce clinically relevant deficits. Thus, it is vital to distinguish these non-critical areas from those that are critical to normal function. The assumption underlying the cortical stimulation technique is that the temporary deactivation induced by electrical interference will identify any such critical areas.

The published studies comparing fMRI and cortical stimulation report encouraging results. These reports have involved relatively small samples (less than 15 patients). Methods for comparing the activation maps have tended to be qualitative and subjective rather than quantitative and objective, with a few exceptions.[23,30] Fitzgerald and colleagues reported an average sensitivity of 81% and specificity of 53% in 11 patients when using fMRI to predict critical language sites on intraoperative cortical stimulation mapping, employing a criterion that the fMRI focus in question must spatially overlap the stimulation site.[23] When the criterion was loosened to include instances in which the fMRI focus was within two centimeters of the stimulation site, sensitivity improved to 92%, but specificity was 0%. Sensitivity and specificity were highly variable across subjects. Rutten and colleagues reported an average sensitivity of 92% and specificity of 61%, but this analysis was performed after removing three patients (out of 11) in whom cortical stimulation mapping showed no language sites.[30] Moreover, the fMRI data appear to have been used during surgery to select the sites for cortical stimulation, so the measurements being compared were not made independently.

Several factors make these comparisons particularly difficult to carry out. One problem is in matching the task characteristics across the two modalities. Functional MRI studies usually employ controls for nonlinguistic aspects of task performance, whereas this is typically not true of stimulation mapping studies. For example, stimulation studies often focus on speech arrest, which can result from disruption of motor or attentional systems, as well as language systems.[12] A second difficulty is the fact that many fMRI activation foci lie buried in the depths of sulci, which are not available for stimulation mapping. Thus, it is reasonable to expect that many foci of activation observed by fMRI simply will not be tested adequately during cortical stimulation mapping. Finally, the assumptions forming the basis for the cortical stimulation technique have yet to be assessed adequately. There is, for example, very little evidence that resection of critical areas detected by cortical stimulation necessarily leads to postoperative language deficits. One study, in fact, showed that the likelihood of finding critical foci in the left anterior temporal lobe was higher among patients with poor language function, even though these patients are less likely to show language decline after left anterior temporal lobectomy.[155,156] Moreover, there is very little evidence that cortical stimulation mapping has any effect on preventing language decline,[157] suggesting that there are critical language areas that may not be detected by focal electrical interference. This lack of sensitivity might occur, for example, if language functions were redundently distributed across a number of nearby zones, several of which fell within the resection area, but none of which produced a language deficit when deactivated in isolation.

## Prediction of Language Outcome

It could be argued that neither the Wada test nor cortical stimulation mapping constitute an ideal gold standard against which to judge fMRI language maps. Both of these tests have recognized limitations, and both differ sufficiently from fMRI in terms of methodology and level of spatial detail that it is probably unreasonable to expect strong concordance with fMRI maps. A more meaningful measure of the validity of fMRI language maps is how well they predict postoperative language deficits. The purpose of preoperative language mapping, after all, is to assess the risk of such deficits and (in the case of cortical stimulation mapping) to minimize their severity. If fMRI can predict postoperative language deficits as well as, or better than, the Wada test, then what need is there to compare fMRI directly with the Wada?

Sabsevitz and colleagues[32] assessed the ability of preoperative fMRI to predict naming decline in 24 consecutively encountered patients undergoing left anterior temporal lobectomy (ATL). Functional MRI employed a Semantic Decision versus Sensory Discrimination protocol. All left ATL patients also underwent Wada testing and intraoperative cortical stimulation mapping, and surgeries were performed blind to the fMRI data. Compared to a control group of 32 right ATL patients, the left ATL group declined postoperatively on the 60-item Boston Naming Test ($p < 0.001$). Within the left ATL group, however, there was considerable variability, with 13 patients (54%) showing significant declines relative to the control group and no decline to the remainder. A laterality index based on fMRI activation in a temporal lobe region of interest was correlated strongly with outcome ($r = -0.64$, $p < 0.001$), such that the degree of language lateralization toward the surgical (left) hemisphere was related to poorer naming outcome, whereas language lateralization toward the non-surgical (right) hemisphere was associated with less or no decline (Figure 10.5). Of note, an LI based on a frontal lobe ROI was considerably less predictive ($r = -0.47$, $p < 0.05$), suggesting that an optimal LI is one that indexes lateralization near the surgical resection area. The fMRI temporal lobe LI showed 100% sensitivity, 73% specificity, and a positive predictive value of 81% for predicting significant decline. By comparison, the Wada language LI showed a somewhat weaker correlation with decline ($r = -0.50$, $p < 0.05$), 92% sensitivity, 43% specificity, and a positive predictive value of 67%.

These results suggest that preoperative fMRI could be used to stratify patients in terms of risk for language decline, allowing patients and physicians to weigh more accurately the risks and benefits of brain surgery. It is crucial to note, however, that these results hold only for the particular methods used in the study and may not generalize to other fMRI protocols, analysis methods, patient populations, or surgical procedures. Future studies should not only confirm these results using larger patient samples, but also test their generalizability to other protocols.

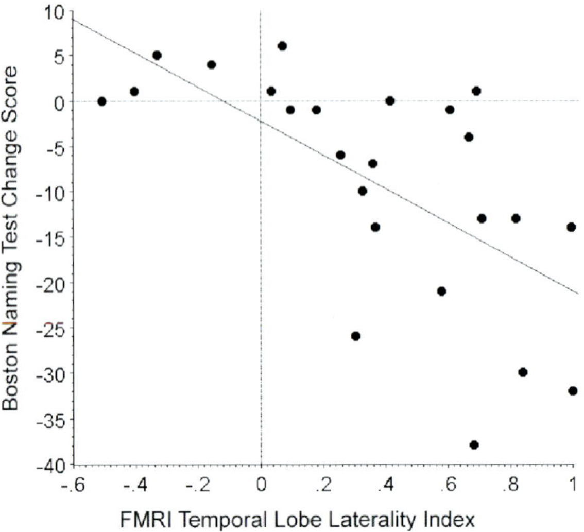


**Figure 10.5.** Scatterplot depicting the relationship between preoperative lateralization of language-related brain activation in a temporal lobe region of interest and postoperative decline in confrontation naming performance. Reprinted with permission from Sabsevitz DS, Swanson SJ, Hammeke TA, Spanaki MV, Possing ET, Morris GL 3rd, et al. Use of preoperative functional neuroimaging to predict language deficits from epilepsy surgery. *Neurology* 2003;60:1788–92.

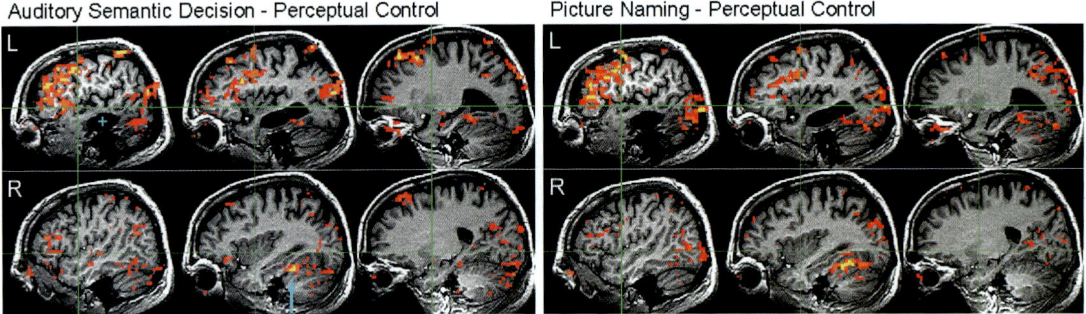


**Figure 10.6.** Language-related activation in a young man considering repeat surgery for intractable left temporal lobe epilepsy. Results from two separate activation protocols are shown in serial sagittal sections through the left (top) and right (bottom) hemispheres. Data are formatted in stereotactic space, with stereotactic axes indicated by green lines. Maps are thresholded at $p < 0.001$ to allow viewing of the background anatomy. A large area of left temporal lobe encephalomalacia (blue cross) is the result of previous epilepsy surgery. Activation in both protocols is strongly left-lateralized in the frontal lobe (frontal LI = 0.54 and 0.79 for the Semantic Decision and Picture Naming protocols, respectively) and modestly right-lateralized in the temporal lobe (temporal LI = –0.27 and –0.13). The Semantic Decision protocol elicits greater activation in the angular gyrus and prefrontal cortex, while the Picture Naming protocol elicits greater activation in ventral visual association areas. The blue arrow indicates activation in the fusiform gyrus ("basal temporal language area"), which has likely undergone a shift to the right hemisphere as the result of longstanding left temporal lobe pathology.

Several clinical examples of language system mapping with fMRI are presented. Figure 10.6 illustrates the use of two distinct activation protocols to determine language dominance and functional status of the left temporal lobe preoperatively in a patient with a large left

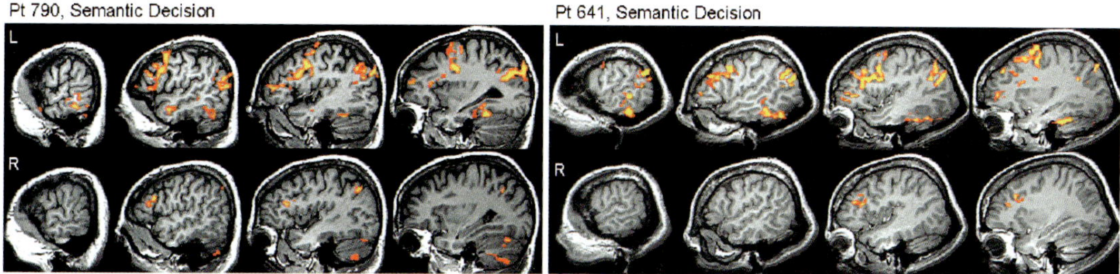


**Figure 10.7.** Presurgical language mapping (semantic decision vs. perceptual control) in two patients with intractable left temporal lobe epilepsy. Both patients had strong leftward lateralization of temporal lobe activity (Patient 790 temporal LI = 0.84, Patient 641 temporal LI = 0.82), and both declined on the Boston Naming Test after left anterior temporal lobectomy (Patient 790 BNT change = –30, Patient 641 BNT change = –13).

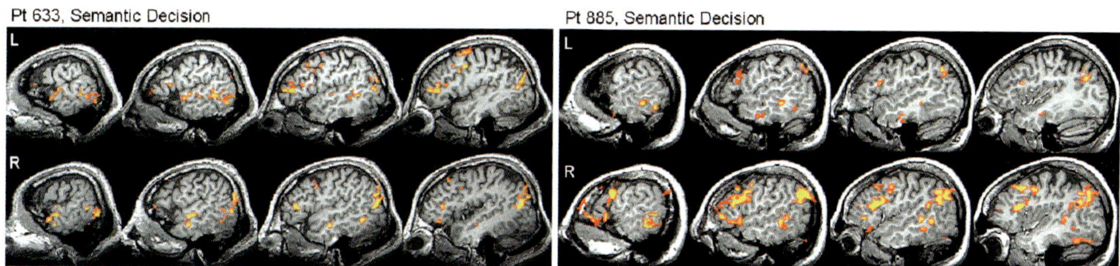


**Figure 10.8.** Presurgical language mapping (semantic decision vs. perceptual control) in two more patients with intractable left temporal lobe epilepsy. Both had clear bilateral temporal lobe activation (Patient 633 temporal LI = 0.03, Patient 885 temporal LI = –0.33), and neither patient declined on the Boston Naming Test after left anterior temporal lobectomy (Patient 633 BNT change = +1, Patient 885 BNT change = +5). In Patient 633, the Wada language asymmetry was strongly left lateralized (Wada LI = 0.87), incorrectly predicting language decline. These cases illustrate the utility of quantitative presurgical fMRI of the temporal lobes for predicting language decline from left ATL surgery.

temporal lesion. Figure 10.7 illustrates preoperative language activation patterns in 2 patients who subsequently underwent left anterior temporal lobectomy complicated by significant declines in object naming performance. Figure 10.8, in contrast, illustrates preoperative language activation patterns in 2 patients who subsequently underwent left anterior temporal lobectomy without any decline in object naming.

## Future Applications: Use of fMRI Language Maps in Surgical Planning

It remains to be established how useful fMRI language activation maps will be for more precise planning of surgical resections. At least three significant problems complicate progress: (i) inconsistencies in language maps produced by different activation protocols, (ii) the failure to date to find an activation protocol that reliably activates the anterior temporal lobe where the majority of epilepsy surgeries are performed,

mapping, and frameless stereotaxy in the resection of lesions in eloquent areas of brain in children. *Pediatr Neurosurg.* 1997;26:68–82.
25. Yetkin FZ, Mueller WM, Morris GL, McAuliffe TL, Ulmer JL, Cox RW, et al. Functional MR activation correlated with intraoperative cortical mapping. *Am J Neuroradiol.* 1997;18:1311–1315.
26. Ruge MI, Victor JD, Hosain S, Correa DD, Relkin NR, Tabar V, et al. Concordance between functional magnetic resonance imaging and intraoperative language mapping. *Stereotact Funct Neurosurg.* 1999;72:95–102.
27. Schlosser MJ, Luby M, Spencer DD, Awad IA, McCarthy G. Comparative localization of auditory comprehension by using functional magnetic resonance imaging and cortical stimulation. *J Neurosurg.* 1999;91:626–635.
28. Lurito JT, Lowe MJ, Sartorius C, Mathews VP. Comparison of fMRI and intraoperative direct cortical stimulation in localization of receptive language areas. *J Comput Assist Tomogr.* 2000;24:99–105.
29. Rutten GJM, van Rijen PC, van Veelen CWM, Ramsey NF. Language area localization with three-dimensional functional magnetic resonance imaging matches intrasulcal electrostimulation in Broca's area. *Ann Neurol.* 1999;46:405–408.
30. Rutten GJM, Ramsey NF, van Rijen PC, Noordmans HJ, van Veelen CW. Development of a functional magnetic resonance imaging protocol for intraoperative localization of critical temporoparietal language areas. *Ann Neurol.* 2002;51:350–360.
31. Rutten GJ, Ramsey N, van Rijen P, van Veelen C. Reproducibility of fMRI-determined language lateralization in individual subjects. *Brain Lang.* 2002;80:421–437.
32. Sabsevitz DS, Swanson SJ, Hammeke TA, Spanaki MV, Possing ET, Morris GL, et al. Use of preoperative functional neuroimaging to predict language deficits from epilepsy surgery. *Neurology.* 2003;60:1788–1792.
33. Binder J. FMRI: Language mapping. *Neurosurg Clin N Am.* 1997;8:383–392.
34. Gaillard WD, Theodore WH. Mapping language in epilepsy with functional neuroimaging. *Neuroscientist.* 2000;6:391–401.
35. Hammeke TA, Bellgowan PSF, Binder JR. FMRI methodology: Cognitive function mapping. *Adv Neurol.* 2000;83:221–233.
36. Detre JA, Floyd TF. Functional MRi and its applications to the clinical neurosciences. *Neuroscientist.* 2001;7:64–79.
37. Binder JR, Achten E, Constable RT, Detre JA, Gaillard WD, Jack CR, et al. Functional MRI in epilepsy. *Epilepsia.* 2002;43 (Suppl 1):51–63.
38. Carpentier A, Pugh KR, Westerveld M, et al. Functional MRI of language processing: dependence on input modality and temporal lobe epilepsy. *Epilepsia.* 2001;42:1241–1254.
39. Fernández G, Specht K, Weis S, Tendolkar I, Reuber M, Fell J, et al. Intrasubject reproducibility of presurgical language lateralization and mapping using fMRI. *Neurology.* 2003;60:969–975.
40. Kertesz A, Harlock W, Coates R. Computer tomographic localization, lesion size, and prognosis in aphasia and nonverbal impairment. *Brain Lang.* 1979;8:34–50.
41. Porch BE, Collins M, Wertz RT, Friden TP. Statistical prediction of change in aphasia. *J Speech Hear Res.* 1980;23:312–321.
42. Selnes OA, Knopman DS, Niccum N, Rubens AB, Larson D. Computed tomographic scan correlates of auditory comprehension deficits in aphasia: A prospective recovery study. *Ann Neurol.* 1983;13:558–566.
43. Metter EJ, Jackson CA, Kempler D, Hanson WR. Temporoparietal cortex and the recovery of language comprehension in aphasia. *Aphasiology.* 1992;6:349–358.

44. Ferro JM. The influence of infarct location on recovery from global aphasia. *Aphasiology*. 1992;6:415–430.
45. Code C, Rowley D, Kertesz A. Predicting recovery from aphasia with connectionist networks: Preliminary comparisons with multiple regression. *Cortex*. 1994;30:527–532.
46. Karbe H, Kessler J, Herholz K, Fink GR, Heiss W-D. Long-term prognosis of poststroke aphasia studied with positron emission tomography. *Arch Neurol*. 1995;52:186–190.
47. Pedersen PM, Jorgensen HS, Nakayama H, Raaschou HO, Olsen TS. Aphasia in acute stroke: Incidence, determinants, and recovery. *Ann Neurol*. 1995;38:659–666.
48. Cao Y, Vikingstad BS, George PK, Johnson AF, Welch KMA. Cortical language activation in stroke patients recovering from aphasia with functional MRI. *Stroke*. 1999;30:2331–2340.
49. Thulborn KR, Carpenter PA, Just MA. Plasticity of language-related brain function during recovery from stroke. *Stroke*. 1999;30:749–754.
50. Calvert GA, Brammer MJ, Morris RG, Williams SCR, King N, Matthews PM. Using fMRI to study recovery from acquired dysphasia. *Brain Lang*. 2000;71:391–399.
51. Rosen HJ, Petersen SE, Linenweber MR, Snyder AZ, White DA, Chapman L, et al. Neural correlates of recovery from aphasia after damage to left inferior frontal cortex. *Neurology*. 2000;55:1883–1894.
52. Eden GF, VanMeter JW, Rumsey JM, Maisog JM, Woods RP, Zeffiro TA. Abnormal processing of visual motion in dyslexia revealed by functional brain imaging. *Nature*. 1996;382:66–69.
53. Demb JB, Boynton GM, Heeger DJ. Brain activity in visual cortex predicts individual differences in reading performance. *PNAS*. 1997;94: 13363–13366.
54. Shaywitz SE, Shaywitz BA, Pugh KR, Fulbright RK, Constable RT, Mencl WE, et al. Functional disruption in the organization of the brain for reading in dyslexia. *PNAS*. 1998;95:2636–2641.
55. Temple E, Deutsch GK, Poldrack RA, Miller SL, Tallal P, Merzenich MM, et al. Neural deficits in children with dyslexia ameliorated by behavioral remediation: Evidence from functional MRI. *PNAS*. 2003;100:2860–2865.
56. Petersen SE, Fox PT, Posner MI, Mintun M, Raichle ME. Positron emission tomographic studies of the cortical anatomy of single-word processing. *Nature*. 1988;331:585–589.
57. Wise R, Chollet F, Hadar U, Friston K, Hoffner E, Frackowiak R. Distribution of cortical neural networks involved in word comprehension and word retrieval. *Brain*. 1991;114:1803–1817.
58. Démonet J-F, Chollet F, Ramsay S, Cardebat D, Nespoulous J-L, Wise R, et al. The anatomy of phonological and semantic processing in normal subjects. *Brain*. 1992;115:1753–1768.
59. Binder JR, Price CJ. Functional imaging of language. In: Cabeza R, Kingstone A, editors. *Handbook of Functional Neuroimaging of Cognition*. Cambridge, MA: MIT Press; 2001:187–251.
60. Macleod CM. Half a century of research on the Stroop effect: an integrative review. *Psychol Bull*. 1991;109:163–203.
61. Reicher GM. Perceptual recognition as a function of meaningfulness of stimulus material. *J Exp Psychol*. 1969;81:274–280.
62. Warren RM, Obusek CJ. Speech perception and phonemic restorations. *Percept Psychophys*. 1971;9:358–362.
63. Ganong WF. Phonetic categorization in auditory word perception. *J Exp Psychol Hum Percept Perform*. 1980;6:110–115.

64. Marslen-Wilson WD, Tyler LK. Central processes in speech understanding. *Philos Trans R Soc London B Biol Sci.* 1981;295:317–332.
65. Carr TH, McCauley C, Sperber RD, Parmalee CM. Words, pictures, and priming: On semantic activation, conscious identification, and the automaticity of information processing. *J Exp Psychol Hum Percept Perform.* 1982;8:757–777.
66. Marcel AJ. Conscious and unconscious perception: Experiments on visual masking and word recognition. *Cognit Psychol.* 1983;15:197–237.
67. Van Orden GC. A ROWS is a ROSE: Spelling, sound, and reading. *Mem Cognit.* 1987;15:181–198.
68. Burton MW, Baum SR, Blumstein SE. Lexical effects on phonetic categorization of speech: The role of acoustic structure. *J Exp Psychol Hum Percept Perform.* 1989;15:567–575.
69. Glaser WR. Picture naming. *Cognition.* 1992;42:61–105.
70. Raichle ME, Fiez JA, Videen TO, MacLeod AM, Pardo JV, Fox PT, et al. Practice-related changes in human brain functional anatomy during nonmotor learning. *Cereb Cortex.* 1994;4:8–26.
71. Buckner RL, Raichle ME, Petersen SE. Dissociation of human prefrontal cortical areas across different speech production tasks and gender groups. *J Neurosci.* 1995;74:2163–2173.
72. Bookheimer SY, Zeffiro TA, Blaxton T, Gaillard T, Theodore W. Regional cerebral blood flow during object naming and word reading. *Hum Brain Mapp.* 1995;3:93–106.
73. Price CJ, Wise RSJ, Frackowiak RSJ. Demonstrating the implicit processing of visually presented words and pseudowords. *Cereb Cortex.* 1996;6:62–70.
74. Damasio H, Grabowski TJ, Tranel D, Hichwa RD, Damasio AR. A neural basis for lexical retrieval. *Nature.* 1996;380:499–505.
75. Binder JR, Frost JA, Hammeke TA, Cox RW, Rao SM, Prieto T. Human brain language areas identified by functional MRI. *J Neurosci.* 1997;17: 353–362.
76. James W. *Principles of Psychology*, vol. 1. New York: Dover Publications; 1890.
77. Hebb DO. The problem of consciousness and introspection. In: Adrian ED, Bremer F, Jasper HH, editors. *Brain Mechanisms and Consciousness: A Symposium.* Springfield, IL: Charles C. Thomas; 1954:402–421.
78. Miller GA, Galanter E, Pribram K. *Plans and the Structure of Behavior.* New York: Holt; 1960.
79. Pope KS, Singer JL. Regulation of the stream of consciousness: Toward a theory of ongoing thought. In: Schwartz GE, Shapiro D, editors. *Consciousness and Self-Regulation.* New York: Plenum Press; 1976:101–135.
80. Antrobus JS, Singer JL, Greenberg S. Studies in the stream of consciousness: Experimental enhancement and suppression of spontaneous cognitive processes. *Percept Mot Skills.* 1966;23:399–417.
81. Teasdale JD, Proctor L, Lloyd CA, Baddeley AD. Working memory and stimulus-independent thought: Effects of memory load and presentation rate. *Eur J Cogn Psychol.* 1993;5:417–433.
82. Révész G, editor. *Thinking and Speaking: A symposium.* Amsterdam: North Holland Publishing; 1954.
83. Weiskrantz L, editor. *Thought without Language.* Oxford: Clarendon; 1988.
84. Vygotsky LS. *Thought and Language.* New York: Wiley; 1962.
85. Karmiloff-Smith A. *Beyond Modularity: A Developmental Perspective on Cognitive Science.* Cambridge, MA: MIT Press; 1992.
86. Andreasen NC, O'Leary DS, Cizadlo T, Arndt S, Rezai K, Watkins GL, et al. Remembering the past: Two facets of episodic memory explored

with positron emission tomography. *Am J Psychiatry.* 1995;152:1576–1585.

87. Shulman GL, Fiez JA, Corbetta M, Buckner RL, Meizin FM, Raichle ME, et al. Common blood flow changes across visual tasks: II. Decreases in cerebral cortex. *J Cogn Neurosci.* 1997;9:648–663.
88. Binder JR, Frost JA, Hammeke TA, Bellgowan PSF, Rao SM, Cox RW. Conceptual processing during the conscious resting state: a functional MRI study. *J Cogn Neurosci.* 1999;11:80–93.
89. Mazoyer B, Zago L, Mellet E, Bricogne S, Etard O, Houdé O, et al. Cortical networks for working memory and executive functions sustain the conscious resting state in man. *Brain Res Bull.* 2001;54:287–298.
90. Raichle ME, McLeod AM, Snyder AZ, Powers WJ, Gusnard DA, Shulman GL. A default mode of brain function. *PNAS.* 2001;98:676–682.
91. Stark CE, Squire LR. When zero is not zero: The problem of ambiguous baseline conditions in fMRI. *PNAS.* 2001;98:12760–12766.
92. McKiernan KA, Kaufman JN, Kucera-Thompson J, Binder JR. A parametric manipulation of factors affecting task-induced deactivation in functional neuroimaging. *J Cogn Neurosci.* 2003;15:394–408.
93. Grabowski TJ, Damasio AR. Investigating language with functional neuroimaging. In: Toga AW, Mazziotta JC, editors. *Brain Mapping: The Systems.* San Diego, CA: Academic Press; 2000:425–461.
94. Binder JR. Wernicke aphasia: A disorder of central language processing. In: D'Esposito ME, editor. *Neurological Foundations of Cognitive Neuroscience.* Cambridge, MA: MIT Press; 2002:175–238.
95. Binder JR, Frost JA, Hammeke TA, Bellgowan PSF, Springer JA, Kaufman JN, et al. Human temporal lobe activation by speech and nonspeech sounds. *Cereb Cortex.* 2000;10:512–528.
96. Scott SK, Blank C, Rosen S, Wise RJS. Identification of a pathway for intelligible speech in the left temporal lobe. *Brain.* 2000;123:2400–2406.
97. Liebenthal E, Binder JR, Piorkowski RL, Remez RE. Short-term reorganization of auditory analysis induced by phonetic experience. *J Cogn Neurosci.* 2003;15:549–558.
98. Belin P, Zatorre RJ, Ahad P. Human temporal-lobe response to vocal sounds. *Cogn Brain Res.* 2002;13:17–26.
99. Cohen L, Lehéricy S, Chochon F, Lemer C, Rivaud S, Dehaene S. Language-specific tuning of visual cortex? Functional properties of the visual word form area. *Brain.* 2002;125:1054–1069.
100. Wise RSJ, Scott SK, Blank SC, Mummery CJ, Murphy K, Warburton EA. Separate neural subsystems within "Wernicke's area". *Brain.* 2001;124:83–95.
101. Mazoyer BM, Tzourio N, Frak V, Syrota A, Murayama N, Levrier O, et al. The cortical representation of speech. *J Cogn Neurosci.* 1993;5:467–479.
102. Price CJ, Wise RJS, Warburton EA, Moore CJ, Howard D, Patterson K, et al. Hearing and saying. The functional neuro-anatomy of auditory word processing. *Brain.* 1996;119:919–931.
103. Zatorre RJ, Evans AC, Meyer E, Gjedde A. Lateralization of phonetic and pitch discrimination in speech processing. *Science.* 1992;256:846–849.
104. Mummery CJ, Ashburner J, Scott SK, Wise RJS. Functional neuroimaging of speech perception in six normal and two aphasic subjects. *J Acoust Soc Am.* 1999;106:449–457.
105. Belin P, Zatorre RJ, Lafaille P, Ahad P, Pike B. Voice-selective areas in human auditory cortex. *Nature.* 2000;403:309–312.

106. Binder JR, Rao SM, Hammeke TA, Frost JA, Bandettini PA, Hyde JS. Effects of stimulus rate on signal response during functional magnetic resonance imaging of auditory cortex. *Cogn Brain Res.* 1994;2:31–38.
107. Eulitz C, Elbert T, Bartenstein P, Weiller C, Müller SP, Pantev C. Comparison of magnetic and metabolic brain activity during a verb generation task. *Neuroreport.* 1994;6:97–100.
108. Warburton E, Wise RJS, Price CJ, Weiller C, Hadar U, Ramsay S, et al. Noun and verb retrieval by normal subjects. Studies with PET. *Brain.* 1996;119:159–179.
109. Ojemann JG, Buckner RL, Akbudak E, Snyder AZ, Ollinger JM, McKinstry RC, et al. Functional MRI studies of word-stem completion: Reliability across laboratories and comparison to blood flow imaging with PET. *Hum Brain Mapp.* 1998;6:203–215.
110. Palmer ED, Rosen HJ, Ojemann JG, Buckner RL, Kelley WM, Petersen SE. An event-related fMRI study of overt and covert word stem completion. *Neuroimage.* 2001;14:182–193.
111. Thompson-Schill SL, D'Esposito M, Kan IP. Effects of repetition and competition on activity in left prefrontal cortex during word generation. *Neuron.* 1999;23:513–522.
112. Malach R, Reppas JB, Benson RR, Kwong KK, Jiang H, Kennedy WA, et al. Object-related activity revealed by functional magnetic resonance imaging in human occipital cortex. *PNAS.* 1995;92:8135–8139.
113. Kanwisher N, Woods R, Iacoboni M, Mazziotta J. A locus in human extrastriate cortex for visual shape analysis. *J Cogn Neurosci.* 1996;91:133–142.
114. Grill-Spector K, Kushnir T, Edelman S, Avidian-Carmel G, Itzchak Y, Malach R. Differential processing of objects under various viewing conditions in the human lateral occipital complex. *Neuron.* 1999;24:187–203.
115. Martin A, Wiggs CL, Ungerleider LG, Haxby JV. Neural correlates of category-specific knowledge. *Nature.* 1996;379:649–652.
116. Price CJ, Moore CJ, Humphreys GW, Frackowiak RSJ, Friston KJ. The neural regions sustaining object recognition and naming. *Proc R Soc London B.* 1996;263:1501–1507.
117. Zelkowicz BJ, Herbster AN, Nebes RD, Mintun MA, Becker JT. An examination of regional cerebral blood flow during object naming tasks. *J Int Neuropsychol Soc.* 1998;4:160–166.
118. Murtha S, Chertkow H, Beauregard M, Evans A. The neural substrate of picture naming. *J Cogn Neurosci.* 1999;11:399–423.
119. Kiasawa M, Inoue C, Kawasaki T, Tokoro T, Ishii K, Ohyama M, et al. Functional neuroanatomy of object naming: A PET study. *Graefes Arch Clin Exp Ophthalmol.* 1996;234:110–115.
120. Vandenberghe R, Price C, Wise R, Josephs O, Frackowiak RSJ. Functional anatomy of a common semantic system for words and pictures. *Nature.* 1996;383:254–256.
121. Müller R-A, Kleinhans N, Courchesne E. Linguistic theory and neuroimaging evidence: an fMRI study of Broca's area in lexical semantics. *Neuropsychologia.* In press.
122. Price CJ, Moore CJ, Humphreys GW, Wise RJS. Segregating semantic from phonological processes during reading. *J Cogn Neurosci.* 1997;9:727–733.
123. Mummery CJ, Patterson K, Hodges JR, Price CJ. Functional neuroanatomy of the semantic system: divisible by what? *J Cogn Neurosci.* 1998;10:766–777.
124. Chee MWL, O'Craven KM, Bergida R, Rosen BR, Savoy RL. Auditory and visual word processing studied with fMRI. *Hum Brain Mapp.* 1999;7:15–28.

125. Roskies AL, Fiez JA, Balota DA, Raichle ME, Petersen SE. Task-dependent modulation of regions in the left inferior frontal cortex during semantic processing. *J Cogn Neurosci.* 2001;13:829–843.
126. Bavelier D, Corina D, Jezzard P, Padmanabhan S, Clark VP, Karni A, et al. Sentence reading: a functional MRI study at 4 tesla. *J Cogn Neurosci.* 1997;9:664–686.
127. Herbster AN, Mintun MA, Nebes RD, Becker JT. Regional cerebral blood flow during word and nonword reading. *Hum Brain Mapp.* 1997;5:84–92.
128. Indefrey P, Kleinschmidt A, Merboldt K-D, Krüger G, Brown C, Hagoort P, et al. Equivalent responses to lexical and nonlexical visual stimuli in occipital cortex: a functional magnetic resonance imaging study. *Neuroimage.* 1997;5:78–81.
129. Chee MW, Caplan D, Soon CS, Sriram N, Tan EWL, Thiel T, et al. Processing of visually presented sentences in Mandarin and English studied with fMRI. *Neuron.* 1999;23:127–137.
130. Pugh KR, Shaywitz BA, Shaywitz SE, Constable RT, Skudlarski P, Fulbright RK, et al. Cerebral organization of component processes in reading. *Brain.* 1996;119:1221–1238.
131. Springer JA, Binder JR, Hammeke TA, Swanson SJ, Frost JA, Bellgowan PSF, et al. Language dominance in neurologically normal and epilepsy subjects: a functional MRI study. *Brain.* 1999;122:2033–2045.
132. Pujol J, Deus J, Losilla JM, Capdevila A. Cerebral lateralization of language in normal left-handed people studied by functional MRI. *Neurology.* 1999;52:1038–1043.
133. Vikingstad EM, George KP, Johnson AF, Cao Y. Cortical language lateralization in right handed normal subjects using functional magnetic resonance imaging. *J Neurol Sci.* 2000;175:17–27.
134. Szaflarski JP, Binder JR, Possing ET, McKiernan KA, Ward DB, Hammeke TA. Language lateralization in left-handed and ambidextrous people: fMRI data. *Neurology.* 2002;59:238–244.
135. Hund-Georgiadis M, Lex U, Friederici AD, von Cramon DY. Non-invasive regime for language lateralization in right- and left-handers by means of functional MRI and dichotic listening. *Exp Brain Res.* 2002;145:166–176.
136. Knecht S, Deppe M, Dräger B, Bobe L, Lohmann H, Ringelstein EB, et al. Language lateralization in healthy right-handers. *Brain.* 2000;123:74–81.
137. Shaywitz BA, Shaywitz SE, Pugh KR, Constable RT, Skudlarski P, Fulbright RK, et al. Sex differences in the functional organization of the brain for language. *Nature.* 1995;373:607–609.
138. Price CJ, Moore CJ, Friston KJ. Getting sex into perspective. *Neuroimage.* 1996;3:S586.
139. Frost JA, Binder JR, Springer JA, Hammeke TA, Bellgowan PSF, Rao SM, et al. Language processing is strongly left lateralized in both sexes: Evidence from FMRI. *Brain.* 1999;122:199–208.
140. Knecht S, Dräger B, Deppe M, Bobe L, Lohmann H, Flöel A, et al. Handedness and hemispheric language dominance in healthy humans. *Brain.* 2000;123:2512–2518.
141. Rasmussen T, Milner B. The role of early left-brain injury in determining lateralization of cerebral speech functions. *Ann N Y Acad Sci.* 1977;299:355–369.
142. Loring DW, Meador KJ, Lee GP, Murro AM, Smith JR, Flanigin HF, et al. Cerebral language lateralization: Evidence from intracarotid amobarbital testing. *Neuropsychologia.* 1990;28:831–838.

143. Grady CL, Maisog JM, Horwitz B, et al. Age-related changes in cortical blood flow activation during visual processing of faces and location. *J Neurosci.* 1994;14:1450–1462.
144. Grady CL, McIntosh AR, Bookstein F, Horwitz B, Rapoport SI, Haxby JV. Age-related changes in regional cerebral blood flow during working memory for faces. *Neuroimage.* 1998;8:409–425.
145. Woods RP, Dodrill CB, Ojemann GA. Brain injury, handedness, and speech lateralization in a series of amobarbital studies. *Ann Neurol.* 1988;23:510–518.
146. Risse GL, Gates JR, Fangman MC. A reconsideration of bilateral language representation based on the intracarotid amobarbital procedure. *Brain Lang.* 1997;33:118–132.
147. Binder JR, Rao SM, Hammeke TA, Frost JA, Bandettini PA, Jesmanowicz A, et al. Lateralized human brain language systems demonstrated by task subtraction functional magnetic resonance imaging. *Arch Neurol.* 1995; 52:593–601.
148. Cohen MS, Dubois RM. Stability, repeatability, and the expression of signal magnitude in functional magnetic resonance imaging. *J Magn Reson Imaging.* 1999;10:33–40.
149. Binder JR, Hammeke TA, Possing ET, Swanson SJ, Spanaki MV, Morris GL, et al. Reliability and validity of language dominance assessment with functional MRI. *Neurology.* 2001;56 (Suppl 3):A158.
150. Xiong J, Rao S, Gao JH, Woldorff M, Fox PT. Evaluation of hemispheric dominance for language using functional MRI: a comparison with positron emission tomography. *Hum Brain Mapp.* 1998;6:42–58.
151. Altenmüller DM, Kriechbaum W, Helber U, Moini S, Dichgans J, Petersen D. Cortical DC-potentials in identification of the language dominant hemisphere: linguistical and clinical aspects. *Acta Neurochir (Wien).* 1993;56 (Suppl.):20–33.
152. Khedr EM, Hamed E, Said A, Basahi J. Handedness and language cerebral lateralization. *Eur J Appl Physiol.* 2002;87:469–473.
153. Deppe M, Knecht S, Papke K, Lohmann H, Fleischer H, Heindel W, et al. Assessment of hemispheric language lateralization: A comparison between fMRI and fTCD. *J Cereb Blood Flow Metab.* 2000;20:263–268.
154. Foundas AL, Leonard CM, Gilmore R, Fennell E, Heilman KM. Planum temporale asymmetry and language dominance. *Neuropsychologia.* 1994;32:1225–1231.
155. Chelune GJ. Using neuropsychological data to forecast postsurgical cognitive outcome. In: Lüders H, editor. *Epilepsy Surgery.* New York: Raven Press; 1991:477–485.
156. Schwartz TH, Devinsky O, Doyle W, Perrine K. Preoperative predictors of anterior temporal language areas. *J Neurosurg.* 1998;89:962–970.
157. Hermann BP, Perrine K, Chelune GJ, Barr W, Loring DW, Strauss E, et al. Visual confrontation naming following left anterior temporal lobectomy: A comparison of surgical approaches. *Neuropsychology.* 1999; 13:3–9.
158. Grabowski TJ, Damasio H, Tranel D, Ponto LL, Hichwa RD, Damasio AR. A role for left temporal pole in the retrieval of words for unique entities. *Hum Brain Mapp.* 2001;13:199–212.
159. Hamberger MJ, Goodman RR, Perrine K, Tamny TR. Anatomic dissociation of auditory and visual naming in the lateral temporal cortex. *Neurology.* 2001;56:56–61.

160. Hermann BP, Wyler AR, Somes G, Clement L. Dysnomia after left anterior temporal lobectomy without functional mapping: frequency and correlates. *Neurosurgery.* 1994;35:52–57.
161. Langfit JT, Rausch R. Word-finding deficits persist after left anterotemporal lobectomy. *Arch Neurol.* 1996;53:72–76.
162. Davies KG, Bell BD, Bush AJ, Hermann BP, Dohan FC, Jaap AS. Naming decline after left anterior temporal lobectomy correlates with pathological status of resected hippocampus. *Epilepsia.* 1998;39:407–419.
163. Bell BD, Davies KG, Hermann BP, Walters G. Confrontation naming after anterior temporal lobectomy is related to age of acquisition of the object names. *Neuropsychologia.* 2000;38:83–92.

# 11

# fMRI Wada Test: Prospects for Presurgical Mapping of Language and Memory

Brenna C. McDonald, Andrew J. Saykin, J. Michael Williams, and Bassam A. Assaf

## Introduction

Since the inception of functional magnetic resonance imaging (fMRI) in the early 1990s, clinicians and researchers have been interested in the potential utility of this technology for replacement of the intracarotid amobarbital test (IAT). The IAT, or Wada test, is an invasive angiographic procedure, with some potential risks, that currently serves as the conventional standard for lateralization of language, memory, and other functions. The IAT is used primarily in patients under consideration for neurosurgery to treat epilepsy, but also in other neurosurgical populations (e.g., motor cortex tumor, arteriovenous malformation in language association cortex, etc.). If a valid assessment paradigm could be created, the advantages of fMRI assessment of memory and language functions over the IAT would be obvious. Functional MRI is a repeatable, noninvasive procedure with no significant known health risks for most individuals. It is also very flexible and can be readily modified to assess the clinical questions at issue for a particular patient. In addition, a recent cost analysis demonstrated considerable savings of total direct costs for fMRI over IAT.[1]

While some patients (e.g., those with ferromagnetic metal in their bodies, or those who are moderately or severely claustrophobic) may be unable or ineligible to undergo fMRI, the number of those who meet these exclusion criteria is no greater than for the IAT. Furthermore, while the IAT can provide information regarding predominant hemispheric lateralization of language functions and, to a lesser degree, memory, it cannot provide information regarding the spatial location of brain regions critical for these tasks. In contrast, fMRI, with typical spatial resolution of two to four millimeters, can provide much more precise information regarding localization of brain regions that are active during memory and language tasks.

Both the IAT and fMRI are possible techniques for representing the location of important cognitive functions that are considered as part of surgery planning. The IAT was invented first and has a long history of use, and therefore has become the gold standard to which fMRI language and memory localization paradigms are compared. Many basic aspects of the IAT's validity and reliability have not been systematically investigated, however, due to the nature of the procedure and the lack of alternative techniques available for this purpose. The present chapter stresses the contrast between the testing methods. It is clear, however, that the same standards of measurement should be applied to both tests. For example, it is possible that both techniques adequately measure the lateralization of language. In contrast, both techniques may not adequately assess the location of memory abilities. The strong focus of the research literature and other discussions has been on replacing the IAT with fMRI, which, if possible, would be a worthy goal, given factors noted throughout this chapter, including the increased time, risk, and cost of the IAT. However, this focus may at times overlook basic measurement issues that apply to both techniques; in the end, the overarching goal is clearly to obtain the most reliable and valid data possible to meet the stated need of localization of language and memory functions.

The conclusions of several studies conducted over the past decade strongly suggest that fMRI paradigms exist that can be used successfully to replace the IAT in terms of language lateralization, although the status of appropriately reliable and valid memory assessment paradigms remains uncertain. Despite the apparent advantages of fMRI in such presurgical assessment, there remain methodological challenges and issues of interpretation that have thus far prevented its widespread use in place of the IAT. This chapter will briefly discuss the background of the IAT and its risks and benefits compared to fMRI. The current status of fMRI protocols aiming to replace the IAT will then be reviewed, along with future steps needed to make this goal a reality.

## The IAT: History and Background

As noted by other authors,[2,3] the first use of selective anesthetization to localize human language function was reported by Gardner in 1941.[4] Gardner utilized intracranial injection of procaine hydrochloride to unilaterally anesthetize frontal brain regions in two left-handed brain tumor patients in order to assess lateralization of hemispheric dominance for language prior to resective surgery and prevent surgically induced aphasia. The model for modern IAT procedures, however, is the work of Juhn Wada,[5] who established the feasibility of selective hemispheric anesthetization using intracarotid injection of sodium amytal.

Wada's original work in the 1940s was designed to attempt to minimize the cognitive side effects of electroconvulsive shock therapy (ECT) by preventing bilateral generalization of ECT-related seizure activity through temporary anesthetization of the language-dominant hemisphere.[3] The utility of this technique for presurgical evaluation of epilepsy quickly became apparent, and Wada pioneered this approach both in Japan and later with colleagues at the Montreal Neurological

Institute. While significant variations can currently be encountered across surgical epilepsy centers in terms of IAT procedures, several standardized methodologies have been published,[2,6,7] and the IAT is considered a critical component of presurgical evaluation of patients with epilepsy, along with clinical neuropsychological assessment, which is important for providing a context within which to interpret IAT results.[8–11] The IAT may also be used much as Gardner originally proposed, to assess the lateralized integrity of cognition prior to resection of nonepileptogenic lesions located in frontal or temporal cortex presumed to be critical to language and/or memory functions.

The need for lateralization and localization of cognitive functions such as language and memory is self-evident. For patients under consideration for resective surgery to treat medically refractory seizures, particularly in the case of temporal lobe epilepsy (TLE), the seizure focus likely to be resected includes brain regions potentially critical to the support of language and memory. It therefore becomes vital to provide as much information as possible regarding the potential deficits that might occur as a result of surgery, should the seizure focus (e.g., a sclerotic hippocampus) also be supporting one or more critical cognitive functions.

For patients whose presumed seizure focus lies adjacent to or within language cortex, detailed presurgical localization of eloquent tissue is needed to assess the feasibility of surgery and define the potential resection margin. The IAT typically is used for hemispheric lateralization of language functioning, while intracranial electrical stimulation can provide more precise mapping of language cortex, either prior to or during epilepsy surgery. While the left hemisphere is the dominant hemisphere for language in virtually all healthy right-handed individuals, the neurodevelopmental abnormalities that can be associated with epilepsy make atypical lateralization or bilateral participation in language more likely in epileptic patients.[12–16] For left-handed individuals, the issue of hemispheric language dominance becomes even more salient given the increased prevalence of right hemisphere dominance for language in left-handed individuals, which has been demonstrated using fMRI.[17,18] In addition, many fMRI studies show some degree of bilateral activation even in right-handed subjects from normal as well as clinical samples,[19–23] although most language-related activation is observed in the dominant hemisphere. Such nondominant hemisphere activation may relate to linguistic task complexity or to nonverbal aspects of language, such as prosody, narrative organization, inference, or language pragmatics.[24–31]

Assessment of hemispheric support of memory functioning is particularly important in TLE patients given the critical role of mesial temporal lobe (MTL) structures, including the hippocampus, entorhinal cortex, and amygdala, in encoding of new information. The IAT does not lateralize memory per se, but rather assesses the potential for unilateral hemispheric support of memory encoding, to prevent an iatrogenic postsurgical amnestic syndrome such as that exhibited in the classic case of patient H.M.[32] For TLE patients, the presence of mesial temporal sclerosis or other hippocampal disease may preclude effective support of memory functions by the region to be resected. Some patients, however, demonstrate memory functioning using the diseased hemisphere on IAT, indicating the potential for acquired postoperative cognitive deficits. This issue becomes even more of a concern in TLE patients with normal MRI scans, who may be more likely to have MTL tissue supporting memory in the presumed epileptogenic region.

Limitations in the use of the IAT include its invasive nature and attendant risk of potential medical complications, such as infarction, carotid artery dissection, potentiation of seizures, and adverse reaction to contrast or anesthetizing agents.[33,34] Surveys have indicated that such IAT morbidity is uncommon. For high-volume epilepsy centers, the typical risk of IAT-related complication is less than one percent.[35] Certain patient risk factors also can increase the risk of angiography, and therefore contraindicate use of the IAT; for example, individuals with significant vascular risk factors or other major medical problems may not be appropriate candidates for such a procedure. Additionally, very young children are also often not considered for IAT given the cognitive demands and medical risks involved in the test. Other limitations of the IAT include invalidation of studies due to aberrant vasculature (e.g., arteriovenous malformations) or to normal neurodevelopmental vascular variations, such as significant cortical crossflow. Given the short-acting nature of sodium amobarbital and the other drugs typically used to anesthetize the cerebral hemispheres, the IAT is a very time-sensitive procedure that can be invalidated by individual variation in sensitivity to sodium amobarbital (e.g., obtundation in some patients), as well as to related delays and nonstandardized administration of test stimuli. The IAT can also can be nondiagnostic due to failure to adequately lateralize language or memory functioning in a given individual. Finally, although some standardized IAT protocols are available,[2,6–8,35,36] comparison of IAT studies across epilepsy surgery centers can be challenging, as methodology and interpretation of the IAT procedure vary considerably from site to site. Efforts to standardize IAT administration across epilepsy centers are ongoing and may permit correlation with fMRI in larger samples in the future.

## Description of a Standardized IAT Protocol

At Dartmouth–Hitchcock Medical Center (DHMC), a standardized IAT protocol is utilized that initially was developed at Graduate Hospital in Philadelphia.[7,36] The procedure is begun on the presumed side of surgery, then repeated on the contralateral side. A catheter is positioned under fluoroscopy into the internal carotid artery (ICA). Following cerebral angiography, the patient is available for cognitive testing. All patients receive studies ipsilateral and contralateral to the seizure focus on the same day with 30 to 45 minutes between injections. The neuropsychological protocol[36] was designed for rapid speech and memory assessment. Emphasis is placed on quantitative memory evaluation for verbal and nonverbal material and for material that can be encoded either verbally or nonverbally (common objects). This provides a continuum of verbal–nonverbal material for encoding. Two forms of equivalent task difficulty were developed by randomization of the original item pool. Our standard dosage is 125 milligrams of sodium amobarbital in five cubic centimeters of saline with slow hand injection over five seconds in each ICA, with injections separated by at least 30 minutes. Occasionally, it is necessary to titrate the dosage of sodium amobarbital up or down (usually in 25-milligram increments) to achieve the goal of unilateral anesthesia as indicated by hemiparesis or electroencephalogram (EEG) without causing global sedation or obtundation. Language testing begins immediately after injection until speech normalizes, and includes: (1) automatic speech (counting, recitation of the alphabet); (2) comprehension (following simple commands, Modified Token Test); (3) word and sentence repetition; (4) visual confrontation naming (3 objects); and (5) reading (three words). Memory testing commences about two minutes postinjection, and overlaps with the language protocol (naming and word reading). During the registration and encoding phase, the patient is shown three common objects (e.g., spoon, glove) one at a time and asked to name and remember them. Each stimulus is exposed for approximately five to ten seconds, with emphasis placed on ensuring that the patient is attending to the stimuli. Special care must be taken to present the stimuli in the intact visual field. The same procedure is followed for three low-imagery words (e.g., random, enough, prefer) and three abstract designs (after Kimura[37]). At ten minutes postinjection, if language and motor functioning have returned to baseline, the free and cued recall phase is begun. Progressively structured recall testing is initiated by asking the patient to recall "everything that you remember from the test." Responses are recorded verbatim. Cued recall is then initiated (e.g., "Did I show you any objects?"). Paper and felt-tip pen are provided for drawings of the abstract designs. During the recognition phase, the patient is shown a series of nine stimuli (separately for objects, words, and designs). Three of the nine are target stimuli and six are distractors, fixing the probability of a chance correct response at 33%. For each item, the patient must determine whether he/she has seen the item during the test. Patients also are asked to provide a confidence rating so that signal detection analysis can be applied for determination of sensitivity and bias in responses.[38] Response alternatives are: "Definitely No" (non-target); "Probably No"; "Probably Yes" (target); "Definitely Yes." Responses are recorded; outcome is total number of targets correct and subscores for each type of material. False-positive responses are considered in the interpretation of the test results. For the designs, a second recognition task is administered, in which all nine designs are shown simultaneously, and the patient is asked to "Select the three that you think you might have seen earlier during the test." To assess emotional change during the IAT, behavioral observations are made regarding affective changes following injection. All patients are interviewed by the attending neuropsychologist after the procedure to elicit any subjective reactions. Interpretation of IAT data includes conclusions regarding language laterality based on the comprehensive language assessment. Memory performance is compared for each injection following adjustment for false-positive responses. Any atypical features of the examination (e.g., cortical crossflow, obtundation) also are noted.

## Replacement of the IAT with Functional Neuroimaging

Given the limitations of the IAT, suggestions for alternative technologies for gathering presurgical data regarding brain regions supporting cognitive functions have included event-related potentials[39] and transcranial magnetic stimulation.[40] Functional MRI[20,23,41,42] and $^{15}$O-water positron emission tomography (PET)[43,44] have been proposed as alternatives to the IAT to localize language and memory cortex more precisely. Disadvantages of $^{15}$O-water PET include invasiveness, lower availability and repeatability than fMRI, and lower spatial resolution. In this chapter, fMRI studies of memory and language functioning as related to the IAT will be the focus, although aspects of relevant PET studies will be addressed where appropriate.

The IAT demonstrates functional lateralization through unilateral hemispheric suppression of neuronal activity by anesthetization of the anterior and middle cerebral arterial distribution, followed by assessment of the cognitive functions of interest. In contrast, as described elsewhere in this volume, fMRI detects blood oxygen level-dependent (BOLD) signal during cognitive processing in an unsedated patient. This BOLD signal serves as an endogenous contrast agent and as a marker of task-related neuronal activity. As with the IAT, fMRI paradigms designed to assess language and memory functioning vary considerably. Although some language tasks (e.g., verbal fluency paradigms) have been more widely used, specific task and scan parameters are rarely consistent across studies, making direct comparison of fMRI activation patterns difficult. Despite this concern, some broad conclusions regarding the status of fMRI assessment of language and memory can be made.

## fMRI Language Paradigms and the IAT

Significant progress has been made in the past decade with regard to the development of language-based fMRI paradigms. Although different tasks have been used to elicit language-related activation, including word generation, naming, and reading paradigms, most studies have found near-perfect agreement between lateralization based on fMRI activation patterns and that based on IAT. In the few studies where discrepancies between fMRI and IAT have been noted, these more typically reflect a nondiagnostic study in one modality, or bilateral language participation in one study, but not in the other, rather than frank disagreement regarding hemispheric language dominance (see Table 11.1 for summary of studies comparing language lateralization using fMRI and IAT).

While replicating IAT language results would require only establishing hemispheric dominance for language, most groups designing fMRI language paradigms to replace the IAT are interested in achieving activation of the broad neural networks subserving various language functions in order not only to lateralize language at the hemispheric level, but to localize specific aspects of language functioning to more focal brain regions. Some groups have used auditory paradigms to activate temporal lobe receptive language cortex in healthy controls and in epilepsy patients.[20,45–49] These tasks often activate primary auditory cortex bilaterally and may show additional activation in posterior superior temporal gyrus.[50–52] As bilateral primary auditory cortex activation is of less utility in assessing hemispheric language dominance, some tasks use auditory control conditions to allow for subtraction of primary auditory cortex activation. However, such strategies may also remove from analysis activation of brain regions important in language processing,[20,45–48] potentially resulting in a reduction of the laterality index many studies have used as a measure of language dominance, thus making dominance appear less marked.[46,53] Reading-based tasks[28–30,53,54] offer an alternative for localization of middle and superior temporal lobe receptive language areas involved in reading decoding and comprehension, as well as frontal regions involved in grammatical language processing or verbal working memory.[55–57] Semantic retrieval aspects of these tasks are thought to engage anterior language regions.[19,23,28,43,58–60]

Desmond and colleagues[61] were the first researchers to publish the results of a group of patients in whom language dominance was studied with both IAT and fMRI. In their series of seven epilepsy patients, 100% concordance was observed between the two methods with regard to language lateralization. In addition, they provided data on intrahemispheric localization, namely activation of frontal lobe language regions (Brodmann's areas 45, 46, and 47) when patients were asked to make semantic as compared to perceptual judgments about visually presented words. While seminal, the use of a reading task prohibited more general conclusions about localization of speech and speech comprehension, which are important for surgical planning. In a series of 22 consecutive epilepsy surgery patients, Binder and colleagues[20] likewise found complete agreement between IAT and fMRI language lateralization and a high concordance ($r = 0.96$) between IAT and fMRI language lateralization indices. These authors also were able to demonstrate intrahemispheric activation of lateral frontal and heteromodal temporo-parieto-occipital cortex during a single-word semantic decision-making task. The study employed a baseline tone discrimination task to control for activation of auditory and attentional systems; this task design permitted elegant localization of areas involved in speech comprehension, but, it could be argued, prohibited examination of language as a multidimensional ability intimately related to both hearing and attention. In a later study, Benbadis and colleagues[62] reanalyzed fMRI and IAT data from the Binder[20] sample to determine whether IAT speech arrest alone constitutes sufficient criteria for determination of language dominance, in comparison to the comprehensive language evaluation cited in Binder and colleagues.[20] They found that a laterality index calculated solely based on speech arrest did not correlate significantly with either the comprehensive IAT laterality index or with fMRI language lateralization. Categorical classification of language dominance as right, left, or bilateral was likewise discordant in several cases when using the speech arrest index, as compared to the complete agreement between IAT and fMRI reported by Binder and colleagues[20] when IAT lateralization was based on comprehensive speech assessment. Therefore, Benbadis and colleagues[62] concluded that IAT speech arrest alone is not a valid indicator of language lateralization, highlighting the importance of the consideration of assessment techniques in the evaluation of IAT and fMRI concordance, as an inappropriate strategy (e.g., a nonspecific measure such as speech arrest) in either modality may lead to spurious conclusions regarding concordance.

Bahn and colleagues[63] reported a series of seven epilepsy patients who received both IAT and fMRI assessment of language functioning. These authors utilized aurally presented covert word generation paradigms in which subjects were asked either to think of words beginning with a certain letter or to think of words that rhymed with a target word. Functional MRI laterality was judged by comparing the number of voxels activated above threshold in language regions (specifically Broca's and Wernicke's areas) of each hemisphere. Intracarotid amobarbital test language laterality was judged using assessment of object naming, reading, and object recall, with dysnomia as a principal measure of language integrity. Intracarotid amobarbital test and fMRI lateralization agreed in all cases, including two right-handed participants with atypical right hemisphere dominance. No disagreement was found in lateralization of fMRI activation patterns between the two language tasks in any case, nor were there any instances of discordant lateralization of frontal and temporal language regions. Overall, however, asymmetric activation of Broca's area was visualized more reliably than activation of posterior language regions, including Wernicke's area. The rhyming task tended to demonstrate more robust activation and clearer hemispheric asymmetry than the naming to letter task, although a potential confound of task order was noted. While these findings were generally consistent with those of previous studies[20,61] demonstrating agreement between IAT and fMRI assessment of language dominance, the authors noted that fMRI conventions for classification of mixed or codominance of language were not well established, requiring further experience with this technique.

In the first extension of this type of research to pediatric populations, Hertz-Pannier and colleagues[23] used fMRI to assess language dominance in 11 children and adolescents with complex partial seizures (CPS) using word generation tasks. In all seven cases where either IAT, electrostimulation mapping, or surgical outcome results were available for comparison, findings regarding language dominance were concordant with fMRI asymmetry indices. All subjects demonstrated highest

Table 11.1. Summary of Concordance between IAT and fMRI Language Lateralization Results and Regions of fMRI Activation[a]

| Authors | Sample (Age range, years)[b] | IAT language tasks | fMRI language tasks | IAT/fMRI concordance | fMRI language regions activated |
|---|---|---|---|---|---|
| Desmond et al., 1995[61] | $n = 7$ (20–53) | Presence of speech arrest, paraphasic errors, and errors in naming, repetition, reading, and aural comp | Visually presented words 1. Semantic encoding: Abstract vs. Concrete 2. Perceptual encoding: Upper vs. Lower case | 100% | Frontal |
| Binder et al., 1996[20] | $n = 22$ (17–64) | Numerical rating of speech arrest, ability to follow commands, paraphasic errors, naming, repetition, reading, and comp | Aurally presented noun-categorization task | 100% | Frontal, temporal, temporo-parieto-occipital junction |
| Bahn et al., 1997[63] | $n = 7$ (mean = 29) | Assessment of naming, reading, and recall | Covert word generation to a target letter and to rhyme with a target word (aural stimuli-au) | 100% | Frontal, temporal |
| Hertz-Pannier et al., 1997[23] | $n = 6$ (10–18) | Not reported | Covert and overt word generation to a target letter and to a target semantic category (au) | 100% | Frontal, temporal |
| Worthington et al., 1997[64] | $n = 12$ (12–56) | Assessment of naming, repetition, reading, and comp | Covert word generation to a target letter | 42%[c] | Not reported |
| Benbadis et al., 1998[62] (subset of patients from Binder et al., 1996)[20] | $n = 21$ (17–64) | Numerical rating of speech arrest, ability to follow commands, paraphasic errors, naming, repetition, reading, and comp | Aurally presented noun-categorization task | 71–100%[d] | Frontal, temporal, temporo-parieto-occipital junction |
| Yetkin et al., 1998[65] | $n = 13$ (22–43) | Numerical rating of speech arrest, ability to follow commands, paraphasic errors, naming, repetition, reading, and comp | Covert word generation to a target letter (aural stimuli) | 100% | Frontal |
| Benson et al., 1999[66] | $n = 12$ (19–70) | Assessment of speech arrest, paraphasic errors, naming, reading and comp | Visually presented verb-generation task | 92%[e] | Not reported[f] |
| Lehéricy et al., 2000[46] | $n = 10$ (18–55) | Assessment of serial speech, naming, reading, spelling, and ability to follow commands | Covert word generation and sentence repetition, story listening (all aural stimuli) | 100%[g] | Frontal, temporal |

| | | | | | |
|---|---|---|---|---|---|
| **Carpentier et al., 2001[67]** | **$n = 10$ (24–51)** | **Assessment of speech arrest, paraphasic errors, comp, repetition, and naming** | **Identification of syntactic and semantic errors in sentences (aural and visual stimuli)** | **80–90%[h]** | **Frontal, temporal** |
| **Baciu et al., 2001[68]** | **$n = 10$ (20–48)** | **Presence/absence of speech arrest followed by transient aphasia** | **Visually presented rhyming/visual task** | **80–100%[i]** | **Frontal, temporal** |
| **Gaillard et al., 2002[29]** | **$n = 20$ (8–56)** | **Not reported** | **Covert naming in response to reading** | **75%[j]** | **Frontal, temporal** |
| **Rutten et al., 2002[100]** | **$n = 18$ (20–54)** | **Assessment of naming, expressive language, and paraphasic errors** | **Visually presented verb-generation, verbal-fluency, picture-naming, and sentence-comp task** | **83%[k]** | **Frontal, temporoparietal** |

[a] Adapted from Baxendale S. The role of functional MRI in the presurgical investigation of temporal lobe epilepsy patients: A clinical perspective and review. *J Clin Exp Neuropsychol* 2002;24(5):664–676. Adapted with permission from Psychology Press Ltd., *http://www.psypress.co.uk/journals.asp*.

[b] excluding healthy control subjects and epilepsy patients who did not receive IAT.

[c] Five patients demonstrated identical language laterality on IAT and fMRI. Three patients had disagreement between IAT and fMRI, one patient had bilateral IAT but lateralized fMRI, and three patients had a nondiagnostic fMRI study.

[d] 71% agreement was found between fMRI lateralization and IAT lateralization based solely on speech arrest; 100% concordance was found when IAT lateralization incorporated comprehensive language assessment.

[e] Eleven patients demonstrated identical language laterality on IAT and fMRI. One patient had equivocal findings on IAT and lateralized fMRI.

[f] While images are presented highlighting activation patterns in selected subjects, discussion of specific language regions activated is not included.

[g] Nine patients demonstrated left hemisphere dominance on both IAT and fMRI language measures, although strength of lateralization varied. One patient showed bilateral IAT, with strong right hemisphere fMRI lateralization of frontal language regions, but weak left lateralization of temporal areas.

[h] IAT and fMRI findings were concordant in eight patients when the whole brain was considered in fMRI analysis, and in nine patients when Brodmann's area 41/42 was excluded from analysis.

[I] Functional fMRI and IAT were entirely consistent in eight patients with conclusive IAT studies. Two patients had inconclusive IAT studies. In one of these, VEEG findings confirmed fMRI language lateralization. In the other, no other data was conclusive with regard to language lateralization.

[j] Five patients demonstrated identical language laterality on IAT and fMRI. One patient had a nondiagnostic IAT study, and another had a nondiagnostic fMRI study. One patient with left hemisphere language dominance on IAT showed bilateral language representation on fMRI and two patients with bilateral language functioning on IAT showed left hemisphere dominance on fMRI. In no case was there frank disagreement between IAT and fMRI.

[k] Of the three patients in whom fMRI and IAT were discordant, one was left dominant on fMRI, but mixed dominant on IAT; one was mixed dominant on fMRI, but left dominant on IAT; and one was right dominant on fMRI but left dominant on IAT.

activation in the vicinity of Broca's area (inferior frontal gyrus), as well as in the middle and superior frontal gyri, and cingulate gyrus activation was observed in all but two subjects. With regard to the technical difficulties inherent in studying children using fMRI, these authors noted that second studies were successful in four children whose initial studies were uninterpretable due to noncompliance or motion artifact. Studies also were repeated in two other children to assess reproducibility of the fMRI findings; language lateralization and spatial extent of activation were comparable across studies. These findings offered promising preliminary evidence that fMRI is a feasible technique for assessing language dominance in pediatric epilepsy surgery candidates without the potential risks of IAT or ESM.

In one of the very few studies demonstrating poor concordance between fMRI and IAT language lateralization, Worthington and colleagues[64] studied frontal and temporal brain regions using an fMRI verbal fluency task in 12 adolescents and adults who had completed IAT. The method used for determining hemispheric laterality appeared to involve counting the number of significantly activated voxels in each hemisphere. Language dominance was concordant in five of 12 patients who completed both IAT and fMRI. Three cases apparently demonstrated overt disagreement between IAT and fMRI lateralization, while one case demonstrated bilateral representation of language on IAT, but lateralized findings on fMRI. Three fMRI studies were nondiagnostic due to motion artifact or unclear activation. While these authors concluded that their findings suggest that fMRI lacks the sensitivity and specificity to be of clinical utility in presurgical evaluation of language dominance, several shortcomings in their study may explain their findings. The task used for some subjects included the requirement that subjects count the number of words generated as a method of monitoring task performance. Such a working memory component is uncommon in fMRI word generation tasks and may have led to atypically broad brain activation patterns, which may have obscured laterality. In addition, it is unclear if data analysis accounted for the different tasks used between subjects. Furthermore, 25% of fMRI data collected in this study was reportedly unusable. The authors do not discuss whether additional motion correction strategies were attempted, if alteration of a statistical significance threshold improved interpretability, or if second fMRI studies were attempted to obtain adequate data. Overall, while the unusually low concordance between fMRI and IAT language lateralization reported in this study should not be dismissed, several technical and methodological issues raise important questions regarding the validity of these findings and suggest that they should not be weighted heavily in general consideration of the research findings in this area.

Yetkin and colleagues[65] also used a word-generation task to compare fMRI and IAT language lateralization in 13 CPS patients. In all subjects, frontal lobe language regions (predominantly inferior frontal gyrus and precentral gyrus) demonstrated activation during fMRI word generation. Functional MRI language lateralization was 100% concordant with IAT results, offering a further contribution to the now-growing evidence that fMRI language lateralization paradigms are a reliable and feasible option for replacement of the IAT. In an attempt to broaden the scope of fMRI language lateralization techniques, Benson and colleagues[66] developed and validated an fMRI language paradigm to determine hemispheric dominance for a group of subjects with potentially resectable brain lesions near language cortex in addition to epilepsy. Using whole-brain fMRI, only a verb generation task (versus object naming and single word reading measures) reliably lateralized language in 19 control subjects. The clinical applications of this task were evaluated in a group of 23 patients who had IAT and/or ESM results available for comparison with fMRI laterality indices. Concordant findings with IAT/ESM were found in 96% of patients. In the sole patient with discordant findings, exclusion of a large tumor and its reflection in the opposite hemisphere from fMRI laterality analysis led to concordance.

Lehéricy and colleagues[46] utilized fMRI semantic verbal fluency, covert repetition, and story listening tasks to assess the reliability of fMRI frontal and temporal language systems activation in evaluating language dominance in ten TLE patients. Laterality indices were calculated for IAT and for several fMRI regions of interest (ROIs). For 90% of patients, language lateralization to the left hemisphere was concordant between IAT and fMRI frontal and temporal lobe activation, although the strength of lateralization varied, and fMRI activation in frontal regions tended to demonstrate a stronger relationship with IAT findings than more posterior brain activation. For the tenth patient, IAT suggested symmetric hemispheric support of language, while fMRI demonstrated strong right hemisphere lateralization for frontal regions and weak left hemisphere dominance for temporal regions. Lehéricy and colleagues concluded that fMRI demonstrated good sensitivity for detection of frontal language lateralization, but was less able to demonstrate lateralization in temporal lobe regions using these tasks. They also concluded, however, that use of multiple fMRI language tasks (i.e., story listening and repetition in addition to verbal fluency) might prove useful in demonstrating activation of posterior language regions in patients under consideration for surgical resection of brain lesions in these areas.

Carpentier and colleagues[67] utilized visual and aural language comprehension fMRI tasks to lateralize language functioning in ten epilepsy surgery candidates with left hemisphere seizure foci in or near presumed language cortex and ten healthy controls. Functional MRI tasks required subjects to make syntactic or semantic decisions regarding sentence accuracy. While fMRI activation was observed in a wide neural network of brain regions involved in language comprehension, Broca's area was the most consistently activated region, demonstrating activation in all subjects for both tasks, with controls demonstrating more robust laterality indices than epilepsy patients. Using whole-brain analysis, 80% concordance was observed between IAT and fMRI language lateralization, which rose to 90% when Brodmann's area 41/42 was excluded from laterality scoring. Functional MRI language lateralization scores demonstrated greater agreement with IAT and neuropsychological testing for the visual versus the auditory task. Strongest agreement was found using an fMRI laterality index including only Brodmann's areas 44/45 and 22, and the conjunction analysis of both fMRI tasks. These authors concluded that application of fMRI to replace the IAT should consider both modality-specific and modality-nonspecific patterns of brain activation. They also noted that their finding of greater bilateral representation of language functioning in epilepsy patients relative to controls supported previous findings and may provide further evidence of language plasticity related to epilepsy.

Baciu and colleagues[68] used an fMRI rhyme-detection task to assess language dominance in 19 epilepsy patients and compared these findings with those obtained using IAT, intracranial EEG stimulation and recording (SEEG), and/or video EEG recording (VEEG). Concordant lateralization was observed in 16 of 17 patients in whom language lateralization could be conclusively determined by both fMRI and one of these alternate methods. In the remaining subject, VEEG suggested left hemisphere language dominance, while fMRI activation during the rhyming task suggested bilateral language participation. These authors noted that, despite low intellectual functioning in some subjects, all patients were able to complete the fMRI task appropriately, and fMRI activation was apparent in frontal and temporal language regions across subjects. Baciu and colleagues[68] concluded that their rhyming paradigm offers a useful method for fMRI lateralization of language functions, and note that, unlike in other language tasks (e.g., covert naming or word generation), subject performance accuracy can be directly assessed.

In a recent study, Gaillard and colleagues[29] assessed hemispheric language dominance in children and adults with partial epilepsy of presumed temporal or frontotemporal origin using a covert naming in response to reading fMRI paradigm, in which subjects silently named an object after reading a sentence describing the object. Functional MRI data analysis included visual inspection and ROI analysis using regional asymmetry indices (AIs) for ROIs in frontal, temporal, and parietal regions. Of 20 patients who had IAT language lateralization data, fMRI demonstrated agreement in 15 cases (75%). In the five cases with disagreement between IAT and fMRI, the discrepancy was that one measure predicted bilateral language participation, whereas the other suggested unilateral dominance. Clinical visual inspection was found to be comparable to statistical ROI analysis. This fMRI paradigm resulted in visualization of both frontal and temporal language regions in the majority of cases, which is a significant finding given that previous studies[17,20,22,23,41,42,66,69–71] reliably demonstrated frontal language activation, but could not typically show task-related activation in more posterior language regions (for exceptions, see Refs. 28, 30, 48, 54). Typically, group averaging has been necessary to demonstrate language-related temporal lobe activation, and reliable findings have been more difficult to achieve in individual subjects.[19,22,72,73] Like Carpentier and colleagues,[67] Gaillard and colleagues[29] showed discrepancies in language lateralization between patients and controls, with all control subjects showing left hemisphere dominance, and greater right hemisphere language activation in patients, which seemed to be accounted for mainly by those with a left hemisphere seizure focus. These findings support previous research suggesting that early localization-related epilepsy can lead to intra- or interhemispheric alteration from normal language representation,[14,74] as well as the possibility that such activation also may reflect compensatory processes, such as atypical use of the intact right hemisphere to support the dysfunctional left hemisphere. Further analysis of this pattern of dominant and nondominant hemisphere language activation may help to identify individuals more likely to recover language functions after an acquired insult to dominant hemisphere language regions.[75–77]

Given the variability of language lateralization indices reported by prior studies, Rutten and colleagues[78] used four language tasks in combination to attempt to locate language cortex reliably in 18 TLE patients in an effort to provide a reliable distinction between patients with unilateral and bilateral language dominance, which they argued had thus far prevented the use of fMRI language assessment to replace the IAT. Through use of combined task analysis (CTA), these authors achieved more robust and reliable results than with any single task, and achieved concordance with IAT findings in 91% (10 out of 11) of patients who were left dominant by IAT, 75% (3 out of 4) of those with bilateral dominance by IAT, and 67% (2 out of 3) of those right dominant by IAT. Consistent with previous studies, verb generation was the most useful task in terms of providing language lateralization concordant with IAT, although it did not demonstrate similar effectiveness in bilateral hemispheric dominant patients. Of note, Rutten and colleagues[78] used a fixed user-independent approach to statistical analysis, which did not allow for individual variability in the threshold set for significant activation. As will be discussed below, this method may not be ideal for all subjects due to significant interindividual variability in the level of fMRI activation. Overall, however, they concluded that CTA offered a more effective means of differentiating typical (left) from atypical (right, bilateral) language dominance in the context of surgical planning than single-task fMRI assessment, and may in the future obviate the need for IAT language assessment in patients with clearly typical hemispheric dominance.

Overall, fMRI paradigms designed to lateralize and localize language functions typically have been successful in demonstrating activation patterns that are concordant with IAT results. Although a few studies have found surprisingly low concordance between IAT and fMRI language assessment, most have demonstrated perfect or near-perfect agreement. In studies with lower concordance rates, typical discrepancies involve technically inadequate or nondiagnostic IAT or fMRI studies, or bilateral representation in one study and unilateral hemispheric dominance in the other. In very few cases was there frank disagreement between fMRI and IAT. These infrequent instances in which IAT and fMRI language lateralization disagree highlight the importance of consideration of all available clinical data in presurgical epilepsy cases, including scalp and intracranial EEG recordings, seizure semiology, neuropsychological assessment, structural MRI, electrostimulation mapping, and other functional neuroimaging techniques such as PET and single photon emission computed tomography (SPECT).

While much remains to be learned regarding the most efficient method of precise fMRI localization of specific language skills, it appears that current fMRI paradigms can consistently lateralize language as effectively as the IAT, and can be used with confidence in place of the IAT in some circumstances. At DHMC, for example, fMRI verb generation tasks have been utilized effectively to determine language dominance and localization of Broca's area in presurgical tumor and arteriovenous malformation (AVM) patients, as well as in epilepsy patients who cannot undergo the IAT (e.g., due to vascular risk factors). In particular, use of fMRI language paradigms provides a potential alternative for language lateralization in epilepsy patients who would not necessarily be considered for IAT, including adults with medical contraindications and young children, who may be trained to tolerate the fMRI procedure, and thus have language laterality assessed without the potential morbidity risks of the IAT. Another potential advantage of fMRI in studying language functions in young patients is the potential to observe intrahemispheric reorganization in cases of early brain injury and recovery, which could not be visualized with the IAT.

While studies have noted technical issues that must be considered in the use of fMRI with children,[23,50,79–81] including tailoring of cognitive paradigms and adjustment of statistical thresholds, results from DHMC and other centers suggest that language can be lateralized successfully using fMRI in pediatric populations. At DHMC, we have achieved successful language lateralization using fMRI word generation paradigms in epilepsy patients as young as six years of age. Our experience has been that children can effectively perform such fMRI tasks following out-of-scanner preparation, including practicing the fMRI tasks and instruction regarding the importance of remaining motionless, and with minimal in-scanner head restraints (i.e., only foam padding and/or tape across the forehead). With modification of fMRI paradigms as appropriate for level of cognitive functioning and additional physical assistance in head stabilization, it seems likely that fMRI may come into wider use for lateralization of language in very young children, in whom the IAT often is considered unfeasible or its attendant medical risks too great.

As noted in a recent review of fMRI paradigms with potential to replace the IAT,[82] future directions for fMRI assessment of language skills in presurgical epilepsy patients should include not only consistent lateralization of language dominance, but also specific localization of regions subserving the cognitive functions most likely to be affected negatively by surgical resection in the dominant hemisphere. Previous research[83] has demonstrated postoperative declines in naming skills following dominant temporal lobe resection, and other complex language functions such as reading and semantic processing also may be disrupted. Therefore, while some of the language paradigms used in the studies discussed above may not provide maximal information regarding overall language lateralization, such tasks may be useful in demonstrating activation of extrafrontal language regions (e.g., temporoparietal association cortex), which may be helpful in assessing the likelihood of postsurgical cognitive impairment and the potential for recovery of function. As TLE patients are those most commonly considered for epilepsy surgery, the importance of delineating temporal lobe language regions, as well as memory circuitry, becomes evident. In addition, it is important to note that the specific fMRI language task used may not be critical to achieving adequate language lateralization. For example, Grandin and colleagues[22] found that the number of pixels activated in frontal and temporal language regions did not differ for semantic versus phonemic verbal fluency tasks. Similarly, both tasks lateralized language functioning to the dominant hemisphere, suggesting no particular advantage to one form of verbal fluency task over the other. This information is particularly useful in the study of children, who may not be able to accurately generate words beginning with a particular letter, but who often can generate words to a semantic category such as animals or foods.

The available literature suggests that functional neuroimaging techniques such as PET and fMRI can reliably identify language dominance in both adults and children, and typically produce findings that agree with results from IAT and electrocortical stimulation.[20,23,41,42,46,61,63,65,66,70,84,85] A small percentage of studies, however, have shown disagreement between IAT and PET,[43,44,46,63,65,66] or only partial agreement between IAT and fMRI in terms of language lateralization,[65,66] with surgery at times confirming the functional imaging findings.[43,44] These findings may reflect difficulties in sensitivity to functional reorganization in individuals with atypical dominance, or dissociation of receptive and expressive language,[86,87] at least for some methods. Therefore, a conservative approach would include IAT or cortical stimulation confirmation of fMRI results at present. In cases of dominant hemisphere resection or where language dominance is unclear, intraoperative language mapping often is essential.

## Case Examples of fMRI Language Activation

At DHMC, patients referred for clinical fMRI language mapping most typically complete an aurally presented verb generation task similar to those described in the previous section. Patients are presented with blocks of nouns alternating with blocks of tones. For each noun presented, the patient is instructed to mentally generate as many verbs as possible that go with that noun (e.g., for "frog", the patient might think "leap", "croak", "hop", etc.). The patient is instructed not to say the words or make any mouth movements. During the control condition (tones), the patient is instructed to simply listen and clear his/her mind. As this task does not involve collection of objective performance data, successful completion of the task is assessed by postscanning debriefing and comparison with performance on similar measures during out-of-scanner neuropsychological testing. Analysis contrasts hemodynamic responses during the two task conditions. The typical pattern of brain activation for this task comprises dominant hemisphere frontal regions, with more posterior temporal lobe activation observed in some patients. Consistent with the literature, cingulate gyrus activation is also often noted. In Figure 11.1, data are presented from a 44-year-old, right-handed female epilepsy patient. This patient displayed a typical pattern of left frontal activation, with cingulate cortex and bilateral cerebellar activation also apparent.

We have observed similar activation patterns in children with epilepsy. Figures 11.2 and 11.3 demonstrate the variation that can be observed in individual patient activation for verb generation. In Figure 11.2, frontal language-related activation is observed bilaterally in a nine-year-old, right-handed boy, in regions approximating Broca's area. Global peak activation is in the left frontal lobe, however, suggesting left hemisphere dominance for language. In addition, posterior temporal task-related activation is observed in the left, but not the right hemisphere. In contrast, in Figure 11.3, activation maps from an 11-year-old, right-handed girl show only left hemisphere task-related activation, but in a more widely distributed network of frontal and temporal regions.

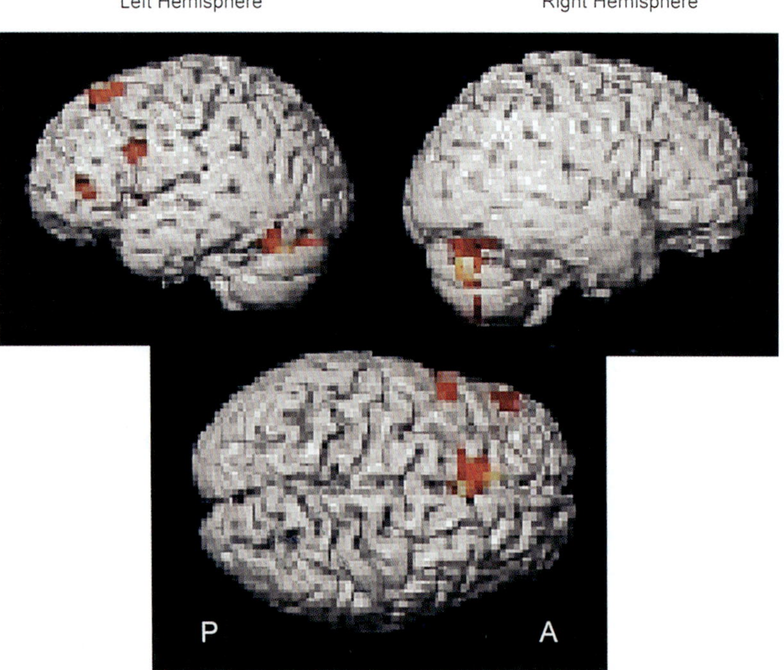


**Figure 11.1.** Functional MRI brain activation ($p_{crit} = 0.01$) during verb generation in a 44-year-old, right-handed female demonstrating strong left frontal fMRI brain activation. Bilateral cerebellar and medial cingulate gyrus activation also were noted. (Neurologic coordinates)

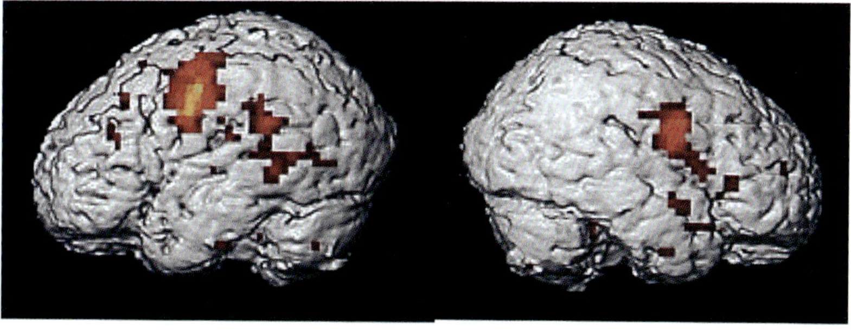


**Figure 11.2.** Functional MRI brain activation ($p_{crit} = 0.0001$) during verb generation in a 9-year-old, right-handed boy with an epileptogenic left orbitofrontal lesion. This patient displayed stronger left than right frontal activation in regions approximating Broca's area, suggesting left hemisphere dominance for language, with some right participation.

## fMRI Memory Paradigms and the IAT

The development of fMRI memory paradigms to replace the IAT is in a state of relative infancy compared to the language lateralization literature. Whereas fMRI memory tasks cannot yet serve the critical IAT function of assessing unilateral support of memory functions on an individual basis, as neither hemisphere is anesthetized during stimulus presentation, research with fMRI and PET has examined episodic memory encoding and retrieval processes in healthy controls and TLE populations (see Table 11.2 for summary of studies assessing memory functioning in TLE using fMRI and IAT).

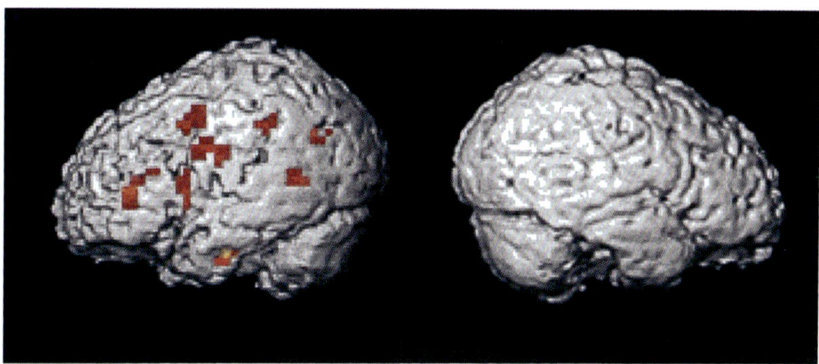


**Figure 11.3.** Functional MRI brain activation ($p_{crit} = 0.01$) during verb generation in an 11-year-old, right-handed girl with left TLE and left hippocampal sclerosis. This patient displayed clear left hemisphere dominance for language (confirmed by IAT), with activation of frontal and temporal language regions, including Broca's area.

Table 11.2. Summary of Studies Assessing Memory Performance in TLE Using fMRI

| Authors | Sample (Age range, years) | IAT memory tasks | fMRI memory tasks | Findings |
|---|---|---|---|---|
| Detre et al., 1998[88] | Left TLE: $n = 6$ (17–48)<br>Right TLE: $n = 3$ (18–37)<br>Controls: $n = 8$ (18–40) | Assessment of free recall and recognition of common objects, low-imagery words, and abstract line drawings | Complex scene-encoding task | Controls demonstrated generally symmetric MTL activation.<br>Patients showed asymmetric MTL activation, which agreed in all cases with memory asymmetry on IAT. |
| Bellgowan et al., 1998[90] | Left TLE: $n = 14$ (20–57)<br>Right TLE: $n = 14$ (28–69) | Not described, although IAT memory lateralization data are presented | Semantic and tone decision task | Right TLE patients: similar activation in left MTL as previously observed in healthy controls in a separate study.<br>Left TLE patients: decreased left MTL activation relative to right TLE patients, but similar whole-brain and left hemisphere activation and task performance. |
| Dupont et al., 2000[91] | Left TLE: $n = 7$ (18–53)<br>Controls: $n = 10$ (23–30) | Not described, only IAT data presented are that all patients are left language dominant | Verbal episodic encoding and retrieval tasks | Bilateral parahippocampal gyrus activation during retrieval in both groups, more so in controls, who had stronger task performance.<br>Patients also activated left prefrontal regions during encoding and retrieval. |
| Dupont et al., 2001[92] | Left TLE: $n = 7$ (18–53)<br>Controls: $n = 10$ (23–31)[a] | Not described, only IAT data presented are that all patients are left language dominant | Verbal retrieval task | Relative to the prior scan:<br>Controls: decreased activation in parahippocampal, occipitotemporal, and ventrolateral frontal regions, but new activation in right posterior hippocampus and bilateral parietal cortex.<br>Patients: slightly poorer task performance, absent MTL activation, and dramatic decrease in previously noted neocortical fMRI activation. |

Table 11.2. *Continued*

| Authors | Sample (Age range, years) | IAT memory tasks | fMRI memory tasks | Findings |
|---|---|---|---|---|
| Jokeit et al., 2001[93] | Left TLE: $n = 16$ (13–55)<br>Right TLE: $n = 14$ (14–54)<br>Controls: $n = 17$ (7–63) | Assessment of free recall and recognition of 20 items (e.g., actual and drawn objects, words, abstract drawings) | Mental navigation and recall task | Both groups showed MTL activation; in controls, no significant asymmetry was evident.<br>Patients: Hemispheric asymmetry in activation lateralized seizure onset in 90% (weaker activation on side of focus); left TLE patients showed correlation between left MTL activation and IAT memory performance using the left hemisphere. |
| Golby et al., 2002[94] | Left TLE: $n = 6$ (26–33)<br>Right TLE: $n = 3$ (42–54) | Assessment of recognition memory for objects, words, and designs | Tasks requiring encoding and processing of words, faces, scenes, and patterns | Functional MRI and IAT memory lateralization concordant in 89% of subjects; in each group, greater encoding-related activation was observed in MTL structures contralateral to seizure focus; material-specific interaction between side of seizure focus and memory for verbal versus nonverbal stimuli. |

[a] Same subjects as Dupont et al.,[91] rescanned 24 hours after scanning session reported in the previous study, and asked to recall words learned during the first scanning session.

In TLE, Detre and colleagues[88] used a complex visual scene-encoding fMRI task, previously demonstrated to activate bilateral mesial temporal lobe structures in healthy controls,[89] to assess functional asymmetry in comparison with IAT memory lateralization in nine TLE patients. A tenth patient participated in fMRI, but IAT results were uninterpretable due to crossflow and subsequent obtundation. The fMRI paradigm involved memorization of novel complex scenes. In controls, comparison of activation during the task condition as compared to a visual control condition demonstrated bilateral posterior temporal and visual association cortex and right frontal activation, with a slight right hemisphere predominance overall in MTL ROIs. Epilepsy patients demonstrated markedly more asymmetric MTL activation. In nine out of ten patients, asymmetry ratios were greater than one standard deviation from the control mean; four out of ten patients showed asymmetry ratios greater than two standard deviations away from the control mean. In all patients, the direction of hemispheric asymmetry was concordant with IAT findings. As two patients demonstrated paradoxically greater fMRI activation and better IAT memory performance ipsilateral to the seizure focus, this pattern was thought not entirely attributable to epilepsy-related structural abnormalities. This finding is clinically significant, as it demonstrates the potential utility of fMRI in demonstrating brain activation patterns that might by extension to the IAT predict memory deficits following temporal lobectomy, and thus inform risk–benefit discussions, or, in the extreme case, serve as a potential contraindication for surgery.

Bellgowan and colleagues[90] were able to discriminate left and right TLE patients based on their fMRI activation patterns on a semantic encoding task. Right TLE patients showed predominant left MTL activation involving the hippocampus, parahippocampal gyrus, and collateral sulcus, whereas those with a left hemisphere seizure focus demonstrated little activation in these regions. In contrast to the studies noted above, this task did not demonstrate bilateral activation of memory structures; neither right nor left TLE patients showed significant right hemisphere activation in MTL regions while completing the task. This is not unexpected, in that semantic tasks do not typically generate right hemisphere activation, and highlights a paradigm potentially useful for preferential activation of the left MTL in presurgical fMRI evaluation of epilepsy patients. The authors hypothesized that the lack of left MTL activation in left TLE patients in spite of relatively intact episodic memory functioning may indicate intra- or interhemispheric reorganization of memory functions in this group, which may be related to factors such as age at seizure onset. Bellgowan and colleagues[90] concluded that further demonstration of the reliability of similar techniques for evoking MTL activation in patients may in the future allow fMRI to replace the IAT for memory assessment.

In another study of fMRI memory patterns in TLE, Dupont and colleagues[91] utilized verbal episodic memory-encoding and retrieval tasks to demonstrate memory functioning in ten healthy control subjects and seven left TLE patients with left hippocampal sclerosis in an attempt to illustrate reallocation of verbal memory functions in left TLE. During fMRI scanning, subjects were asked to encode a supraspan list of 17 words over repeated presentations, then to covertly recall the words. In addition to activation across broader neural networks, both patients and controls demonstrated bilateral parahippocampal gyrus activation (right greater than left) during retrieval, although this effect was more marked in controls. Patients also recruited left prefrontal regions for encoding and retrieval, which were not activated in controls. Controls demonstrated significantly stronger memory for the word list on postscanner testing. Given the performance deficit noted in patients, Dupont and colleagues[91] hypothesized that this frontal cortex recruitment reflects ineffective reallocation of memory functions (i.e., cortical dysfunction rather than efficient reorganization) in the patient group due either to hippocampal dysfunction or epileptogenesis. In a later study,[92] this group analyzed differences in brain activation in the same subjects for 24-hour delayed retrieval of the verbal material. At the follow-up fMRI session, subjects were asked only to retrieve the words memorized the day before (i.e., the word list was not presented again). Memory was tested again through free recall following the scanner session. For controls, retrieval was similar to prior performance, whereas patient performance was slightly poorer. Analysis of changes in fMRI brain activation patterns in controls revealed decreases in parahippocampal, occipitotemporal, and ventrolateral frontal activation, and emergence of a new focus of activation in the right posterior hippocampus and bilateral parietal cortex. In the epilepsy patients, no MTL activation was apparent, and activation in neocortical brain regions observed at the previous session was dramatically decreased. The authors concluded that these findings support the assertion that MTL structures play a critical role in the neural networks involved in episodic verbal memory, including retrieval of stored information, and that dysfunction of these regions in TLE patients likely underlies the memory deficits and alterations in fMRI activation they observed in patients relative to controls.

Jokeit and colleagues[93] utilized fMRI to lateralize declarative memory functioning in a group of 30 TLE (16 left TLE, 14 right TLE) patients and 17 healthy control subjects using a mental navigation task involving mental recall and navigation of the subject's hometown, contrasted with a covert counting baseline condition. Both controls and patients (including children, older subjects, and some subjects with lower intellectual functioning) reliably activated MTL structures. Hemispheric asymmetry in MTL activation lateralized seizure onset in 90% of TLE patients, with diminished activation observed on the side of seizure focus. Controls did not demonstrate significant fMRI MTL activation asymmetry. The authors concluded that these activation patterns were related specifically to memory rather than to visuospatial abilities based on correlations between out-of-scanner neuropsychological testing of memory functions and fMRI MTL activation. Examination of fMRI activation patterns and IAT results demonstrated a significant correlation between number of activated voxels in the left MTL and left hemisphere IAT performance. Unfortunately, too few

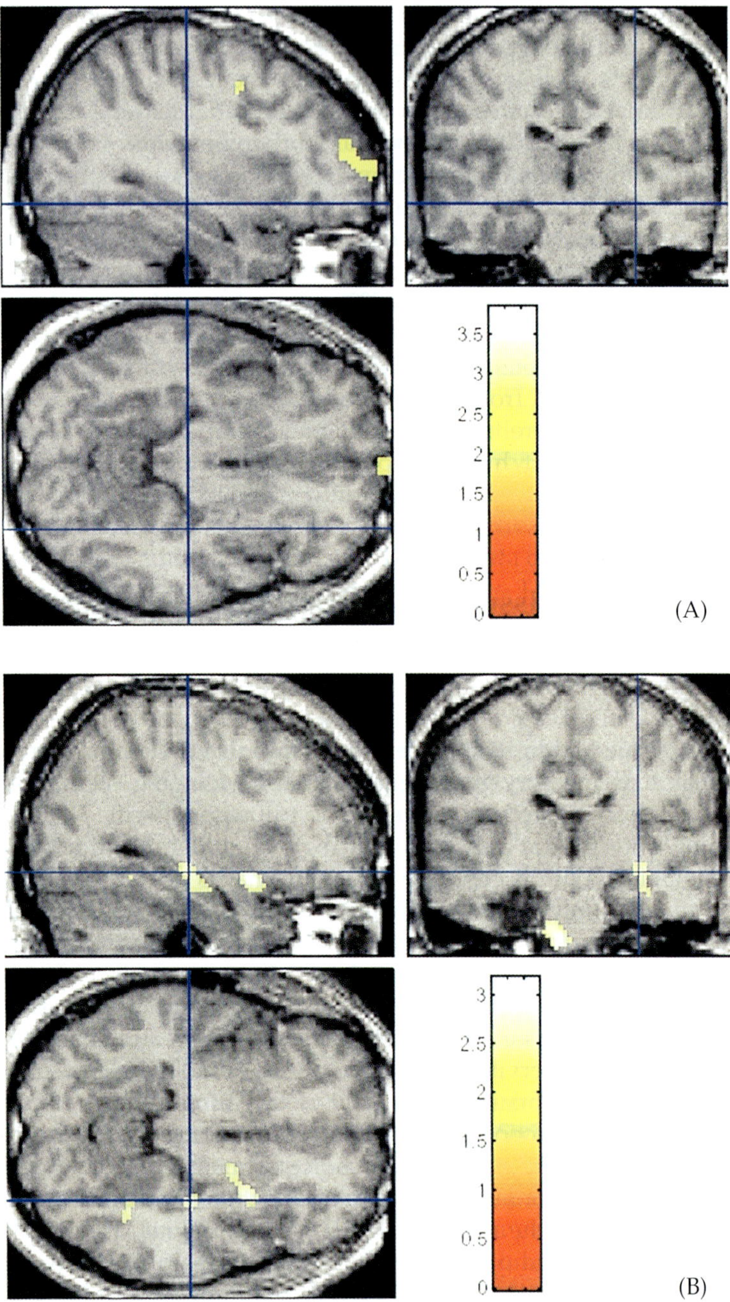


**Figure 11.4.** Right hippocampal activation ($p_{crit} = 0.01$) in a 25-year-old, right-handed male during verbal encoding before (A) and after (B) left selective amygdalohippocampectomy. Right MTL activation observed after, but not before, surgery in the nonepileptic hippocampus suggests a possible functional release from the irritative seizure focus (see McDonald and colleagues[95]). (Neurologic coordinates)

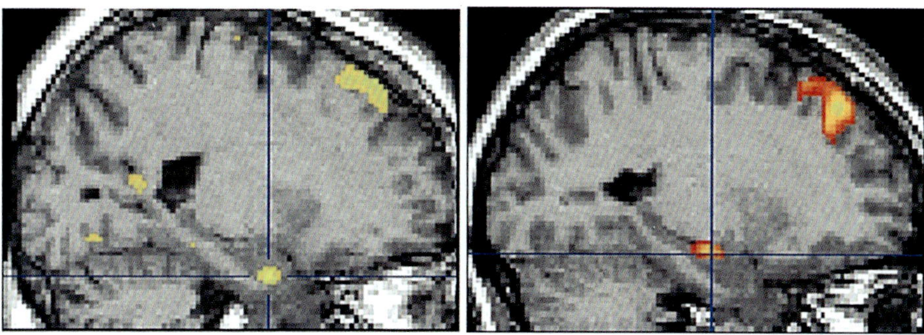

**Figure 11.5.** Left medial temporal lobe activation ($p_{crit} = 0.05$) in two female right temporal lobe resection patients (both right-handed and left hemisphere dominant for language on IAT), during encoding of novel words showing contralateral memory functioning after surgery (fMRI conducted 2.8 and 4.8 years after surgery, see McDonald and colleagues.[95])

lateralization. In some cases, however, lowering the significance threshold can lead to a spurious increase in regionally nonspecific activation and loss of a significant AI. The need to lower the threshold for significant activation may be greater in younger subjects due to developmental differences in overall levels of observed activation, although such a technique in these subjects could likewise lower the AI due to increased spurious activation or activation in homologous regions in the contralateral hemisphere.

The question of whether or not fMRI measures of cognition produce reproducible results is also of direct relevance whenever surgical intervention is under consideration. In a sophisticated statistical approach to analyzing the reproducibility of fMRI activation patterns, Fernandez and colleagues[99] examined the reliability of fMRI lateralization of language functions within and between individual subjects, and within and between scanning sessions. They administered a semantic judgment task to 34 epilepsy patients on one occasion and to 12 other patients at two separate scanning sessions on the same day using alternate task forms. Results demonstrated good within-test and test–retest reliability of task-related activation patterns. For test–retest patients, a significant amount of overlap was noted between the first and second evaluations on a voxel-by-voxel basis, with higher significance levels for activation in frontal (e.g., Broca's area, premotor region) than more posterior regions (temporoparietal cortex). This method provided similarly reliable activation patterns for patients with right or mixed hemisphere dominance for language as those with left hemisphere dominance. The authors concluded that fMRI holds great promise for replacing the IAT in terms of language lateralization for lateralizing frontal language regions. They pointed out, however, that fMRI may activate some, but not necessarily all, brain regions participating in a given function; consequently, they recommend caution in replacing deactivation procedures (e.g., cortical stimulation mapping) entirely for planning surgical resection margins. Furthermore, they noted that their data cannot speak to the definition of such surgical margins, as the normalization paradigm required for group statistical analysis introduces spatial distortion of individual activation data. It should be noted, however, that such spatial normalization is not required for fMRI, and analyses can be performed in native brain space, as is typically done at DHMC for individual presurgical cases. With regard to setting the surgical margin, the statistical threshold chosen will necessarily affect degree and extent of activation observed. As the overall level of observed fMRI brain activation varies between individuals, it generally is not considered appropriate or feasible to set the same a priori threshold for all subjects. Rutten and colleagues[100] examined fMRI activation patterns in the temporal lobes in nonnormalized scans as compared to cortical stimulation mapping. Their study demonstrated a specificity of 61% of subjects, and false-positive activation in 51%, suggesting that fMRI cannot yet be used for direct delineation of the surgical resection margin. Fernandez and colleagues[99] suggest that one method to alleviate this difficulty would be to create individualized normalization of language regions in relation to brain regions with known, quantifiable relationships between fMRI task stimulation and activation response (e.g., primary visual cortex, where a linear relationship has been demonstrated between changes in neural activity and fMRI signal[101]).

### Clinical Concerns

Future fMRI studies of cognition in epilepsy patients attempting to replace the IAT also will need to address issues related to neurodevelopmental abnormalities in cognition due to factors unique to epilepsy patients. For example, previous research[83,102–104] has demonstrated an interaction between factors such as age at seizure onset and age at first risk factor for epilepsy (e.g., febrile convulsions, traumatic brain injury, meningitis, encephalitis) and cognitive outcomes following temporal lobectomy. In a study of eight TLE patients, Killgore and colleagues[105] reported that presurgical fMRI memory lateralization predicted postsurgical seizure freedom as effectively as IAT, with asymmetry of fMRI MTL activation favoring the nonepileptogenic hemisphere, demonstrating an association with seizure freedom one year postsurgery. Similarly, Sabsevitz and colleagues[106,107] demonstrated that presurgical activation during an fMRI semantic decision-making task in a group of left TLE patients showed a significant relationship with performance on an out-of-scanner naming task postsurgery, suggesting that fMRI might be a useful tool in predicting postsurgical cognitive outcome. Another study from this group[108] showed that earlier age of seizure onset is associated with greater atypical language lateralization, and that subjects with a left hemisphere seizure focus whose language skills appear to have undergone reorganization demonstrated poorer naming skills. These findings point to the need for further investigation of the relationship of early risk factors for epilepsy and related abnormalities in neurodevelopment to later brain organization of cognitive functions such as language and memory. Functional MRI may be an ideal tool to study the reorganization suggested by earlier neuropsychological[83,109] and IAT studies.[110]

To date, fMRI studies of cognition in epilepsy generally have not explicitly addressed the potential contribution of antiepileptic drugs (AEDs) to observed activation patterns. Antiepileptic drugs have known or presumed effects on cerebral blood flow and metabolism[111–116], although, at present, these effects remain unelucidated or poorly understood for many AEDs. Direct or indirect effects on cortical blood flow may differentially affect the observed BOLD response in epilepsy patients in comparison to healthy medication-free control subjects. There are differences between AEDs in the nature and extent of influence on neural activity, cortical blood flow, and metabolism, and the role these mechanisms play in the BOLD response requires systematic investigation. This potential confound has not been addressed directly in fMRI studies of epilepsy patients. Sex differences in brain language organization also merit consideration when using presurgical IAT results to assess feasibility of surgery or predict postsurgical risk for cognitive deficits.[117,118] Baxter and colleagues[119] have utilized fMRI to examine brain activation during a semantic processing task in healthy adult subjects to assess the applicability of models of intra- versus interhemispheric sex differences in language organization. The results of this study offered some support for both models of language organization; females showed greater bilateral representation of language functions than did males, while males demonstrated more diffuse activation within the left hemisphere than did females. These findings are consistent with previous studies demonstrating sex differences in language lateralization, which may affect predictions regarding cognitive outcome following epilepsy surgery and warrant consideration in presurgical evaluation.

As noted previously, it can be difficult to directly compare fMRI and IAT results, as different aspects of language and memory functioning typically are measured in these paradigms. In addition, given the current state of fMRI technology, observed activation patterns may reflect not only activation of regions critical for the function under examination, but also activation of areas related to other functions tapped by a particular fMRI task; for example, some language tasks may reflect brain activation related to attention and planning functions rather than language per se.[84] Therefore, it may be possible to include some activated areas within the resection margin to increase the likelihood of obtaining seizure control without leading to impairment in language and/or memory (though such resection may affect other cognitive functions). Furthermore, brain regions important for a given function may fail to activate during a particular task, suggesting that appropriate caution must be used when interpreting fMRI findings as they relate to surgical intervention.

## Conclusions and Future Directions: Can We Replace the IAT with fMRI?

At present, the potential for replacement of the IAT with fMRI is quite different for language versus memory. Using the simple standard of language lateralization, it appears that fMRI paradigms are poised to replace the IAT, and that they can reliably lateralize language in children and adults, even in subjects with atypical (right or mixed) dominance. Functional MRI also has the advantage of providing information beyond that of the IAT in terms of intrahemispheric localization of language regions, although it does not yet have the proven reliability and validity required to replace current techniques used for setting the surgical margin, including electrostimulation mapping. For memory, while the few available fMRI studies provide promising data that suggest that IAT might eventually be able to be replaced, further investigation is necessary to ascertain the functional utility of these data with regard to surgical planning and outcome, as well as to extend the applicability to pediatric populations. Evidence-based standards for the recommendation of new diagnostic tests and treatments have been articulated by relevant professional organizations,[120] with the highest (Class I) standard being prospective, randomized controlled clinical trials (RCTs), with masked outcome assessment. Clearly, none of the fMRI research discussed above meets these stringent standards, but instead falls at the Class IV level (reports of case series). The IAT has likewise never undergone Class I trials, but has become the de facto clinical standard due to its long history and the lack of available alternatives. As with fMRI, a few case studies (e.g., Ref. 121) are available demonstrating reproducibility of IAT results and offering evidence towards reliability and validity. Based on the currently available data, it seems unlikely that the field will reach consensus in terms of the acceptability of replacing the IAT with fMRI, particularly for memory. The early results are promising, however, and much more systematic research is needed, including RCTs. A true gold standard for language and memory localization will only be ascertained through systematic assessment of postsurgical outcome data in relation to presurgical localization data, a task that has not yet been adequately completed for the IAT or for fMRI.

Overall, it seems certain that fMRI prardigms designed to replace the IAT will include multiple language and memory tasks in order to elicit activation of broad neural networks, including frontal and temporal language and memory circuitry. Future directions in the development of an fMRI paradigm to replace the IAT may be similar to work recently conducted by Deblaere and colleagues.[122] In a study unique in its attempt to include fMRI measures for both language and memory functioning, these authors utilized a group of activation paradigms, including complex scene encoding, picture naming, reading, word generation, and semantic decision-making tasks. While this study included only healthy control subjects, its findings are promising for future research, as these investigators were able to demonstrate bilateral MTL activation consistent with prior studies[88,89] during memory encoding, as well as robust language lateralization. While IAT results are obviously not available for comparison, the authors noted their intention to utilize this group of fMRI tasks with epilepsy patients to attempt to determine its feasibility in replicating, and eventually replacing, the IAT.

The next decade of clinical research is likely to establish fMRI firmly as a valuable tool for preoperative assessment of language and memory, as well as other eloquent cortical functions, in various neurosurgical contexts. Functional MRI is expected to be seen combined with structural imaging and other advanced diagnostic modalities. Further technical advances in field strength, gradient and radiofrequency coils, software, and cognitive paradigms will improve the sensitivity and specificity of fMRI. In the not too distant future, accurate results of preoperative fMRI mapping will be registered in the neurosurgeon's computer and microscope and routinely used to guide surgery.

## Acknowledgments

The authors thank Barbara C. Jobst, MD, Jennifer D. Schoenfeld, PhD, the Department of Diagnostic Radiology, and the Epilepsy and Epilepsy Surgery Programs at Dartmouth-Hitchcock Medical Center for their contributions to the data presented in this chapter.

## References

1. Medina LS, Aguirre E, Bernal B, Altman NR. Functional MR imaging versus Wada test for evaluation of langauge lateralization: Cost analysis. *Radiology.* 2004;230(1):49–54.
2. Loring DW, Meador KJ, Lee GP, King DW. *Amobarbital Effects and Lateralized Brain Function: The Wada Test.* New York: Springer-Verlag; 1992.
3. van Emde Boas W, Juhn A. Wada and the sodium amytal test in the first (and last?) 50 years. *J Hist Neurosci.* 1999;8(3):286–292.
4. Gardner WJ. Injection of procaine into the brain to locate speech area in left-handed persons. *Arch Neurol Psychiatry.* 1941;46:1035–1038.
5. Wada J, Rasmussen T. Intracarotid injection of sodium amytal for the lateralization of cerebral speech dominance. *J Neurosurgery.* 1960;17:266–282.
6. Milner B, Branch C, Rasmussen T. Study of short-term memory after intracarotid injection of sodium amytal. *Trans Am Neurol Assoc.* 1962;87:224–226.
7. Sperling MR, Saykin AJ, Glosser G, Moran M, French JA, Brooks M, et al. Predictors of outcome after anterior temporal lobectomy: The intracarotid amobarbital test. *Neurology.* 1994;44(12):2325–2330.
8. Rausch R. Role of the neuropsychological evaluation and the intracarotid sodium amobarbital procedure in the surgical treatment for epilepsy. *Epilepsy Res Suppl.* 1992;5:77–86.
9. Tatum WO, IV, Benbadis SR, Vale FL. The neurosurgical treatment of epilepsy. *Arch Fam Med.* 2000;9(10):1142–1147.
10. Assessment: Neuropsychological testing of adults. Considerations for neurologists. Report of the Therapeutics and Technology Assessment Subcommittee of the American Academy of Neurology. *Neurology.* 1996;47(2): 592–599.
11. Surgery for epilepsy. NIH Consensus Statement Online 1990;8(2):1–20.
12. Devinsky O, Perrine K, Llinas R, Luciano DJ, Dogali M. Anterior temporal language areas in patients with early onset of temporal lobe epilepsy. *Ann Neurol.* 1993;34(5):727–732.
13. Mizrahi EM, Kellaway P, Grossman RG, Rutecki PA, Armstrong D, Rettig G, et al. Anterior temporal lobectomy and medically refractory temporal lobe epilepsy of childhood. *Epilepsia.* 1990;31(3):302–312.

14. Rasmussen T, Milner B. The role of early left-brain injury in determining lateralization of cerebral speech functions. *Ann N Y Acad Sci.* 1977;299: 355–369.
15. Satz P, Strauss E, Wada J, Orsini DL. Some correlates of intra- and inter-hemispheric speech organization after left focal brain injury. *Neuropsychologia.* 1988;26(2):345–350.
16. Woods RP, Dodrill CB, Ojemann GA. Brain injury, handedness, and speech lateralization in a series of amobarbital studies. *Ann Neurol.* 1988;23(5):510–518.
17. Pujol J, Deus J, Losilla JM, Capdevila A. Cerebral lateralization of language in normal left-handed people studied by functional MRI. *Neurology.* 1999;52(5):1038–1043.
18. Szaflarski JP, Binder JR, Possing ET, McKiernan KA, Ward BD, Hammeke TA. Language lateralization in left-handed and ambidextrous people: fMRI data. *Neurology.* 2002;59(2):238–244.
19. Binder JR, Rao SM, Hammeke TA, Frost JA, Bandettini PA, Jesmanowicz A, et al. Lateralized human brain language systems demonstrated by task subtraction functional magnetic resonance imaging. *Arch Neurol.* 1995; 52(6):593–601.
20. Binder JR, Swanson SJ, Hammeke TA, Morris GL, Mueller WM, Fischer M, et al. Determination of language dominance using functional MRI: A comparison with the Wada test. *Neurology.* 1996;46(4):978–984.
21. Gaillard WD, Hertz-Pannier L, Mott SH, Barnett AS, LeBihan D, Theodore WH. Functional anatomy of cognitive development: fMRI of verbal fluency in children and adults. *Neurology.* 2000;54(1):180–185.
22. Grandin CB, Gaillard WD, Hunter KE, Petrella JR, Braniecki SH, Whitnah JR, et al. Comparison of phonemic and semantic verbal fluency tasks: An fMRI study. *Neuroimage.* 1998;7:S133.
23. Hertz-Pannier L, Gaillard WD, Mott SH, Cuenod CA, Bookheimer SY, Weinstein S, et al. Noninvasive assessment of language dominance in children and adolescents with functional MRI: A preliminary study. *Neurology.* 1997;48(4):1003–1012.
24. Beauregard M, Chertkow H, Bub D, Murtha S, Dixon R, Evans A. The neural substrate for concrete, abstract, and emotional word lexica: A positron emission tomography study. *J Cogn Neurosci.* 1997;9(4):441–461.
25. Beeman M. Semantic processing in the right hemisphere may contribute to drawing inferences from discourse. *Brain Lang.* 1993;44(1):80–120.
26. Beeman M, Friedman RB, Grafman J, Perez E, Diamond S, Lindsay MB. Summation priming and coarse coding in the right hemisphere. *J Cogn Neurosci.* 1994;6:26–45.
27. Fletcher PC, Happe F, Frith U, Baker SC, Dolan RJ, Frackowiak RS, et al. Other minds in the brain: A functional imaging study of "theory of mind" in story comprehension. *Cognition.* 1995;57(2):109–128.
28. Gaillard WD, Pugliese M, Grandin CB, Braniecki SH, Kondapaneni P, Hunter K, et al. Cortical localization of reading in normal children: An fMRI language study. *Neurology.* 2001;57(1):47–54.
29. Gaillard WD, Balsamo L, Xu B, Grandin CB, Braniecki SH, Papero PH, et al. Language dominance in partial epilepsy patients identified with an fMRI reading task. *Neurology.* 2002;59(2):256–265.
30. Just MA, Carpenter PA, Keller TA, Eddy WF, Thulborn KR. Brain activation modulated by sentence comprehension. *Science.* 1996;274:114–116.

31. Ross ED, Mesulam MM. Dominant language functions of the right hemisphere? Prosody and emotional gesturing. *Arch Neurol.* 1979;36(3): 144–148.
32. Scoville W, Milner B. Loss of recent memory after bilateral hippocampal lesions. *J Neurol Neurosurg Psychiatry.* 1957;20:11–21.
33. Loddenkemper T, Morris HH, 3rd, Perl J, 2nd. Carotid artery dissection after the intracarotid amobarbital test. *Neurology.* 2002;59(11):1797–1798.
34. Morris P. *Practical Neuroangiography.* Baltimore: Williams & Wilkins; 1997.
35. Rausch R, Silfvenius H, Wieser H-G, Dodrill CB, Meador KJ, Jones-Gotman M. Intraarterial amobarbital procedures. In: Engel J Jr, ed. *Surgical Treatment of the Epilepsies.* 2nd ed. New York: Raven Press, Ltd.; 1993:341–357.
36. Saykin AJ, Sussman NM, Gur RC. Neuropsychological methods in temporal lobectomy: Comparison of traditional batteries and specialized procedures. *J Clin Exp Neuropsychol.* 1987;9(1):33–34.
37. Kimura D. Right temporal damage. *Arch Neurol.* 1963;8:264–271.
38. Green D, Swets J. *Signal Detection Theory and Psychophysics.* New York: Krieger: 1974.
39. Gerschlager W, Lalouschek W, Lehrner J, Baumgartner C, Lindinger G, Lang W. Language-related hemispheric asymmetry in healthy subjects and patients with temporal lobe epilepsy as studied by event-related brain potentials and intracarotid amobarbital test. *Electroencephalog Clin Neurophysiol.* 1998;108(3):274–282.
40. Epstein CM, Woodard JL, Stringer AY, Bakay RA, Henry TR, Pennell PB, et al. Repetitive transcranial magnetic stimulation does not replicate the Wada test. *Neurology.* 2000;55(7):1025–1027.
41. Fitzgerald DB, Cosgrove GR, Ronner S, Jiang H, Buchbinder BR, Belliveau JW, et al. Location of language in the cortex: A comparison between functional MR imaging and electrocortical stimulation. *AJNR Am J Neuroradiol.* 1997;18(8):1529–1539.
42. Stapleton SR, Kiriakopoulos E, Mikulis D, Drake JM, Hoffman HJ, Humphreys R, et al. Combined utility of functional MRI, cortical mapping, and frameless stereotaxy in the resection of lesions in eloquent areas of brain in children. *Pediatr Neurosurg.* 1997;26(2):68–82.
43. Hunter KE, Blaxton TA, Bookheimer SY, Figlozzi C, Gaillard WD, Grandin C, et al. (15)O water positron emission tomography in language localization: A study comparing positron emission tomography visual and computerized region of interest analysis with the Wada test. *Ann Neurol.* 1999;45(5):662–665.
44. Pardo JV, Fox PT. Preoperative assessment of the cerebral hemispheric dominance for language with CBF PET. *Hum Brain Mapp.* 1993;1:57–68.
45. Dehaene S, Dupoux E, Mehler J, Cohen L, Paulesu E, Perani D, et al. Anatomical variability in the cortical representation of first and second language. *Neuroreport.* 1997;8(17):3809–3815.
46. Lehéricy S, Cohen L, Bazin B, Samson S, Giacomini E, Rougetet R, et al. Functional MR evaluation of temporal and frontal language dominance compared with the Wada test. *Neurology.* 2000;54(8):1625–1633.
47. Mazoyer BM, Tzourio N, Frak V, Syrota A, Murayama N, Levrier O, et al. The cortical representation of speech. *J Cogn Neurosci.* 1993;5(4):467–479.
48. Schlosser MJ, Aoyagi N, Fulbright RK, Gore JC, McCarthy G. Functional MRI studies of auditory comprehension. *Hum Brain Mapp.* 1998;6(1):1–13.
49. Schlosser MJ, Luby M, Spencer DD, Awad IA, McCarthy G. Comparative localization of auditory comprehension by using functional magnetic resonance imaging and cortical stimulation. *J Neurosurg.* 1999;91(4):626–635.

50. Bookheimer SY, Dapretto M, Karmarkar U. Functional MRI in children with epilepsy. *Dev Neurosci.* 1999;21(3–5):191–199.
51. Booth JR, Macwhinney B, Thulborn KR, Sacco K, Voyvodic J, Feldman HM. Functional organization of activation patterns in children: Whole brain fMRI imaging during three different cognitive tasks. *Prog Neuropsychopharmacol Biol Psychiatry.* 1999;23:669–682.
52. Howard D, Patterson K, Wise R, Brown WD, Friston K, Weiller C, et al. The cortical localization of the lexicons. Positron emission tomography evidence. *Brain.* 1992;115:1769–1782.
53. Gaillard WD, Xu B, Balsamo LM, Grandin CB, Papero PH, Weinstein S, et al. fMRI identification of language dominance in patients with complex partial epilepsy using an auditory based language comprehension task. *Epilepsia.* 2000;41(Suppl 7):83.
54. Bavelier D, Corina D, Jezzard P, Padmanabhan S, Clark VP, Karni A, et al. Sentence reading: A functional MRI study at 4 Tesla. *J Cogn Neurosci.* 1997;9(5):664–686.
55. Dapretto M, Bookheimer SY. Form and content: Dissociating syntax and semantics in sentence comprehension. *Neuron.* 1999;24(2):427–432.
56. Embick D, Marantz A, Miyashita Y, O'Neil W, Sakai KL. A syntactic specialization for Broca's area. *Proc Nat Acad Sci U S A.* 2000;97(11):6150–6154.
57. Gabrieli JD, Poldrack RA, Desmond JE. The role of left prefrontal cortex in language and memory. *Proc Nat Acad Sci U S A.* 1998;95(3):906–913.
58. Bookheimer SY, Zeffiro TA, Blaxton TA, Gaillard WD, Malow B, Theodore WH. Regional cerebral blood flow during auditory responsive naming: Evidence for cross-modality neural activation. *Neuroreport.* 1998;9(10): 2409–2413.
59. Demb JB, Desmond JE, Wagner AD, Vaidya CJ, Glover GH, Gabrieli JD. Semantic encoding and retrieval in the left inferior prefrontal cortex: A functional MRI study of task difficulty and process specificity. *J Neurosci.* 1995;15(9):5870–5878.
60. Poldrack RA, Wagner AD, Prull MW, Desmond JE, Glover GH, Gabrieli JD. Functional specialization for semantic and phonological processing in the left inferior prefrontal cortex. *Neuroimage.* 1999;10(1):15–35.
61. Desmond JE, Sum JM, Wagner AD, Demb JB, Shear PK, Glover GH, et al. Functional MRI measurement of language lateralization in Wada-tested patients. *Brain.* 1995;118(Pt 6):1411–1419.
62. Benbadis SR, Binder JR, Swanson SJ, Fischer M, Hammeke TA, Morris GL, et al. Is speech arrest during Wada testing a valid method for determining hemispheric representation of language? *Brain Lang.* 1998;65(3): 441–446.
63. Bahn MM, Lin W, Silbergeld DL, Miller JW, Kuppusamy K, Cook RJ, et al. Localization of language cortices by functional MR imaging compared with intracarotid amobarbital hemispheric sedation. *AJR Am J Roentgenol.* 1997;169(2):575–579.
64. Worthington C, Vincent DJ, Bryant AE, Roberts DR, Vera CL, Ross DA, et al. Comparison of functional magnetic resonance imaging for language localization and intracarotid speech amytal testing in presurgical evaluation for intractable epilepsy. Preliminary results. *Stereotact Funct Neurosurg.* 1997;69(1–4 Pt 2):197–201.
65. Yetkin FZ, Swanson S, Fischer M, Akansel G, Morris G, Mueller W, et al. Functional MR of frontal lobe activation: Comparison with Wada language results. *AJNR Am J Neuroradiol.* 1998;19(6):1095–1098.
66. Benson RR, FitzGerald DB, LeSueur LL, Kennedy DN, Kwong KK, Buchbinder BR, et al. Language dominance determined by whole brain

functional MRI in patients with brain lesions. *Neurology.* 1999;52(4): 798–809.
67. Carpentier A, Pugh KR, Westerveld M, Studholme C, Skrinjar O, Thompson JL, et al. Functional MRI of language processing: Dependence on input modality and temporal lobe epilepsy. *Epilepsia.* 2001;42(10): 1241–1254.
68. Baciu M, Kahane P, Minotti L, Charnallet A, David D, Le Bas JF, et al. Functional MRI assessment of the hemispheric predominance for language in epileptic patients using a simple rhyme detection task. *Epileptic Disord.* 2001;3(3):117–124.
69. Cuenod CA, Bookheimer SY, Hertz-Pannier L, Zeffiro TA, Theodore WH, Le Bihan D. Functional MRI during word generation, using conventional equipment: A potential tool for language localization in the clinical environment. *Neurology.* 1995;45(10):1821–1827.
70. Springer JA, Binder JR, Hammeke TA, Swanson SJ, Frost JA, Bellgowan PS, et al. Language dominance in neurologically normal and epilepsy subjects: A functional MRI study. *Brain.* 1999;122(Pt 11):2033–2046.
71. Yetkin FZ, Mueller WM, Morris GL, McAuliffe TL, Ulmer JL, Cox RW, et al. Functional MR activation correlated with intraoperative cortical mapping. *AJNR Am J Neuroradiol.* 1997;18(7):1311–1315.
72. Fiez JA, Petersen SE. Neuroimaging studies of word reading. *Proc Nat Acad Sci U S A.* 1998;95(3):914–921.
73. Price CJ, Moore CJ, Humphreys GW, Wise RJS. Segregating semantic from phonological processes during reading. *J Cogn Neurosci.* 1997;9(6):727–733.
74. Ojemann G, Ojemann J, Lettich E, Berger M. Cortical language localization in left, dominant hemisphere. An electrical stimulation mapping investigation in 117 patients. *J Neurosurg.* 1989;71(3):316–326.
75. Heiss WD, Kessler J, Thiel A, Ghaemi M, Karbe H. Differential capacity of left and right hemispheric areas for compensation of poststroke aphasia. *Ann Neurol.* 1999;45(4):430–438.
76. Warburton E, Wise RJ, Price CJ, Weiller C, Hadar U, Ramsay S, et al. Noun and verb retrieval by normal subjects. Studies with PET. *Brain.* 1996;119(Pt 1):159–179.
77. Weiller C, Isensee C, Rijntjes M, Huber W, Muller S, Bier D, et al. Recovery from Wernicke's aphasia: A positron emission tomographic study. *Ann Neurol.* 1995;37(6):723–732.
78. Rutten GJ, Ramsey NF, van Rijen PC, Alpherts WC, van Veelen CW. fMRI-determined language lateralization in patients with unilateral or mixed language dominance according to the Wada test. *Neuroimage.* 2002; 17(1):447–460.
79. Benson RR, Logan WJ, Cosgrove GR, Cole AJ, Jiang H, LeSueur LL, et al. Functional MRI localization of language in a 9-year-old child. *Can J Neurol Sci.* 1996;23(3):213–219.
80. Gaillard WD, Grandin CB, Xu B. Developmental aspects of pediatric fMRI: Considerations for image acquisition, analysis, and interpretation. *Neuroimage.* 2001;13(2):239–249.
81. Hertz-Pannier L, Chiron C, Vera P, Van de Morteele PF, Kaminska A, Bourgeois M, et al. Functional imaging in the work-up of childhood epilepsy. *Childs Nerv Syst.* 2001;17(4–5):223–228.
82. Baxendale S. The role of functional MRI in the presurgical investigation of temporal lobe epilepsy patients: A clinical perspective and review. *J Clin Exp Neuropsychol.* 2002;24(5):664–676.
83. Saykin AJ, Stafiniak P, Robinson LJ, Flannery KA, Gur RC, O'Connor MJ, et al. Language before and after temporal lobectomy: Specificity of acute

changes and relation to early risk factors. *Epilepsia.* 1995;36(11):1071–1077.
84. Bookheimer SY, Zeffiro TA, Blaxton T, Malow BA, Gaillard WD, Sato S, et al. A direct comparison of PET activation and electrocortical stimulation mapping for language localization. *Neurology.* 1997;48(4):1056–1065.
85. Muller RA, Rothermel RD, Behen ME, Muzik O, Mangner TJ, Chugani HT. Differential patterns of language and motor reorganization following early left hemisphere lesion: A PET study. *Arch Neurol.* 1998;55(8): 1113–1119.
86. Kurthen M, Helmstaedter C, Linke DB, Solymosi L, Elger CE, Schramm J. Interhemispheric dissociation of expressive and receptive language functions in patients with complex-partial seizures: An amobarbital study. *Brain Lang.* 1992;43(4):694–712.
87. Staudt M, Grodd W, Niemann G, Wildgruber D, Erb M, Krageloh-Mann I. Early left periventricular brain lesions induce right hemispheric organization of speech. *Neurology.* 2001;57(1):122–125.
88. Detre JA, Maccotta L, King D, Alsop DC, Glosser G, D'Esposito M, et al. Functional MRI lateralization of memory in temporal lobe epilepsy. *Neurology.* 1998;50(4):926–932.
89. Stern CE, Corkin S, Gonzalez RG, Guimaraes AR, Baker JR, Jennings PJ, et al. The hippocampal formation participates in novel picture encoding: Evidence from functional magnetic resonance imaging. *Proc Nat Acad Sci U S A.* 1996;93(16):8660–8665.
90. Bellgowan PS, Binder JR, Swanson SJ, Hammeke TA, Springer JA, Frost JA, et al. Side of seizure focus predicts left medial temporal lobe activation during verbal encoding. *Neurology.* 1998;51(2):479–484.
91. Dupont S, Van de Moortele PF, Samson S, Hasboun D, Poline JB, Adam C, et al. Episodic memory in left temporal lobe epilepsy: A functional MRI study. *Brain.* 2000;123(Pt 8):1722–1732.
92. Dupont S, Samson Y, Van de Moortele PF, Samson S, Poline JB, Adam C, et al. Delayed verbal memory retrieval: A functional MRI study in epileptic patients with structural lesions of the left medial temporal lobe. *Neuroimage.* 2001;14(5):995–1003.
93. Jokeit H, Okujava M, Woermann FG. Memory fMRI lateralizes temporal lobe epilepsy. *Neurology.* 2001;57(10):1786–1793.
94. Golby AJ, Poldrack RA, Illes J, Chen D, Desmond JE, Gabrieli JD. Memory lateralization in medial temporal lobe epilepsy assessed by functional MRI. *Epilepsia.* 2002;43(8):855–863.
95. McDonald BC, Saykin AJ, Jobst BC, Williamson PD, Roberts DW, Thadani VM, et al. Brain activation patterns in frontal and temporal memory circuitry following temporal lobe resection for intractable epilepsy: An fMRI study. *J Neuropsychiatry Clin Neurosci.* 2003;15(2):282.
96. Saykin AJ, Weaver JB, Burr RB, Riordan HJ, Roberts DW, Williamson PD, et al. Functional magnetic resonance imaging in the evaluation of epilepsy surgery patients: A memory activation study. *Epilepsia.* 1994;35:86.
97. Swick D, Knight R. Contributions of prefrontal cortex to recognition memory: Electrophysiological and behavioral evidence. *Neuropsychology.* 1999;13(2):155–170.
98. Martin A. Automatic activation of the medial temporal lobe during encoding: Lateralized influences of meaning and novelty. *Hippocampus.* 1999;9(1):62–70.
99. Fernandez G, Specht K, Weis S, Tendolkar I, Rueber M, Fell J, et al. Intrasubject reproducibility of presurgical language lateralization and mapping using fMRI. *Neurology.* 2003;60:969–975.

100. Rutten GJ, Ramsey NF, van Rijen PC, Noordmans HJ, van Veelen CW. Development of a functional magnetic resonance imaging protocol for intraoperative localization of critical temporoparietal language areas. *Ann Neurol.* 2002;51(3):350–360.
101. Boynton GM, Engel SA, Glover GH, Heeger DJ. Linear systems analysis of functional magnetic resonance imaging in human V1. *J Neurosci.* 1996; 16(13):4207–4221.
102. Saykin AJ, Gur RC, Sussman NM, O'Connor MJ, Gur RE. Memory deficits before and after temporal lobectomy:effect of laterality and age of onset. *Brain Cogn.* 1989;9:191–200.
103. Saykin AJ, Robinson LJ, Stafiniak P, Kester DB, Gur RC, O'Connor MJ, et al. Neuropsychological changes after anterior temporal lobectomy: Acute effects on memory, language, and music. In: Bennett TL, ed. *The Neuropsychology of Epilepsy.* New York: Plenum Press; 1992.
104. Stafiniak P, Saykin AJ, Sperling MR, Kester DB, Robinson LJ, O'Connor MJ, et al. Acute naming deficits following dominant temporal lobectomy: Prediction by age at 1st risk for seizures. *Neurology.* 1990;40(10):1509–1512.
105. Killgore WD, Glosser G, Casasanto DJ, French JA, Alsop DC, Detre JA. Functional MRI and the Wada test provide complementary information for predicting post-operative seizure control. *Seizure.* 1999;8(8):450–455.
106. Sabsevitz DS, Swanson SJ, Hammeke TA, Possing ET, Spanaki MV, Morris GL, et al. Predicting naming deficits following left anterior temporal lobectomy using fMRI. *J Int Neuropsychol Soc.* 2002;8(2):317.
107. Sabsevitz DS, Swanson SJ, Hammeke TA, Spanaki MV, Possing ET, Morris GL, 3rd, et al. Use of preoperative functional neuroimaging to predict language deficits from epilepsy surgery. *Neurology.* 2003;60(11):1788–1792.
108. Swanson SJ, Binder JR, Possing ET, Hammeke TA, Sabsevitz DS, Spanaki M, et al. fMRI language laterality during a semantic task: Age of onset and side of seizure focus effects. *J Int Neuropsychol Soc.* 2002;8(2):222.
109. Hermann BP, Seidenberg M, Haltiner A, Wyler AR. Relationship of age at onset, chronologic age, and adequacy of preoperative performance to verbal memory change after anterior temporal lobectomy. *Epilepsia.* 1995;36(2):137–145.
110. Glosser G, Saykin A, Deutsch G, Sperling M, O'Connor M. Patterns of reorganization of memory functions within and between cerebral hemispheres as assessed by the intracarotid amobarbital test. *Neuropsychology.* 1995;9(4):449–456.
111. Ketter TA, Kimbrell TA, George MS, Willis MW, Benson BE, Danielson A, et al. Baseline cerebral hypermetabolism associated with carbamazepine response, and hypometabolism with nimodipine response in mood disorders. *Biol Psychiatry.* 1999;46(10):1364–1374.
112. Matheja P, Weckesser M, Debus O, Lottgen J, Schuierer G, Schober O, et al. Drug-induced changes in cerebral glucose consumption in bifrontal epilepsy. *Epilepsia.* 2000;41(5):588–593.
113. Roberts MA, Manshadi FF, Bushnell DL, Hines ME. Neurobehavioural dysfunction following mild traumatic brain injury in childhood: A case report with positive findings on positron emission tomography (PET). *Brain Inj.* 1995;9(5):427–436.
114. Theodore WH. Antiepileptic drugs and cerebral glucose metabolism. *Epilepsia.* 1988;29(Suppl 2):S48–S55.
115. Theodore WH, Bromfield E, Onorati L. The effect of carbamazepine on cerebral glucose metabolism. *Ann Neurol.* 1989;25(5):516–520.

116. Theodore WH. Therapeutics: Pharmacologic. In: Mazziotta JC, Toga AW, Frackowiak RSJ, eds. *Brain Mapping: The Disorders.* San Diego, CA: Academic Press; 2000:599–612.
117. Kimura D. Sex differences in cerebral organization for speech and praxic functions. *Can J Psychol.* 1983;38:19–35.
118. McGlone J. Sex differences in the cerebral organization of verbal functions in patients with unilateral brain lesions. *Brain.* 1977;100(4):775–793.
119. Baxter LC, Saykin AJ, Flashman LA, Johnson SC, Guerin SJ, Babcock DR, et al. Sex differences in semantic language processing: A functional MRI study. *Brain Lang.* 2003;84(2):264–272.
120. American Academy of Neurology. *AAN Clinical Practice Handbook.* St. Paul, MN: American Academy of Neurology; 1995–2003.
121. Bramham J, Morris RG. Pre- and postoperative intracarotid amytal procedure: An assessment of validity. *Epilepsy Behav.* 2003;4(5):556–563.
122. Deblaere K, Backes WH, Hofman P, Vandemaele P, Boon PA, Vonck K, et al. Developing a comprehensive presurgical functional MRI protocol for patients with intractable temporal lobe epilepsy: A pilot study. *Neuroradiology.* 2002;44(8):667–673.

# 12

# fMRI of Epilepsy

Karsten Krakow

## Introduction

Since the demonstration a decade ago that functional magnetic resonance imaging (fMRI) is able to provide high spatial resolution maps of brain function, considerable effort has been directed at applying this technique to the study of patients with epilepsy, in particular, patients with intractable epilepsy considered for epilepsy surgery. Successful epilepsy surgery is vitally dependent on the accurate determination of the epileptogenic zone and of the risks of postoperative neurological deficits. Functional MRI can be used to address these issues in different ways. First, through determination of eloquent cortical areas, fMRI may predict deficits in cognitive (e.g. language and memory) or sensorimotor functions that might arise from surgical intervention. Second, functional asymmetries in activation may facilitate the lateralization and localization of an epileptogenic focus. Lastly, fMRI may provide evidence for the localization of focal epileptogenic regions through ictal or interictal blood oxygenation level-dependent (BOLD) signal changes.

## Special Issue in Patients with Epilepsy

Only in the last few years has fMRI been increasingly applied to larger numbers of neurological patients. Working with clinical populations in general and patients with epilepsy in particular requires special considerations. The issue of task compliance and difficulty has to be addressed carefully in neurological patients. Patients may be less motivated than normal volunteers to perform well on tasks. If the epilepsy is associated with intellectual impairment, patients may be less able to perform cognitive tasks that were developed for neurologically normal subjects. Emotional distress from MRI scanning is reported to interfere with completion of the procedure in as many as 20% of patients.[1,2] Although these situations often are managed with tranquilizing agents in standard MRI studies, use of such drugs in fMRI complicates interpretation of cognitive activation pattern. The effects of medication on the BOLD signal response have not yet been systematically studied. In a recent study by Jokeit and colleagues,[3] the extent of fMRI activation of the mesial temporal lobes (MTLs) induced by a task based on the retrieval of individually visuo-spatial knowledge[4] was correlated with the carbamazepine serum level in 21 patients with refractory temporal lobe epilepsy (TLE). Compared to normal controls, the activation over the supposedly normal MTL (i.e., contralateral to the seizure onset) was smaller in patients. In the patient group, the extent of the BOLD activation over the MTLs was correlated inversely to the carbamazepine drug level. The reduction of fMRI cluster size was most marked when the drug levels were close to toxic levels. There was no behavioral data concerning memory function described for the patient group, and a possible bias of the study was the possibility that a high carbamazepine level is associated with more severe epilepsy. However, these preliminary data provide some evidence that antiepileptic drug (AED) treatment may significantly influence fMRI activation of cognitive tasks.

Another consideration with epilepsy patients relates to the effects of epileptic activity to fMRI activation. A recent case report described a patient in whom fMRI falsely lateralized language cortex to the right hemisphere when performed after a cluster of left temporal lobe seizures.[5] The interaction between ictal and interictal activity with fMRI activation tasks is unclear and requires further investigation. In patients with frequent seizures or epileptiform discharges, results of fMRI activation studies should be interpreted carefully, and in some patients, electroencephalogram (EEG) monitoring before or during the fMRI study might be necessary.

## fMRI Applications in the Definition of Eloquent Cortical Areas in Epilepsy

No technique used in the identification of eloquent cortical areas is without a limiting sensitivity and specificity, including the gold standard direct cortical stimulation. Whereas cortical stimulation is essentially a lesion study, fMRI measures endogenous function. Thus, these modalities may be expected to differ somewhat in functional localization. Functional MRI has the advantage of being able to acquire functional and anatomic maps concurrently and preoperatively; it is equally sensitive to superficial and deep regions, non-invasive, cost effective, and easy to employ, even using routine clinical scanners.[6]

### Lateralization and Localization of Language

Just three years after the first reports on fMRI, a preliminary study showed that the BOLD signal contrast obtained in simple tests of language and motor function was very similar between subjects with epilepsy and normal controls, demonstrating the feasibility of the technique in studies of patients with epilepsy.[7] Since then, fMRI of language processing has become one of the most clinically relevant applications in the field of epilepsy. The main aim of localizing language functions is to predict and minimize postoperative language deficits in patients considered for epilepsy surgery, who are mainly patients with TLE.[8] In these patients, fMRI is predominantly used for language lateralization (i.e., determination of hemispheric dominance), and only to a lesser extent for intrahemispheric distribution of eloquent cortex. Numerous studies have demonstrated fMRI to identify language hemispheric dominance reliably.[9–22] However, the areas identified in different studies of language processing have varied markedly, likely relating to use of different linguistic activation or control tasks and imaging and postprocessing techniques, among other factors. There is no single fMRI paradigm that identifies language cortex. Language is a complex process that involves specialized sensory systems for speech, text, and object recognition, access to whole-word information, access to word meaning, and processing of syntax and multiple mechanisms for written and spoken language production.[23] Hence, the activation pattern is crucially dependent on the chosen fMRI task design. Hearing words—whether the task involves passive listening, repeating, or categorizing—activates the superior temporal gyrus bilaterally when compared with a resting state.[19,24,25] The symmetry of this activation can be explained by the task contrast (complex sounds compared with no sounds). The rest condition contains no control for prelinguistic auditory processing that engage auditory cortex in both superior temporal gyri. These activation patterns bear almost no relation to language dominance measured by Wada testing.[26] A further problem of such word-listening tasks is that brain areas associated with semantic processing also might be activated during the rest state, and hence reduce sensitivity for the activation task.[27]

Similar problems occur in designs that contrast reading or naming tasks with a resting or visual-fixation baseline. In a study consisting mostly of patients with lateralized lesions but not epilepsy, Benson and colleagues[28] found that such procedures did not reliably produce lateralized activation and did not correlate with language dominance measured by Wada testing.

The most common types of tasks successfully used for lateralization purpose are word-generation tasks (also called verbal-fluency tasks) and semantic decision-making, the former tending to show relatively consistent activation of anterior language areas and the latter demonstrating a more widely distributed network, including anterior and posterior hemispheric regions.[20]

In word-generation tasks, subjects are given a beginning letter, a semantic category (e.g., animal, food), and must retrieve a phonologically or semantically associated word. In verb-generation tasks, the subject generates a verb in response to seeing or hearing a noun. These tasks reliably activate the dominant inferior and dorsolateral frontal lobe, including prefrontal and premotor areas,[25,29–31] and lateralization measures obtained from this frontal activation agree well with Wada language lateralization.[9,26,28,32] There is evidence that semantic language tasks such as verb generation in response to nouns, noun categorization, or noun generation within specific categories may be more effective in lateralizing than phonologically based generation tasks such as covert repetition.[26]

Word-generation tasks usually are performed silently in fMRI studies to avoid movement artifacts. The resulting absence of task-performance data usually is not a problem when clear activation is observed, but bars the investigator from assessing the contribution of poor task performance in cases with poor activation.

A semantic decision task was used by Springer and colleagues to address the issue of language dominance in patients with epilepsy.[33] Fifty right-handed patients with epilepsy were compared with 100 right-handed normal controls. Language activation was accomplished by contrasting a semantic decision task with a tone discrimination test. For the semantic task, subjects listened to animal names and responded to those animals that met the semantic criteria of being "native to the United States" and "commonly used by humans." The contrast task required patients to listen to sequences of 500 and 750 hertz pure tones and identify those sequences that contained two high tones. The tone-discrimination task was developed to control for nonlinguistic components of the task (e.g., attention, sound processing, manual response). Using a categorical dominance classification, 94% of the normal control subjects were considered left hemisphere dominant, six percent had bilateral language representation, and none of the subjects had rightward dominance. In the epilepsy group, there was greater variability of language dominance, with 78% showing left hemisphere dominance, 16% showing a roughly symmetric pattern, and six percent showing right hemisphere dominance. Atypical language dominance in the epilepsy patients was associated with an earlier age of brain injury and with weaker right-hand dominance. The relatively high prevalence of atypical language representation in epilepsy patients stresses the importance of assessment of hemispheric dominance before interventional procedures are performed in areas potentially relevant for language in either cerebral hemisphere.[34] Further studies with the paradigm described above were performed by Binder and colleagues.[20–22] The activation pattern was, in general, strongly left lateralized and involved both prefrontal and posterior association areas. In patients with epilepsy, the activation was correlated strongly with Wada language lateralization.[22] Another study using a semantic decision task by Desmond and colleagues came to the same result. Seven postoperative patients with TLE were examined and the BOLD signal correlates were compared with a preoperative Wada test. In all cases, using a region of interest (ROI) based analysis looking only at inferior frontal regions, the lateralization by fMRI was the same as by the Wada test.[35] An attractive feature of semantic decision tasks is that measured behavioral responses consisting of simple button presses for stimuli that meet response criteria permit task performance to be precisely quantified.

As mentioned above, both word-generation and semantic decision tasks identify mainly frontal lobe language areas, but are less consistent activators of temporal language regions. An fMRI paradigm with a consistent temporal lobe activation was recently reported by Gaillard and colleagues.[36] The paradigm consisted of silent naming of items in response to silent reading of item description. The authors found language lateralization in 27 of 30 patients with TLE. The fMRI dominance was in agreement with the Wada test in 15 of 20 patients.

There are several fMRI studies reported in children with epilepsy.[11,14,37,38] Successful fMRI lateralization paradigms have been reported on children with epilepsy as young as six years.[37] The hemodynamic response appears to be similar in children and adults.[14,39] Word-generation tasks are the most commonly used tasks for evaluation of pediatric epilepsy surgery candidates, and, as in adults, show general agreement with Wada testing and electrocortical stimulation.[11,14,38] There is some evidence that young children activate more widely than adults, at least in verbal-fluency tasks.[40] Other fMRI studies in children were performed with reading tasks or naming to description.[41] Special considerations in children, like choice of suitable experimental and control conditions, have been reviewed recently.[42,43]

In addition to information on lateralization, fMRI has the potential to provide detailed maps of the intrahemispheric localization of critical language areas. There are a number of studies suggesting a close spatial relation between fMRI activation and intraoperative electrocortical stimulation.[10,44–50] A recent study by Rutten and colleagues compared the results of fMRI quantitatively with intraoperative electrocortical stimulation mapping (ESM) in thirteen patients with temporal lobe epilepsy.[51] In eight patients, critical language areas were detected by electrocortical stimulation, and in seven of eight patients, sensitivity of fMRI was 100% (i.e., fMRI correctly detected all critical language with high spatial accuracy). This indicates that such areas could be resected safely without the need for intraoperative electrocortical resection. A combination of three different fMRI language tasks (verb generation, picture naming, and sentence processing) was needed to ensure this high sensitivity, as no single task was sufficient for this purpose. On the other hand, on average, only 51% of fMRI activations were confirmed by electrocortical stimulation, resulting in a low specificity of fMRI. Both sensitivity and specificity are strongly dependent on the statistical threshold. This study illustrates the current problems of basing clinical decisions (e.g., surgical strategies) on fMRI activation maps. Different language-related paradigms activate a different set of brain regions, and a combination of different tasks is necessary to achieve high sensitivity in identifying critical areas.[52] However, a generally accepted standard protocol has not yet been established. Furthermore, the extent of the activation is critically dependent on the applied statistical threshold. An observer-independent statistical methodology (i.e., a fixed statistical threshold) would be necessary to standardize fMRI for clinical use. Finally, the presence of fMRI activation at noncritical language sites limits the predictive value of fMRI for the presence of critical language areas. Some regions activated during language tasks obviously play a minor, supportive role for language function, and resection of these areas may not necessarily produce clinically relevant deficits. Still, because of these problems, the clinical role of fMRI in identifying eloquent cortical areas of cognitive function needs to be investigated further. Currently, it can be useful to compliment intraoperative electrocortical stimulation rather than replace this method.[53]

## Language fMRI Compared with Wada Testing

One primary goal of fMRI is to displace Wada testing as the standard of care for determining language and memory dominance in candidates for epilepsy surgery. If established as a valid and reliable technique, fMRI will either render the Wada test obsolete, or at least reduce its role to a secondary procedure to be used only when fMRI is not practical because of either technical considerations or patient variables. In the Wada test [intracarotid amobarbital test (IAT)], the portions of one hemisphere supplied by the anterior circulation are transiently anesthetized using a bolus of short-acting amobarbital, allowing the contralateral hemisphere to be assessed independently.[54] The Wada test is invasive, carries significant risks, and the validity of individual Wada test results can be compromised by acute drug effects, which may produce behavioral confounds of sedation and agitation. Although the Wada test is commonly designated as the gold standard in language lateralization tests,[55] it is not a single standardized procedure. Differences in almost every aspect of methodology and design can be found in the Wada test protocols described in the literature and make between-center comparisons of the results difficult.

In a recent review by Baxendale[56], 70 patients were found in the literature who have undergone both fMRI language studies and Wada testing.[9,14,16,22,26,28,32,35,45,57,58] With the exception of one study[16] that showed a comparatively low concordance of only 75% with a verbal fluency task used as fMRI paradigm, all other studies report impressive concordance rates between the two techniques despite the use of different language tasks and Wada test protocols. A study by Binder and colleagues correlated the Wada test and fMRI assessment of language laterality using a laterality index for the Wada test (a continuous variable) and a laterality index from fMRI calculated as an asymmetry in the voxels activated in each hemisphere by a semantic decision task.[22] The correlation was extremely strong ($r = 0.96$, $p < 0.0001$), and all 22 subjects were classified to the same laterality by the two tests. Concordance at or near 100% also was found in the other studies that have employed categorial analyses to classify language representation.[32,58] While these findings are promising, there are reasons to be cautious about replacing the Wada test with fMRI procedures at this time. In all of the Wada–fMRI comparison studies reviewed above, there were less than thirty cases collectively with crossed or atypical cerebral dominance patterns as defined by Wada, an extremely limited sample on which to base clinical decisions. As mentioned above, there is evidence for a greater variability of language dominance in epilepsy subjects compared to normal controls.[33,45] Atypical language representation is the very condition that is, perhaps, the most important to detect, and the small numbers currently available do not allow any firm conclusions to be drawn about sensitivity or specificity of the various fMRI tests. Moreover, the incidence of significant discrepancy between fMRI and Wada lateralization measures is not known, nor have the reasons for the occasional discrepancies been investigated. For example, Hammeke and colleagues reported a significant discrepancy between fMRI and Wada lateralization indices in approximately one in ten patients.[59] In particular, temporal tumors of the dominant hemisphere have been reported to lead to false-negative activation of the dominant hemisphere.[60,61]

Finally, it has to be emphasized that the Wada test is not only undertaken to determine language dominance only, but also, and perhaps more importantly, to reveal the ability of each hemisphere to sustain verbal memory. Before fMRI can fully displace the Wada test, further large scale studies are necessary to establish its equivalence to the Wada test, which has been validated repeatedly with respect to memory function, language representation, and prediction of both cognitive and seizure outcome.[23] Moreover, acceptance of fMRI will depend largely on the perceived clinical need for the lesion test aspect of the Wada test, which provides more direct information about how well language and memory functions can be supported after functional removal of the contralateral hemisphere Presently, the diagnostic value of fMRI and the Wada test seems to be rather complementary. Killgore and colleagues found that, when combined, fMRI and the Wada test provided complementary data that resulted in improved prediction of postoperative seizure control compared with either procedure alone.[62]

## Memory

In addition to the investigation of language functions, the study of long-term memory systems is central to the presurgical evaluation of patients with TLE. There is long-standing evidence from animal and clinical lesional studies that memory function depends on the functional integrity of the hippocampus and parahippocampal regions in the MTL.[63–65] Whereas the hippocampus proper is the brain region most commonly associated with episodic memory function,[66] fMRI studies have often demonstrated activation more posteriorly in the parahippocampal formation. The explanation for this is poorly understood.

Functional imaging studies of these structures are potentially useful in two ways. First, identification of functionally hypoactive temporal lobe structures may have predictive value for lateralization of seizure

invasive electrocortical stimulation.[50,76,77,79,86,89,98,99] The differences in fMRI versus cortical stimulation localization varied from zero to 20 millimeters and are typically below 10 millimeters. The greatest differences were found in tumors surrounded by significant perilesional edema.

The most frequent causes for fMRI failure in sensorimotor mapping are stimulus-correlated head movement, inability to move adequately because of existing neurological deficit, and altered hemodynamic response, therefore due to arteriovenous malformations or vascular tumors.[84]

## Malformations of Cortical Development

Malformations of cortical development are an important cause for refractory epilepsy in adults and children.[100] Results of surgical treatment are less favorable compared with mesial temporal lobe epilepsy (MTLE), with about 40% of patients rendered seizure-free over a minimum two-year follow-up period. Space-occupying lesions of the brain primarily displace functional cortex. For this reason, resection within the boundaries of a lesion should not directly damage eloquent cortex and result in a significant deficit. In contrast, cortical stimulation studies showed functional reorganization within dysplastic cortex, as well as functional overlap between dysplastic cortex and normal brain tissue. Over the last years, fMRI has shown its ability to demonstrate coactivation of malformations of cortical development during physiological activation tasks.[101] Two studies on patients with subcortical laminar heterotopia[102,103] showed fMRI activation both in the outer cortex and the subcortical band heterotopia during performance of a motor task. In another patient with epilepsy and a microgyric visual cortex, the dysplastic cortex was activated by visual stimulation.[104]

In contrast, another case report found a common cortical representation of both hands on the unaffected hemisphere and no activation in the hemisphere with a complex malformation.[105] Cortical reorganization and participation of ectopic neuronal tissue in physiologic cerebral functions are of clinical importance in patients who are considered for epilepsy surgery with resection of cortical dysplasia. In addition to localized physiological activation, fMRI has the potential to identify epileptogenicity of dysplastic cortex by imaging ictal or interictal events.[106–108]

## Localization of the Epileptic Focus

Beside the identification of eloquent cortices and the prediction of functional deficits caused by epilepsy surgery, fMRI is also capable of providing evidence for the localization of the epileptic focus by identifying ictal or interictal epileptic activity, as described in the next section.

## Ictal fMRI

Ictal fMRI activation has the advantage that it can be expected to reflect changes within the epileptogenic region itself (and propagation sites). Currently, only a few anecdotal reports on ictal fMRI have been published. The section provides a brief review of the literature.

The first attempt to use fMRI for localization of epileptic activity was reported in 1994 by Jackson and colleagues.[109] This case report dealt with a 4-year old patient with the diagnosis of Rasmussen's encephalitis. A standard MRI of the patient's brain showed widespread right hemispheric atrophy primarily over the more dorsal lateral frontal region and inferior Rolandic Area. The patient was prone to frequent and prolonged focal motor seizures that involved the left arm, hand, and face. These bouts of epilepsia partialis continua were then targeted for investigation using a FLASH sequence to obtain susceptibility-weighted images every eight seconds from a single slice only. This study demonstrated a seizure-related perfusion change over the right inferior motor cortex, corresponding to the area of maximum atrophy seen on the conventional MRI and to the region of maximum abnormality as identified with an ictal single photon emission tomography (SPECT) study.[109] Another case was reported by Warach and colleagues.[110] The patient in this study had prolonged focal status epilepticus and demonstrated a perfusion MRI abnormality over the left parieto-frontal region using a susceptibility-weighted sequence and dynamic enhancement with gadolinium. This abnormal region was in keeping with the localization of the spike focus of scalp EEG and the hyperperfusion defect detected with ictal SPECT. The EEG, perfusion-based MRI abnormality, and SPECT findings normalized after more aggressive medical management.[110] Further case reports with equal findings were subsequently published.[106,111,112] In not one of these report was EEG recording available during MR image acquisition; seizure detection was only possible by clinical observation of the patient in the MR scanner. The first ictal fMRI with simultaneous EEG recording was reported by Salek-Haddadi and colleagues.[113] A patient with partial and generalized tonic–clonic seizures showed ictal EEG changes (rhythmic delta and theta activity maximum over F7/T3 lasting for about 40 seconds) in the EEG recorded inside the MR scanner. A continuous BOLD-fMRI series was simultaneously acquired and revealed an two and a half percent signal increase mainly over the left temporal lobe peaking at around six seconds into the seizure, followed later by a prolonged undershoot.[113]

In summary, ictal fMRI studies have demonstrated that fMRI, analogous to ictal SPECT, is capable of imaging reversible perfusion or BOLD abnormalities associated with epileptic seizures, with the abnormality localized closely to the site of maximum electric abnormality. However, in contrast to ictal SPECT, which is costly but feasible in specialized epilepsy units, ictal fMRI is not routinely practicable for a number of reasons: Most ictal events are associated with head and body movement and impairment of consciousness usually to a degree that the required level of cooperation for an MRI scan cannot be achieved.

Furthermore, BOLD-fMRI is not sensitive to detecting low-frequency state-related changes due to large intersessional effects and scanner noise characteristics. Together with the slow hemodynamic response function (HRF), this limits detection power to a narrow frequency band and will tend to necessitate capturing both seizure onset and termination. Seizures, however, are usually of short duration and unpredictable. It is impracticable for a patient, even with frequent seizures, to lie for hours in a MR scanner awaiting the onset of one or several seizures. Functional MRI studies with concurrent EEG recording are complicated further by the extra time involved in attaching electrodes and equipment set up. For these practical reasons, the investigation of ictal activity will be limited to selected patients who have very frequent seizures without gross head movement, in particular, seizure series, status epilepticus, or epilepsia partialis continua, or have epilepsy syndromes with seizures occurring predictably, therefore, reflex epilepsy.[114]

## Interictal fMRI

Like physiological brain activity (and epileptic seizures), interictal epileptiform discharges (IED) are associated with alterations of cerebral blood flow (CBF) and deoxyglobin concentration in the venous bed. Hence, fMRI should be able to identify the sources of IED in the same way that it can identify sources of functional activation from movement or cognitive processing. This is in contrast to methods such as dipole modeling, which can find only possible intracerebral sources of surface potentials and rely on assumptions that are not always easy to justify.

Compared with ictal fMRI, mapping of interictal activity has several advantages: (1) IED are a common phenomenon in patients with epilepsy; (2) IED are not associated with stimulus-correlated motion; and (3) fMRI activation associated with single discharges are less likely to be confounded with propagation effects compared with ongoing ictal activity. On the other hand, fMRI correlated with IED localizes brain areas involved in generating these particular EEG events. The area of cortex that generates IED is labelled as the irritative zone, which is not necessarily indicatory for the epileptogenic zone, the area of cortex that is indispensable for the generation of epileptic seizures.[115]

As IED are by definition a sub-clinical phenomenon, a second modality is necessary to identify these events. Hence, this approach was only made possible by recording EEG inside the MR scanner (EEG-correlated fMRI).

### *Methodological Aspects of EEG Correlated fMRI*

The MRI scanner is a hostile environment for EEG recordings. Magnetic resonance-compatible EEG recording equipment must ensure patient safety, sufficient quality of the EEG signals and avoid compromising MR image quality. Since the first report on EEG recording during MRI 10 years ago,[116] these issues have been addressed by several studies and technical solutions have been proposed.[117–119] Several commercial systems for intra-MR EEG recordings are now available. The main additional features implemented in these systems are a battery-powered nonmagnetic amplifier with a fiberoptic link, a high dynamic range of the amplifier, and careful choice of materials for the electrode assembly. The most crucial practical difficulty that must be overcome before useful functional data can be acquired is EEG quality. The two most relevant artifact obscuring the EEG recorded inside the MR scanner are (1) pulse artifact (or cardioballistogram) and (2) image-acquisition artifact (Figure 12.1).[120]

Cardioballistic and other movment-related artifacts are caused by movements of the body and EEG leads relative to the magnetic field of the MR scanner. It can be reduced by minimizing the area of the EEG wire loops, lead fixation, and bipolar montage of the EEG with small inter-electrode distances. Remaining pulse artifact can be removed by averaging and subtraction of the artifacts synchronized to the ECG.[120–122] These methods provide a degree of EEG quality sufficient for the accurate identification on IED,[123] sleep stages,[124] or physiological EEG rhythms.[125] During MR image acquisition, the EEG is obscured completely by large artifacts, mainly due to induced voltages in the EEG leads subjected to the rapidly changing gradient fields.

Two solutions to the problem of EEG-imaging artifact removal have been proposed.[122,126] Both rely on amplification with sufficient dynamic range to avoid saturation of the EEG amplifier due to the artifact. The method developed by Allen and colleagues[126] uses a scanner-generated slice-timing pulse. For each channel, online subtraction of a running time-averaged waveform, followed by adaptive noise cancellation, reduced any residual artifact. Hoffmann and colleagues[122] proposed a postprocessing filtering method based on the Fast Fourier transform (FFT); segments of EEG without MR activity are compared with the FFT of the EEG recorded during imaging. Frequencies with amplitudes over a threshold determined based on the FFT of the normal EEG are then discarded. The inverted FFT gives the corrected EEG.

The ability to remove image artifacts determines the data acquisition of EEG-correlated fMRI experiments. Without image artifact removal, the EEG is obscured during imaging and interleaved data acquisition has to be applied. In epilepsy studies, this approach was introduced as spike-triggered fMRI (Figure 12.2). This method takes advantage of the delayed BOLD response after a neuronal event. This makes it possible to observe the EEG recording on-line (which requires the presence of an experienced electroencephalographer during data acquisition), and to start image acquisitions manually at a fixed interval after the event of interest (usually three seconds, as the BOLD response peaks at two to seven seconds after an event) or during control periods. However, spike-triggered fMRI suffers from two main limitations, both linked to the obliteration of the EEG during the image acquisition. First, there are constraints on the scanning rate and the duration of each scan. The minimum time gap between successive image acquisitions must be of the order of 15 seconds to avoid signal variations due to the T1 signal decay, and the maximum duration of each image acquisition must be less than the expected duration of the BOLD response in order to

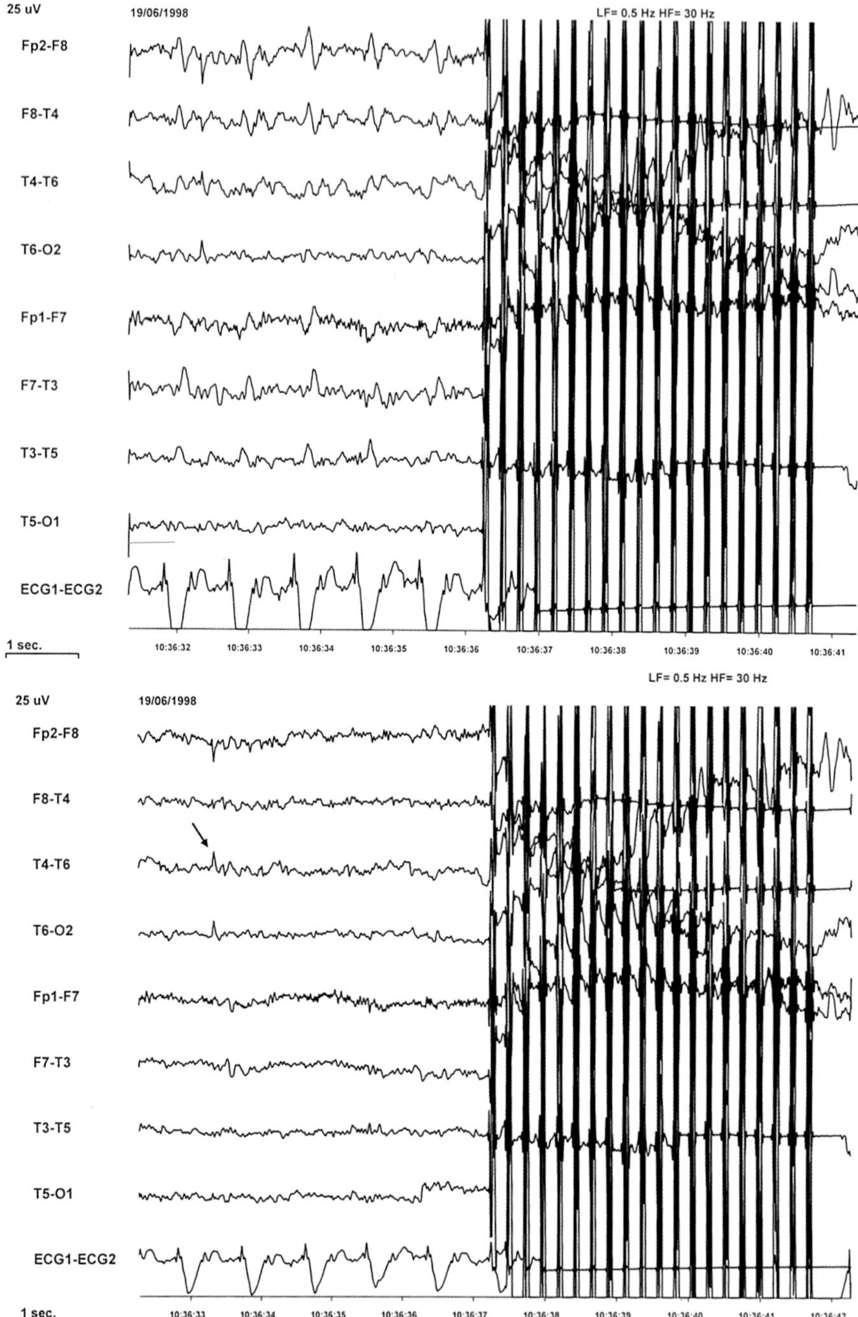


**Figure 12.1.** Electroencephalogram recorded inside a 1.5T scanner. In (a), an ECG-related artifact is obscuring the EEG activity (pulse artifact, cardioballistogram), making the identification of IED difficult; (b) shows the identical EEG sequence after on-line pulse artifact subtraction. A small amplitude spike is clearly detectable over the right hemisphere. Three and a half seconds after the spike, a 20 slice EPI sequence is triggered, leading to a large EEG artifact (image acquisition artifact). The result of the spike-triggered fMRI experiment is demonstrated in Figure 12.2.

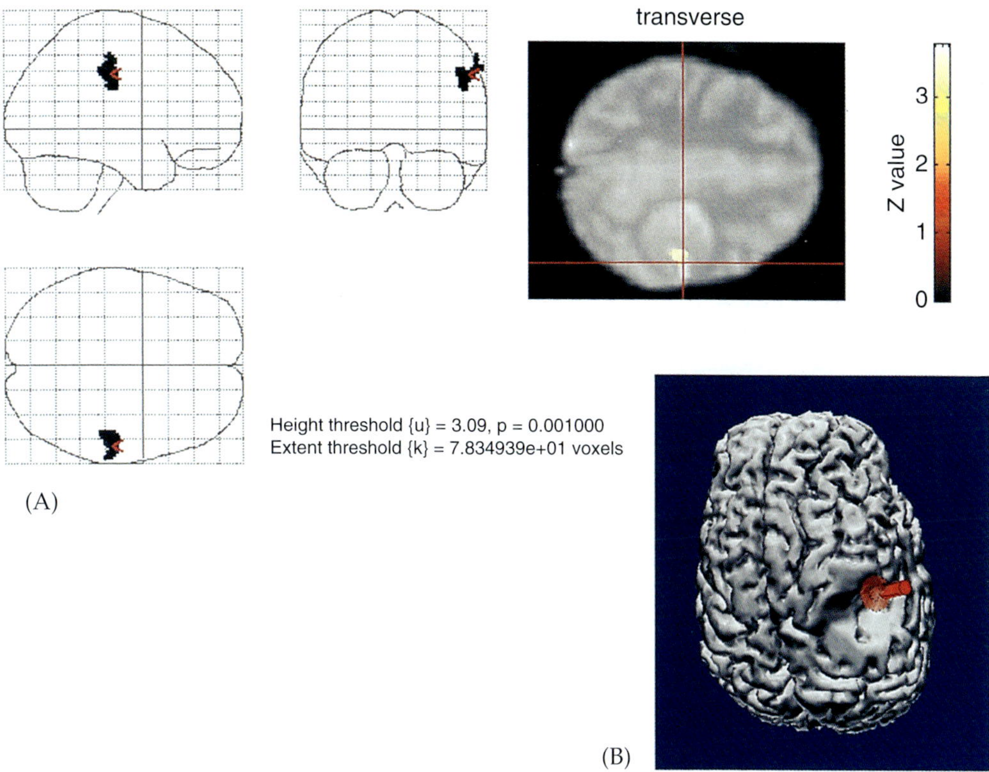


**Figure 12.2.** (A) The statistical parametric mapping BOLD activation map of a spike-triggered fMRI experiment, which was performed on an 22-year-old patient with refractory partial and secondarily generalized seizures. Standard MRI showed subcortical nodular heterotopia of the right hemisphere with a large mass in the central region. Interictal EEG demonstrated frequent focal IED over the temporal and parasagittal region of the right hemisphere. Functional MRI result shows an axial image with crosshair through the center of the activation (overlaid in yellow) in the center of the nodular heterotopia of the right hemisphere. (B) Result of a 64-channel EEG source analysis (multiple unconstrained moving dipole model, CURRY 3.0), superimposed on a T1-weighted anatomical scan, showing co-localization with the result of the spike-triggered fMRI. (Neurologic coordinates).

ensure proper separation of the responses from events that may occur during image acquisition, and therefore be undetected. Second, as mentioned above, the spike-triggered approach relies on assumptions about the BOLD response peak time and duration. However, spike-triggered fMRI is not able to reveal the hemodynamic response function due to a delayed image acquisition and the lack of preactivity baseline images.

With the possibility of image artifact subtraction, these limitations can be overcome by continuous and simultaneous EEG and fMRI. In principle, continuous EEG/fMRI should be more sensitive than the spike-triggered approach for the following reasons: a larger amount of data can be acquired per time unit, and the time course of the response in individual subjects can be measured. Furthermore, it should allow more flexibility in patient selection concerning the frequency of IED (Figure 12.3).

## EEG Correlated fMRI in Patients with Epilepsy

Most of the studies used spike-triggered fMRI,[108,123,127–132] only since 2001 have several cases and small scale studies with continuous EEG/fMRI been reported.[133–135]

In summary, the studies showed that EEG-correlated fMRI is a practicable method to be applied to patients with epilepsy showing frequent IED on scalp EEG. The EEG quality was sufficient to detect spontaneous IED off- or on-line. Discomfort or injuries of the patients due to the EEG recording were not reported and the MR image quality was not significantly compromised by the EEG recording. In the studies listed, a total number of 75 patients was reported. Most of the patients had intractable focal epilepsy, some of the patients were considered for epilepsy surgery, and in a few, surgery was carried out after the EEG/fMRI experiment.[130] Patients for EEG/FMRI experiments were, in general, highly selected, particularly with regard to the frequency of their IED. Nevertheless, in many patients, the EEG/fMRI experiments failed, mainly because of absence of IED or due to motion artifacts. In the lager studies, fMRI activation was reported in about 50% of patients.[108,129–131] In general, the activations were anatomically related to the proposed epileptic focus (as defined by interictal EEG, EEG source analysis, structural MRI, ictal video-EEG, or, in less than 10 patients, intracranial EEG).

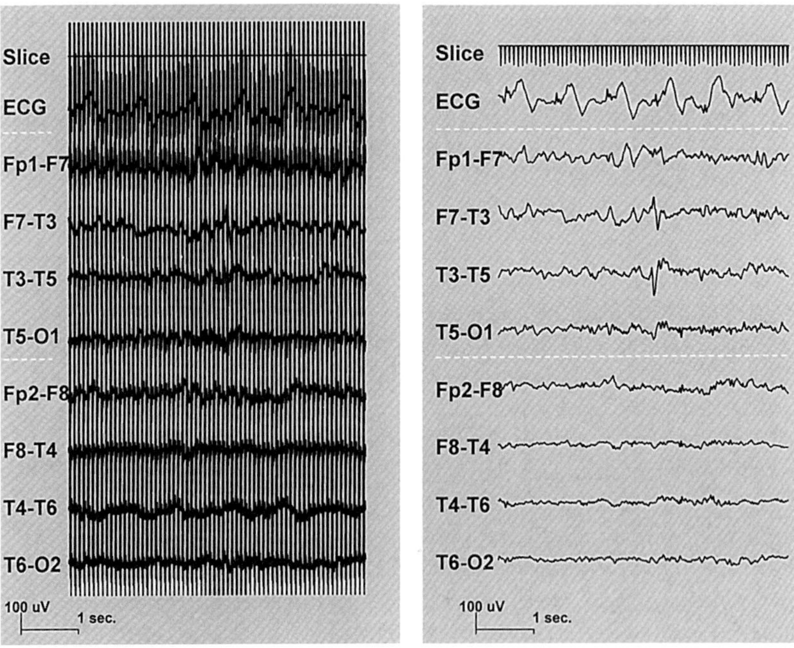


**Figure 12.3.** Two segments of an EEG recording made during a continuous EEG/fMRI experiment before and after image artifact subtraction. The possibility of removing image acquisition artifact enables continuous and simultaneous EEG/fMRI in contrast to spike-triggered fMRI. (Neurologic coordinates).

While the studies mentioned above dealt predominantly with patents with focal epilepsy, there exists only one study applying EEG-correlated fMRI to a patient with idiopathic generalized epilepsy and absence seizures. A 36-year old patient with intractable juvenile absence epilepsy had four prolonged runs (from 31 to 60 seconds) of three hertz generalized spike-wave discharges during continuous and simultaneous EEG/fMRI. There were two highly significant patterns of seizure-related BOLD changes. Positives changes of around three percent relative to baseline were seen exclusively within the thalamus bilaterally (three percent signal change relative to the baseline). Negative signal changes were present symmetrically over large areas of cortical grey matter with a frontal emphasis and a maximum of around minus eight percent relative to baseline. This result suggests the reciprocal participation of focal thalamic and widespread cortical networks during human absence seizures. The negative cortical BOLD response may be interpreted as an inactive cortical state with low mean synaptic activity during absence seizures.[136]

The possible clinical application of EEG-correlated fMRI would be contributing to the accurate localization of the epileptogenic zone, which is the basis for successful epilepsy surgery in patients with medically refractory focal seizures. Information on the epileptogenic zone is derived from the convergence of diverse investigations. In some patients, particularly with neocortical cryptogenic epilepsy, additional intracranial EEG recordings often have to be applied to reliably identify the epileptic focus. It remains unclear whether EEG-correlated fMRI has the potential to replace invasive techniques, or at least provide additional information to guide the placement of invasive intracranial electrodes where necessary. The clinical interpretation of the fMRI activation maps is difficult for various reasons:

1. The size of the fMRI activation cluster is greatly variable between studies and between subjects in individual studies. Some patients have a widespread, multifocal activation, others show a circumscribed activation (Figure 12.4). The extent of the activation is critically dependent on the applied statistical threshold, which partly explains differences between studies. However, the reason for the variability between patients who were studied with identical methodology and thresholds remains unclear. No significant correlations were found between clinical characteristics (e.g., epilepsy syndrome, spike amplitude) and the size of the fMRI activation. The same applies for the number of IED that have been analyzed. In some patients, even individual IED are associated with large activations;[137] in other patients, as many as 50 IED are not associated with significant activations. Hence, EEG-correlated fMRI may contribute to localize the source of IED, but currently it cannot provide information about its extent.

In patients with widespread fMRI activation, another problem is to distinguish the primary sources from activation, which may represent areas of propagation. In such cases with equivocal information on localization, a combination of fMRI data with EEG source analysis may provide complementary information.[128]

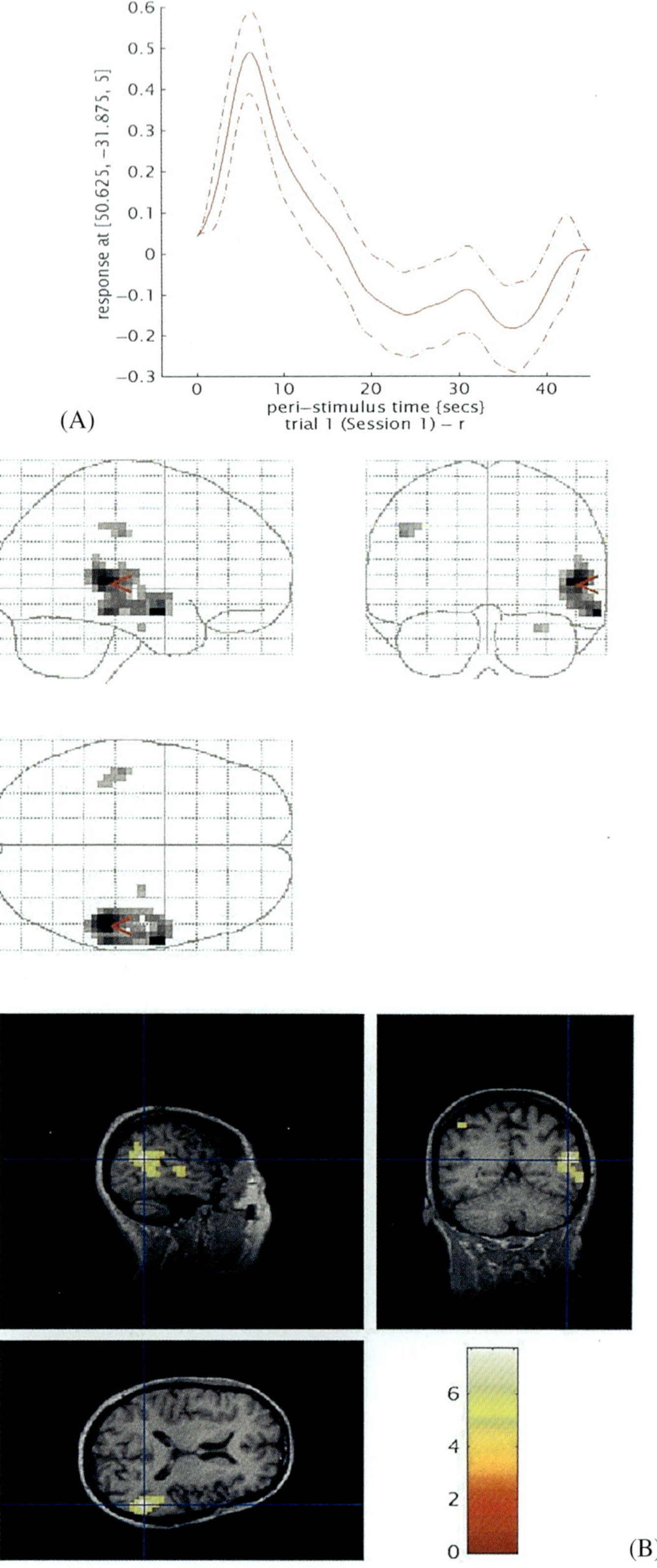


**Figure 12.4.** (A) Result of a continuous and simultaneous EEG/FMRI experiment in a patient with partial seizures due to a right tempro-parietal malformation of cortical development and frequent right temporal spikes. The time course of the event-related response at location of the cross-hair. (B) The fMRI activation is located within the subtle cortical dysplasia. (Neurologic coordinates).

2. Until now, the results of EEG-correlated fMRI have not been validated systematically with a gold standard, which are intracranial recordings and outcomes after epilepsy surgery. Before EEG-triggered fMRI can be used as a decisive method in the presurgical assessment of epilepsy patients, the relation between fMRI results, invasive EEG recordings, and surgical outcome in relation to resection of the activated area has to be established.

3. The high percentage of negative results (up to fifty percent in studies using spike-triggered fMRI,) currently hinders the wider clinical application of EEG-correlated fMRI. In spike-triggered fMRI, the physiological explanation of a negative fMRI result is most likely that a non-significant difference in the blood oxygenation exists between activation and control states. This might be due to there being only a modest cerebral hyperperfusion following an IED, or due to an absence of a true control state, therefore, such as ongoing epileptic activity not detected on scalp EEG. In both cases, the relative signal change within the spike generator may not achieve significance.

As mentioned above, it is conceivable that continuous and simultaneous EEG/fMRI will increase the sensitivity of the method; however, this has to be proven by larger scale studies using this technique and comparative studies between spike-triggered and simultaneous EEG/fMRI. Furthermore, the use of higher-strength magnets will increase the signal-to-noise ratio, and hence, fMRI sensitivity. Multichannel EEG has already been recorded in a four Tesla MR scanner on humans and in a seven Tesla MR scanner in animals.[138] An improved signal-to-noise ratio may not only increase the proportion of fMRI-positive experiments, but also may reduce the number of analyzed IED necessary for a significant fMRI activation, thus rendering this method applicable to patients with less-frequent IED. In summary, EEG-correlated fMRI has to be considered a research tool providing insights to the pathophysiological processes underlying epileptic disorders and in the future may be used in the clinical work-up of epilepsy patients.

## References

1. Melendez JC, McCrank E. Anxiety-related reactions associated with magnetic resonance imaging examinations. *JAMA.* 1993;270:745–747.
2. Thorp D, Owens RG, Whitehouse G, Dewey ME. Subjective experiences of magnetic resonance imaging. *Clin Radiol.* 1990;41:276–278.
3. Jokeit H, Okujava M, Woermann FG. Carbamazepine reduces memory induced activation of mesial temporal lobe structures: a pharmacological fMRI-study. *BMC Neurol.* 2001;1:6.
4. Jokeit H, Okujava M, Woermann FG. Memory fMRI lateralizes temporal lobe epilepsy. *Neurology.* 2001;57:1786–1793.
5. Jayakar P, Bernal B, Santiago Medina L, Altman N. False lateralization of language cortex on functional MRI after a cluster of focal seizures. *Neurology* 2002;58:490–492.
6. Fernandez G, de Greiff A, von Oertzen J, et al. Language mapping in less than 15 minutes: real-time functional MRI during routine clinical investigation. *Neuroimage.* 2001;14:585–594.

44. Yetkin FZ, Mueller WM, Morris GL, et al. Functional MR activation correlated with intraoperative cortical mapping. *AJNR Am J Neuroradiol.* 1997; 18:1311–1315.
45. Carpentier A, Pugh KR, Westerveld M, et al. Functional MRI of language processing: dependence on input modality and temporal lobe epilepsy. *Epilepsia.* 2001;42:1241–1254.
46. Rutten GJ, van Rijen PC, van Veelen CW, Ramsey NF. Language area localization with three-dimensional functional magnetic resonance imaging matches intrasulcal electrostimulation in Broca's area. *Ann Neurol.* 1999; 46:405–408.
47. Lurito JT, Lowe MJ, Sartorius C, Mathews VP. Comparison of fMRI and intraoperative direct cortical stimulation in localization of receptive language areas. *J Comput Assist Tomogr.* 2000;24:99–105.
48. Schlosser MJ, Luby M, Spencer DD, Awad IA, McCarthy G. Comparative localization of auditory comprehension by using functional magnetic resonance imaging and cortical stimulation. *J Neurosurg.* 1999;91:626–635.
49. Ruge MI, Victor J, Hosain S, et al. Concordance between functional magnetic resonance imaging and intraoperative language mapping. *Stereotact Funct Neurosurg.* 1999;72:95–102.
50. Mueller WM, Yetkin FZ, Hammeke TA, et al. Functional magnetic resonance imaging mapping of the motor cortex in patients with cerebral tumors. *Neurosurgery.* 1996;39:515–520; discussion 520–521.
51. Rutten GJ, Ramsey NF, van Rijen PC, Noordmans HJ, van Veelen CW. Development of a functional magnetic resonance imaging protocol for intraoperative localization of critical temporoparietal language areas. *Ann Neurol.* 2002;51:350–360.
52. Ramsey NF, Sommer IE, Rutten GJ, Kahn RS. Combined analysis of language tasks in fMRI improves assessment of hemispheric dominance for language functions in individual subjects. *Neuroimage.* 2001;13: 719–733.
53. Deblaere K, Backes WH, Hofman P, et al. Developing a comprehensive presurgical functional MRI protocol for patients with intractable temporal lobe epilepsy: a pilot study. *Neuroradiology.* 2002;44:667–673.
54. Wada J, Rasmussen T. Intracarotid injection of sodium amytal for the lateralization of cerebral speech dominance. Experimental and clinical observations. *J Neurosurg.* 1960;17:266–282.
55. Rausch R, Silfvenious H, Wieser HG, Dodrill CB, Meador KJ, Jones-Gotman M. Intra-arterial amobarbital procedures. In: Engel JJ, ed. *Surgical Treatment of the Epilepsies.* New York: Raven Press; 1993:341–357.
56. Baxendale S. The role of functional MRI in the presurgical investigation of temporal lobe epilepsy patients: a clinical perspective and review. *J Clin Exp Neuropsychol.* 2002;24:664–676.
57. Bazin B, Cohen L, Lehericy S, et al. [Study of hemispheric lateralization of language regions by functional MRI. Validation with the Wada test]. *Rev Neurol (Paris).* 2000;156:145–148.
58. Benbadis SR, Binder JR, Swanson SJ, et al. Is speech arrest during wada testing a valid method for determining hemispheric representation of language? *Brain Lang.* 1998;65:441–446.
59. Hammeke TA, Bellgowan PS, Binder JR. fMRI: methodology–cognitive function mapping. *Adv Neurol.* 2000;83:221–233.
60. Gaillard WD, Bookheimer SY, Cohen M. The use of fMRI in neocortical epilepsy. *Adv Neurol.* 2000;84:391–404.

61. Westerveld K, Stoddard K, McCarthy K. Case report of false lateralization using fMRI: comparison of language localization, Wada testing, and cortical stimulation. *Arch Clin Neuropsychol.* 1999;14:162–163.
62. Killgore WD, Glosser G, Casasanto DJ, French JA, Alsop DC, Detre JA. Functional MRI and the Wada test provide complementary information for predicting post-operative seizure control. *Seizure.* 1999;8:450–455.
63. McGaugh JL. Memory—a century of consolidation. *Science.* 2000;287: 248–251.
64. Sass KJ, Spencer DD, Kim JH, Westerveld M, Novelly RA, Lencz T. Verbal memory impairment correlates with hippocampal pyramidal cell density. *Neurology.* 1990;40:1694–1697.
65. Scoville WB, Milner B. Loss of recent memory after bilateral hippocampal lesions. 1957. *J Neuropsychiatry Clin Neurosci.* 2000;12:103–113.
66. Squire LR. Memory and the hippocampus: a synthesis from findings with rats, monkeys, and humans. *Psychol Rev.* 1992;99:195–231.
67. Fernandez G, Weyerts H, Schrader-Bolsche M, et al. Successful verbal encoding into episodic memory engages the posterior hippocampus: a parametrically analyzed functional magnetic resonance imaging study. *J Neurosci.* 1998;18:1841–1847.
68. Gabrieli JD, Brewer JB, Desmond JE, Glover GH. Separate neural bases of two fundamental memory processes in the human medial temporal lobe. *Science.* 1997;276:264–266.
69. Stern CE, Corkin S, Gonzalez RG, et al. The hippocampal formation participates in novel picture encoding: evidence from functional magnetic resonance imaging. *Proc Natl Acad Sci U S A.* 1996;93:8660–8665.
70. Bellgowan PS, Binder JR, Swanson SJ, et al. Side of seizure focus predicts left medial temporal lobe activation during verbal encoding. *Neurology.* 1998;51:479–484.
71. Detre JA, Maccotta L, King D, et al. Functional MRI lateralization of memory in temporal lobe epilepsy. *Neurology.* 1998;50:926–932.
72. Dupont S, Samson Y, Van de Moortele PF, et al. Delayed verbal memory retrieval: a functional MRI study in epileptic patients with structural lesions of the left medial temporal lobe. *Neuroimage.* 2001;14:995–1003.
73. Dupont S, Van de Moortele PF, Samson S, et al. Episodic memory in left temporal lobe epilepsy: a functional MRI study. *Brain.* 2000;123:1722–1732.
74. Golby AJ, Poldrack RA, Illes J, Chen D, Desmond JE, Gabrieli JD. Memory lateralization in medial temporal lobe epilepsy assessed by functional MRI. *Epilepsia.* 2002;43:855–863.
75. Roland PE, Eriksson L, Stone-Elander S, Widen L. Does mental activity change the oxidative metabolism of the brain? *J Neurosci.* 1987;7:2373–2389.
76. Jack CR Jr., Thompson RM, Butts RK, et al. Sensory motor cortex: correlation of presurgical mapping with functional MR imaging and invasive cortical mapping. *Radiology.* 1994;190:85–92.
77. Puce A, Constable RT, Luby ML, et al. Functional magnetic resonance imaging of sensory and motor cortex: comparison with electrophysiological localization. *J Neurosurg.* 1995;83:262–270.
78. Cosgrove GR, Buchbinder BR, Jiang H. Functional magnetic resonance imaging for intracranial navigation. *Neurosurg Clin N Am.* 1996;7:313–322.
79. Yousry TA, Schmid UD, Schmidt D, Hagen T, Jassoy A, Reiser MF. The central sulcal vein: a landmark for identification of the central sulcus using functional magnetic resonance imaging. *J Neurosurg.* 1996;85: 608–617.

80. Roux FE, Ranjeva JP, Boulanouar K, et al. Motor functional MRI for presurgical evaluation of cerebral tumors. *Stereotact Funct Neurosurg.* 1997;68:106–111.
81. Roux FE, Boulanouar K, Ranjeva JP, et al. Cortical intraoperative stimulation in brain tumors as a tool to evaluate spatial data from motor functional MRI. *Invest Radiol.* 1999;34:225–229.
82. Dymarkowski S, Sunaert S, Van Oostende S, et al. Functional MRI of the brain: localisation of eloquent cortex in focal brain lesion therapy. *Eur Radiol.* 1998;8:1573–1580.
83. Krings T, Reul J, Spetzger U, et al. Functional magnetic resonance mapping of sensory motor cortex for image-guided neurosurgical intervention. *Acta Neurochir (Wien).* 1998;140:215–222.
84. Krings T, Reinges MH, Erberich S, et al. Functional MRI for presurgical planning: problems, artefacts, and solution strategies. *J Neurol Neurosurg Psychiatry.* 2001;70:749–760.
85. Nitschke MF, Melchert UH, Hahn C, et al. Preoperative functional magnetic resonance imaging (fMRI) of the motor system in patients with tumours in the parietal lobe. *Acta Neurochir (Wien).* 1998;140:1223–1229.
86. Pujol J, Conesa G, Deus J, Lopez-Obarrio L, Isamat F, Capdevila A. Clinical application of functional magnetic resonance imaging in presurgical identification of the central sulcus. *J Neurosurg.* 1998;88:863–869.
87. Schulder M, Maldjian JA, Liu WC, et al. Functional image-guided surgery of intracranial tumors located in or near the sensorimotor cortex. *J Neurosurg.* 1998;89:412–418.
88. Wildforster U, Falk A, Harders A. Operative approach due to results of functional magnetic resonance imaging in central brain tumors. *Comput Aided Surg.* 1998;3:162–165.
89. Achten E, Jackson GD, Cameron JA, Abbott DF, Stella DL, Fabinyi GC. Presurgical evaluation of the motor hand area with functional MR imaging in patients with tumors and dysplastic lesions. *Radiology.* 1999; 210:529–538.
90. Bittar RG, Olivier A, Sadikot AF, Andermann F, Pike GB, Reutens DC. Presurgical motor and somatosensory cortex mapping with functional magnetic resonance imaging and positron emission tomography. *J Neurosurg.* 1999;91:915–921.
91. Fandino J, Kollias SS, Wieser HG, Valavanis A, Yonekawa Y. Intraoperative validation of functional magnetic resonance imaging and cortical reorganization patterns in patients with brain tumors involving the primary motor cortex. *J Neurosurg.* 1999;91:238–250.
92. Lee CC, Ward HA, Sharbrough FW, et al. Assessment of functional MR imaging in neurosurgical planning. *AJNR Am J Neuroradiol.* 1999;20: 1511–1519.
93. Atlas SW, Howard RS 2nd, Maldjian J, et al. Functional magnetic resonance imaging of regional brain activity in patients with intracerebral gliomas: findings and implications for clinical management. *Neurosurgery.* 1996;38:329–338.
94. Rao SM, Binder JR, Bandettini PA, et al. Functional magnetic resonance imaging of complex human movements. *Neurology.* 1993;43:2311–2318.
95. Kleinschmidt A, Nitschke MF, Frahm J. Somatotopy in the human motor cortex hand area. A high-resolution functional MRI study. *Eur J Neurosci.* 1997;9:2178–2186.
96. Maldjian JA, Gottschalk A, Patel RS, Detre JA, Alsop DC. The sensory somatotopic map of the human hand demonstrated at 4 Tesla. *Neuroimage.* 1999;10:55–62.

97. Lotze M, Erb M, Flor H, Huelsmann E, Godde B, Grodd W. fMRI evaluation of somatotopic representation in human primary motor cortex. *Neuroimage.* 2000;11:473–481.
98. Schlosser MJ, McCarthy G, Fulbright RK, Gore JC, Awad IA. Cerebral vascular malformations adjacent to sensorimotor and visual cortex. Functional magnetic resonance imaging studies before and after therapeutic intervention. *Stroke.* 1997;28:1130–1137.
99. Chapman PH, Buchbinder BR, Cosgrove GR, Jiang HJ. Functional magnetic resonance imaging for cortical mapping in pediatric neurosurgery. *Pediatr Neurosurg.* 1995;23:122–126.
100. Sisodiya SM. Surgery for malformations of cortical development causing epilepsy. *Brain.* 2000;123:1075–1091.
101. Salek-Haddadi A, Lemieux L, Fish DR. Role of functional magnetic resonance imaging in the evaluation of patients with malformations caused by cortical development. *Neurosurg Clin N Am.* 2002;13:63–69, viii.
102. Spreer J, Martin P, Greenlee MW, et al. Functional MRI in patients with band heterotopia. *Neuroimage.* 2001;14:357–365.
103. Pinard J, Feydy A, Carlier R, Perez N, Pierot L, Burnod Y. Functional MRI in double cortex: functionality of heterotopia. *Neurology.* 2000;54:1531–1533.
104. Innocenti GM, Maeder P, Knyazeva MG, Fornari E, Deonna T. Functional activation of microgyric visual cortex in a human. *Ann Neurol.* 2001;50: 672–676.
105. Staudt M, Pieper T, Grodd W, Winkler P, Holthausen H, Krageloh-Mann I. Functional MRI in a 6-year-old boy with unilateral cortical malformation: concordant representation of both hands in the unaffected hemisphere. *Neuropediatrics.* 2001;32:159–161.
106. Schwartz TH, Resor SR Jr., De La Paz R, Goodman RR. Functional magnetic resonance imaging localization of ictal onset to a dysplastic cleft with simultaneous sensorimotor mapping: intraoperative electrophysiological confirmation and postoperative follow-up: technical note. *Neurosurgery.* 1998;43:639–644; discussion 644–645.
107. Krakow K, Wieshmann UC, Woermann FG, et al. Multimodal MR imaging: functional, diffusion tensor, and chemical shift imaging in a patient with localization-related epilepsy. *Epilepsia.* 1999;40:1459–1462.
108. Krakow K, Lemieux L, Messina D, et al. Spatio-temporal imaging of focal interictal epileptiform activity using EEG-triggered functional MRI. *Epileptic Disord.* 2001;3:67–74.
109. Jackson GD, Connelly A, Cross JH, Gordon I, Gadian DG. Functional magnetic resonance imaging of focal seizures. *Neurology.* 1994;44:850–856.
110. Warach S, Levin JM, Schomer DL, Holman BL, Edelman RR. Hyperperfusion of ictal seizure focus demonstrated by MR perfusion imaging. *AJNR Am J Neuroradiol.* 1994;15:965–968.
111. Detre JA, Sirven JI, Alsop DC, O'Connor MJ, French JA. Localization of subclinical ictal activity by functional magnetic resonance imaging: correlation with invasive monitoring. *Ann Neurol.* 1995;38:618–624.
112. Krings T, Topper R, Reinges MH, et al. Hemodynamic changes in simple partial epilepsy: a functional MRI study. *Neurology.* 2000;54:524–527.
113. Salek-Haddadi A, Merschhemke M, Lemieux L, Fish DR. Simultaneous EEG-Correlated Ictal fMRI. *Neuroimage.* 2002;16:32–40.
114. Archer JS, Briellmann RS, Syngeniotis A, Abbott DF, Jackson GD. Spike-triggered fMRI in reading epilepsy: Involvement of left frontal cortex working memory area. *Neurology.* 2003;60:415–421.

115. Rosenow F, Luders H. Presurgical evaluation of epilepsy. *Brain.* 2001;124: 1683–1700.
116. Ives JR, Warach S, Schmitt F, Edelman RR, Schomer DL. Monitoring the patient's EEG during echo planar MRI. *Electroencephalogr Clin Neurophysiol.* 1993;87:417–420.
117. Lemieux L, Allen PJ, Franconi F, Symms MR, Fish DR. Recording of EEG during fMRI experiments: patient safety. *Magn Reson Med.* 1997;38: 943–952.
118. Krakow K, Allen PJ, Symms MR, Lemieux L, Josephs O, Fish DR. EEG recording during fMRI experiments: image quality. *Hum Brain Mapp.* 2000;10:10–15.
119. Krakow K, Allen PJ, Lemieux L, Symms MR, Fish DR. Methodology: EEG-correlated fMRI. *Adv Neurol.* 2000;83:187–201.
120. Allen PJ, Polizzi G, Krakow K, Fish DR, Lemieux L. Identification of EEG events in the MR scanner: the problem of pulse artifact and a method for its subtraction. *Neuroimage.* 1998;8:229–239.
121. Bonmassar G, Purdon P, Jaaskelainen I, et al. Motion and Ballistocardiogram Artifact Removal for Interleaved Recording of EEG and EPs during MRI. *Neuroimage.* 2002;16:1127.
122. Hoffmann A, Jager L, Werhahn KJ, Jaschke M, Noachtar S, Reiser M. Electroencephalography during functional echo-planar imaging: detection of epileptic spikes using post-processing methods. *Magn Reson Med.* 2000;44:791–798.
123. Krakow K, Woermann FG, Symms MR, et al. EEG-triggered functional MRI of interictal epileptiform activity in patients with partial seizures. *Brain.* 1999;122:1679–1688.
124. Portas CM, Krakow K, Allen P, Josephs O, Armony JL, Frith CD. Auditory processing across the sleep-wake cycle: simultaneous EEG and fMRI monitoring in humans. *Neuron.* 2000;28:991–999.
125. Goldman RI, Stern JM, Engel J Jr., Cohen MS. Simultaneous EEG and fMRI of the alpha rhythm. *Neuroreport.* 2002;13:2487–2492.
126. Allen PJ, Josephs O, Turner R. A method for removing imaging artifact from continuous EEG recorded during functional MRI. *Neuroimage.* 2000; 12:230–239.
127. Warach S, Ives JR, Schlaug G, et al. EEG-triggered echo-planar functional MRI in epilepsy. *Neurology.* 1996;47:89–93.
128. Seeck M, Lazeyras F, Michel CM, et al. Non-invasive epileptic focus localization using EEG-triggered functional MRI and electromagnetic tomography. *Electroencephalogr Clin Neurophysiol.* 1998;106:508–512.
129. Patel MR, Blum A, Pearlman JD, et al. Echo-planar functional MR imaging of epilepsy with concurrent EEG monitoring. *AJNR Am J Neuroradiol.* 1999;20:1916–1919.
130. Lazeyras F, Blanke O, Perrig S, et al. EEG-triggered functional MRI in patients with pharmacoresistant epilepsy. *J Magn Reson Imaging.* 2000;12: 177–185.
131. Jager L, Werhahn KJ, Hoffmann A, et al. Focal epileptiform activity in the brain: detection with spike-related functional MR imaging—preliminary results. *Radiology.* 2002;223:860–869.
132. Archer JS, Briellman RS, Abbott DF, Syngeniotis A, Wellard RM, Jackson GD. Benign epilepsy with centro-temporal spikes: spike triggered FMRI shows somato-sensory cortex activity. *Epilepsia.* 2003;44:200–204.
133. Lemieux L, Salek-Haddadi A, Josephs O, et al. Event-related fMRI with simultaneous and continuous EEG: description of the method and initial case report. *Neuroimage.* 2001;14:780–787.

134. Baudewig J, Bittermann HJ, Paulus W, Frahm J. Simultaneous EEG and functional MRI of epileptic activity: a case report. *Clin Neurophysiol.* 2001;112:1196–1200.
135. Benar CG, Gross DW, Wang Y, et al. The BOLD response to interictal epileptiform discharges. *Neuroimage.* 2002;17:1182–1192.
136. Salek-Haddadi A, Lemieux L, Merschhemke M, Friston K, Duncan JS, Fish DR. Functional MRI of human absence seizures. *Ann Neurol.* In press.
137. Krakow K, Messina D, Lemieux L, Duncan JS, Fish DR. Functional MRI activation of individual interictal epileptiform spikes. *Neuroimage.* 2001;13:502–505.
138. Sijbers J, Michiels I, Verhoye M, Van Audekerke J, Van der Linden A, Van Dyck D. Restoration of MR-induced artifacts in simultaneously recorded MR/EEG data. *Magn Reson Imaging.* 1999;17:1383–1391.

# 13

# fMRI of the Visual Pathways

Atsushi Miki, Grant T. Liu, and Scott H. Faro

## Introduction

Visual cortex activation was a frequent topic of initial functional magnetic resonance imaging (fMRI) investigations,[1,2] and since then, fMRI has had a great impact on visual neuroscience as it relates to the human brain. The reasons for this are severalfold. Firstly, visual cortical areas occupy a large portion of cerebral cortex; their localization, for the most part, is relatively well-known from animal, lesion, and positron emission tomography (PET) and single-photon emission computed tomography (SPECT) studies. Secondly, robust activation can be obtained within many of the visual areas because of their relatively large changes in blood flow and/or blood oxygenation level-dependent (BOLD) responses following visual stimuli, and thirdly, visual stimuli can be presented easily to subjects inside the MR scanner. Although simple experiments can use photic flash goggles, reversing checkerboards or even more complicated computer-generated psychophysical stimuli can be shown to subjects using a video projector/mirror setup or fiberoptic system.

The variety and information gained from visual fMRI research studies has been rich with regards to human brain mapping, psychophysics, and physiology. For instance, the retinotopic organization and the borders of early visual areas (V1, V2) in human visual cortex[3] have been demonstrated using retinotopic stimuli. Efforts to image ocular dominance columns in primary visual cortex have been made with high-resolution fMRI at high field MR scanners.[4] Color-sensitive V4/V8 areas[5,6] and motion-sensitive MT/V5 areas[7] have now been well characterized with fMRI. Additionally, the lateral geniculate nucleus of the thalamus has been imaged with high field MR scanners,[8,9] and even 1.5 Tesla scanners.[10] In the visual cortex, young children may have signal decreases during visual stimulation,[11] as opposed to the signal increases observed in adults. Eye movements produce activation in cortical areas such as the frontal eye field, parietal eye field, and supplementary eye fields.[12]

Unfortunately, despite these research advances, fMRI has not yet become a widely used clinical tool in the evaluation and management of patients with visual disorders. Roadblocks consist primarily of technical challenges and patient limitations.

This chapter will first review recent ophthalmologic and neuro-ophthalmologic applications of fMRI,[13,14] then discuss the limitations for the routine use of fMRI in the clinical setting.

## Review of Current Clinical Applications of fMRI in Patients with Visual Disturbances

### Normal Pathways

In patients with normal vision and visual pathways, there is no clinical indication for an fMRI study.

### fMRI in Structural Lesions

#### *Visual Field Defects*

Initially, the relationship between cerebral lesions and visual deficits was explored in pathologic studies of patients with head injury from, for instance, strokes, tumors, or gunshot wounds. Anatomical neuroimaging techniques such as computed tomography (CT) and MRI have become indispensable tools for determining the localization and extent of such lesions[15] in vivo.

More recently, investigators have used MRI techniques to study cortical activation in patients with visual field defects (Table 13.1). In patients with lesions of the visual cortex, fMRI might be able to disclose a patient's visual field defects objectively by correlating cortical activation with the known retinotopic organization map,[3] at least theoretically.

In this regard, most studies have been done in patients with retrochiasmal lesions. In the majority of cases, some correlation between visual field deficits and cortical activation patterns was found.[16–19] Early studies used single-slice acquisition. However, multislice acquisition is more desirable for evaluating left–right asymmetry of activation because cortical structures are rarely symmetric, and therefore the same regions on both hemispheres cannot always be precisely included within one slice. When BOLD fMRI, T2-weighted images, and relative cerebral blood volume (CBV) were compared with each patient's visual fields, the best correlation was found in the BOLD activation map of patients with homonymous hemianopia/quadrantanopia.[16] Sorensen and colleagues suggested that fMRI might be more sensitive than conventional imaging techniques that sometimes failed to show the responsible lesions.[16]

Children with unilateral optic radiation damage showed unilateral or markedly asymmetric activation that was more robust on the unaffected side.[20] Although perimetric correlation was not performed in that study, fMRI was thought to be a promising method for young patients as an objective method for visual assessment because they often cannot cooperate with standard visual field testing.

However, there are several reports suggesting that fMRI might not be a reliable tool in this clinical setting. Firstly, disagreements between

**Table 13.1.** Highlighted fMRI Research in Patients with Visual Disorders

| Paper | Subjects | Results |
|---|---|---|
| Werring et al., 2000[25] | Seven patients with a single episode of unilateral optic neuritis | Stimulation of the affected eye induced extensive extraoccipital activation that was not observed in normal control subjects. |
| Goodyear et al., 2000[41] | Four patients with strabismic/anisometropic amblyopia | A good relationship between fMRI response and psychophysical measurements was found. Stimulation of the amblyopic eye was associated with a decreased number of activated voxels compared with stimulation of the good eye. |
| Barnes et al., 2001[44] | Ten patients with strabismic amblyopia | Functional MRI during visual stimulation with LCD shutter glasses was used. Decreased cortical activation in both V1 and V2 was found when the amblyopic eyes were stimulated regardless of the spatial frequency of the visual stimulus. No close correlation was found between fMRI responses and psychophysical deficits. |
| Goebel et al., 2001[53] | Two patients with hemianopia | Responsiveness of dorsal and ventral stream areas was investigated with fMRI during the stimulation of cortically blind visual fields. The stimulation to the blind fields produced strong responses in ipsilesional extrastriate cortex (but not in the early visual areas) without patients' awareness of the stimuli. |
| Faro et al., 2002[40] | Nine patients with multiple sclerosis and a history of optic neuritis | The patients showed a significantly lower number of activated voxels as compared with healthy controls. When luminance contrast was modulated, different patterns of activation were observed between the controls and the patients. |

visual fields and fMRI have been reported. In patients with abnormalities (stenosis or dissection of arteries) in vascular imaging (MR angiography or conventional catheter angiography), fMRI showed decreased visual cortex activation on the same side regardless of abnormality of visual fields or T2-weighted images.[21] In a patient with moyamoya disease and cerebral atrophy, unilateral activation of visual cortex was found despite preserved perfusion bilaterally demonstrated by SPECT.[22] Visual fields of this patient showed only a slight depression contralateral to the cortical atrophy, and thus did not correlate with the fMRI finding.[22] It is problematic to assume that the BOLD effect has not been altered, as the balance between regional cerebral blood flow (CBF) and metabolism may be changed. Accordingly, fMRI results should not be used for clinical management of visual function in stroke patients in whom hypoperfusion of the area is suspected.

There are other problems, as even the detection of dense homonymous hemianopias with fMRI may not be straightforward. Normal control subjects without any visual field defects may have asymmetric activation of visual cortex mimicking hemianopic activation patterns (ref. 19, Figure 2). In addition, because the fovea is represented in a large area of visual cortex posteriorly, it is inherently difficult to detect hemianopias with macular sparing by fMRI, even when only a few degrees are spared.[17] Functional MRI also does not seem to be very sensitive for detecting peripheral visual field defects/depression, as the reduced activation would only appear within a small cortical area in the anterior visual cortex. Further attempts to improve specificity and sensitivity need to be done before fMRI is used clinically for objective assessment of hemianopias.

Furthermore, does lack of visual cortex activation always imply that the patient cannot see in the portion of the visual field that the defective region subserves? Conversely, does activation necessarily imply that the patient has intact vision in the portion of the visual field that the region subserves? Interpreting extrastriate cortex activation is even more complicated. While patients with visual disturbance generally show reduced activation in primary visual cortex corresponding to visual field defects,[17,23] they may have increased activity of extrastriate cortex[24] or extraoccipital cortex.[25,26] Therefore, it is not clear whether decreased visual input actually results in decreased fMRI activation.

A visual field plot, which was fairly consistent with the actual visual field plot, was constructed from fMRI data after brain flattening and retinotopic mapping.[27] Although this is a good example of the use of fMRI as objective perimetry, it is noteworthy that the plot created from fMRI was only for the central five degrees. It may require enormous effort and time to construct a whole visual field plot from fMRI data. In addition, in our experience, determining V1 regions of interest (ROIs) is difficult in individual patients. In general, patients cannot cooperate for multiple studies if retinotopic mapping is desired. The only practical way may be to hand draw the ROIs based upon the anatomical images (see discussion below). Thus, fMRI is not currently a reliable method for correlating visual field defects with cortical function, particularly in patients with homonymous hemianopias.

### *Lateral Geniculate Activation*

Although the lateral geniculate nucleus (LGN) is a small thalamic structure, fMRI activation of this area has been demonstrated (Figure 13.1). In addition to retinal visual stimulation, visual imagery also can activate the LGN.[28] Although initial studies used relatively high field scanners, LGN activation can be shown using conventional 1.5 T scanners.[10,10A,10B] Using high-resolution fMRI during hemifield, upper-field, and lower-field stimulation, the retinotopic organization of human LGN was found to be similar to that of primate LGN.[29] The hemifield stimulation activated the contralateral LGN, and the lower-field and upper-field stimulation activated the superior and inferior portions of LGN, respectively.

The signal increase in LGN is fairly small (about one percent), and detection of activation in this area is still technically difficult.[8,9] In contrast to the signal decrease observed in the visual cortex, consistent

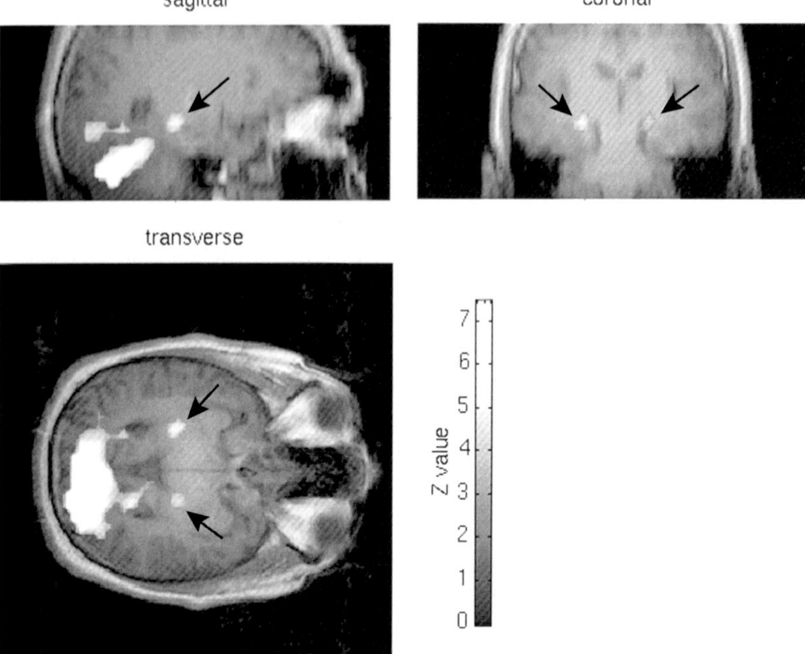


**Figure 13.1.** Functional MRI maps of a normal volunteer at 4 Tesla showing bilateral activation of visual cortex and lateral geniculate nucleus (arrows). The area was activated by a diffuse flashing visual stimulus. Reprinted from *Survey of Ophthalmology*, Vol. 47(6), 562–579, Miki A, Haselgrove JC, Liu GT. Functional MRI and its clinical utility in patients with visual disturbances. Copyright © 2002, with permission from Elsevier. (Neurologic coordinates)

signal increases in the LGN have been observed in children regardless of the subjects' age,[30] perhaps reflecting earlier developmental changes in LGN as compared with visual cortex.

Activation of LGN and visual cortex have been evaluated in patients with retrochiasmal lesions to investigate whether fMRI can be helpful for the localization of the lesions (i.e., pregeniculate or postgeniculate hemianopia).[31,31A]

### *Presurgical Mapping*

Attempts to use fMRI for presurgical mapping to preserve functioning areas have been reported.[32] Such presurgical mapping could be useful when the brain structure is distorted by the disease or the area is buried deep inside the brain for which intraoperative mapping is difficult. However, false-negative activation is a major problem because visual loss may result if the surgery is performed based on the fMRI results.

Patients with dysplastic cortical areas in or near the visual cortex may present with seizures. If the seizures do not respond to medical management, surgery (removal or cortectomy) to these regions may be required. However, preserved function within these dysplastic regions has been been demonstrated in some instances with fMRI (Figure 13.2).[33,34]

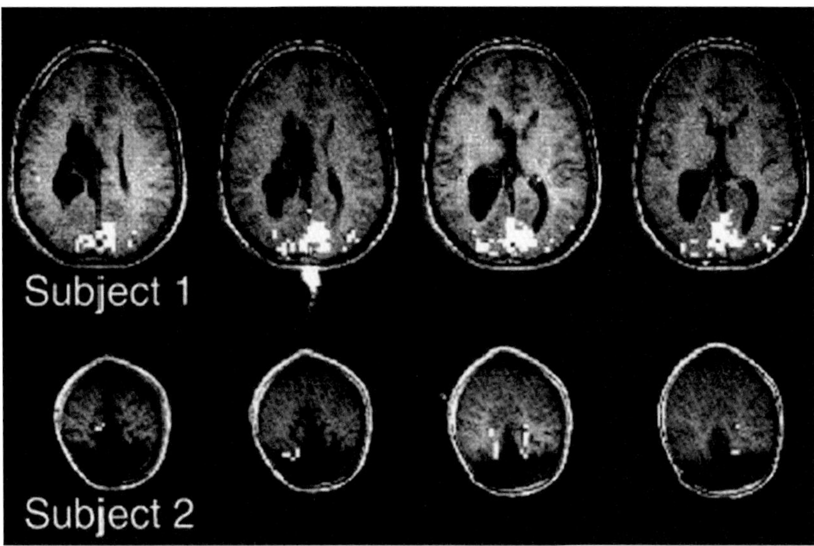


**Figure 13.2.** Demonstration of visually activated areas in visual cortex for both subjects. The data, depicted as white pixels, are superimposed upon each subject's $T_1$-anatomical axial MR images, each parallel to the calcarine sulcus, and four continguous slices containing visual cortex are shown for each subject. The most dorsal image is left, and in each image, the left side of the brain is on the right, and the right side on the left. The white pixels represent the activated areas with a $t$-statistic above a treshold corresponding to a Bonferroni-corrected $p$-value of 0.05. Thus, the corresponding $t$-statistic thresholds are 4.99 for Subject 1 and –4.82 for Subject 2. From Liu GT, Hunter J, Miki A, et al. Functional MRI in children with congenital structural abnormalities of occipital cortex. *Neuropediatrics* 2000;31:13–15. Reprinted by permission.

### *Optic Neuritis*

Cortical activation in patients with optic neuritis (associated with demyelination and multiple sclerosis) has been studied with fMRI. In most studies, unilateral optic neuritis has been studied,[25,35–37] but patients with bilateral optic neuritis also have been examined.[38] The stimulation of affected eyes produced reduced volume of visual cortex activation[35] compared to stimulation of the unaffected eye. Additionally, stimulation of the clinically unaffected eyes showed decreased volume of activation compared with controls. The finding supports the notion that fMRI may be sensitive for early detection of demyelination in the contralateral clinically unaffected eye. A portion of patients with unilateral optic neuritis represent a form fruste of multiple sclerosis. In the future, if fMRI can accurately and reliable diagnosis demyelination within in the optic pathway, then a patient at risk for multiple sclerosis would benefit from early treatment. In patients with unilateral optic neuritis, the interocular difference in visual evoked potential latency correlated with the interocular difference in fMRI activation.[36]

In another fMRI report, patients with recovered unilateral optic neuritis[25] were studied. Extraoccipital activation was found when recovered eyes were stimulated and the volume of extraoccipital activation correlated with VEP latency. The authors suggested that this extraoccipital activation may underly part of the mechanism of visual recovery in optic neuritis. Another study in patients with unilateral optic neuritis showed no significant relationship between fMRI variables and visual acuity.[39] Correlations between VEP variables (P 100 latency and amplitude) and fMRI variables also were found to be significant, although VEP was more sensitive than fMRI in the discrimination of affected and unaffected eyes.[39]

One study examined the number of activated voxels in patients with a history of optic neuritis and healthy volunteers when luminance contrasts of the visual stimulus were varied[40] whereas another study tested various checkerboard reversal frequencies.[39] Modulation of the luminance contrast or checkerboard reversal rate may be useful in showing different patterns of activation between patients and normal subjects (Figure 13.3). In patients with previous optic neuritis (some patients showed decreased visual acuity), the activated volume associated with stimulation of each eye of the patients correlated with the contrast sensitivity, and the BOLD signal increase correlated with the contrast sen-

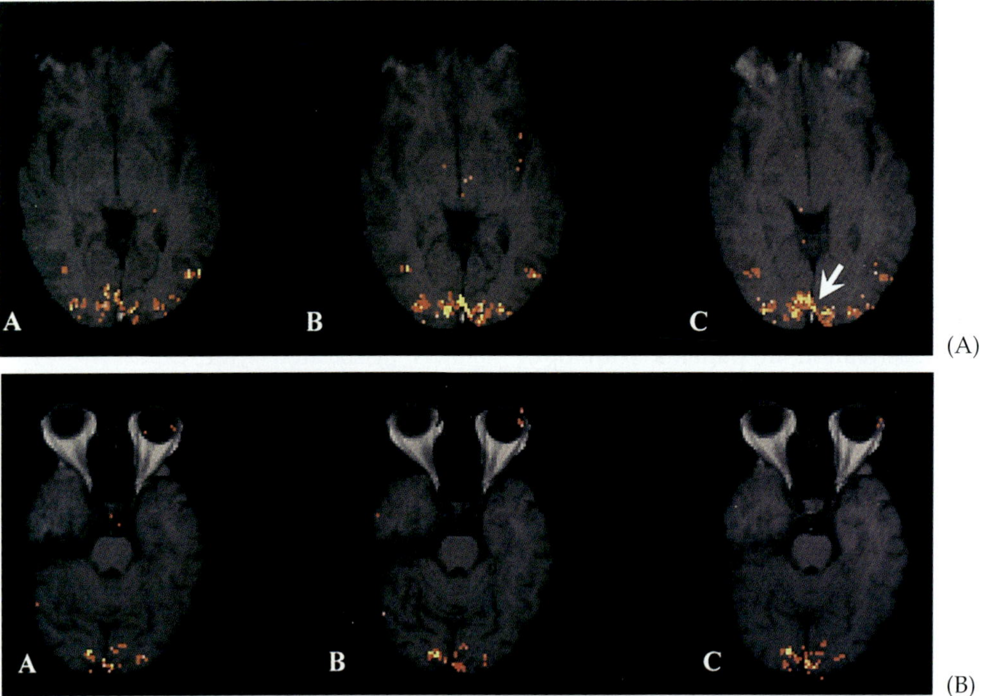


**Figure 13.3.** (A) Composite, axial T1-weighted image and fMRI imaging activation map at the level of the primary visual cortex in a healthy volunteer at three luminance contrast levels: (*A*) lowest (baseline), (*B*) intermediate, (*C*) highest. Activation in the ROI, which represents the primary visual cortex within the medial portion of the occipital lobes (*arrow*, *C*), is shown in red and yellow, with yellow corresponding to the relatively more significantly activated voxels. (B) Composite, axial T1-weighted image and fMRI imaging activation map at the level of the primary visual cortex in a patient with MS at three luminance contrast levels: (*A*) lowest (baseline), (*B*) intermediate, (*C*) highest. Activation in the primary visual cortex is shown in red and yellow. There is low-level fMRI imaging activation in *A*, no significant change in activation in *B*, and prominent activation in *C*. Reprinted with permission from Faro SH, Mohamed FB, Tracy JI, et al. Quantitative functional MR imaging of the visual cortex at 1.5T as a function of luminance contrast in healthy volunteers and patients with multiple sclerosis. *AJNR Am J Neuroradiol*. 2002;23:59–65.

sitivity and the visual acuity.[38] The former correlation did not seem to be strong because of the large variation within the group, and the visual acuity did not correlate with the activated volume. As activation volume may differ considerably between right and left eye stimulation even in control subjects,[35] it may not be a sensitive measure of visual function.

Thus, fMRI has offered some insights into the cortex's possible role in visual loss and recovery associated with optic neuritis. However, the current role of fMRI is uncertain at this time in relation to the other clinical methods, such as the routine clinical examination, visual fields, or visual evoked potentials in the diagnosis or management of optic neuritis.

### *Amblyopia*

Amblyopia is a condition in which unilateral loss of vision occurs in an early critical period in childhood without an obvious funduscopic abnormality. Causes include strabismus (ocular misalignment), anisometropia (asymmetric refractive errors), or deprivation (from congenital cataract or corneal opacities, for instance). Animal studies have suggested that a lack of competition for connections in striate cortex is responsible, but this mechanism has not been proven in humans. Currently, the evaluation of patients with amblyopia consists of the routine ophthalmological examination, including measurement of visual acuity and refractive error, and a dilated funduscopic examination. However, clinicians have been seeking an objective tool for following amblyopia. Visual evoked potentials, in part because they are insensitive to changes in visual acuity, are not widely used in amblyopia. Anatomical neuroimaging is normal in patients with amblyopia.

Previous functional imaging studies with PET or SPECT revealed that reduced regional CBF and glucose metabolism in visual cortex for stimulation of the amblyopic eyes compared with the contralateral eye. Patients with unilateral strabismic/anisometropic amblyopia have been studied with fMRI by alternately stimulating the eyes within one testing session or each eye separately in different sessions.[41–46] Patients with severe unilateral amblyopia were chosen in these studies probably because the sensitivity to detect amblyopic change by fMRI had been unknown. The number of activated voxels and percentage signal change within regions of interest are reduced during stimulation of the amblyopic eyes than during stimulation of the contralateral eye, in primary visual cortex,[41,42,44,46] (Figure 13.4), as well as in higher visual areas.[44]

Not only stimuli visible to the amblyopic eyes, but also stimuli invisible to those eyes were used to examine primary visual cortex activation in amblyopia.[44] In some patients, extrastriate activation was observed when the amblyopic eyes were stimulated with the invisible stimulus in the affected eyes.

In one study, primary visual cortex activation was found to correlate with psychophysical measurements of contrast perception,[41] but another study found no close relationship between fMRI response and psychophysical deficits such as contrast sensitivity.[44] The lack of correlation in the latter case may be explained by the contrast level used.[44]

| A | B | C | D |
|---|---|---|---|
| S2, n=112, m.t. = +0.22 | S1, n=112, m.t. = +0.92 | S1, n=175, m.t. = +2.47 | S1, n=124, m.t. = +0.213 |
| 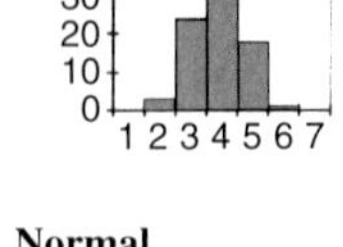 | 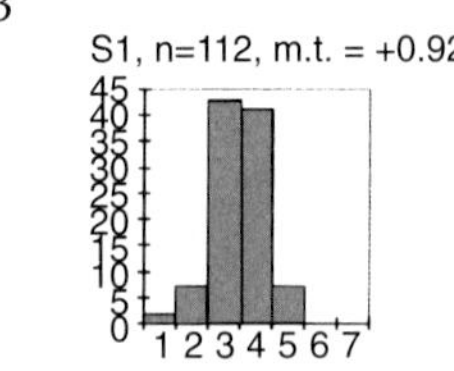 | 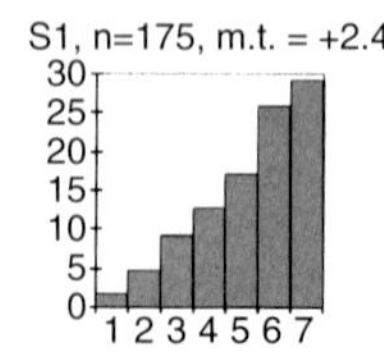 | 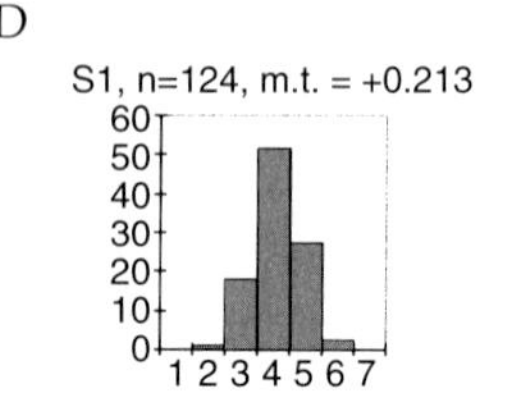 |
| **Normal** | **Anisometropic amblyopia OD** | **Anisometropic amblyopia OS** | **Accommodative esotropia and monocular suppression OS** |
| Normal individual 20/20 OU. | 11 year old boy. Visual acuities: 20/70+ OD, 20/15 OS. No afferent pupillary defect. Cycloplegic refraction: +3.50+1.50×0.93 OD, +0.50 OS. | 13 year old girl. Visual acuities: 20/20+ OD, 20/800 OS. No afferent pupillary defect. Cycloplegic refraction: +0.50+0.50×086 OD, +4.75+4.75×095 OS. | 33 year old man. Poor stereopsis. Visual acuities: 20/20-2 OD, 20/25+ OS. No afferent pupillary defect. Cycloplegic refraction: +3.00+0.25×115 OD, +2.25+0.25×107 OS. |

**Figure 13.4.** Eye dominance distributions in visual cortex using fMRI at 1.5T in amblyopia. A 1.5T Siemens MR scanner was used to obtain T2*-weighted EP images (voxel size 3.75 × 3.75 × 5 cubic millimeters) of V1. Epochs consisted of RE, LE, and BE stimulation with a 1 c/d checkerboard (8Hz), and rest periods. Monocular stimulation was achieved by using a red filter RE and a green filter LE and alternating identical filters over the video projector lens. A 0.9log neutral density filter LE was used to make the stimuli to each eye equiluminant. The eye dominance of each voxel within the individual's V1 was determined using their Student *t*-statistics during the LE versus RE contrast. Their eye dominance distribution was plotted, and the mean *t*-statistic was used to describe the histogram asymmetry (S = subject number, *n* = number of voxels analyzed, m.t. = mean *t*-statistic, *y*-axis: percentage of *n*, *x*-axis: eye dominance number (1 = left eye dominant, 7 = right eye dominant)). (A) Normal subject, with relatively symmetric distribution. (B, C) Anisometropic amblyopia. (D) Accommodative esotropia. In the two patients with anisometropic amblyopia (B,C), the eye dominance histogram is shifted towards the good eye, and the shift is more pronounced in the patient with the worse acuity. In the patient with accommodative esotropia, monocular suppression OS and relatively normal visual acuities (D) had no relative shift in the histogram. Thus, from these data, it seems that in amblyopia the ocular dominance histogram shifts towards the good eye, and the amount of shift is acuity dependent. (A) *Source*: *Journal of AAPOS*, Vol. 6(1), 40–8, Liu GT, Miki A, Goldsmith Z, et al. Eye dominance in visual cortex using functional MRI at 1.5T. An alternative method. Copyright © 2002 American Association for Pediatric Ophthalmology and Strabismus. (B–D) *Source*: *Journal of AAPOS*, Vol. 8(2), 184–186, Liu GT, Miki A, Francis E, et al. Eye dominance in visual cortex in amblyopia using functional MRI (fMRI). Copyright © 2004 American Association for Pediatric Opthalmology and Strabismus.

A lower proportion of the voxels in the primary visual cortex activated by both eyes during monocular stimulation in strabismic amblyopia than in anisometropic amblyopia was attributed to the loss of binocular interaction.[45] On the other hand, anisometropic amblyopes had reduced primary visual cortex activation for the stimulation with higher spatial frequencies as compared with strabismic amblyopes,[45,46] and this finding seems to be in agreement with previous animal studies. Functional MRI may be useful in differentiating between these two types of amblyopia.

Functional MRI at a spatial resolution of the cortical columns revealed that patients with amblyopia developed during infancy showed a reduced number of pixels within the visual cortex activated by stimulation of the affected eyes.[47] In contrast, patients with late-onset amblyopia (developed after two years of age) showed lack of the shift in ocular dominance in the unaffected eye. The finding suggests that the effect of early onset and late-onset amblyopia on ocular dominance columns may be different.

Thus, fMRI has been helpful in studying cortical mechanisms in amblyopia. However, fMRI has not become part of the routine evaluation of patients with amblyopia. The reasons are as follows. Firstly, the fMRI studies mentioned above were performed mostly in amblyopic adolescents and adults who could cooperate with the testing. Amblyopia develops during a critical period within the first few years of life. Treatments such as patching or atropine blur need to be administered during this period as well. In order for fMRI to make a difference in their management, fMRI would need to be performed while they are young. However, these children cannot cooperate for an fMRI study without sedation. Most doctors and parents would be unwilling to have their child undergo a sedated MRI study with amblyopia as their only diagnosis. Furthermore, their eyes would be closed during such tests, making only flash stimuli practical, and precluding the use of checkerboards or contrast gratings.

### *Chiasmal Anomalies*

Chiasmal miswiring syndromes are very rare. Functional MRI is particularly suitable for demonstrating visual pathway miswiring, such as in chiasmal anomalies. In albinos, for instance, a large majority of fibers from temporal retina crosses at the optic chiasm. In normal subjects, only slightly more then half the fibers cross. This can be shown as predominant contralateral visual cortex activation and a small area of anterior visual cortex activation on the ipsilateral hemisphere to the stimulated eye during monocular full-field flash stimulation[48] or visual cortex activation contralateral to the stimulated eye regardless of the stimulated side during monocular hemifield stimulation with a central checkerboard stimulus.[49] In a comparative study with VEP, fMRI appears to show the misrouting in albinism more clearly than VEP.[50] On the other hand, non-decussating retinal–fugal fiber syndrome is a congenital malformation of the optic chiasm, and the patient's optic nerves are projected solely to the ipsilateral optic tracts. Monocular checkerboard stimulation results in activation of ipsilateral primary visual cortex.[51]

### *Residual Vision after Brain Damage (Blindsight)*

Patients with brain damage in visual areas sometimes exhibit a rare unconscious visual ability, termed blindsight. Several studies have investigated neural correlates of such residual vision by stimulating the blind portion of patients' visual fields. Whether such residual vision depends on preserved V1 is a matter of debate, and several fMRI studies have focused on this subject. Cortical activation was found even when patients did not consciously perceive the stimuli. Among patients with a complete homonymous hemianopia stimulated within their hemianopic fields, activation of ipsilateral extrastriate cortex was found only in a patient with blindsight.[52] A rotating spiral stimulus and colored images of natural objects (fruit and vegetables) placed in the supposed blind field of a patient with blindsight activated ipsilesional extrastriate cortex without evoking the patient's awareness of the stimuli.[53] Patients with relative blindness (i.e., with some conscious vision) also were studied.[54] The literature seems to suggest that the presence of V1 is not necessary for unconscious vision.

#### *Subjective and Positive Visual Symptoms*

Patients with subjective photophobic symptoms in one eye after laser in situ keratomikeusis (LASIK) theoretically due to flap abnormalities were tested with fMRI during monocular visual stimulation.[55] Comparison between the affected eyes and the contralateral (control) eye revealed activation of visual cortex (both striate and extrastriate cortex) and extra-occipital areas in some cases. Particularly, stimulation of the affected eyes showed activation of the ventral visual system, which is associated with object vision. Therefore, it is possible that the identification of the visual stimulus with photophobic symptoms led to the amplified activation of such areas, but this is conjecture.

Patients with migraine may have visual aura, thought to reflect cortical spreading depression. During the visual aura in patients studied with fMRI, a suppression of stimulus-induced visual cortex activation by a flickering checkerboard progressed over the visual cortex on the contralateral hemisphere to the aura in a manner consistent with cortical retinotopic organization.[56] That is, the perturbation of BOLD signal moved from the posterior occipital cortex to more anterior areas during the progression of the aura from central to peripheral visual fields. The mean BOLD signal increased at the beginning, followed by decrease later in the aura, perhaps reflected vasodilatation then vasoconstriction. The source of the aura-related BOLD changes was identified in extrastriate cortex, V3A.

Spontaneous visual hallucinations may be observed in patients with ophthalmologic diseases such as optic neuritis, glaucoma, and macular degeneration (Charles Bonnet syndrome). During the hallucinations, signal intensity increases were seen in the ventral occipital lobe.[57] In addition, a visual stimulus, which evoked activation of the ventral occipital lobe in control subjects, did not produce activation of that area in the patients, suggesting a tonic increase in activity of the ventral visual system.

#### *Reorganization after Brain Damage or Congenital Abnormality*

Reorganization of the brain, such as receptive field size change, has been shown in animal models. Functional MRI may be a useful tool to investigate reorganization of the cerebral cortex. In a patient with primary visual cortex damage, different (abnormal) retinotopic organization of the remaining visual cortex was found when the stimulation was limited to the blind portion of the visual field.[58] Rod monochromats, who lack functioning cone photoreceptors, responded to stimulation thought preferentially to activate rods within the cortical areas normally corresponding to the rod-free foveola.[49,59] The absence of visual input from cones may have reorganized the retinotopic topography of the visual cortex. The effect of the occipital stroke on visual cortex activation was investigated with hemifield stimulation.[24] Activation of ipsilateral extrastriate cortex activation to the hemifield stimulation was stronger in patients with incomplete homonymous hemianopia compared with normal controls,[24] suggesting an association between the altered activation and clinical recovery after stroke.

*Clinical Examples of Field Deficit and Occipital Lobe Lesions*

The presence or absence of visual field deficits in association with an occipital lobe lesion is an important clinical question. Additionally, the association of fMRI visual field activation and the patients visual field may be clinically significant. Figure 13.5 shows a patient with a normal visual field and a right occipital lobe arterial venous malformation (AVM) with bilateral and symmetric medial occipital lobe primary visual field activation. The close association and intact nature of the right primary visual cortex and the right occipital lobe lesion would lead the intervention away from a surgical approach more towards an endovascular therapy. A second example is a patient with a right

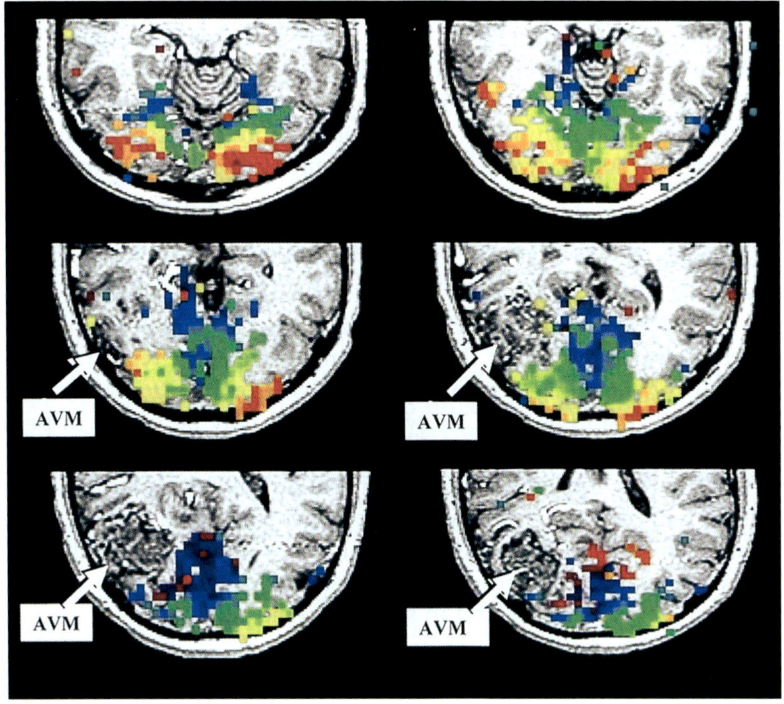


**Figure 13.5.** A 41-year-old with an right occipital AVM and no visual field deficits. The AVM nidus is closest to visual cortex responding to peripheral visual field stimulation (Courtesy of Edgar A. DeYoe, PhD, and John L. Ulmer, MD).

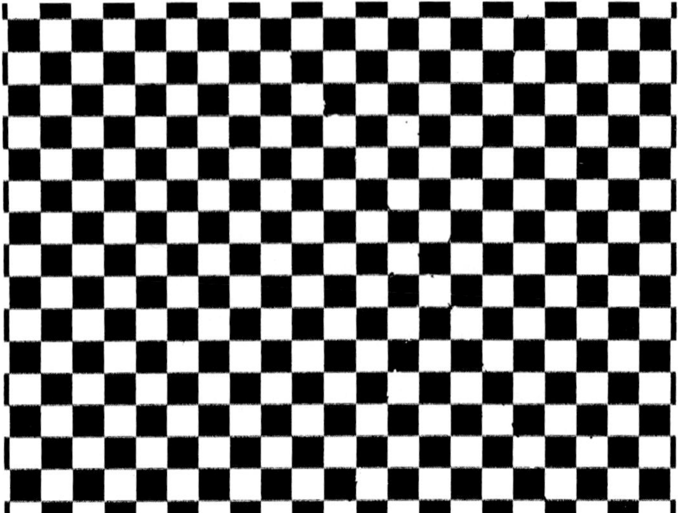

**Figure 13.7.** Checkerboard visual stimulus. Each check subtends a visual angle of 0.5 degrees (one cycle per degree), and in the current setup, the entire checkerboard subtends 10.6 × 8.0 degrees.

Ten scans of visual stimulation of both eyes (epochs 1, 3, 5, 7, 9, and 11) are alternated with 10 scans of darkness (epochs 2, 4, 6, 8, 10, and 12). Relatively brief periods of visual stimulation are considered to be better for accurate localization of activated areas because the vascular response may be saturated by a prolonged visual stimulus.[67]

For monocular visual stimulation, liquid-crystal shutter glasses,[68] special visual stimulation devices,[69] or red/green filters[70] may used.

## Data Analysis

Data analysis is performed on UNIX workstations with IDL (Interactive Data Language) and SPM (Wellcome Department of Cognitive Neurology, London, UK) packages. The first five scans of echo planar imaging (EPI) images are discarded before the postprocessing of the data to eliminate magnetic saturation effects. Functional images of each subject are corrected for the delay associated with slice acquisition timing and then realigned to the first volume. The images are transformed into the anatomical space of Talairach and Tournoux with the voxel size of $2 \times 2 \times 2$ cubic millimeters. Data is smoothed with a Gaussian filter (full width at half maximum = $4 \times 4 \times 4$ millimeters). A boxcar convolved with the hemodynamic response function is used as a reference wave form. $T$ statistics are calculated for each voxel for the contrast of the condition with the stimulation versus the fixation-only condition. The statistical $t$-maps are overlaid on the SPM T-1 template to identify activation of visual cortex. The statistical threshold is set at $P < 0.001$ (uncorrected).

### Comment: Region of Interest (ROI) Determination and Retinotopic Mapping in Clinical Settings

How the ROI is chosen is particularly important; for instance, for calculating percent signal changes within a given cortical area. Inappropriate selection of the ROI invalidates the data. There are several ways in defining ROIs: suprathreshold areas of activation, anatomically defined areas on structural images, or functionally defined areas. In vision-related experiments, retinotopic mapping is ideal (for instance, without retinotopic mapping, it is not straightforward to differentiate between V1 and surrounding V2/V3) for defining an ROI of early visual areas. However, it cannot be readily carried out in most institutes, and the procedures for data analysis are complicated. In addition, retinotopic mapping requires an additional testing session with visual stimulation of rotating rings and expanding rings. Patients find it difficult to tolerate multiple testing sessions. Oftentimes it is hard to define an exact border due to noisy results, especially when the patient cannot fixate centrally.

A more practical approach uses a predetermined anatomically defined ROI, such as the one for V1 along the calcarine fissure using the standard SPM T-1 template.[70]

## fMRI Technical Challenges Involved in the Applications Pertaining to the Authors' Expertise

### Subject Cooperation

Not all patients are able to cooperate for an fMRI study, either because they cannot stay still or alert in the magnet, or they may be claustrophobic. It is often very difficult for patients with neurologic problems due to strokes, brain tumors, and degenerative diseases to remain awake and motionless despite the testers' best efforts. Sedating patients precludes the ability to perform many of the visual studies. Furthermore, many of the visual paradigms require maintenance of central fixation, and in uncooperative patients or those with severe visual deficits, fixation instability is likely to be a problem.

### Potential Confounding Factors

In most fMRI studies, control subjects have either volunteered or are paid to participate in the experiment. On the other hand, clinical subjects may not be as motivated and may not be as attentive to the visual task. Lack of attention may be problematic in visual fMRI studies, as it has been demonstrated that increased visual attention may increase activation in visual cortex.[71]

In addition, control subjects tend to be younger than patients who may be evaluated for visual loss, particularly those with strokes. For instance, the patients were older than the control subjects in all the previous studies on optic neuritis except one, in which the subjects' ages were not described. It has been shown that age influences fMRI activation (the activation decreases with aging),[72] so the interpretation of the data should be done with care if the patients are significantly older or younger than the controls.

Refractive correction should be performed in each subject when necessary. Defocus may have an effect on cortical activation.[70]

## Reproducibility

The reproducibility of visual activation has been studied by repeating measurements of the same subjects on different occasions.[73–76] The results have been variable, that is, some studies reported favorable reproducibility, but others did not, in part because of the difference in the acquisition and analysis used. In one study,[75] good reproducibility was found in some subjects, but in others, test results from different sessions varied widely (Figure 13.8). Poor reproducibility hinders interpretation of the results of single and longitudinal studies.

## Altered BOLD Response

Blood oxygenation level-dependent effects may be different from subject to subject. This could be a problem because BOLD fMRI assumes that the regional CBF is normally regulated. Patients with perfusion deficits may have decreased BOLD signal change, even if the corresponding brain function is normal.[21,22,77] This makes it difficult to evaluate visual function from fMRI findings in patients with brain damage due to stroke, for instance, within and around visual areas.

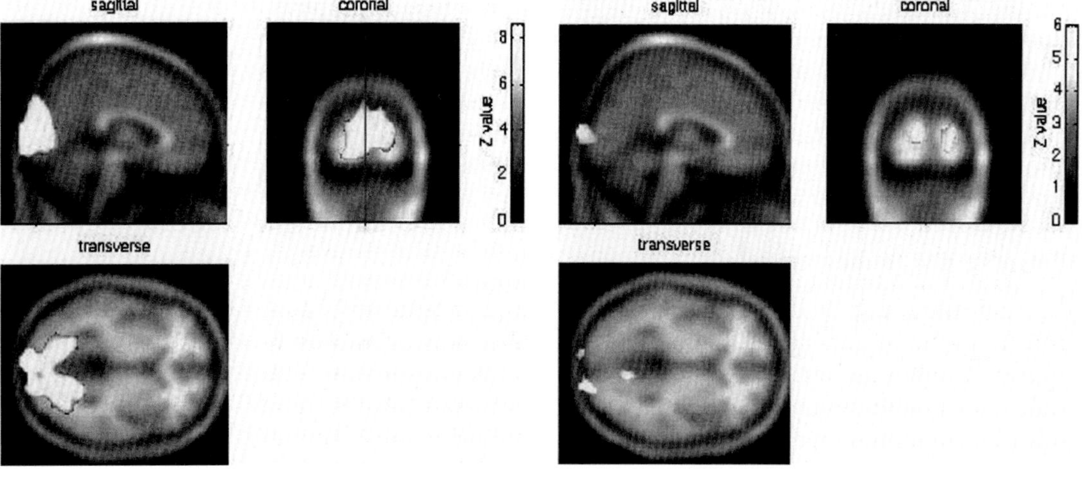


**Figure 13.8.** Reproducibility of visual cortex activation by flash stimulation in a normal volunteer. This subject was tested twice with an interval of few days and with the identical condition, however, the subject had fewer activated voxels on the second experiment. Reprinted from *Survey of Ophthalmology*, Vol. 47(6), 562–579, Miki A, Haselgrove JC, Liu GT. Functional MRI and its clinical utility in patients with visual disturbances. Copyright © 2002, with permission from Elsevier. (Neurologic coordinates)

### Group Analyses

Although group data generally allow for more powerful inferences than individual data, special care should be taken if the visual function of patients differs within the group; for example, when patients with optic neuritis are studied, their visual field defects are typically variable. Therefore, the group activation may be underestimated because the common activated areas may be small. More homogeneous group data would show greater activation.

## Future Applications

Advances in fMRI technique will improve test–retest reliability and sensitivity. Potential future applications include studying functional reorganization and longitudinal follow-up of patients with damage to visual pathway structures. Stimulus parameters (such as check size[78]) and analysis methods may be manipulated to enhance the quality of fMRI in this setting. In younger patients with amblyopia and anisometropia fMRI may contribute to earlier diagnosis and characterization of improving acuity helping in treatment planning. In the future in patients with unilateral optic neuritis if fMRI can reliably demonstrate decreased activation of the contralateral eye. This may lead to early diagnosis and treatment for multiple sclerosis.

## References


1. Kwong KK, Belliveau JW, Chesler DA, et al. Dynamic magnetic resonance imaging of human brain activity during primary sensory stimulation. *Proc Natl Acad Sci U S A.* 1992;89:5675–5679.
2. Ogawa S, Tank DW, Menon R, et al. Intrinsic signal changes accompanying sensory stimulation: functional brain mapping with magnetic resonance imaging. *Proc Natl Acad Sci U S A.* 1992;89:5951–5955.
3. Sereno MI, Dale AM, Reppas JB, et al. Borders of multiple visual areas in humans revealed by functional magnetic resonance imaging. *Science.* 1995;268:889–893.
4. Menon RS, Ogawa S, Strupp JP, et al. Ocular dominance in human V1 demonstrated by functional magnetic resonance imaging. *J Neurophysiol.* 1997;77:2780–2787.
5. McKeefry DJ, Zeki S. The position and topography of the human colour centre as revealed by functional magnetic resonance imaging. *Brain.* 1997;120:2229–2242.
6. Hadjikhani N, Liu AK, Dale AM, et al. Retinotopy and color sensitivity in human visual cortical area V8. *Nature Neurosci.* 1998;1:235–240.
7. Tootell RBH, Reppas JB, Kwong KK, et al. Functional analysis of human MT and related visual cortical areas using magnetic resonance imaging. *J Neurosci.* 1995;15:3215–3230.
8. Buchel C, Turner R, Friston K. Lateral geniculate activations can be detected using intersubject averaging and fMRI. *Magn Reson Med.* 1997;38:691–694.
9. Chen W, Kato T, Zhu X-H, et al. Mapping of LGN activation during visual stimulation in human brain using fMRI. *Magn Reson Med.* 1998;39:89–96.

10. Miki A, Raz J, Haselgrove JC, et al. Functional magnetic resonance imaging of lateral geniculate nucleus at 1.5 Tesla. *J Neuroophthalmol.* 2000;20:285–287.
10A. Miki A, Liu C-SJ, Liu GT. Effects of voxel size on detection of lateral geniculate nucleus activation in functional magnetic resonance imaging. *Jpn J Ophthalmol.* 2004;48:558–564.
10B. Miki A, Liu GT, Goldsmith ZG, et al. Decreased activation of the lateral geniculate nucleus in a patient with anisometropic amblyopia demonstrated by functional magnetic resonance imaging. *Ophthalmologica* 2003; 217:365–369.
11. Born P, Leth H, Miranda MJ, et al. Visual activation in infants and young children studied by functional magnetic resonance imaging. *Pediatr Res.* 1998;44:578–583.
12. Berman RA, Colby CL, Genovese CR, et al. Cortical networks subserving pursuit and saccadic eye movements in humans: an FMRI study. *Hum Brain Mapp.* 1999;8:209–225.
13. Miki A, Liu GT, Modestino EJ, et al. Functional magnetic resonance imaging of the visual system. *Curr Opin Ophthalmol.* 2001;12:423–431.
14. Miki A, Haselgrove JC, Liu GT. Functional MRI and its clinical utility in patients with visual disturbances. *Surv Ophthalmol.* 2002;47:562–579.
15. Horton JC, Hoyt WF. The representation of the visual field in human striate cortex. *Arch Ophthalmol.* 1991;109:816–824.
16. Sorensen AG, Wray SH, Weisskoff RM, et al. Functional MR of brain activity and perfusion in patients with chronic cortical stroke. *AJNR Am J Neuroradiol.* 1995;16:1753–1762.
17. Miki A, Nakajima T, Fujita M, et al. Functional magnetic resonance imaging in homonymous hemianopsia. *Am J Ophthalmol.* 1996;121: 258–266.
18. Kollias SS, Landau K, Khan N, et al. Functional evaluation using magnetic resonance imaging of the visual cortex in patients with retrochiasmatic lesions. *J Neurosurg.* 1998;89:780–790.
19. Roux F-E, Ibarrola D, Lotterie J-A, et al. Perimetric visual field and functional MRI correlation: implications for image-guided surgery in occipital brain tumors. *J Neurol Neurosurg Psychiatry.* 2001;71:505–514.
20. Born AP, Miranda MJ, Rostrup E, et al. Functional magnetic resonance imaging of the normal and abnormal visual system in early life. *Neuropediatrics.* 2000;31:24–32.
21. Lee Y-J, Chung T-S, Yoon YS, et al. The role of functional MR imaging in patients with ischemia in the visual cortex. *AJNR Am J Neuroradiol.* 2001;22:1043–1049.
22. Miki A, Nakajima T, Takagi M, et al. Functional magnetic resonance imaging of visual cortex in a patient with cerebrovascular insufficiency. *Neuroophthalmol.* 2000;23:83–88.
23. Miki A, Nakajima T, Takagi M, et al. Detection of visual dysfunction in optic atrophy by functional magnetic resonance imaging during monocular visual stimulation. *Am J Ophthalmol.* 1996;122:404–415.
24. Nelles G, Widman G, de Greiff A et al. Brain representation of hemifield stimulation in poststroke visual field defects. *Stroke.* 2002;33:1286–1293.
25. Werring DJ, Bullmore ET, Toosy AT, et al. Recovery from optic neuritis is associated with a change in the distribution of cerebral response to visual stimulation: a functional magnetic resonance imaging study. *J Neurol Neurosurg Psychiatry.* 2000;68:441–9.
26. Rausch M, Widdig W, Eysel UT, et al. Enhanced responsiveness of human extravisual areas to photic stimulation in patients with severely reduced vision. *Exp Brain Res.* 2000;135:34–40.

27. Morland AB, Baseler HA, Hoffmann MB, et al. Abnormal retinotopic representations in human visual cortex revealed by fMRI. *Acta Psychologica.* 2001;107:229–247.
28. Chen W, Kato T, Zhu X-H, et al. Human primary visual cortex and lateral geniculate nucleus activation during visual imagery. *Neuroreport.* 1998;9: 3669–3674.
29. Chen W, Zhu X-H, Thulborn KR, et al. Retinotopic mapping of lateral geniculate nuclues in humans using functional magnetic resonance imaging. *Proc Natl Acad Sci U S A.* 1999;96:2430–2434.
30. Morita T, Kochiyama T, Yamada H, et al. Difference in the metabolic response to photic stimulation of the lateral geniculate nucleus and the primary visual cortex of infants: a fMRI study. *Neurosci Res.* 2000;38: 63–70.
31. Miki A, Liu GT, Modestino EJ, et al. Functional magnetic resonance imaging of lateral geniculate nucleus and visual cortex at 4 Tesla in a patient with homonymous hemianopia. *Neuroophthalmol.* 2001;25: 109–114.

31A. Miki A, Liu GT, Modestino EJ, et al. Decreased lateral geniculate nucleus activation in retrogeniculate hemianopia demonstrated by functional magnetic resonance imaging at 4 Tesla. *Ophthalmologica.* 2005;219: 11–15.

32. Hirsch J, Ruge MI, Kim KHS, et al. An integrated functional magnetic resonance imaging procedures for preoperative mapping of cortical areas associated with tactile, motor, language, and visual functions. *Neurosurgery.* 2000;47:711–722.
33. Liu GT, Hunter J, Miki A, et al. Functional MRI in children with congenital structural abnormalities of occipital cortex. *Neuropediatrics.* 2000;31: 13–15.
34. Innocenti GM, Maeder P, Knyazeva MG, et al. Functional activation of microgyric visual cortex in a human. *Ann Neurol.* 2001;50:672–676.
35. Rombouts SARB, Lazeron RHC, Scheltens P, et al. Visual activation patterns in patients with optic neuritis: an fMRI pilot study. *Neurology.* 1998;50:1896–1899.
36. Gareau PJ, Gati JS, Menon RS, et al. Reduced visual evoked responses in multiple sclerosis patients with optic neuritis: comparison of functional magnetic resonance imaging and visual evoked potentials. *Mult Scler.* 1999;5:161–164.
37. Toosy AT, Werring DJ, Bullmore ET, et al. Functional magnetic resonance imaging of the cortical response to photic stimulation in humans following optic neuritis recovery. *Neurosci Lett.* 2002;330:255–259.
38. Langkilde AR, Frederiksen JL, Rostrup E, et al. Functional MRI of the visual cortex and visual testing in patients with previous optic neuritis. *Eur J Neurol.* 2002;9:277–286.
39. Russ MO, Cleff U, Laufermann H, et al. Functional magnetic resonance imaging (fMRI) in acute unilateral optic neuritis. *J Neuroimaging.* 2002; 12:339–350.
40. Faro SH, Mohamed FB, Tracy JI, et al. Quantitative functional MR imaging of the visual cortex at 1.5T as a function of luminance contrast in healthy volunteers and patients with multiple sclerosis. *AJNR Am J Neuroradiol.* 2002;23:59–65.
41. Goodyear BG, Nicole DA, Humphrey GK, et al. BOLD fMRI response of early visual areas to perceived contrast in human amblyopia. *J Neurophysiol.* 2000;84:1907–1913.
42. Liu GT, Miki A, Francis E, et al. Eye dominance in visual cortex in amblyopia using functional MRI (fMRI). *J AAPOS* 2004;8:184–186.

43. Bonhomme GR, Liu GT, Miki A, et al. Decreased cortical activation in response to a motion stimulus in anisometropic amblyopic eyes. *Invest Ophthalmol Vis Sci.* 2000;41:S703.
44. Barnes GR, Hess RF, Dumoulin SO, et al. The cortical deficit in humans with strabismic amblyopia. *J Physiol.* 2001;533:281–297.
45. Lee K-M, Lee S-H, Kim N-Y, et al. Binocularity and spatial frequency dependence of calcarine activation in two types of amblyopia. *Neurosci Res.* 2001;40:147–153.
46. Choi MY, Lee K-M, Hwang J-M, et al. Comparison between anisometropic and strabismic amblyopia using functional magnetic resonance imaging. *Br J Ophthalmol.* 2001;85:1052–1056.
47. Goodyear BG, Nicolle DA, Menon RS. High resolution fMRI of ocular dominance columns within the visual cortex of human amblyopes. *Strabismus.* 2002;10:129–136.
48. Hedera P, Lai S, Haacke EM, et al. Abnormal connectivity of the visual pathways in human albinos demonstrated by susceptibility-sensitized MRI. *Neurology.* 1994;44:1921–1926.
49. Morland AB, Baseler HA, Hoffmann MB, et al. Abnormal retinotopic representations in human visual cortex revealed by fMRI. *Acta Psychologica.* 2001;107:229–247.
50. Morland AB, Hoffmann MB, Neveu M, et al. Abnormal visual projection in a human albino studied with functional magnetic resonance imaging and visual evoked potentials. *J Neurol Neurosurg Psychiatry.* 2002;72: 523–526.
51. Victor JD, Apkarian P, Hirsch J, et al. Visual function and brain organization in non-decussating retinal-fugal fibre syndrome. *Cereb Cortex.* 2000;10:2–22.
52. Bittar RG, Ptito M, Faubert J, et al. Activation of remaining hemisphere following stimulation of the blind hemifield in hemispherectomized subjects. *Neuroimage.* 1999;10:339–346.
53. Goebel R, Muckli L, Zanella FE, et al. Sustained extrastriate cortical activation without visual awareness revealed by fMRI studies of hemianopic patients. *Vision Res.* 2001;41:1459–1474.
54. Kleiser R, Wittsack J, Niedeggen M, et al. Is V1 necessary for conscious vision in areas of relative cortical blindness? *Neuroimage.* 2001;13:654–661.
55. Malecaze FJ, Boulanouar KA, Demonet JF, et al. Abnormal activation in the visual cortex after corneal refractive surgery for myopia. Demonstration by functional magnetic resonance imaging. *Ophthalmology.* 2001;108: 2213–2218.
56. Hadjikhani N, Sanchez del Rio M, Wu O, et al. Mechanisms of migraine aura revealed by functional MRI in human visual cortex. *Proc Natl Acad Sci U S A.* 2001;98:4687–4692.
57. ffytche DH, Howard RJ, Brammer MJ, et al. The anatomy of conscious vision: an fMRI study of visual hallucinations. *Nature Neurosci.* 1998;1: 738–742.
58. Baseler HA, Morland AB, Wandell BA. Topographic organization of human visual areas in the absence of input from primary cortex. *J Neurosci.* 1999;19:2619–2627.
59. Baseler HA, Brewer AA, Sharpe LT, et al. Reorganization of human cortical maps caused by inherited photoreceptor abnormalities. *Nature Neurosci.* 2002;5:364–370.
60. Moritz CH, Rowley HA, Haughton VM, et al. Functional MR imaging assessment of a non-responsive brain injured patient. *Magn Reson Imaging.* 2001;19:1129–1132.

61. Sie LTL, Rombouts SA, Valk IJ, et al. Functional MRI of visual cortex in sedated 18 month-old infants with or without periventricular leukomalacia. *Dev Med Child Neurol.* 2001;43:486–490.
62. Tsubota K, Kwong KK, Lee T-Y, et al. Functional MRI of brain activation by eye blinking. *Exp Eye Res.* 1999;69:1–7.
63. Renshaw PF, Yurgelun-Todd DA, Cohen BM. Greater hemodynamic response to photic stimulation in schizophrenic patients: an echo planar MRI study. *Am J Psychiatry.* 1994;151:1493–1495.
64. Thulborn KR, Martin C, Voyvodic JT. Functional MR imaging using a visually guided saccade paradigm for comparing activation patterns in patients with probable Alzheimer's disease and in cognitively able elderly volunteers. *AJNR Am J Neuroradiol.* 2000;21:524–531.
65. McDowell JE, Brown GG, Paulus M, et al. Neural correlates of refixation saccades and antisaccades in normal and schizophrenia subjects. *Biol Psychiatry.* 2002;51:216–223.
66. Noll DC, Genovese CR, Nystrom LE, et al. Estimating test-retest reliability in functional MR imaging 2: application to motor and cognitive activation studies. *Magn Reson Med.* 1997;38:508–517.
67. Goodyear BG, Menon RS. Brief visual stimulation allows mapping of ocular dominance in visual cortex using fMRI. *Hum Brain Mapp.* 2001;14: 210–217.
68. Menon RS, Goodyear BG. Submillimeter functional localization in human striate cortex using BOLD contrast at 4 Tesla: implications for the vascular point-spread function. *Magn Reson Med.* 1999;41:230–235.
69. Nishida Y, Hayashi O, Iwami T, et al. Development of a new binocular visual stimulation device using image guides for functional MRI. *J Neuroophthalmology.* 2000;24:343–348.
70. Liu GT, Miki A, Goldsmith Z, et al. Eye dominance in visual cortex using functional MRI at 1.5T. An alternative method. *J AAPOS.* 2002;6:40–48.
71. Watanabe T, Sasaki Y, Miyauchi S, et al. Attention-regulated activity in human primary visual cortex. *J Neurophysiol.* 1998;79:2218–2221.
72. Ross MH, Yurgelun-Todd DA, Renshaw PF, et al. Age-related reduction in functional MRI response to photic stimulation. *Neurology.* 1997;48: 173–176.
73. Rombouts SARB, Barkhof F, Hoogenraad FGC, et al. Within-subject reproducibility of visual activation patterns with functional magnetic resonance imaging using multislice echo planar imaging. *Magn Reson Imaging.* 1998;16:105–113.
74. McGonigle DJ, Howseman AM, Athwal BS, et al. Variability in fMRI: an examination in intersession differences. *Neuroimage.* 2000;11:708–734.
75. Miki A, Raz J, van Erp TGM, et al. Reproducibility of visual activation in functional MR imaging and effects of postprocessing. *AJNR Am J Neuroradiol.* 2000;21:910–915.
76. Miki A, Raz J, Englander SA, et al. Reproducibility of visual activation in functional magnetic resonance imaging at very high field strength (4 Tesla). *Jpn J Ophthalmol.* 2001;45:1–4.
77. Holodny AI, Schulder M, Liu W-C, et al. The effect of brain tumors on BOLD functional MR imaging activation in the adjacent motor cortex: implications for image-guide neurosurgery. *AJNR Am J Neuroradiol.* 2001; 21:1415–1422.
78. Miki A, Liu GT, Goldsmith ZG, et al. Effects of check size on visual cortex activation studied by functional magnetic resonance imaging. *Ophthalmic Res.* 2001;33:180–184.

# 14

# fMRI of the Auditory Cortex

Deborah A. Hall

## Introduction

During the last two decades, auditory neuroscience has made significant progress in understanding the functional organization of the auditory system in both normally hearing listeners and patients with sensorineural hearing impairments. Modern brain imaging techniques have made an enormous contribution to that progress by enabling the in vivo study of human central auditory function. Significant contributions have come from positron emission tomography (PET), functional magnetic resonance imaging (fMRI), electroencephalography (EEG), and magnetoencephalography. Of these four, fMRI has become the tool of choice for addressing many research questions for three reasons. First, fMRI is suitable for research use with children, as well as adults. Second, because multiple observations can be made on the same individual, fMRI permits the investigation of longer-term dynamic processes, such as functional plasticity after disease, damage, retraining, or therapy. Third, the need for averaging data across individuals is reduced, further improving the accuracy with which activations can be mapped onto subject-specific brain structure. Thus, fMRI has become one of the key imaging techniques for human auditory neuroscience.

To date, auditory fMRI has not been widely implemented for routine clinical purposes. However, there is a growing literature on its potential clinical application. To enhance the clinical use of auditory fMRI, standardized protocols are required that are easy and quick to use with patients and yield robust replicable results. From the auditory fMRI research with normally hearing subjects, the most efficient protocols can now be transferred to study patients with hearing impairment. For example, it is known which acoustic stimuli generate robust activation of the central auditory system [such as temporally varying, wideband sounds presented at 70 to 90 decibels sound pressure level (SPL)]. In addition, it has been shown that patients are able to comply more easily with a passive listening task rather than one that requires an active response decision, particularly if the patient is liable to make errors. A material obstacle for efficient auditory fMRI in general is the intense acoustic scanner noise generated during image acquisition. The noise reduces the sensitivity for detecting stimulus-evoked activation and can be particularly troublesome for those patients who are averse to noisy environments. Noise-reduction methods have been developed for auditory fMRI, and the availability of these methods is now facilitating clinical fMRI applications.

This chapter discusses some of the theoretical and technical challenges of auditory fMRI and some of the major clinical applications within this field. Challenges include the intense acoustic noise and the effects of the magnetic field on sound presentation equipment and on implanted hearing devices. Clinical applications of auditory fMRI embrace the preoperative or intraoperative mapping of functional areas relevant to spoken language (for example, for planning surgical intervention to relieve chronic epileptic seizures) in the study of involuntary auditory hallucinations in schizophrenia and in the investigation of reorganization of spoken language processing after temporal lobe lesions. This research often evaluates patterns of distributed brain activation, including amodal language areas, as well as unimodal auditory areas. Here, only those major clinical applications that investigate the processing of basic (i.e., non-linguistic) acoustic features in sound will be reviewed. The focus will be on those areas of clinical auditory research in which fMRI techniques have been used in preference to other brain imaging techniques. There are a number of promising applications such as studies of the functional reorganisation of the auditory cortex as a consequence of adaptation to hearing loss, investigations of tinnitus, and the assessment of candidature for cochlear implantation.

## Anatomical Organization of the Central Auditory System

### Subcortical Organization

The auditory system is composed of the outer and middle ear, the cochlea, the auditory nerve, a chain of subcortical nuclei, and multiple cortical areas (Figure 14.1). Sound is picked up by the outer ear, transformed by the middle ear, and is converted by the hair cells of the cochlea into neural signals that are transmitted along the auditory nerve. The cochlea acts like a mechanical spectrum analyzer, where the sensory hair cells at its apex are excited by low frequencies, and by high frequencies at its base. The conversion of sound frequency to coding in terms of the position of excitation is called tonotopic mapping. Tonotopy is the main organizing principle throughout the auditory system.

Auditory nerve fibers terminate within the cochlear nucleus (CN) in the lower brainstem, where excitatory and inhibitory interactions transform the signal both spatially and temporally. Parallel pathways transmit the output of the CN to the higher auditory nuclei. Pathways from the left and right CN converge in the superior olivary complex (SOC), where a combination of the information from the two ears enables encoding of the spatial characteristics of the signal. Other pathways project from the CN via the lateral lemniscus (LL) to the inferior

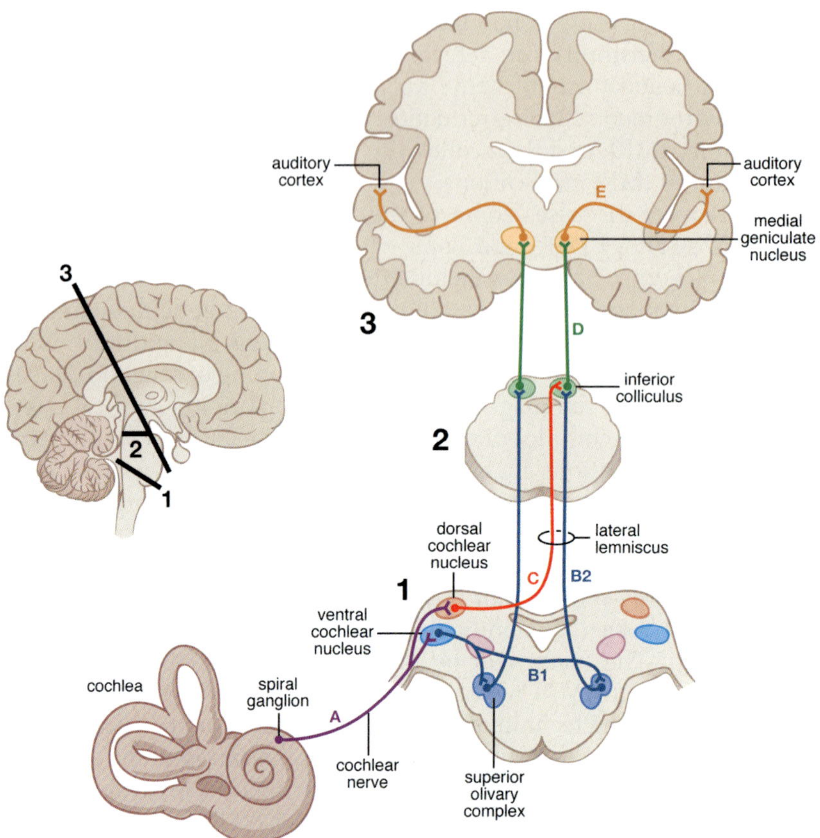


**Figure 14.1.** Schematic diagram of the bilateral ascending auditory pathway from the cochleae, lower pons (1), midbrain (2), and cortex (3). Unilateral auditory pathway: cochlear nerve (A), ventral cochlear nucleus to contralateral and ipsilateral superior olivary complex (B1), superior olivary complex to inferior colliculus (B2), dorsal cochlear nucleus to contralateral inferior colliculus (C), inferior colliculus to medial geniculate nucleus (D), medial geniculate nucleus to auditory cortex (E).

colliculus (IC) in the midbrain. At the IC and above, the activity in the auditory pathway generally is dominated by the responses to the opposite (contralateral) ear. The IC represents an obligatory relay for information analyzed in the lower brainstem nuclei; inputs from these brainstem nuclei (including the CN, SOC, and LL) reconverge in the IC, where further processing and transformation of the signal takes place. In turn, the IC projects to the medial geniculate nucleus (MGN) in the thalamus, which is the main relay station to the auditory cortex. Throughout this central auditory system, information is distributed over divergent and convergent pathways. This arrangement allows for serial and parallel processing of ascending information, where descending connections also modify the signal.

## Cortical Organization

Kaas and Hackett[1,2] presented a model of auditory cortical organization in non-human primates in which a primary core region, located

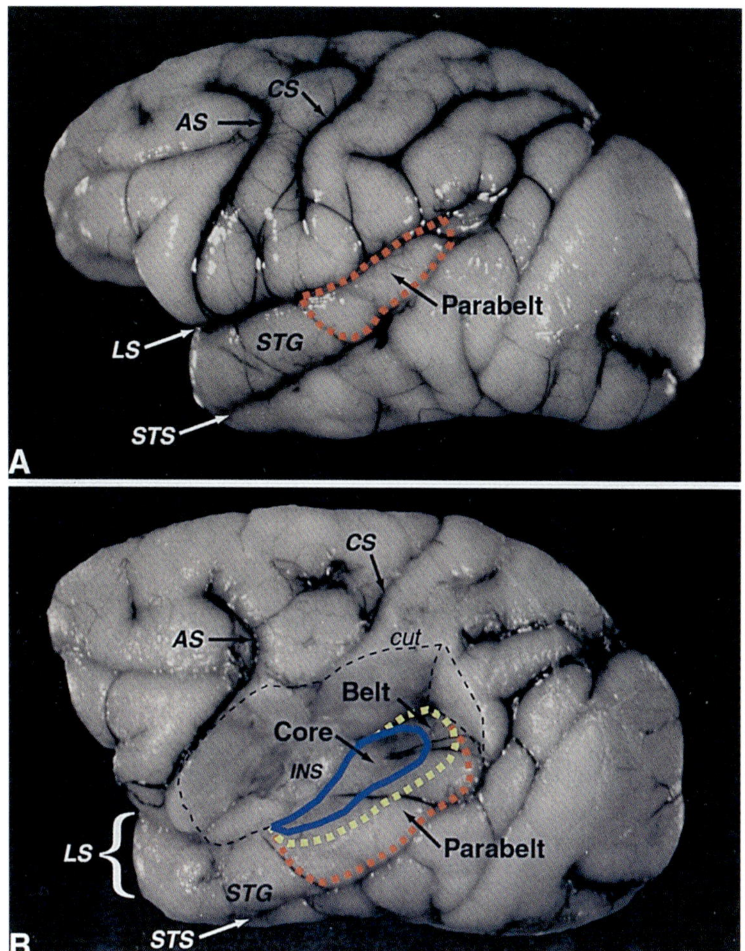


**Figure 14.2.** A lateral view of the left hemisphere of the macaque brain. (A) The approximate location of the parabelt region on the lateral aspect of the superior temporal gyrus (dashed red line). (B) Dorsolateral view of the same brain after removal of the overlying frontal and parietal cortex, exposing the ventral bank of the lateral sulcus and insula. The dashed black line defines the portion of cortex cut away. The approximate location of the core region (solid blue line), posterior and lateral portions of the belt region (dashed yellow line), and the parabelt region (dashed red line) are shown. The medial portion of the belt region and the anterior part of the core are not visible. AS, arcuate sulcus; CS, central sulcus; INS, insula; LS, lateral sulcus; STG, superior temporal gyrus; STS superior temporal sulcus. Reprinted with permission from Kaas JH, Hackett TA. Subdivisions of auditory cortex and processing streams in primates. Proceedings of the National Academy of Sciences 2000;97:11793-11799. Copyright © 2000 National Academy of Sciences, U.S.A.

upon the lower bank of the lateral sulcus, is encircled by nonprimary belt regions. These core and belt regions are predominantly hidden from view by the overlying frontal lobe. Parabelt nonprimary auditory regions extend onto the lateral aspect of the superior temporal gyrus (STG) (Figure 14.2). The organization of primate auditory cortex is generally thought to be a good model for the organization of the auditory areas of the human brain. Again, in humans, the arrangement of auditory fields is localized to the surface of the STG, along the inferior margin of the lateral sulcus (Sylvian sulcus). Although different authors have proposed a variety of classification schemes of the human auditory cortex (in terms of the number and location of areas, and nomenclature), they all identify an elongated primary area, surrounded by numerous nonprimary auditory fields.[3–5]

*Primary Core Region*

The core has a granular and densely myelinated appearance and is highly metabolically active. The core receives ascending inputs from the ventral MGN and projects to ipsilateral and contralateral core areas, as well as to adjacent belt areas. Neurons in the core respond well and with short latencies to pure tones, with narrow frequency tuning at their characteristic frequency.[6,7] Neurons with a similar characteristic frequency are arranged in rows that are organized along a frequency gradient.[8] Three distinguishable frequency gradients have been reported in the core region of the macaque monkey (Figure 14.3). These subdivisions are referred to as A1, R, and RT. Subdivisions A1 and R share a common low-frequency border, and R and RT may share a high-frequency border.[9]

In humans, the core region extends about 15 millimeters and is generally located on the medial two-thirds of the anterior-most long axis of Heschl's gyrus (HG). In some studies, architectonic criteria have been used to subdivide the core area. Galaburda and Sanides[3] distinguished a medial and a lateral zone in six hemispheres, whereas Morosan and colleagues[10] identified three core fields in 20 hemispheres. In both studies, boundaries were perpendicular to the long axis of HG.

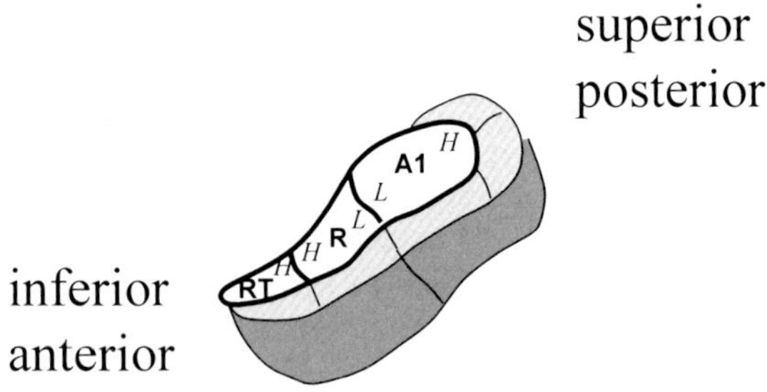


**Figure 14.3.** Further subdivisions of the macaque auditory cortex illustrated in Figure 14.2B. Auditory core fields (A1, R, RT) are surrounded by belt (light grey) and parabelt (dark grey) fields. The core fields A1 and R are tonotopically organized. High-frequency (H) acoustic stimuli are represented posteromedially in A1, anteromedially in R. Low-frequency (L) stimuli are represented anterolaterally in A1 and posterolaterally in R. Tonotopic organization in RT is uncertain, but may mirror that found in R. Putative borders within belt and parabelt regions are depicted by the black lines.

### *Nonprimary Belt and Parabelt Regions*

In the macaque, the belt region includes seven or eight nonprimary fields. Relative to the core, belt areas have reduced cell density and columnar spacing, larger pyramidal cells, and less dense myelination. Each belt field receives major inputs from the adjacent core field and from the dorsal and medial divisions of the MGN. Belt neurons respond less well to pure tones, but sufficiently to indicate tonotopic gradients.[6,8] Neurons in the belt region generally have broader frequency tuning than those in the core.[11] Activation results from integration between converging inputs; consequently, neurons have complex receptive field properties. For example, in the lateral belt region (on the STG), neurons respond vigorously to spectrally complex stimuli such as vocalizations.[6,12,13] The parabelt contains at least two fields that receive inputs from the adjacent belt and the dorsal and medial divisions of the MGN. The physiological characteristics of the parabelt are not established and subdivisions between nonprimary regions are poorly specified by architectonic markers; as a result, the definition of parabelt borders is made on the basis of differences in cortico-cortical connectivity.[2] The belt and parabelt connect with multiple areas in the superior temporal sulcus and anterior and posterior zones of the STG, which may have a polymodal function. Thus, at least four hierarchically organized levels of processing have been described in non-human primate auditory cortex.

In the human brain, between five and six nonprimary regions have been proposed on the basis of histochemical staining criteria (see Figure 14.4).[4,5] Like the primate, these areas surround the primary core region and extend to the convexity of the STG. The distinction between belt and parabelt nonprimary regions has been, so far, also difficult to ascertain in humans, partly because there is a lack of information about the cortico-cortical connections.

## Imaging Auditory Anatomy

One of the principal aims of current neuroimaging research in normally hearing listeners is to seek evidence for the anatomical and physiological systems known from studies in other mammals (particularly primates). Thus, the interpretation of imaging data often relates the patterns of brain activation to the underlying anatomy and draws links with what is known from animal neurophysiological studies. The small anatomical volumes of the auditory nuclei pose challenges for the detectability of fMRI activation. Approximate sizes in humans are 0.02 cubic centimeters for the CN, 0.01 cubic centimeters for the SOC, 0.25 cubic centimeters for the IC, and 0.08 cubic centimeters for the MGN. Given that the spatial resolution of fMRI is 0.03 cubic centimeters (for a typical voxel size of $3 \times 3 \times 3$ cubic millimeters), only the IC and MGN are above this spatial scale. Subcortical activity has not been readily imaged using fMRI. In addition to their small size, difficulties also may be due to the characteristics of the metabolic activity or of the neurovasculature in these areas, or the fact that the brain moves with each arterial pulsation. Such cardiac-related motion can be eliminated by

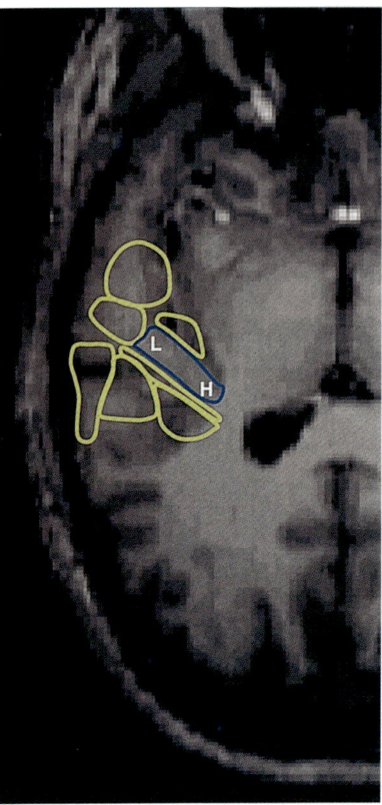


**Figure 14.4.** Multiple auditory areas on the superior surface of the temporal lobe of left hemisphere in humans. The core auditory area is shown in blue with the tonotopic gradient from low (L) to high (H) frequency gradient. Surrounding the core region, seven nonprimary areas have been identified by Wallace and colleagues[5] on the basis of histochemical staining. (Neurologic coordinates)

synchronizing image acquisition with a fixed point in the cardiac cycle,[14] and robust activation in the IC has been achieved in single subjects using this gating technique.[15] Auditory activation also can be detected in the subcortical nuclei with multisubject averaging, without the use cardiac gating.[16]

Auditory cortical activation in humans studied using fMRI has been widely reported. However, relatively little is known about the functional organization along the STG; for example, there is no general consensus about the number and spatial arrangement of tonotopic fields. Neither EEG nor PET have sufficient spatial resolution to segregate frequency-specific responses within HG. Single-unit electrophysiology has provided the most direct demonstration of a frequency gradient along HG. Using electrodes implanted in epileptic patients to detect the foci of seizures, a lateral progression in frequency sensitivity from high frequency (3360 hertz) to lower frequency (1480 hertz) has been measured along HG.[17] High-precision magnetoencephalography techniques have shown that the source of the response in HG again moves more laterally as tone frequency decreases, and that there is a second tonotopic gradient in a nonprimary region posterior to HG.[18] Functional MRI has revealed multiple frequency-dependent areas on the STG, indicating at least four tonotopic fields.[19] Two of these tonotopic areas were located on HG and abutted at their low isofrequency contours—a tonotopic arrangement that could be the human homologue of two of the core fields reported in the macaque.

## Technical Challenges Involved in Auditory fMRI

The MR environment has three different types of electromagnetic fields. For 3 Tesla MR systems, the static magnetic field is 60 000 times stronger than the earth's magnetic field. Weaker magnetic fields include the time-varying gradient magnetic fields and the pulsed radiofrequency fields. These electromagnetic fields pose three technical challenges; 1) for developing suitable equipment for the presentation of auditory signals to listeners in the scanner bore, 2) for the safe scanning of patients who have implant devices in their brain, and 3) for the intense acoustic noise generated by the flexing of the gradient coils in the static magnetic field.

### Sound Presentation in the MR Scanner

Studies of auditory function require the presentation of low-distortion acoustic signals for which the frequency spectrum and intensity at the ear can be calibrated. Many systems have utilized loudspeakers, placed away from the high-static magnetic field, from which sound is delivered through plastic tubes inserted into the subjects' ear canal through a protective ear defender. However, the tubing affects both the phase and amplitude of the different frequency components of a stimulus most commonly imposing a severe ripple on the spectra. Electronic systems for psychophysical research deliver high-quality signals, but these systems are generally unsuitable for use in the MR environment. Ordinary headphones use an electromagnet to push and pull on a diaphragm to vibrate the air and generate sound, but this does not work in the high-static magnetic field. Headphone components constructed from ferromagnetic material also disrupt the magnetic fields locally and induce signal loss or spatial distortion in areas close to the ears. In addition, the electronic components can be damaged by the static magnetic field, whereas electromagnetic interference generated by the equipment is detected by the MR receiver coil. Electronic sound-delivery systems for MR research must be designed specifically to overcome these difficulties. An MR-compatible sound-delivery system has been developed for research in our laboratory.[20] Digital audio signals are delivered to the headset via resistive carbon fiber cabling rather than copper wire. The headset is based on commercially available electrostatic headphones modified to remove or replace their ferromagnetic components and combined with standard industrial ear defenders to provide acoustic isolation (Figure 14.5). Electrostatic headphones generate sound using a conductive diaphragm placed next to a fixed conducting panel. A high voltage polarizes the fixed panel, and the audio signal passing through the diaphragm rapidly switches between a positive and a negative signal, attracting or repelling it to the fixed panel and thus vibrating the air. The personal computer (PC), electronics, and power supply that drive the system are housed outside

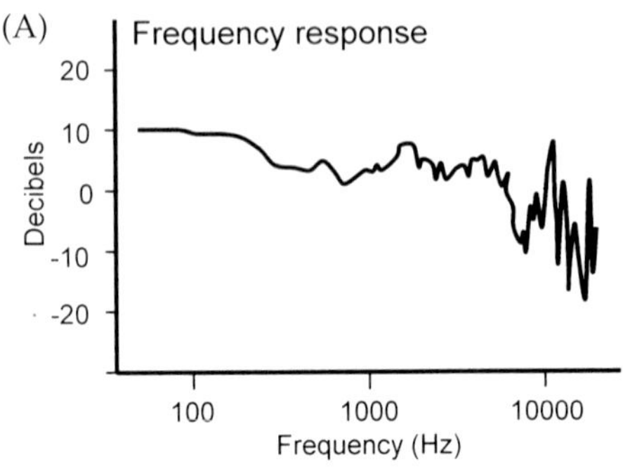


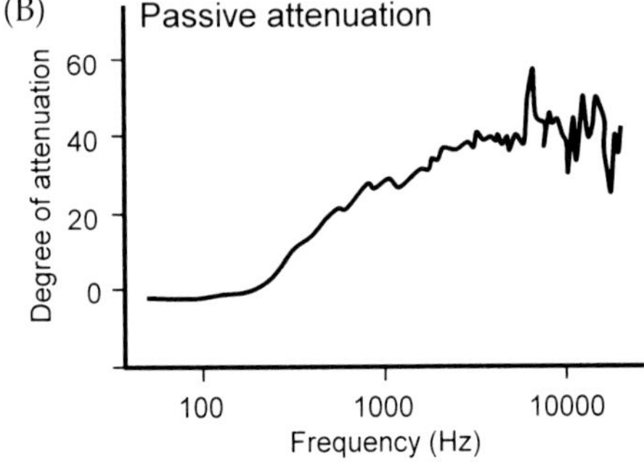


**Figure 14.5.** Frequency response plot for a modified electrostatic headset combined with industrial ear defenders for high-quality sound presentation in the MR scanner. A polypropylene protective grill is inside the headset to protect the front of the electrostatic capsule. Signals are delivered using carbon fiber leads with thick plastic cable protection. (A) The headset is capable of delivering frequencies over a 24 kilohertz bandwidth (which is limited by the digital sampling rate). The frequency response does not differ materially from that of the unmodified Seinheiser headphone and is relatively flat between 50 hertz and 10 kilohertz. (B) The headset reduces free-field noise by 30 decibels between 500 hertz and 10 kilohertz. Measurements were taken using a KEMAR manikin equipped with a microphone at the ear drum to simulate real head listening. Plots have been corrected for the frequency response of the manikin.

the radiofrequency screened magnet hall to avoid electromagnetic interference with MR scanning. All electrical signals passing into the screened room are radiofrequency filtered. In an alternative and novel design for an MR-compatible headset, the electromagnetic components of the headphones are removed and their function replaced by the scanner's static magnetic field.[21]

## Safe Scanning of Patients Who Have Brain Implant Devices

The strong static magnetic field and time-varying magnetic fields pose certain hazards for scanning patients who have received auditory brainstem and cochlear implants because most conventional implants are not specifically designed to meet MR compatibility criteria. For the patient, risks include movement of the device and localized heating of brain tissue, whereas, for the device, the electronic components may be damaged.

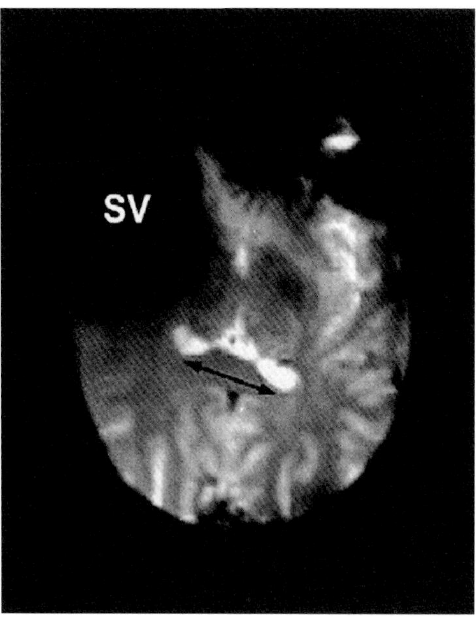


**Figure 14.6.** Magnetizable elements in the electrode preparation causing a signal void (SV) can be seen in the right frontal region. The right ventricle is distorted (compare with the black arrow between the right and left ventricle). The artifact remains ipsilateral. Reprinted with permission from Obler R, Köstler H, Weber B-P, Mack KF, Becker B. Safe electrical stimulation of the cochlear nerve at the promontory during functional magnetic resonance imaging. *Magn Reson Med* 1999;42:371–378.

The static magnetic field exerts forces on implanted ferromagnetic materials, risking displacement of the device and soft tissue trauma. The implant can be stimulated by voltages within the conducting loop, caused directly by the time-varying gradient magnetic fields or the radiofrequency pulse, or as the conducting loop moves in the static field with head movements. If two electrodes from a conducting loop are connected, the current path between them will flow through the brain tissue and may cause local heating in proximity to the implant. For further discussion of the risks in using a nerve-stimulating device in the MR environment see Obler and colleagues.[22]

Magnetizable elements induce artifacts in the brain images that are visible as areas of signal loss or spatial distortion (see Figure 14.6). However, induced current in the electronics is the main hazard to the device, causing either damage to the electronics or uncontrolled stimulation of the patient. The majority of implants also contain a magnet to hold the external transmitter coil in place, which should be removed before scanning. In modern implants, this magnet is reasonably easy to remove under local anesthetic to permit MR scanning. The issue of MR compatibility is particularly important given the number of adults and children receiving implants who should not be excluded from MR scanning for the rest of their lives. Some implant designs have been proven to be MR compatible,[23–26] but they have not been routinely provided in clinical practice. For these safety reasons, clinical imaging research of implantees has generally used other imaging methods, particularly PET.

### Intense Acoustic Noise

The time-varying gradient magnetic fields are switched rapidly on and off during image acquisition and are central to the formation of each image slice through the brain. Currents through three sets of coiled wire induce small magnetic field gradients that are orthogonal and parallel to the long axis of the static magnetic field. The currents are rapidly switched within a large magnetic field, and interactions between the gradient coils and the static magnetic field induce pulsed Lorentz forces that act upon the gradient coils to deform them. These abrupt flexing movements generate a compression wave in the air that is heard as acoustic noise during imaging (Figure 14.7). The acoustic noise is at least as intense as 115 decibels (A).[27] Secondary acoustic noise can be produced if the vibration of the coils and the core on which they are wound conducts through the core supports to the rest of the structure.

The acoustic properties of the scanner noise (e.g., bandwidth, fundamental frequency, spectral envelope) depend on the mechanical resonances of the coil assemblies, on the type of imaging sequence used, and on its switching frequency. The dominant components of the

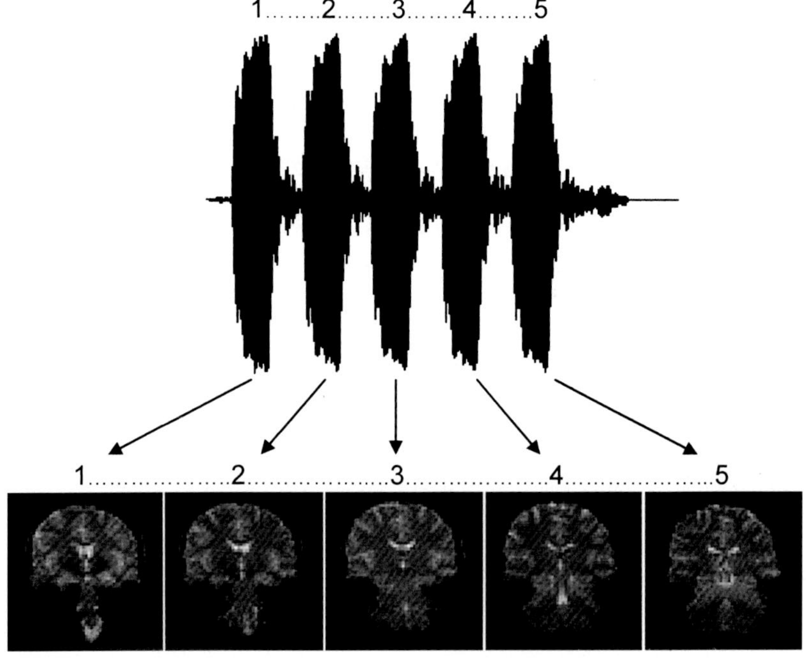


**Figure 14.7.** A sample waveform showing the pulses of acoustic energy generated during the acquisition of a set of five brain slices. The electrical driving signal to the gradient coils is an EPI sequence where a whole slice is acquired for each RF excitation.

noise are spectral peaks at the switching frequency and its higher harmonics, mostly within the frequency range of zero to three kilohertz (Figure 14.8). In fast functional imaging sequences [e.g., echoplanar imaging (EPI)], one brain slice is acquired in one radiofrequency excitation. Echoplanar imaging sequences tend to have extremely fast gradient switching times and high gradient amplitudes, and thus produce high levels of acoustic noise. The aggregate noise dosage for EPI studies can be reduced by acquiring a single, or very few, brain slices, but at the expense of only a partial view of brain activity.[28] The noise exposure is potentially damaging without hearing protection.[29]

The scanner noise can affect the pattern of brain activation that is measured within the auditory cortex. Areas of stimulus-evoked activation are those that show a statistically significant difference between two experimental conditions. The simplest case is one in which one condition contains a sound stimulus and the other does not. Because the scanner noise is present throughout, the sound condition contains both stimulus and scanner noise and the baseline condition contains scanner noise (i.e., it is not silent). The processing of the scanner noise can affect the stimulus-evoked activation pattern in two ways. First, even with hearing protection, scanner noise makes the stimulus more difficult to hear, therefore increasing the demands on attention. In particular, the frequency range of the scanner acoustic noise is crucial for speech intelligibility; thus, the activation pattern can include a cognitive component that reflects the attention cost of filtering out the back-

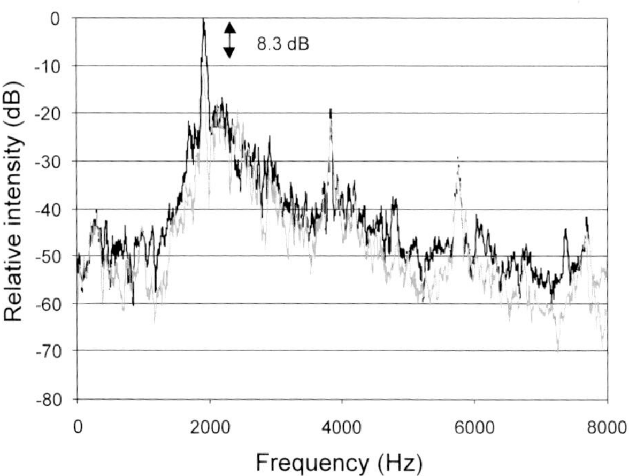


**Figure 14.8.** Sample spectrum of the scanner acoustic noise computed by performing a Fourier transform on one acoustic pulse that corresponds to the acquisition of a single slice. The black line represents the frequency spectrum for the scanner noise measured within the center of the head coil. The grey line represents the frequency spectrum for the same pulse sequence after installing energy-absorbing foam on the entire inner surface of the scanner bore. Values on the upper horizontal axis mark the frequencies of the prominent spectral peaks in hertz at 1921, 3842, 5763, and 7684 hertz. On the intensity axis, zero decibel corresponds to 129 decibels SPL, which is the sound level of the most dominant frequency. The foam installation reduces this dominant peak by 8.3 decibels.

ground acoustical noise. Second, stimulus-induced activations tend to be on the order of one to three percent from baseline; thus, higher levels of baseline activation, caused by the ambient noise, are likely to make the experimentally induced auditory activation more difficult to detect statistically. Indeed, several studies have reported a reduced activation signal (i.e., the difference between stimulation and baseline conditions) in the auditory cortex when the amount of prior scanner noise is increased, indicating that the noise does mask the detection of auditory activation.[30,31]

Ravicz and colleagues[32] have investigated the effectiveness of passive treatments applied to the most dominant routes of noise transmission. Wearing sound-attenuating ear defenders substantially reduced the acoustic noise at the location of the subject's ear by 31 to 38 decibels. Lining the bore inside the scanner with a sound-energy absorbing material reduced the acoustic noise by 12 decibels. This material is constructed from two foam layers that have different densities, giving an abrupt change in acoustic impedance. Figure 14.8 shows an example of an eight-decibel reduction in sound level of the dominant scanner acoustic frequency achieved as a result of installing sound-absorbing foam inside the bore of the 3T scanner at the Magnetic Resonance Center, Nottingham University. The eight-decibel reduction is comparable to that achieved by Ravicz and colleagues.[32]

A combination of ear defenders and energy-absorbing foam is insufficient to eliminate the acoustic noise, and auditory stimuli remain partly masked by the background acoustic noise. Other treatment methods have been investigated. Active treatment includes active noise cancellation using an anti-phase sound presented using the sound-delivery system.[33] If used in combination with the wearing of ear defenders, noise conduction through the head and body may be the more dominant mode of hearing than air-borne transmission; consequently, active cancellation may not reduce the perception of the scanner noise. In this case, gains can be made to reduce the acoustic noise at source by either hardware or software modifications. Novel designs for the MR system hardware include the construction of quiet gradient coils in which the net Lorentz force is compensated between current pathways[34,35] and a vacuum-based acoustic noise-reduction system in which the gradient coils are encased in an evacuated chamber and mounted directly on the floor. Price and colleagues[36] reported that, for a fast imaging sequence, the MR system with the vacuum-sealed gradient coils emitted scanner noise at 84 decibels, whereas comparable MR systems without this modification exceeded 105 decibels. Software modifications principally slow down the gradient switching to reduce acoustic noise. This approach is based on the premise that the spectrum of the acoustic noise is determined by the product of the frequency spectrum of the gradient waveforms and the frequency response function of the gradient system.[37] The frequency response function is generally substantially reduced at low frequencies (below 200 hertz); consequently, the acoustic noise level can be reduced by using gradient pulse sequences whose spectra are band-limited to this low frequency range using soft or sinusoidally ramped pulse shapes.[38]

Using such a low-noise sequence, a peak noise level sound of 58 decibel SPL at the position of the ear has been used for neuroimaging of central auditory function.[39] However, the low noise is achieved at the expense of slower gradient switching, making the acquisition time longer. Low-noise sequences are not suitable for EPI in which the fundamental of the gradient waveform is greater than 200 hertz. In the next section, an experimental protocol will be discussed that avoids these limitations to minimize the effect of the scanner acoustic noise on the measured patterns of auditory cortical activation for whole brain, multi-slice EPI.

## Example fMRI Paradigms

The auditory fMRI response to a single burst of noise is smoothed and delayed in time. It typically rises to a peak by four to five seconds after stimulus onset and decays by five to eight seconds after stimulus offset (see Figure 14.9)[40]; therefore, a brief burst of sound does not generate its maximal auditory response until a few seconds after the stimulus event. Typical functional imaging paradigms measure state-related responses for a stimulus that is presented repeatedly over a period of time. These experiments generally consist of cycles of stimulation and baseline epochs, throughout which whole brain slices are acquired at regular intervals. This imaging protocol produces a burst of scanner noise that is repeated at a rate determined by the time between volume acquisitions. The auditory system is therefore subject to continuous quasi-tonal stimulation, resulting in an elevated baseline level of activation.

During a functional imaging experiment, the scanner noise induces an auditory response that spans two different temporal scales. First, the scanner noise generated by the acquisition of one slice early in the brain volume may induce activation in an imaging slice that covers the audi-

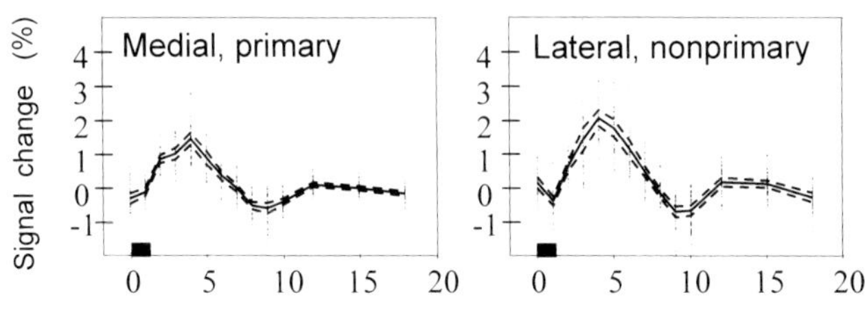


**Figure 14.9.** Example of the mean time course of the auditory response to a one-second burst of EPI scanner noise (16 slices with a 67 millisecond inter-slice interval) within two auditory cortical areas for a single subject. The acoustic stimulus is denoted by the black square on the time axis. Within each plot, dots indicate the signal change at each voxel within the region of interest. The solid line indicates the mean signal change across all voxels within the region of interest and the dashed lines indicate the 95% confidence limits for the mean response. Data taken from Hall DA, Summerfield AQ, Gonçalves MS, Foster JR, Palmer AR, Bowtell RW. Time course of the auditory BOLD response to scanner noise. *Magn Reson Med.* 2000;43:601–606. Magnetic Resonance in Medicine © 2000.[40]

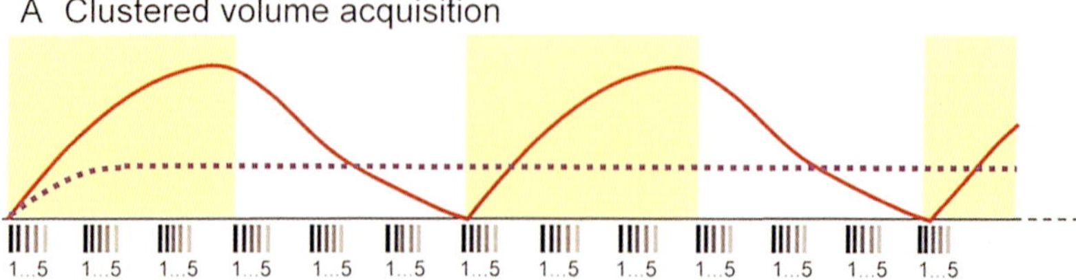


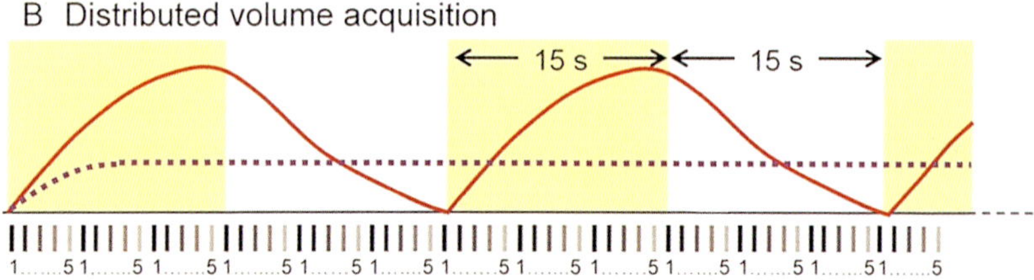


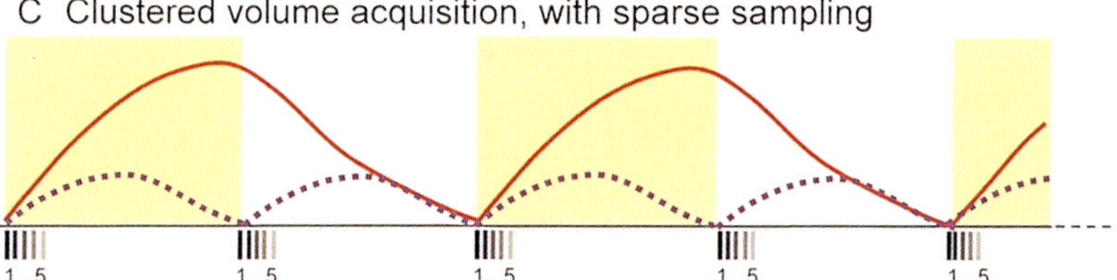


**Figure 14.10.** Comparison of the temporal acquisition of sets of five brain slices for three different image-acquisition protocols. Each slice acquisition is illustrated by a line and numbered 1 . . . 5. The experiment involves 30-second cycles of stimulus (denoted by the yellow shaded areas), followed by a baseline (shown in white). The estimated auditory response evoked by the scanner noise is shown by the dotted lines, while the solid red line shows the response to the stimulus. (A) The clustered volume acquisition sequence in which the five slices are acquired at a rate of 0.6 seconds, generating a three-second burst of pulses, followed by a two-second silent gap. (B) A distributed volume-acquisition sequence in which the five slices are evenly distributed throughout the five-second TR period. This sequence generates scanner noise that is characterized by a train of acoustic pulses at one hertz. Note that the same number of slices are acquired in both (A) and (B). (C) A combination of clustered volume acquisition with sparse sampling so that each three-second burst of pulses is followed by 12 seconds of silence. Sparse sampling permits the auditory response evoked by the scanner noise to decay to baseline level before the next acquisition.

tory cortex and is acquired later in the same volume. This is be called inter-slice noise interference. Second, scanner noise may induce auditory activation that extends across time to subsequent volumes. This second effect is called inter-volume noise interference. By manipulating the timing intervals of the slice and the volume acquisitions in the scanning protocol, the inter-slice and inter-volume noise interference, respectively, can be reduced independently of one another. The inter-slice interval is shortest using a clustered volume-acquisition sequence in which all slices are acquired in rapid succession, followed by a gap (Figure 14.10A). Somewhat longer slice timing is achieved using a distributed volume-acquisition sequence in which slices are acquired at slower, equally spaced intervals (Figure 14.10B). The relative amount of inter-slice noise interference has been compared for clustered volume- and distributed volume-acquisition sequences, when the inter-volume interval is fixed. Edmister and colleagues found that the clustered volume-acquisition sequence was more sensitive to the detection of stimulus-evoked activation over a range of inter-volume intervals.[41] In addition, using a clustered volume-acquisition sequence preceded by scanner acoustic noise, Talavage and colleagues found that the inter-slice interference can be maximally reduced when the duration of each volume acquisition (and hence, the burst of scanner acoustic noise) was two seconds or less.[31] Reducing the inter-volume noise interference can be achieved by prolonging the inter-volume interval (Figure 14.10C). Effectively, this approach acquires single sets of images using clustered volume acquisition at the end of stimulus and baseline conditions. Hall and colleagues[42] showed that this sparse sampling is actually more effective at detecting sound-evoked activation than the clustered volume-acquisition protocol shown in Figure 14.10B, despite the many fewer data samples (see Figure 14.11). A sparse sampling technique has been used by many groups to identify auditory cortical evoked responses in the absence of scanner noise.[43,44]

Clustered volume acquisition

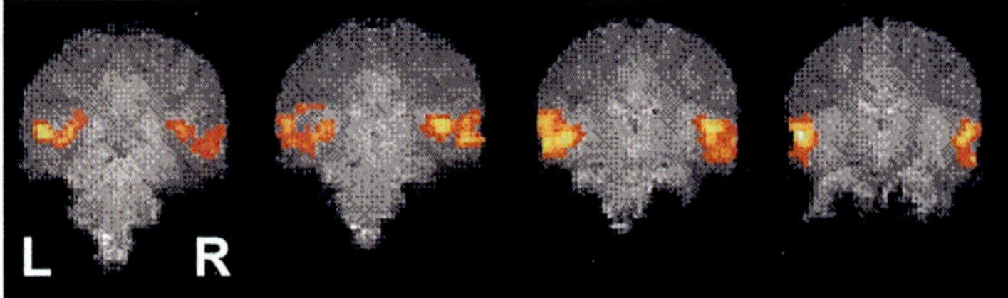


Clustered volume acquisition, with sparse sampling

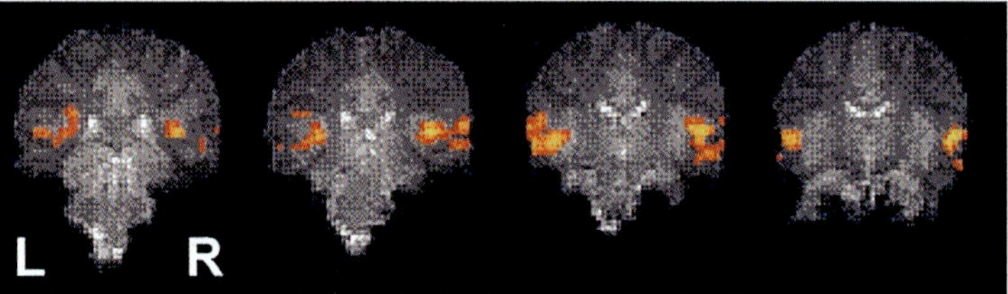


**Figure 14.11.** Pattern of activation in a single subject who was scanned using the two types of temporal sampling for clustered volume acquisition. The first used an inter-volume interval of 2.33 seconds and the second of 14 seconds (sparse sampling). Activation maps were thresholded at $P < 0.001$, uncorrected for multiple comparisons, and regions of activation are shown whose size exceeds 100 voxels. Both techniques succeeded in detecting auditory activation in Heschl's gyrus, superior and middle temporal gyri. Adapted from Hall DA, Haggard MP, Akeroyd MA, Palmer AR, Summerfield AQ, Elliott MR, Gurney E, Bowtell RW. Sparse temporal sampling in auditory fMRI. *Hum Brain Mapp*. 1999;10:471–429. Copyright © 1999 John Wiley & Sons, Inc. With permission of Wiley-Liss, Inc.[42] (Neurologic coordinates)

## Major Clinical Applications of Auditory fMRI

Functional MRI of the auditory system has not yet been widely implemented for routine clinical purposes. However, over the past few years, the number of clinical research studies has grown rapidly. Here, interesting developments in the field will be reported and those clinical applications to which fMRI has made a valuable contribution will be highlighted.

### Functional Adaptation to Hearing Loss

Rather than being fixed in functional organization, the mature brain can show significant neural changes as a result of learning or trauma. Functional reorganization of the auditory system occurs following disruption to its normal input from the periphery, such as after cochlear damage or cochlear nerve resection, and a number of studies are reported in this section. Neuronal adaptations also can occur as a result of increased exposure to sound; for example, in normally hearing volunteers, an improvement in frequency discrimination after training has been associated with a decrease in auditory fMRI activation.[45] To date, there is a paucity of brain imaging studies of improved auditory ability in clinical populations, for example, following surgical intervention, although one magnetoencephalography study has demonstrated a reorganization of the tonotopic map in HG following recovery from conductive hearing loss.[46]

Functional MRI has been used to measure the cortical representation of monaural and binaural sound stimulation in normally hearing and deaf groups. Due to the greater numbers of crossing than noncrossing fibers in the ascending pathways of the auditory system, monaural signals predominantly project to the contralateral hemisphere. Scheffler and colleagues[44] have shown that the extent of the auditory activation on the STG for monaural stimulation was approximately three to five times greater in the contralateral than in the ipsilateral hemisphere in 10 out of 10 normally hearing volunteers, whereas activation for binaural stimulation was almost balanced between the two hemispheres (Table 14.1). They further observed that the binaural activation was approximately one-third larger than the sum of both monaural components. This difference between monaural and binaural responses indicates binaural summation, probably as a result of interaural interaction at some level of the auditory pathway.

The pattern of brain responses to monaural stimulation in deaf patients is quite different and indicates reorganization either of the ascending input or its cortical representation. For all five patients with complete unilateral hearing loss reported by Scheffler and colleagues,[44] monaural stimulation of the healthy ear revealed a rather symmetrical pattern of bilateral activation on the STG (Table 14.1). Furthermore, the monaural activation pattern was comparable to that of binaural stimulation, indicating an absence of interaural summation for the binaural sounds. A similar pattern of monaural symmetry has been shown in a larger cohort of 14 patients with unilateral deafness.[47]

**Table 14.1. Mean Lateralization Ratios for 10 Normally Hearing Volunteers and 5 Monaural Deaf Patients***

| Stimulation paradigm | Lateralization ratio |
|---|---|
| **Normally hearing volunteers** | |
| Binaural | 1.3 ± 0.66 |
| Monaural left | 5.2 ± 3.1 |
| Monaural right | 3.4 ± 1.9 |
| **Monaural deaf patients** | |
| Binaural | 1.0 ± 0.56 |
| Monaural (healthy ear) | 1.3 ± 0.2 |
| Monaural (deaf ear) | – |

* Ratios are calculated using left–right for binaural stimulation and contralateral–ipsilateral for monaural stimulation. A lateralization ratio of 1.0 indicates symmetrical activation in the two hemispheres. Data reproduced from Scheffler K, Bilecen D, Schmid N, Tschopp K, Seelig J. Auditory cortical responses in hearing subjects and unilateral deaf patients as detected by functional magnetic resonance imaging. *Cerebr Cortex*. 1998;8:156–163. By permission of Oxford University Press.

The increase in the ipsilateral activation for monaural stimulation may be a general central auditory compensation process following reduced unilateral peripheral input. The precise neurophysiological mechanisms underlying functional plasticity are unknown, but one explanation is that ipsilateral connections, which are normally suppressed, become disinhibited when contralateral inhibitory inputs are removed. The time dependence of such changes has been explored in a single case using a repeated-measures design.[48] On initial fMRI testing, the patient had preserved bilateral hearing, but hearing was completely lost in the right ear after surgery for acoustic neuroma resection that destroyed the auditory nerve. For sounds presented to the left ear at four weeks before the surgery, the patient showed the normal pattern with greater activation in the contralateral auditory cortex. At one week after surgery, greater contralateral activation was still observed. However, after one year, the response to left ear stimulation was almost the same in both hemispheres (Figure 14.12). Again, as for the deaf patients reported above, the emergence of symmetry was largely the result of an increase in ipsilateral activity, rather than a decrease in contralateral activity.

## Tinnitus: Pathophysiology and Treatment Evaluation

Tinnitus is a phantom auditory sensation in either one ear, both ears, or the center of the head. Tinnitus occurs without any external physical representation that can be objectively measured. To date, psychophysical studies have estimated the perceptual properties of tinnitus, such as its pitch, loudness, spatial lateralization, and the type of effective maskers. Tinnitus patients cannot always achieve a satisfying match between tinnitus and external sounds, and psychophysical measures can vary over time. Tinnitus also has been related to clinical findings such as abnormalities of the audiogram, otoacoustic emissions, the cerebellopontine angle, or the soft tissues of the head or neck. Many cases of tinnitus can be associated with a disturbed cochlear function, like sudden-onset hearing loss or acoustic trauma, but a significant number of cases have no quantifiable cochlear dysfunction. The variability in etiology indicates that tinnitus may not have a single underlying basis. Although many researchers agree that the cochlear is the principal peripheral site involved in tinnitus, numerous findings suggest that central neural mechanisms also play a role in the generation and/or maintenance of tinnitus. Functional imaging has opened new possibilities for objectively measuring these neurophysiological and psychological effects of tinnitus. By comparing tinnitus patients with unaffected controls, brain imaging can identify the underlying pathophysiology associated with tinnitus. It is proposed that tinnitus can result from abnormal neural activity arising at some point along the auditory pathway, and these signals are interpreted as sound at a cortical level; for example, tinnitus may be accompanied by a reorganization of the tonotopic map in the auditory cortex caused by a loss of peripheral input within a particular frequency region of the cochlear. The psychological distress that is experienced as a result of tinnitus also may play a role in maintaining the auditory sensations. Brain imaging studies have identified a tinnitus-related network of areas involved in attention and emotional processing. This network includes prefrontal and parietal cortex and subcortical limbic structures. The attention-related processing can enhance the subjective perception of tinnitus that, in turn, increases the amount of attention that the patient gives to their tinnitus. This behavior may result in a vicious cycle of reinforcement that strengthens the tinnitus-related neuronal activity. In addition, the initial tinnitus can be perceived as an emotionally arousing stimulus that evokes a persistent negative emotional response.

The first neuroimaging study of tinnitus was published in 1996 using [$^{18}$F] deoxyglucose PET.[49] These findings showed an increased resting metabolic activity in the primary auditory cortex relative to non-tinnitus controls. Brain imaging has been applied more generally to tinnitus research using three classes of paradigm. Each paradigm applies a manipulation that modulates the loudness of the tinnitus percept, or suppresses the tinnitus, thus providing two experimental

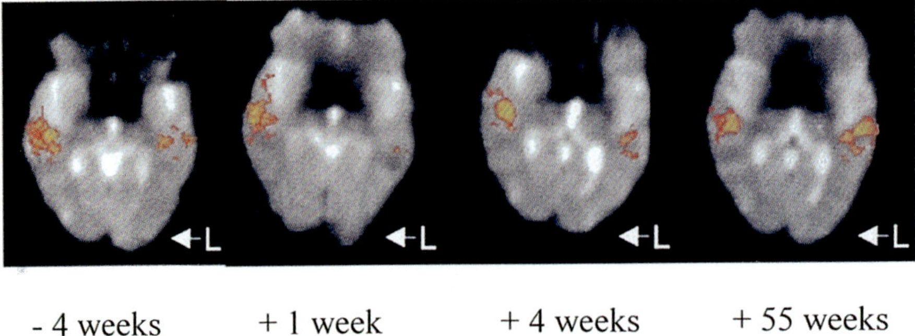


**Figure 14.12.** Auditory activation pattern evoked by unilateral (left) presentation of a one-kilohertz tone. Before surgery (at –4 weeks), a chiefly contralateral response pattern was found. After surgery, stimulation of the left healthy ear produced a progressively more-balanced bilateral activation pattern. Reprinted with permission from Bilecen D, Seifritz E, Radü EW, Schmid N, Setzel S, Probst R, Scheffler K. Cortical reorganization after acute unilateral hearing loss traced by fMRI. *Neurology*. 2000;54:765.[48]

conditions in which tinnitus-related differences in brain activation can be measured. One paradigm has used the fact that tinnitus can sometimes be influenced by performing overt behaviors in other sensory or motor domains, such as making oral facial movements or deviations in eye position, or by touching the hand. A second paradigm has been to modulate tinnitus using an acoustic masker and then to localize the corresponding changes in brain activity patterns. A third approach has quantified the outcome of pharmacological treatments, in particular, a potential tinnitus-suppressing drug, lidocaine, which acts as a local anesthetic agent. This broad range of research has been implemented using PET, magnetoencephalography, and fMRI techniques. Below, this work will be illustrated using three examples from the fMRI literature.

Cacace and colleagues reported two adults for whom cutaneous stimulation of the upper hand and fingertips evoked unilateral (left) tinnitus following neurosurgical intervention.[50] Hearing was somewhat impaired preoperatively, but postoperatively, hearing was completely lost on the operated side. Functional MRI involved a resting baseline condition and two movement tasks; one that elicited the tinnitus and one involving finger-to-thumb tapping that did not elicit tinnitus. One subject showed tinnitus-related activity in the left superior temporal cortex following right-handed cutaneous stimulation, plus contralateral motor and premotor activation, whereas left-handed finger tapping evoked only contralateral motor and premotor activation. These results demonstrate the role of central auditory processes in phantom auditory sensations, as well as implicating interactions between the auditory and somatosensory systems. Functional MRI was unsuccessful for the second patient because she was too nervous to comply with the task instructions and was unable to remain still. The difficulty of conducting fMRI with tinnitus patients who have a general elevated level of anxiety is a material problem.

Melcher and her colleagues hypothesized that patients with a lateralized tinnitus percept may show an abnormal asymmetrical pattern of activation that is related to the asymmetry of their tinnitus percept.[51] A masking noise was used to change the tinnitus loudness. The rationale for the experiments proposes that if tinnitus produces an elevated level of neural activity, then the activation evoked by an externally presented noise will be reduced relative to nontinnitus controls. The fMRI focused on the IC, rather than the cortex, because it is a major site of convergence for ascending and descending fibers in the auditory pathway, and both ICs can be imaged in a single slice (thus reducing the overall scanner noise dosage). The binaural sound produced abnormally asymmetric IC activation in four out of four lateralized tinnitus patients, which was not present in four out of four nontinnitus controls (see Figure 14.13A). Activation was weak in the IC contralateral, but not ipsilateral, to the tinnitus percept. The monaural sound also produced abnormally asymmetric activation in patients with lateralized tinnitus (see Figure 14.13B and C). For patients with tinnitus in the right ear, the sound presented to the right ear generated less contralateral activation than did the sound presented to the left ear. For nontinnitus

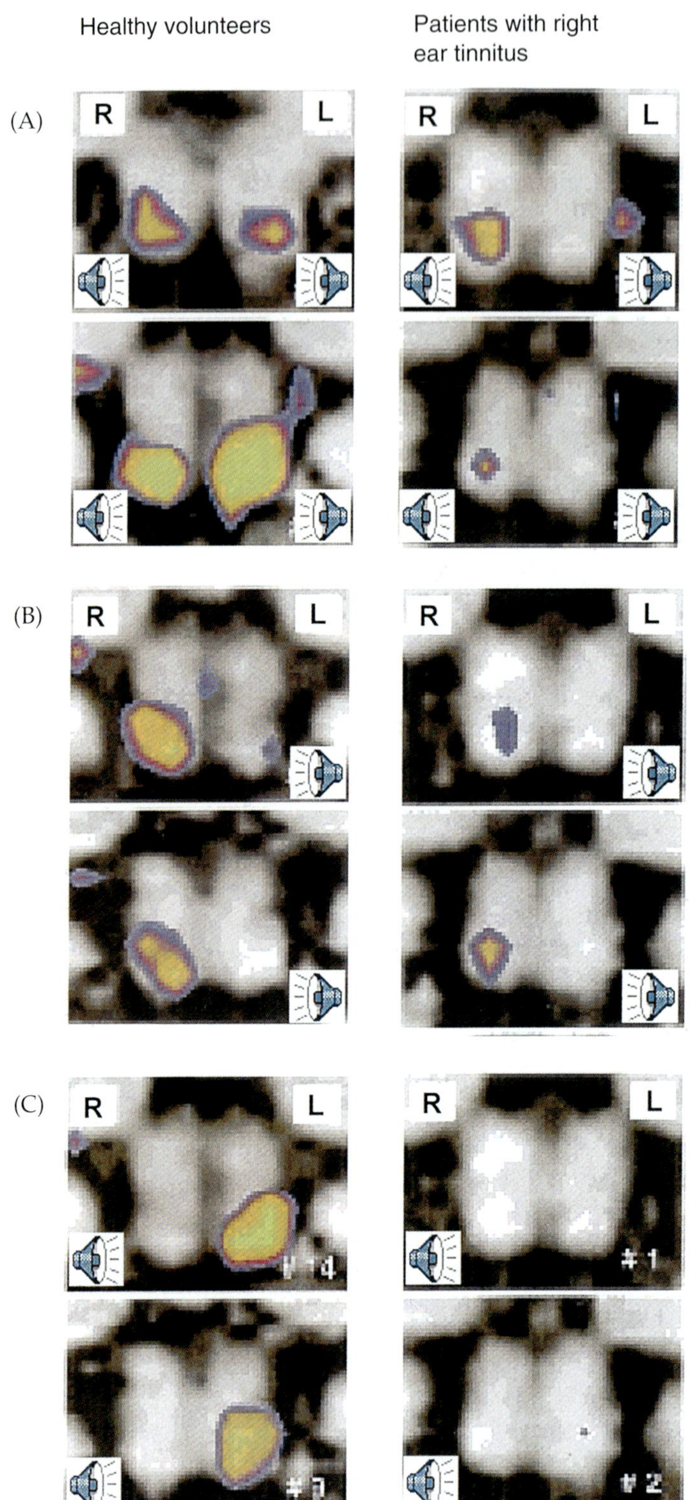


**Figure 14.13.** Inferior colliculus activation for binaural and monaural noise stimulation conditions in healthy volunteers and in patients with right ear tinnitus. Each panel shows an anatomical image of the IC for an individual subject and their superimposed activation map, thresholded at $P < 0.001$. Images are displayed in radiological convention, and the side of sound presentation is denoted by the schematic picture of the speaker. (A) Activation evoked by binaural noise; (B) activation evoked by left monaural stimulation; and (C) by right monaural stimulation. Reprinted with permission from Melcher JR, Sigalovsky IS, Guinan JJ, Levine RA. Lateralized tinnitus studied with functional magnetic resonance imaging: Abnormal inferior colliculus activation. *J Neurophysiol.* 2000;83:1058–1072.

controls, the sound evoked contralateral activation that was equivalent for both monaural sounds. Melcher and colleagues proposed first that the tinnitus percept corresponds to abnormally elevated neural activity that results in weak sound-evoked activation, and second, that the tinnitus percept is like an external sound in terms of its spatial representation of neural activity.[51] They drew an analogy between the lateralized tinnitus sensation and the percept of an external monaural sound, which, due to the dominant crossover organization of the ascending auditory pathway, both produce greater neural activity in the contralateral rather than the ipsilateral IC.

As brain imaging tells us more about the pathophysiology of tinnitus, it also can provide a quantitative measure for the effects of any treatments for tinnitus. Lidocaine is an experimental treatment that may give relief from tinnitus in approximately 60% of patients.[52] Lidocaine has a very short half-life, making the relief temporary, and is effective in injected rather than oral administration. Both these issues render the drug inappropriate for general clinical use. However, if the site of the drug's action can be determined, then those sites could be studied intensively in animals to understand the mechanisms by which lidocaine is effective. Drugs that act by similar mechanisms, but which are longer lasting and do not require intravenous administration, could then be developed. A preliminary fMRI study by Levine and Melcher[53] investigated the time course of lidocaine effects in a patient with right ear tinnitus (Figure 14.14). A baseline measure taken during binaural stimulation revealed that IC activation was abnormally weaker in the left (contralateral) hemisphere than in the right. Shortly after the injec-

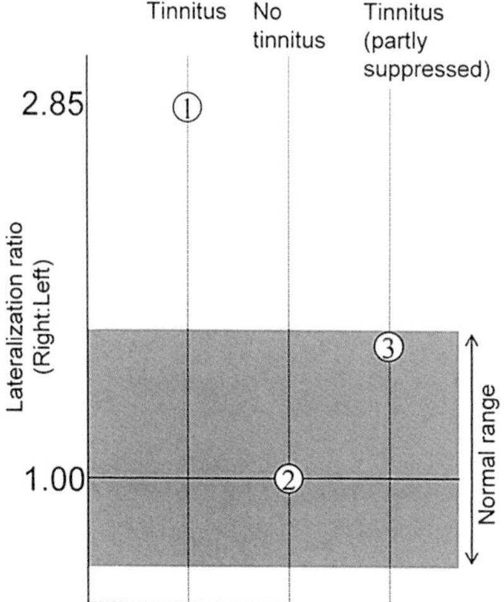


**Figure 14.14.** Lidocaine-suppressed tinnitus and the IC activation in a patient with left ear tinnitus in response to binaural stimulation. The lateralization ratio for activation in IC is plotted for three time intervals; (1) before the injection, (2) 15 to 30 minutes after the injection, and (3) 75 to 85 minutes after the injection. A lateralization ratio of 1.00 indicates symmetrical activation in the two hemispheres and is within the normal range. Adapted with permission from Levine RA, Melcher JR. Editorial: Imaging tinnitus. *J Audiol Med.* 2000;9:v–x.

tion of lidocaine, the patient's tinnitus percept was suppressed and IC activation during binaural stimulation had become normally symmetrical. As the effects of lidocaine wore off and the tinnitus was only partly suppressed, the asymmetry in IC activation reappeared. Thus, the pattern of activation in IC was shown to be directly coupled with the presence or absence of tinnitus.

### Cochlear Implantation: Assessment of Candidature and Evaluation of Hearing Recovery

A cochlear implant is an artificial hearing device for profoundly deaf people and is designed to produce useful auditory sensations by electrically stimulating the cochlear nerve. The system consists of an external microphone and a speech-processing and battery unit, which transmits its signal to an electrode array that is inserted into the cochlea of the inner ear. As has already been discussed, cochlear implants are not generally compatible with MRI; conseqeuntly, PET is generally the neuroimaging tool of choice in such studies. Positron emission tomography has been used to address two general questions (see Giraud and colleagues,[54] for a review). First, the effects of the preceding deafness on functional brain organization have been investigated by studying the effects of cochlear implantation on prelingually and postlingually deaf patients. Second, the manifestations of cortical reorganization after implant switch-on have been measured in the same patients imaged at different stages in their aural rehabilitation.

Functional MRI has also been used prior to implantation to evaluate whether brain imaging can provide an additional objective diagnostic tool for measuring the potential benefit of cochlear implantation in patients.[22,55–58] The basic requirements for a positive outcome of cochlear implantation are a sufficient number of spiral ganglion cells in the medial wall of the cochlear (where the implant electrode is placed), a functional auditory nerve, and an intact central auditory pathway. To assess the integrity of the neural pathway, and hence the potential for benefit from cochlear implantation, patients are sometimes tested preoperatively using direct electrical stimulation applied to the promontory of the cochlea to elicit the perception of auditory sensations. The test has several drawbacks. First, it is generally is conducted only with adults, not children. Second, electrical stimulation occurs some way away from the ganglion cells, and pain receptors may be stimulated before auditory receptors, leading to somewhat inconsistent results. It is possible that the patient cannot report a subjective auditory sensation, and yet their cochlear nerve is intact. Thus, the absence of a promontory response is not, by itself, a contraindication for cochlear implantation. Functional MRI mapping of the evoked auditory cortical response would provide an objective method of verifying the functional integrity of primary and/or nonprimary auditory cortical regions. Auditory cortical activation in deaf patients has so far been identified using both ear-canal[58] and transtympanic.[55–57] stimulation. Functional MRI mapping of direct electrical stimulation is not without technical challenge, as the electrodes that are routinely used in

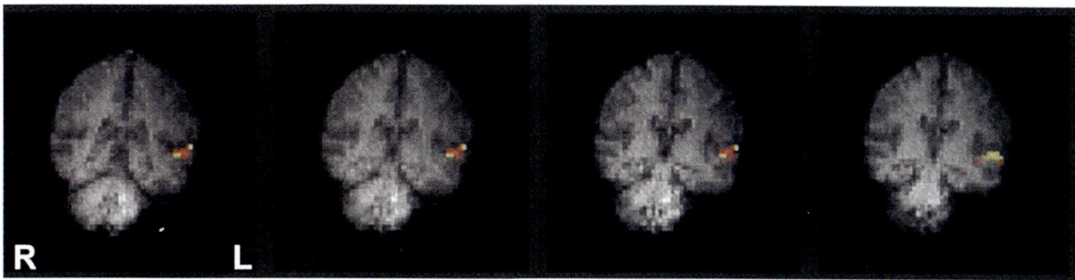


**Figure 14.15.** A 38-year-old man who had profound congenital hearing loss in both ears. A needle electrode was inserted through the tympanic membrane of the right ear and the functional activation map shown was obtained by *t*-test comparison between electrical stimulation and no stimulation conditions. Reprinted with permission from Alwatban AZ, Ludman CN, Mason SM, O'Donoghue GM, Peters AM, Morris PG. A method for the direct electrical stimulation of the auditory system in deaf subjects: A functional magnetic resonance imaging study. *J Magn Reson Imaging*. 2002;16:6–12.

clinical practice are ferromagnetic and the electrode currents can cause ipsilateral image artifacts (see Obler et al.,[22] for a discussion). These image artifacts can be eliminated by using a gold-plated tungsten electrode and carbon fiber cables, thus enabling the imaging of both hemispheres.[55] The fMRI results indicate that monaural stimulation activates the contralateral auditory cortex only (see Figure 14.15). Schmidt and colleagues[56] estimated that fMRI can detect auditory cortical activation in approximately 85% of patients who reported auditory sensations; consequently fMRI may aid the decision for or against an implant and with the decision on which side to place the implant (Figure 14.16).

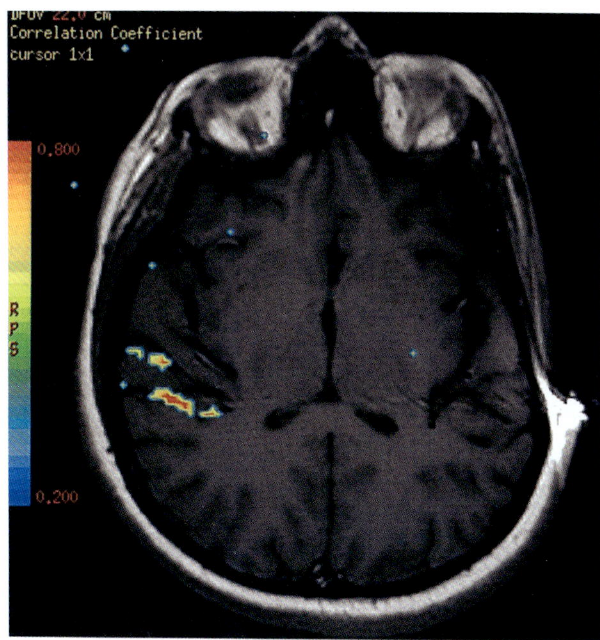


**Figure 14.16.** A 31-year-old woman with congenital blindness exhibited progressive and profound hearing loss since age 12. Promontory testing revealed weak but positive responses at 50, 100, and 200 hertz. Stimulating the left ear elicited a large activation in the vicinity of the secondary auditory cortex on the right side. Implantation was carried out on the left ear with a satisfactory outcome. Reprinted from *Neuroimaging Clinics of North America*, Vol. 11, Schmidt Am, Weber BP, Becker H. Functional magnetic resonance imaging of the auditory cortex as a diagnostic tool in cochlear implant candidates. 2000;11:297–304. Copyright © 2000, with permission from Elsevier.

## Future Applications

To date, auditory fMRI has not been widely implemented for routine clinical purposes. However, with the rapid evolution in commercial MR technology and its decreasing cost, more hospitals are becoming equipped with imaging facilities that have functional capabilities. In addition, solutions to the technical challenges involved in fMRI are being implemented in commercial MR systems. For example, several manufacturers offer MR systems in which the gradient coil noise is attenuated by dampening foam and vacuum-sealed gradient coils. When combined with ear protection, these methods provide an effective reduction of the scanner sound at source, thus increasing patient comfort, as well as enhancing the detectability of sound-evoked brain activation for auditory fMRI. Further improvements will be gained using active control of the scanner acoustic noise to additionally reduce the scanner sound at the ear.[33] Active noise cancellation can be incorporated into electronic systems that are now available for presenting high-fidelity, calibrated sounds in the high magnetic field of the MR scanner. An understanding of the underlying human auditory cortical anatomy also will allow greater precision in identifying the pattern of auditory activation (e.g., in terms of distinguishing primary from nonprimary activated regions). This is a necessary step for interpreting the clinical imaging data in an informative and meaningful way.

The high magnetic field still poses a problem for scanning patients with brain implant devices. Whereas this obviates fMRI measures of hearing in cochlear implantees, fMRI has the potential to be a useful diagnostic tool preimplantation. In cases when the results from promontory testing are not sufficiently compelling to guide clinical judgements, fMRI can aid the decision to choose the better ear for implantation. For patients with multiple sensory impairments such as congenital blindness and acquired deafness, or for patients with congenital deafness, fMRI can be used to evaluate the degree of any functional brain reorganization of the auditory cortex that may have occurred early in life to ensure that acoustical stimulation activates the auditory cortex and that the representation of visual stimuli has not taken over. Technical advances to eliminate the image artifacts caused by the needle stimulation protocol will permit future fMRI research to measure both ipsilateral and contralateral activations in the auditory cortex.

Because volunteers can be scanned safely on multiple occasions, fMRI will prove to be an invaluable clinical tool for measuring changes in the spatial pattern of auditory activation as a result of a change in the patient's auditory experience. Further work will provide more detail about the reorganization of the auditory system that occurs as a result of hearing loss. While recruitment of the auditory cortex ipsilateral to the monaural stimulation has been described,[44,47,48] whether this functional plasticity is restricted to the cortex or whether it arises in brainstem and midbrain auditory nuclei is not fully understood.

The time course of this reorganization is also an important issue. Immediate reorganization of auditory networks indicates some redundancy within the normal system, where new regions can undertake novel processing requirements. In contrast, slower changes indicate different recovery mechanisms, perhaps mediated by physiological adaptations within the neural system. Finer temporal sampling of the fMRI measures over weeks rather than months is required to determine more precisely the nature of cortical reorganization, and also to ascertain whether the time course of cortical reorganization is mirrored or preceded by any reorganization within the brainstem and midbrain nuclei.

Functional MRI has several promising future applications in tinnitus research because it provides the only objective and quantitative measure of the phantom auditory sensations. Functional imaging may provide some insight into the physiological basis of tinnitus and how this relates to the type of percept; for example, whether lateralized tinnitus has an asymmetrical auditory representation throughout the auditory system. A range of tinnitus treatments are available (using acoustic, psychological, pharmacological, and even surgical techniques), but no single type of therapy is effective for the majority of patients. The effect of specific treatments for alleviating tinnitus could be investigated by scanning the same patients across numerous sessions, before, during, and after treatment. As well as providing new objective criteria for distinguishing potential subtypes of tinnitus, functional imaging may elucidate whether certain subtypes of tinnitus respond better to particular treatments; for example, psychological treatments may be most effective for those patients whose tinnitus-related activation involves attention- and emotion-processing networks. The development of new treatments can be informed by fMRI research; for example, fMRI could identify the sites of action of lidocaine in the human brain, and those sites could then be studied using other techniques in animals to understand the mechanism of action of the drug. Alternative drugs that act by similar mechanisms, but are longer lasting and do not require intravenous administration, could then be developed. Another potential use for fMRI is as a biological marker for tinnitus in animals to explore animal models of tinnitus. Animal models are important because they can be used to study tinnitus in ways that are not possible in humans, but a limitation in this field has been the lack of an objective validation that an animal actually experiences tinnitus. Although at an early stage, the development of auditory fMRI in animals opens possibilities of using this imaging tool to determine whether the animal shows tinnitus-related brain activation and to identify the pattern of that activation.

## References

1. Kaas JH, Hackett TA. Subdivisions of auditory cortex and levels of processing in primates. *Audiol Neurootol.* 1998;3:73–85.

2. Kaas JH, Hackett TA. Subdivisions of auditory cortex and processing streams in primates. *Proc Natl Acad Sci.* 2000;97:11793–11799.
3. Galaburda AM, Sanides F. Cytoarchitectonic organisation of the human auditory cortex. *J Comp Neurol.* 1980;221:169–184.
4. Rivier F, Clarke S. Cytochrome oxidase, acetylcholinesterase, and NADPH-diaphorase staining in human supratemporal and insular cortex: evidence for multiple auditory areas. *Neuroimage.* 1997;6:288–304.
5. Wallace MN, Johnston PW, Palmer AR. Histochemical identification of cortical areas in the auditory region of the human brain. *Exp. Brain Res.* 2002;143:499–508.
6. Rauschecker JP, Tian B, Hauser M. Processing of complex sounds in the macaque nonprimary auditory cortex. *Science.* 1995;268:111–114.
7. Rauschecker JP, Tian B, Pons T, Mishkin M. Serial and parallel processing in rhesus monkey auditory cortex. *J Comp Neurol.* 1997;382:89–103.
8. Merzenich MM, Brugge JF. Representation of the cochlear partition on the superior temporal plane of the macaque monkey. *Brain Res.* 1973;50: 275–296.
9. Morel A, Garraghty PE, Kaas JH. Tonotopic organisation, architectonic fields, and connections of auditory cortex in macaque monkeys. *J Comp Neurol.* 1993;335:437–459.
10. Morosan P, Rademacher J, Schleicher A, Amunts K, Schormann T, Zilles K. Human primary auditory cortex: Cytoarchitectonic subdivisions and mapping into a spatial reference system. *Neuroimage.* 2001;13:684–701.
11. Recanzone GH. Spatial processing in the auditory cortex of the macaque monkey. *Proc Natl Acad Sci.* 2000;97:11829–11835.
12. Rauschecker JP, Tian B. Mechanisms and streams for processing of "what" and "where" in auditory cortex. *Proc Natl Acad Sci.* 2000;97:11800–11806.
13. Tian B, Reser D, Durham A, Kustov A, Rauschecker JP. Functional specialisation in rhesus monkey auditory cortex. *Science.* 2001;292:290–293.
14. Guimaraes AR, Melcher JR, Talavage TM, Baker JR, Ledden P, Rosen BR, Kiang NYS, Fullerton BC, Weiskoff RM. Imaging subcortical auditory activity in humans. *Hum Brain Mapp.* 1998;6:33–41.
15. Melcher JR, Sigalovsky IS, Guinan JJ, Levine RA. Lateralised tinnitus studied with functional magnetic resonance imaging: Abnormal inferior colliculus activation. *J Neurophysiol.* 2000;83:1058–1072.
16. Griffiths TD, Uppenkamp S, Johnsrude I, Josephs O, Patterson RD. Encoding of the temporal regularity of sound in the human brainstem. *Nature Neurosci.* 2001;4:633–637.
17. Howard MA, Volkov IO, Abbas PJ, Damasio H, Ollendieck MC, Granner MA. A chronic microelectrode investigation of the tonotopic organisation of human auditory cortex. *Brain Res.* 1996;724:260–264.
18. Lütkenhöner B, Steinsträter O. High-precision neuromagnetic study of the functional organisation of the human auditory cortex. *Audiol Neurootol.* 1998;3:191–213.
19. Talavage TM, Ledden PJ, Benson RR, Rosen BR, Melcher JR. Frequency-dependent responses exhibited by multiple regions in human auditory cortex. *Hearing Res.* 2000;150:225–244.
20. Palmer AR, Bullock DC, Chambers JD. A high-output, high-quality sound system for use in auditory fMRI. *Neuroimage.* 1998;7:S359.
21. Baumgart F, Kaulisch T, Tempelmann C, Gaschler-Markefski B, Tegeler C, Schindler F, Stiller D, Scheich H. Electrodynamic headphones and woofers

for application in magnetic resonance imaging scanners. *Med Phys.* 1998;25:2068–2070.

22. Obler R, Köstler H, Weber B-P, Mack KF, Becker B. Safe electrical stimulation of the cochlear nerve at the promontory during functional magnetic resonance imaging. *Magn Reson Med.* 1999;42:371–378.
23. Heller JW, Brackmann DE, Tucci DL, Nyenhuis JA, Chou C-K. Evaluation of MRI compatibility of the modified nucleus multichannel auditory brainstem and cochlear implants. *Am J Otol.* 1996;17:724–729.
24. Weber BP, Neuberger J, Battmer RD, Lenarz T. Magnetless cochlear implant: relevance of adult experience for children. *Am J Otol.* 1997;18: S50–S51.
25. Chou CK, McDougall JA, Chan KW. Absence of radiofrequency heating from auditory implants during magnetic resonance imaging. *Bioelectromagnetics.* 1995;16:307–316.
26. Shellock FG, Morisoli S, Kanal E. MR procedures and biomedical implants, materials and devices: 1993 update. *Radiology.* 1993;189:587–599.
27. Shellock FG, Ziarati M, Atkinson D, Chen D-Y. Determination of gradient magnetic field-induced acoustic noise associated with the use of echo planar and three-dimensional fast spin echo techniques. *J Magn Reson Imaging.* 1998;8:1154–1157.
28. Harms MP, Melcher JR. Sound repetition rate in the human auditory pathway: representations in the waveshape and amplitude of fMRI activation. *J Neurophysiol.* 2002;88:1433–1450.
29. Foster JR, Hall DA, Summerfield AQ, Palmer AR, Bowtell RW. Sound-level measurements and calculations of safe noise dosage during EPI at 3T. *J Magn Reson Imaging.* 2000;12:157–163.
30. Bandettini PA, Jesmanowicz A, Van Kylen J, Birn RA, Hyde J. Functional MRI of brain activation induced by scanner acoustic noise. *Magn Reson Med.* 1998;39:410–416.
31. Talavage TM, Edmister WB, Ledden PJ, Weisskoff RM. Quantitative assessment of auditory cortex responses induced by imager acoustic noise. *Hum Brain Mapp.* 1999;7:79–88.
32. Ravicz ME, Melcher JR, Kiang NYS. Acoustic noise during functional magnetic resonance imaging. *J Acoust Soc Am.* 2000;108:1683–1696.
33. Chambers J, Akeroyd MA, Summerfield AQ, Palmer AR. Active control of the volume acquisition noise in functional magnateic resonance imaging: Method and psychoacoustical investigation. *J Acoust Soc Am.* 2001;110: 3041–3054.
34. Mansfield P, Chapman BLW, Bowtell R, Glover P, Coxon R, Harvey PR. Active acoustic screening: reduction of noise in gradient coils by Lorentz force balancing. *Magn Reson Med.* 1995;33:276–281.
35. Bowtell R, Mansfield P. Quiet transverse gradient coils: Lorentz force balanced designs using geometric similitude. *Magn Reson Med.* 1995;34: 494–497.
36. Price DL, De Wilde JP, Papadaki AM, Curran JS, Kitney RI. Investigation of acoustic noise on 15 MRI scanners from 0.2 T to 3 T. *J Magn Reson Imaging.* 2001;13:288–293.
37. Hedeen RA, Edelstein WA. Characterisation and prediction of gradient acoustic noise in MR imagers. *Magn Reson Med.* 1997;37:7–10.
38. Hennel F, Girard F, Loenneker T. "Silent" MRI with soft gradient pulses. *Magn Reson Med.* 1999;42:6–10.
39. Scheich H, Baumgart F, Gashler-Markefski B, Tegeler C, Templemann C, Heinze HJ, Schindler F, Stiller D. Functional magnetic resonance imaging

of a human auditory cortex area involved in foreground–background decomposition. *Eur J Neurosci.* 1998;10:803–809.

40. Hall DA, Summerfield AQ, Gonçalves MS, Foster JR, Palmer AR, Bowtell RW. Time-course of the auditory BOLD response to scanner noise. *Magn Reson Med.* 2000;43:601–606.
41. Edmister WB, Talavage TM, Ledden PJ, Weisskoff RM. Improved auditory cortex imaging using clustered volume acquisitions. *Hum Brain Mapp.* 1999; 7:89–97.
42. Hall DA, Haggard MP, Akeroyd MA., Palmer AR, Summerfield AQ, Elliott MR Gurney E, Bowtell RW. Sparse temporal sampling in auditory fMRI. *Hum Brain Mapp.* 1999;7:213–223.
43. Belin P, Zatorre RJ, Hoge R, Evans AC, Pike B. Event-related fMRI of auditory cortex. *Neuroimage.* 1999;10:417–429.
44. Scheffler K, Bilecen D, Schmid N, Tschopp K, Seelig J. Auditory cortical responses in hearing subjects and unilateral deaf patients as detected by functional magnetic resonance imaging. *Cerebr Cortex.* 1998;8:156–163.
45. Jäncke L, Gaab N, Wüstenberg T, Scheich H, Heinze HJ. Short-term functional plasticity in the human auditory cortex: an fMRI study. *Cogn Brain Res.* 2001;12:479–485.
46. Tecchio F, Bicciolo G, De Campora E, Pasqualetti P, Pizzella V, Indovina I, Cassetta E, Romani GL, Rossini PM. Tonotopic cortical changes following stapes substitution in otosclerotic patients: a magnetoencephalographic study. *Hum Brain Mapp.* 2000;10:28–38.
47. Tschopp K, Schillinger C, Schmid N, Rausch M, Bilecen D, Scheffler K. Evidence of central auditory compensation in unilateral deaf patients detected by functional MRI. *Laryngorhinootol.* 2000;79:753–757.
48. Bilecen, D, Seifritz E, Radü EW, Schmid N, Wetzel S, Probst R, Scheffler K. Cortical reorganization after acute unilateral hearing loss traced by fMRI. *Neurology.* 2000;54:765.
49. Arnold W, Bartenstein P, Oestreicher E, Römer W, Schwaiger M. Focal metabolic activation in the predominant left auditory cortex in patients suffering from tinnitus: A PET study with [$^{18}$F]deoxyglucose. *ORL J Otorhinolaryngol Relat Spec.* 1996;58:195–199.
50. Cacace AT, Cousins JP, Parnes SM, Semenoff D, Holmes T, McFarland DJ, Davenport C, Stegbauer K, Lovely TJ. Cutaneous-evoked tinnitus.1. Phenomenology, psychophysics and functional imaging. *Audiol Neurootol.* 1999;4:247–257.
51. Melcher JR, Sigalovsky IS, Guinan JJ, Levine RA. Lateralized tinnitus studied with functional magnetic resonance imaging: Abnormal inferior colliculus activation. *J Neurophysiol.* 2000;83:1058–1072.
52. Schmidt H, Davis A, Stasche N, Hormann K. The lidocaine test in the determination of tinnitus—evaluation of results. *HNO.* 1994;42:677–684.
53. Levine RA, Melcher JR. Editorial: Imaging tinnitus. *J Audiol Med.* 2000; 9:v–x.
54. Giraud AL, Truy E, Frackowiak R. Imaging plasticity in cochlear implant patients. *Audiol Neurootol.* 2001;6:381–393.
55. Alwatban AZ, Ludman CN, Mason SM, O'Donoghue GM, Peters AM, Morris PG. A method for the direct electrical stimulation of the auditory system in deaf subjects: A functional magnetic resonance imaging study. *J Magn Reson Imaging.* 2002;16:6–12.
56. Schmidt AM, Weber, BP, Becker, H. Functional magnetic resonance imaging of the auditory cortex as a diagnostic tool in cochlear implant candidates. *Neuroimaging Clin N Am.* 2001;11:297–304.

57. Berthezène Y, Truy E, Morgon A, Giard HM, Hermier M, Franconi JM, Froment JC. Auditory cortex activation in deaf subjects during cochlear electrical stimulation. *Invest Radiol.* 1997;32:297–301.
58. Hofmann E, Preibisch C, Knaus C, Muller J, Kremser C, Teissl C. Noninvasive direct stimulation of the cochlear nerve for functional MR imaging of the auditory cortex. *Am J Neuroradiol.* 1999;20:1970–1972.

# 15

# Pediatric Applications of fMRI

Nolan R. Altman and Byron Bernal

## Introduction

Magnetic resonance imaging (MRI), which is generated from the protons of the body, has provided a new perspective and detail of the anatomy of the body, and particularly of the brain and spinal cord. Anatomic images not previously possible were obtained by this procedure with high spatial resolution and without the risk of ionizing radiation. Functional magnetic resonance imaging (fMRI) using the BOLD technique has provided major advances in the evaluation of the child, particularly in the exploration of human brain function.

Functional studies have evolved from the electroencephalogram (EEG), which is a graphic representation of the electrocortical activity of the brain, to exams that show regional increase of blood flow or metabolism related to a given task. Positron emission tomography (PET), single-photon emission computed tomography (SPECT), and functional magnetic resonance imaging (fMRI) are examples of these procedures. The advent of these tools allowed clinicians to see brain function. Electroecephalography and evoked potentials provided graphic information related to changes in time domain. Functional MRI, PET, and SPECT provide images with information in the space domain.

Positron emission tomography and SPECT are based on ionizing radiation, and therefore carry risks and limitations for research. In 1936, Linus Carl Pauling[1] discovered that deoxyhemoglobin had paramagnetic characteristics. Kwong and colleagues[2] described how this feature can be utilized to provide endogenous contrast in MRI procedures, coining the acronym BOLD (blood oxygen level-dependant) to describe the technique. Subtle changes yielded by local activity of brain cortex coupled to a functional motor, sensory, or cognitive tasks were revealed.

Functional MRI has been utilized to investigate numerous aspects of brain function from the most simple motor tasks to complex cognitive functions involved with memory in recognition of faces, exploration of language reception and expression, calculation, spatial perception, and psychiatric disorders. The mapping of motor and cognitive functions for presurgical planning with fMRI is gaining an important role in the adult and pediatric patient.

The unique role of fMRI in the pediatric patient has the potential for the investigation of normal neurologic development. Functional MRI demonstrates the regions of brain activation involved in cognition and will potentially lead to an understanding of the development of language and learning. The connectivity in relationship to the maturational stages of white matter, cortical pruning, brain plasticity, and normal brain asymmetry also will be studied.

Functional MRI shows promise in the investigation and follow up of children with a variety of neurological and psychiatric disorders. These include autism, dyslexia, speech delay, and attention deficit hyperactive disorder (ADHD). These disorders have challenged medicine because no definitive or typical anatomical changes in the brain have been described. Cortical or sub-cortical volumetric analysis have shown subtle differences in patients with ADHD, dyslexia, and autism,[3–5] but these changes do not demonstrate a relationship to the degree of the disease or offer a predictive value of the condition. New insights gained from fMRI may one day result in better diagnoses and monitoring of treatments of these conditions.

In children, elucidation of the relationship between neural development, brain maturation, connectivity, and cortical organization is crucial to understanding normal development and the response of the brain to injury. Children undergo many changes in the first few years of life. The brain increases in volume in the first five years to 95% of the adult size.[6,7] Myelination is almost completed by the end of the second year.[8,9] The brain synapse number peaks around eight months of age and is followed by selective synaptic regression in which sprouts are pruned until the age of 16 years.[10] Begining at birth, the number of neurons significantly decrease in number with time. At the age of 19 months, neurons are reduced to less than one-third of that which we are born with.[11] These dynamic structural changes result in higher metabolism in the younger brain, which peaks at three to four years, and reaches adult levels by the end of the second decade.[12] This is the reason that blood volume is higher and the vascular response is greater in children. Children activate between 60% and 400% more voxels than adults using standard fMRI postprocessing techniques.[13,14]. This difference is related to an increased metabolism in children, resulting in better signal-to-noise ratio of the activated voxels.[13] The finding that stimulants such as d-amphetamine increases voxel activation seems to support this.[15] The increase of activation takes place without changes of onset time, rise, and peak amplitude of the hemodynamic response.[14] Children, however, are similar to adults in the variance of the MR signal.[16] These neurobiological facts influence brain activation in children; for example, language tasks in children generate a greater number of activated voxels and frequently bilateral activation compared with adults.[17]

Changes in neuronal population, synapse density, and myelin stage may partially explain age-related differences. Other changes include intra-subject variations that, in part, are due to the normal maturation of myeline. Myelination of the human brain proceeds from inferior to superior, posterior to anterior, from central loci to the lobar poles, and proximal to distal pathways.[18] The frontal lobes mature in the last stages of myelination (after five years of age), which may explain the finding of hypofrontality in children and adolescents.[19] The right frontal lobe seems to mature first.[19,20] Synapse accretion and pruning proceeds at different rates from region to region. It peaks at eight months in the visual cortex, and at four years in auditory and frontal cortices.[21] Despite that pruning peaks at these ages, an adult pattern may be acquired at earlier ages; for example, the auditory cortex has an adult pattern in the infant. The frontal lobes will acquire an adult pattern by the third or fourth month of life.[21] In contrast, the visual cortex shows a different pattern of activation in children between seven weeks and five to seven years, and this is mostly likely related to maturational milestones. These children show negative BOLD signal in the anterior area of the visual cortex coupled with the stimulus frequency.

Maturational changes start at birth, but very little is known of newborn brain function. This paucity of data is due to the constrains of the fMRI environment, which requires complete motion restriction. In infants and small children, sedation is often required, and the medications may have a direct effect on cerebral blood flow (CBF) and cortical metabolism.

## fMRI Technical Challenges in Children

### Overview

The feasibility of performing fMRI in children has been debated. However, it has currently gained acceptance at major children's centers worldwide. Special considerations and constraints must be evaluated in the performance of these exams in children.

As in anatomic imaging, patient motion is a significant challenge in the fMRI examination of children. The imaging usually takes several minutes per task, and the postprocessing methods used require minimal motion for accurate results. Based on previous pediatric radiology experience and of over 500 fMRI paradigms applied in children at Miami Children's Hospital, it is felt that children younger than five years usually can not perform the exam without sedation. Children between five and seven years of age with appropriate training may be successful in completing a short study of five to ten minutes, and those between seven and nine years of age may tolerate a longer exam. Children older than nine years of age usually will cooperate to allow four to six paradigms, plus the anatomical sequences required for co-registration. Girls tend to stay still longer than do boys. As with all exams, there are some children that, despite careful instruction and preparation, still cannot perform the study. These numbers are higher in the child who is mentally challenged. Postprocessing motion correction is only helpful with motion less than three to four millimeters.

Study design in children is also critical. Areas of activation result from technical factors such as T2* effect; magnetic field stength and methods of statistical postprocessing, however, can be equally affected by the subject's education and skillfulness. Activation is lower when the task is too easy or too difficult.[22] Increased difficulty and practice alter the magnitude of signal and pattern of activation; for example, a subject who activated the left inferior frontal gyrus in a verb-generation task may show a change of the activation toward the anterior aspect of the insula if the same task is practiced.[23] This variability of brain activation has implications on study design, application, and interpretation when performing fMRI in children. The more complicated the study, the more likely it will be to obtain spurious activation. Varying the rate of presentation of a stimulus may produce a region-specific parametric response.[24] Response may be seen in a step-like function, as in Wernicke's Area in response to real versus nonsense words.[24]

These concerns are more relevant in research than in clinical exams. In clinical cases, it is best to keep the tasks as simple as possible because children may get confused when complexities are added to the paradigms. Attempts to control too many variables may subtract out activation in brain regions critical for a target function.[22] There may be a trade-off between varying the task to match the patient performance and keeping the task simple. For clinical purposes, the preference is to keep the task constant. Degree of task difficulty must be considered with different ages and a practical approach has been taken using two or three paradigms with different degrees of difficulty depending on the child's ability. Passive paradigms allow the most consistency and are included when feasible.

## Patient Movement

A significant challenge in evaluation of children with fMRI is patient movement. Children have great difficulty remaining still in the MRI magnet.[25] This is a demanding proactive function requiring working memory to store the command, frontal inhibition, and ability to monitor small body movements. The bore of the magnet is a confining space and may be frightening to children. Each child undergoes an evaluation before the exam to determine their ability to cooperate. This is best accomplished by the use of a simulator that consists of a mock-up of the magnet using an MRI table, head coil, magnet housing, and any hardware specific to the task, such as earphones, video screen, or finger buttons (Figure 15.1). Taped scanner noise also can be added. Electronic devices that track head movement have been coupled to video projectors, setting up a feedback in which head movement beyond a given threshold turns off the video display. The child learns how to control head movement as the tolerance for the feedback is narrowed.[26] Use of these techniques greatly improves the likelihood of successful exams.[27] Training is also given of the requested task to guarantee understanding and performance.

Immobilization aids used are bite bars, external cushions, and tape. The bite bar is uncomfortable, resulting in poor tolerance by the chil-

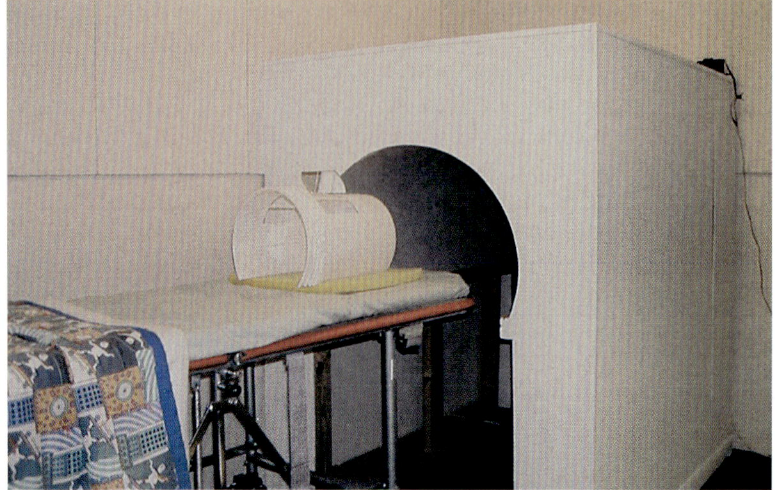

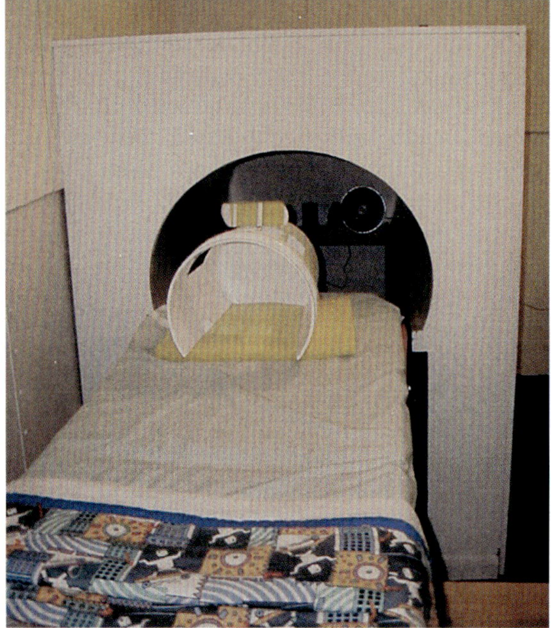

**Figure 15.1.** Picture of a mock scanner. (Courtesy of Dr. Jill Hunter)

dren. The head holder is packed with cushions surrounding the head and support is provided with cloth medical tape between the borders of the head holder and forehead. This results in a somatosensory feedback of the forehead skin, resulting in easier detection by the child of head motion. Despite training and immobilization, motion can not usually be controlled in children less than seven years of age. Sedation may be required with concomitant use of passive paradigms. Neonates and sleep-deprived children may be examined sleeping; however, this technique is limited.

## Sedation

Sedation has been successfully utilized in pediatric fMRI studies.[27–32] Pentobarbital is the most commonly used sedative, followed by chloral hydrate. The paradigms used are limited to presentation of light, sounds, human voice, rubbing of the skin, or passive movement of the hand or foot. Light is delivered through the closed eyes, most frequently by goggles directly placed over the eyelids. Sounds vary from tones to a mother's voice.

There appears to be an age-related pattern with visual activation. The expected positive BOLD response is seen in the occipital cortex of infants less than four to seven weeks that are sleeping or sedated.[29] Children over two months of age show a negative BOLD response to presentation of light. This occurs along the anterior aspect of the calcarine fissure (Figure 15.2). In some cases, there may be concomitantly positive and negative voxels of activation in the visual cortex.[30] The negative BOLD response of the visual cortex is not well understood. Some researchers feel that this is due entirely to an age factor of oxygen metabolism and vasculariity along the visual cortex, whereas others feel that this may be due to the effects of sedation. According to the BOLD mechanism, a reduction in signal may be related to local decrease of cerebral blood flow (CBF), increase of deoxyhemoglobin, relative decrease of oxyhemoglobin, or a sum of these. Measurement of blood flow done in children performing the visual task with near infrared spectroscopy shows that deoxyhemoglobin and oxyhemoglobin increase with photic stimulation.[33] This suggests that increased

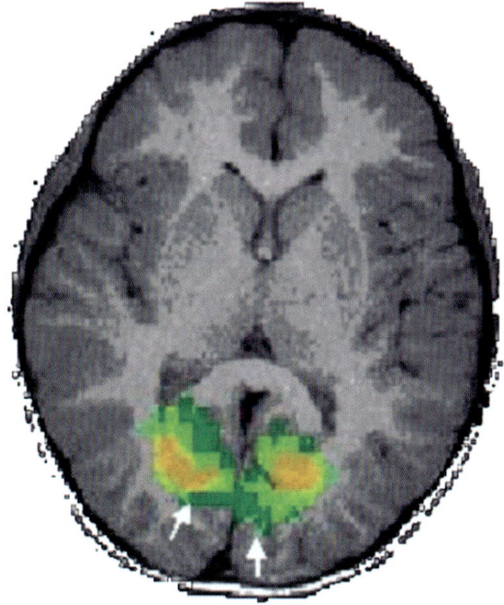

**Figure 15.2.** Visual activation. Axial fMRI images of a sedated child that demonstrate activation along the anterior calcarine cortex (white arrows).

local metabolism on an immature vascular response cannot provide the same increase in blood flow as a mature vasculature.

Negative BOLD response has been reported to be due to sedation or sleeping state. A recent study was performed that examined 10 adults who underwent fMRI with photic stimulation during sleep and monitored with EEG.[34] A control group of patients underwent a PET study under waking and sleep conditions to determine the regional CBF. A BOLD signal decrease during visual stimulation was found in the anterior visual cortex in five of six examinations in sleeping patients. The PET demonstrated regional CBF decrease in the same area in control sleeping subjects. This study suggests that the negative response of the anterior visual cortex in sedated and sleeping patients may be related to the loss of alertness.

Thus, it is not clear if the change from positive BOLD to negative BOLD observed at seven to eight weeks of age reflects a change in the state of alertness or response of the visual cortex. Auditory activation in nonsedated newborns results in negative BOLD response,[35] indicating a dissociated specific age-related pattern of reaction between visual and auditory systems.

Other studies disagree with this claim. No statistical differences in the fMRI responses of sedated and nonsedated infants were documented by Martin and colleagues.[36] A positive BOLD response has been shown in 10 newborns less than five weeks of age despite the fact that they were sedated with pentobarbital.[28] A negative BOLD response has been demonstrated in the visual cortex and a positive BOLD response in the auditory cortex in sedated children.[30]

Other difficulties of sedation are the inconsistency in the response of the child to the medication. The authors have had their best results with single drug protocols and preforming the fMRI exam at the start of the imaging session.

## Image Processing

### Motion Correction

Sedated cases, and those patients with motion less than 20% of the voxel inplane diameter, do not require motion correction. Postprocessing motion-correction tools and surface algorithms may correct for patient motion not task correlated. When there is a movement associated with the task (Graph 15.1), the correction is very difficult and most of these algorithms fail. Inclusion of motion parameters in the statistical postprocessing often results in a decrease of the overall level of activation, although an increase may be observed when motion is random and not correlated with the task.[25]

### Spatial Normalization

Due to the intrinsic variability of the maturing brain, pediatric fMRI studies require group comparisons with other child groups that may be normal, abnormal, or of different age. Comparison may be per-

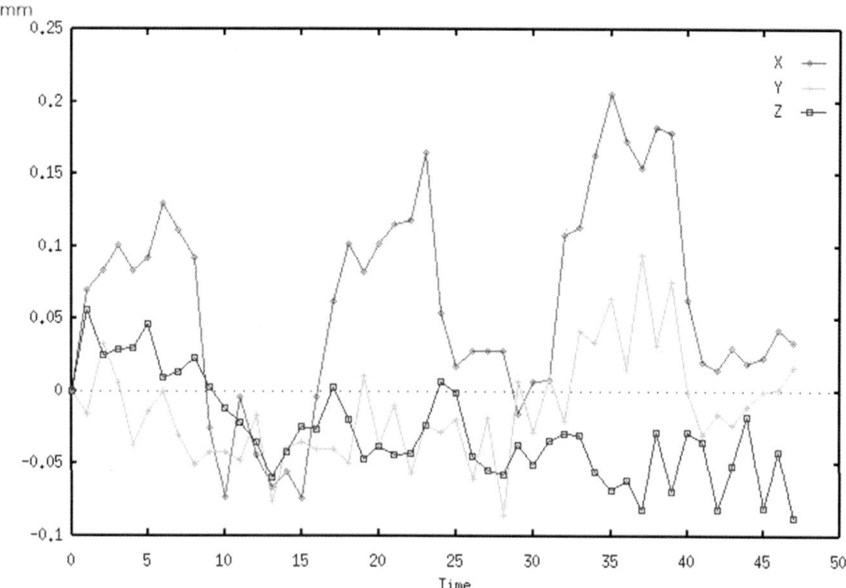


**Graph 15.1.** Motor task-related phasic movement. Graph of patient head motion in the three orthogonal axes: $x$ (red), $y$ (green), and $z$ (blue). $Y$ axis scale is in millimeters; $X$ axis is in timepoints (TP). Patient is performing a tapping task with the right hand. The paradigm consists of 48 TP (TP 0 is the first), starting in OFF and switching every 8 timepoints. The graph shows weak phasic movement, less than 0.2 millimeters in the $x$ axis (red). Changes are seen at 8, 16, 24, 32, and 40 timepoints, correlating the paradigm frequency. This produces a spurious activation and ring-shaped artifacts that are difficult to correct with postprocessing.

formed on the basis of anatomical landmarks; however, many investigators prefer to use a stereotactic three-dimensional (3D) template. This procedure is called spatial normalization and requires a combination of linear and nonlinear basic functions, scaling and coregistration with an atlas template. The most popular atlas is that of Talairach and Tournoux.[37] This atlas is based on the adult brain. Ongoing projects funded by the National Institutes of Health aim to provide brain atlases for different age groups more appropriate use in for children.

Gray white matter contrasts vary throughout adolescence, which can produce errors of subcortical normalization. False-positive areas of activation may arise from different normalization of similar activation areas. A new alternative has been proposed based on high-resolution brain surface registration[38] that negates the effects of subcortical normalization.

## Statistical Analysis

The standard methods of statistical analysis utilized in adult fMRI are also useful in children. The most popular are correlation coefficient, $t$-test, and general linear model. Correlation coefficient analysis looks at variation of the time-course intensities in relation to a predefined function, *t*-tests compare mean distributions of different groups of images such as ON epochs and OFF epochs. The general linear model technique looks at the variation of the BOLD signal at each voxel compared to the baseline. This model may include covariate-confounding effects such as motion estimates or low-frequency fluctuations of the BOLD signal. This also may include the hemodynamic response function of the BOLD technique, and changes related to infant and child brain development. Little is currently known of the differences of the hemodynamic response in infants as compared to adults. In addition, variability of subject performance is a significant challenge that is difficult to incorporate into these models. The degree of difficulty may be manifested by an increase in regional blood flow as seen in motor,[39] sensory,[24] and cognitive tasks.[16,40,41] However, too difficult a task may produce poor activation.[22]

Comparison of activation of different age groups is difficult. The number of voxels activated over a given threshold of different age groups is not a reliable measure of response magnitude.[42] A more valid approach may be magnitude measurements of actual change in signal intensity as percent change from baseline. Another alternative is to have a primary cortex activation as an internal reference; therefore, the occipital activation elicited by a standarized flashing light technique, compared to the activation of cognitive tasks.

## Thresholding

The physiological and developmental, differences in infants and children are important variables that influence fMRI analysis in children. Increased synaptic density, metabolism, and regional blood flow may yield a greater signal activation ratio per unit cortex activated in children.[17] The higher resting levels of CBF and neuronal metabolism found in children compared to adults[43] may explain why a true statistical activation seen in an adult does not reach the statistical significance in a child utilizing equal techniques.[44] The synaptic redundancy of the infant brain may result in more widespread distribution of activation that may mask focal regions of lower signal. Typically, thresholds are set high to avoid false-positive activation; however, significant areas of true activation may go undetected.[44] For practical purposes in children, a lower threshold and re-examination of the raw Z-score map is looked at if no activation is seen using the accepted higher threshold. Activation seen in expected regions as dictated by the clinical picture is then evaluated on a case-by-case basis. This technique has been utilized by different authors investigating language function in adults and children with epilepsy.[43,45,46] Broad comparisons between age groups regarding the general location of brain areas activated may be more justified than interpretation based upon extent and magnitude of activation. This approach is useful in sedated children, where the resting state is more reliable and the vascular responses less pronounced. There are no established guidelines on thresholds for postprocessing analysis except what is regarded by sta-

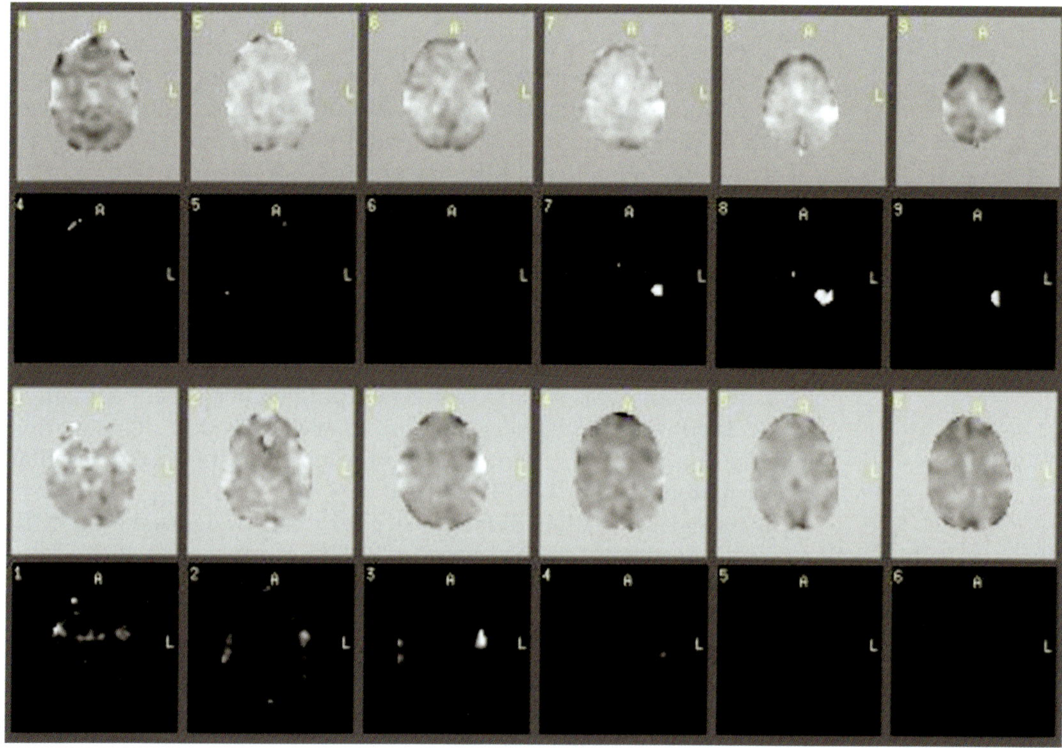

**Figure 15.3.** Activation detection using raw Z-score maps for motor and listening to a story tasks. Gray images are the composite echoplanar imaging (EPI) images with raw Z-score statistical activation far below-maximum Z value of 2.33 ($p < 0.05$), which would not survive any acceptable statistical analysis, however, well-defined clusters of activation from the tasks are present—upper rows are for motor tasks, lower rows for listening to a story—are seen in the expected areas without any other areas demonstrating activation. The black rows demonstrate only positive values that can be superimposed on the anatomic images.

tisticians as appropriate. Additionally, some studies may show significant areas of activation not demonstrated by conventional statistical methods. These areas can be mined by a practical empirical approach. This requires three criteria. The first one looks for well-defined clusters located in task-related areas that match expected group activation maps established in normal children; second, these clusters are then evaluated to see if there are areas of central high activation that would differentiate them from random clusters; and finally, appropriate thresholding is then utilized to produce a clean map of activation (Figure 15.3).

## Current and Future Applications

### Studies with Sedation

Functional MRI provides a window to view the developmental changes in infants and children. These may be associated with specific structural, metabolic, and congenital conditions. Evaluation of developmental processes often require the examinations to be performed under sedation.

The visual cortex of children less than two years of age show a linear relationship between the number of voxels activated and age. Unilateral damage of the optic radiations produces strong asymmetrical activation.[29] Functional MRI has been used to identify visual cortex functionality in patients with Sturge–Weber syndrome prior to hemispherectomy. The activation does not appear related to the size of the vascular malformation. An fMRI performed with sedation on a six-month-old Sturge–Weber patient with a large vascular lesion shows bilateral symmetrical activation of the anterior visual cortex (Figure 15.4A). An additional Sturge–Weber patient with a much smaller vascular lesion who was scanned while sleeping shows absent activation of the involved hemisphere (Figure 15.4B). The lack of activation appears due to dysfunction of the cortex and not due to the vascular malformation.

Functional information of the visual cortex may be derived from fMRI exams. Contralateral eye dominance is observed in adults of the anterior striate cortex, where the calcarine sulcus merges with the parieto-occipital sulcus.[47] Similar results have been demonstrated in a five-year-old boy under sedation as negative BOLD signal.[47] The stimulus was delivered monocularly, alternating the eyes, using light-emitting diode goggles through the patient's eyelids, at eight hertz. Negative BOLD activation of the right anterior visual cortex for the left eye and vice versa for the right eye is seen. This finding may provide a test in

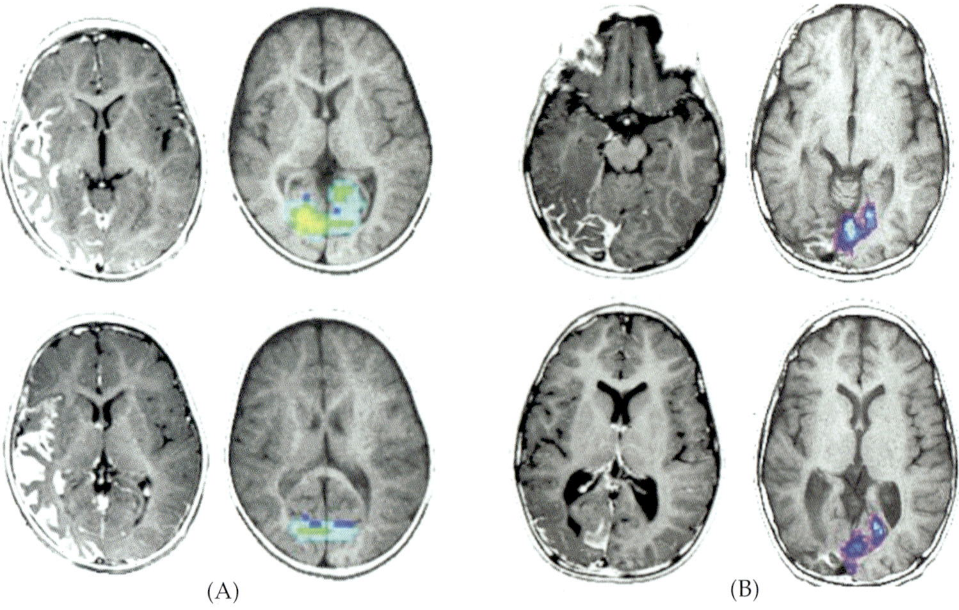


**Figure 15.4.** Sturge–Weber. (A) Sedated six-month-old child with large malformation and fMRI that shows symmetrical activation of the visual cortex. (B) Sleeping 12-year-old child with small malformation that shows absent activation of the involved right hemisphere.

infants and children who cannot cooperate to perform formal visual field testing. Clinical evaluation of visual fields in infants and children is difficult and limited. Functional MRI evaluation of the visual cortex in premature infants is underway. One study conducted in 28 sedated 18-month-old infants with and without periventricular leukomalacia (PVL) revealed no correlation between functional activation and the presence of the white matter abnormality.[48] Strikingly, those infants with higher amounts of PVL tended to have larger regions of activation.

Amblyopic eyes show reduced calcarine activation compared with the contralateral normal eye. Differentiation between anisometric and strabismic amblyopic eyes have been described.[49] Functional MRI has also been shown to be useful in objectively documenting residual visual function in children with severe visual loss.[47]

Passive auditory paradigms show great promise for the evaluation of infants and children. These have been performed in sedated children.[30,32] Activation is obtained in close to 70% of cases in the auditory temporal lobes and in frontal lobes, or both (Figure 15.5).[30] In some cases, the activation is of the secondary auditory cortex predominantly more posterior toward the angular gyrus or the inferior parietal lobule. In pre-verbal infants, there is significant extension toward secondary auditory areas. This is supported by the fact that cognition development appears based on a biological preprogramming of the newborn.[50]

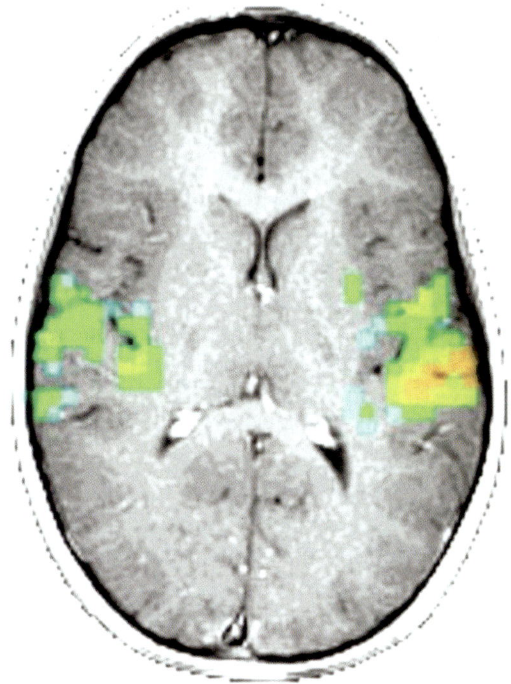

**Figure 15.5.** Passive auditory fMRI. Axial fMRI image that shows bilateral primary auditory cortex activation and secondary auditory cortex lateralized to the left using a passive listening to a story task in a sedated child.

Lateralization trends supporting this assumption have been found, but more investigation is needed. Functional MRI may provide an important tool for assessing language development and organization in infants and children. This has important implications for early diagnosis, intervention, and treatment of children with language delay. There is often a delay in diagnosis of language delay in children who benefit from early identification and treatment of these disorders. Human hearing starts at 27 weeks of gestation.[51] Auditory fMRI could be performed prenatally, as shown in a recent fMRI study of auditory activation in the fetal human brain.[52] In term neonates, auditory activation is obtained in 70% of cases utilizing a frequency-modulated pure tone centered at 1.3 kilohertz at a rate of seven hertz.[35] The auditory cortex activation is frequently accompanied by frontal activation in children over 18 months of age.

Evaluation of motor and sensory function in the sedated infant and child has met with limited success. Sensorimotor areas can be activated using passive movement of the hands.[32] This activation task has not been replicated reliably in sedated patients. The main obstacle is from task-related motion that occurs while the extremity is manipulated. Activation of the central cortex has been obtained in adults with electrical stimulation of the median nerve.[53] This technique holds promise for mapping the sensorimotor areas of children under sedation.

## Surgical Planning

Currently, the primary principal clinical application of fMRI in children is the presurgical mapping of the brain for neurosurgical planning. Particular importance is in the determination of motor areas of the dominant hand and language localization.

Brain function is distributed in specific centers or modules whose boundaries differ from anatomic landmarks. Motor cortical mapping is straightforward and shows good correlation to cortical stimulation. Boundaries may blurr between motor and sensory regions.

Language is more difficult as variation is encountered. Broca's Area is located primarily in the left inferior frontal gyrus, but also includes part of the ipsilateral middle frontal gyrus, precentral gyrus, and insular cortex.[54] These centers are located in similar areas among normal subjects, with some variation associated with dominant handedness. Variations also may be found in patients with anatomical or functional lesions.[55]

Essential centers of speech and motor function may be altered in patients with tumors, vascular malformations, cortical dysgenesis, and epilepsy.[56–58] These functions may be transferred to the contralateral hemisphere, ipsilateral neighboring areas, or scattered in one or both hemispheres. For the appropriate tailoring of elective surgery, the neurosurgeon should have knowledge of at least the lateralization of language.

Lateralization of language has classically been determined by assessing the cognitive deficit following injection of amobarbital into an internal carotid artery (Wada test). Neuropsychological evaluation is carried out during and after the transient period of hemispheric anesthesia. The procedure is invasive, expensive, and nonlocalizing. Patients may show speech arrest without language dominance after injection of amobarbital.[59] Electrocortical stimulation, also used to localize and lateralize language, is a procedure that requires the placement of electrodes on the cortex. It can be performed as an initial procedure with surgical placement of subdural grids and electrodes or during the definitive surgical resection. The procedure usually is performed with the child awake if language is to be determined. This is extremely invasive and has significant limitations, the most significant in that only one hemisphere can be evaluated.

Functional MRI can noninvasively determine the lateralization and localization of the language centers. The procedure is safe, cost-effective, and replicable. Several studies conducted in adults and children have compared language mapping with fMRI to Wada tests and electrocortical mapping (Table 15.1). A further review of fMRI and Wada testing may be found in Chapter 11.

The Wada test has been compared to fMRI utilizing a quantitative approach based in lateralization indexes of both tests, with a positive correlation of 0.96 ($p < 0.0001$).[45] Similar findings were reported more recently.[60–62] Electrocortical stimulation has been also compared with fMRI in adults, confirming the fMRI findings with rare exceptions.[63,64] Possible discrepancies may be due to failure of the Wada test to account for interhemispheric dissociation of receptive and expressive language areas.

Functional MRI appears to be a unique tool for the mapping of cerebral functions in children due to its noninvasiveness and the lack of radiation. Pitfalls can be avoided with knowledge of limitations.

Blood oxygenation level-dependent responses are transitory and severely diminished in the post-ictal temporal lobe (Figure 15.6).[65] The timing of the exam in seizure patients is critical. The exam should be performed preferably before the patient is taken off antiseizure medication, or at least 24 hours following a seizure.

**Table 15.1. Concordance of Language Lateralization by fMRI and Either Wada or Electrocortical Stimulation**

| Reference | Task | Wada test | ECoE |
|---|---|---|---|
| Desmond et al., 1995 | Semantic | 7/7 | NA |
| Binder et al., 1996[45] | Semantic | 22/22 | NA |
| Worthington et al., 1997 | Word generation | 5/9 | NA |
| Bahm et al., 1997 | Word generation, rhyming | 7/7 | NA |
| Hertz-Pannier et al., 1997[113] | Word generation | 6/6 | 1/1 |
| Schlosser et al., 1998 | Passive listening | NA | 12/14 |
| Yetkin et al., 1998[61] | Word generation | 13/13 | NA |
| Benson et al., 1999 | Word generation | 12/12 | 10/11 |
| Spreer et al., 2002[60] | Semantic | 22/22 | NA |
| Total | | 94/98 | 23/26 |
| % | | (96%) | (88%) |

ECoE = Electrocortical stimulation. Numbers: $n/N$ = number of patients with fMRI results concordant with $N$ number of patients. * = All cases concordant when lateralization indexes where extracted from frontal activation.

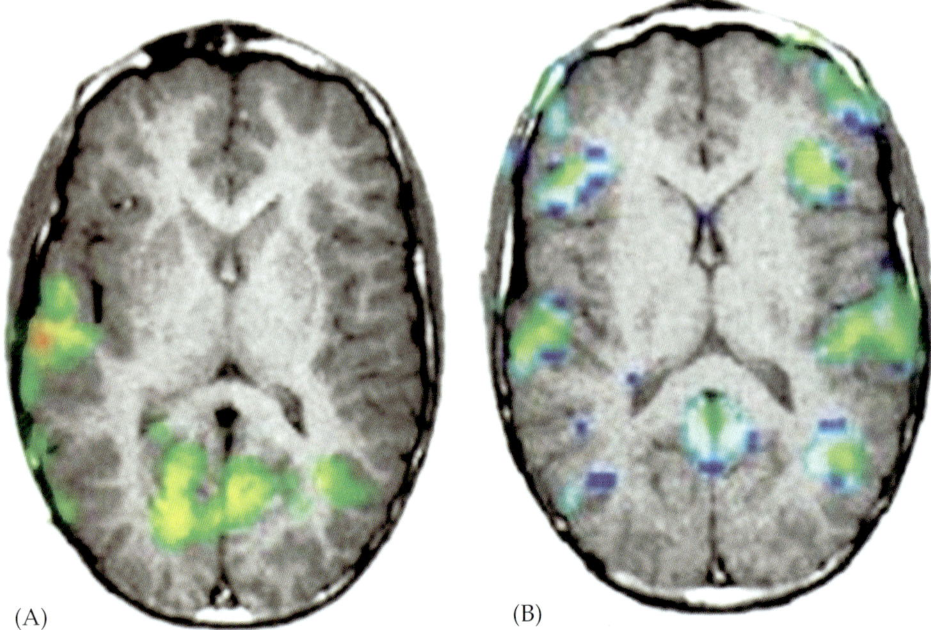


**Figure 15.6.** Post ictal versus interictal fMRI. Functional MRI of a right-handed patient performing a listening to a story task post ictal (A) and interictal (B). The post-ictal image, obtained a few hours following the seizure, shows right temporal lobe dominance. The same procedure, performed seizure-free for 24 hours several days later (inter ictal), revealed bilateral frontal and temporal lobe activation with left sided dominance.

Vascularity related to tumors or vascular malformations also may affect the BOLD response. This is crucial in the accurate mapping of motor or eloquent cortex adjacent to these lesions. Loss of activation in areas adjacent to tumors is related to tumor-induced changes in cerebral hemodynamics or to direct loss of cortical neurons.[66]

Presentation of the fMRI data is usually displayed on coregistered two-dimensional axial images. Surgical guidance and navigation may be better performed with 3D presentations.

## Language Mapping

### Language Mapping at Early Ages

Normal language onset and development occur during the first years of infancy, which makes fMRI evaluation difficult. There appears to be at birth preexisting specific skills of the auditory system for language.[67,68] Minimal phonemic discrimination allows for future phonemic and lexical analysis that permits speech repetition. Maturational events create associations that underlie the appearance of semantic processing. These processes occur in concert with the development of expressive language. Atypical language localization is more frequent in patients with early established cerebral lesions and epilepsy.[53]

Early stages of language have been assessed with fMRI using passive paradigms in sedated infants and children. Left-sided brain lateralization of language areas may be obtained by listening to the mother's voice.[32] Lateralization is less well defined in children less than three years of age. It has been found that lateralization appears more toward the right hemisphere in those less than three years of age (Figure 15.7A). After four years of age, sedated patients hearing their mother or father's voice tend to lateralize to the left temporal lobe (Figure 15.7B). In some cases, this passive-receptive paradigm demonstrates activation of Broca's Area (inferior, posterior, and lateral left frontal lobe). This is most likely explained by automatic antidromic connections via the *arcuate fasciculus*.

## Language Mapping of Cooperative Children

Mapping of expressive and receptive language in cooperative awake preschoolers and older children has also been performed. Language is best mapped with the use of multiple task paradigms to evaluate expressive and receptive functions. Expressive tasks demonstrate inferior and middle frontal gyrus activation. Tasks consist of Phonological fluency, thinking of words that start with specified letters;[43,69] semantic fluency, thinking of specific groups of items such as clothes, animals, toys, etc. (Figure 15.8);[43] silent spelling,[70] verb generation,[17,71] and reading.[17,71] Receptive language paradigms include listening to a

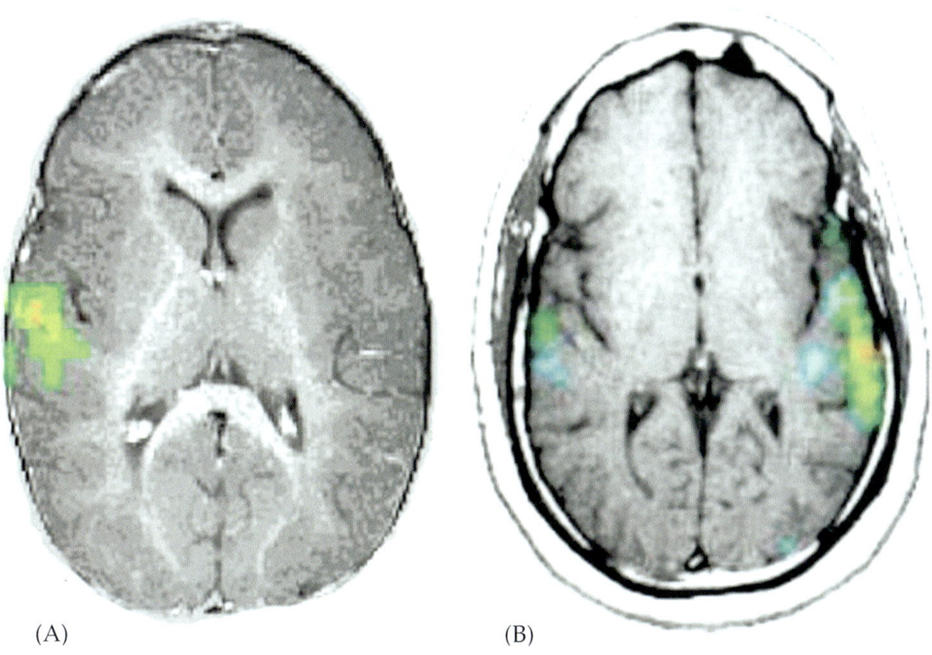


**Figure 15.7.** Functional MRI of changing language lateralization with aging of the child. (A) Sedated two-year-old infant with right lateralization of language. (B) Nonsedated 11-year-old with left lateralization of language.

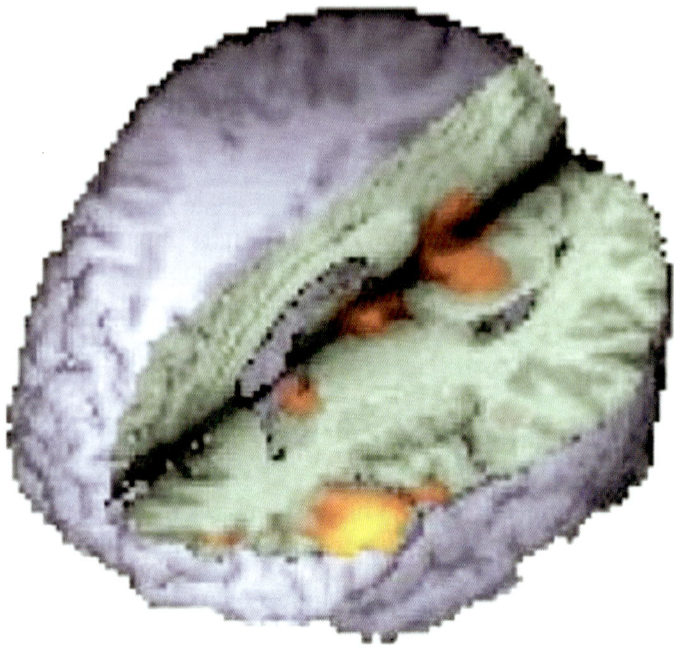

**Figure 15.8.** Three-dimensional fMRI image with coregistration of language mapped by semantic fluency task. The yellow cluster corresponds to the highest intensities located in Broca's Area (left inferior frontal gyrus). Activation of left caudate nucleus, thalamus, and occipital cortex are also seen. The 3D representation can aid the neurosurgeon in localization of deeper areas related to cognitive task.

story,[62] auditory comprehension, naming objects presented visually,[72] and reading. Areas of activation include the posterior third of the superior and middle temporal gyrus, the supramarginal gyrus, the fusiform gyrus, and angular gyrus. Expressive paradigms may produce activation of receptive areas, and vice versa. The verb-generation task most frequently activates Broca's and Wernicke's Areas.

Listening to a story is an important task in evaluation of language in children. This task is so familiar to children that it is readily accepted, particularly when performed by a parent, even in the unusual and uncomfortable environment of the MR scanner. This task has been instrumental in the evaluation of receptive language. The passive nature of the task lends itself to the evaluation of the sedated or sleeping child. Initially, early investigators, did not find lateralization on this passive task comparing number of voxels activated of each side.[73] However, more recent work indicates lateralization to the left supramarginal and angular gyri in both sexes with listening to a story.[74] Primary and secondary auditory activation with lateralization in Wernicke's region has been consistently found with fMRI and has proven to be a good indicator of receptive language representation (Figure 15.5).

When evaluating language in children, the age and academic achievement must be taken into account when designing the task paradigm. A redundant approach for targeting expressive and receptive language areas in pediatric cases has been performed.[32] Children were studied using two tasks that consisted of naming and listening to nouns. By combining these two tasks Wernicke's and Broca's Areas were demonstrated in 91% and 77% of cases, respectively. A study of Gaillard and colleges[75] evaluated other language fMRI studies utilizing two tasks that consisted of reading Aesop's Fables and a Read–Response–Naming task that consists of the subject naming an object described by a sentence, that is, what is a purring house pet? These tasks predominantly activated the left middle temporal gyrus, left middle frontal gyrus, and inferior occipital cortex, including fusiform and lingual gyrus.[75] Reading the fable activates the left inferior frontal gyrus, as well as produces more activation of the left superior temporal gyrus. The primary auditory area also was left dominant in all of these subjects when low thresholds were utilized.

Prior to fMRI, cortical mapping was limited to the cortical surface. Recently, fMRI in adults and children has demonstrated activation occurring deep in the sulci, extending from areas on the cortical surface. An example of the significance of this complex language localization was shown in a 14-year-old girl with a tumor in Broca's Area, with demonstration of eloquent language activation deep in an associated sulci, confirmed with intraoperative electrocortical stimulation.[72] Functional MRI, frameless stereotaxy, and direct cortical stimulation may be utilized together to reduce morbidity in the resection of vascular, neoplastic, and congenital lesions in children.[46] These procedures allow aggressive resection of lesions about the eloquent cortex.

Despite the experience accumulated with language mapping in adults and children, it is important to stress that, in those cases where results are divergent or activation is highly atypical or absent, it would seem prudent to repeat the study to confirm the results. Additionally, these patients may be assessed with Wada testing and intraoperative cortical electrical stimulation if there are important surgical planning issues.

## Motor Mapping

Currently, the most experience with fMRI mapping is of the motor cortex. This is due to the ease and reproducibility of the tasks. The majority of the work has been in adults; however, to date, no differences in findings have been ascribed specifically in children.

Mapping of the motor cortex has focused on the exploration of the hand, given its importance. Two tasks form the typical paradigm. These consist of finger tapping[76] or squeezing a foam pad.[77] Other tasks used consist of flexing and extending the fingers (hand clenching) repetitively.[78] Expected activation of the contralateral areas of the precentral gyrus in the hand knob is identified (Figure 15.9). Additional regions also may be activated, such as the bilateral supplemental motor areas, ipsilateral cerebellum, and basal ganglia. There may be sensory cortex

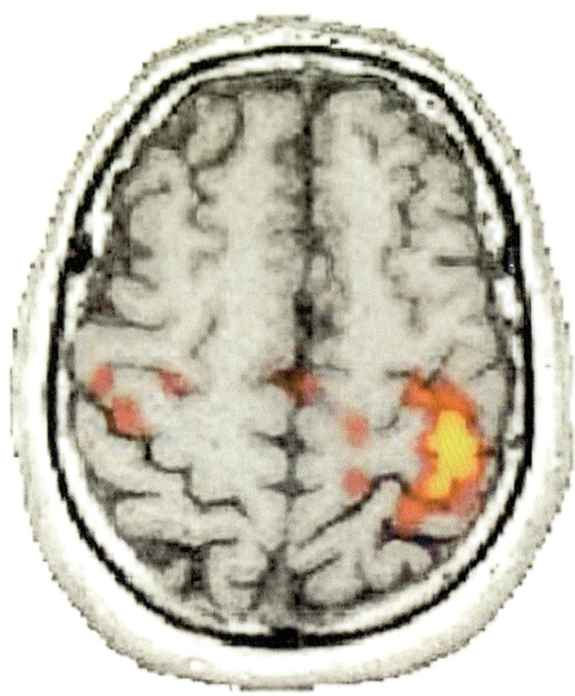

**Figure 15.9.** Motor cortex mapping of right hand finger-tapping task. Functional MRI axial image that shows dominant activation of the left precentral gyrus. Small amount of activation is seen of the ipsilateral motor cortex, contralateral SMA, and sensory area.

activation due to somatosensory and tactile input. Activation is usually isolated to the contralateral hemisphere, but frequently some activation may be seen on the ipsilateral hemisphere. The nondominant hand is more frequently associated with bilateral activation (Figure 15.10). Finger-tapping tasks promote more activation than hand-squeezing tasks. Young children and hemiparetic patients, however, appear to better tolerate the squeezing task. Patients with hemiparesis have decreased activation in primary motor areas with significant increase of activation in secondary motor areas, including contralateral or ipsilateral supplemental motor areas and basal ganglia.[66]

Patients with tumors or dysgenesis may show displacement of the motor cortex (Figure 15.11). In addition to displacement, activation may be reduced or transferred to the contralateral hemisphere. Children with congenital malformations such as schizencephaly performing a finger-tapping task demonstrate increased and wider areas of activation in the unaffected hemisphere.[70] Extreme examples of reorganization are encountered in severe cases of hemimegalencephaly where both hands may show activation in the normal hemisphere.[79] Motor mapping in the young sedated infant is possible utilizing a modified

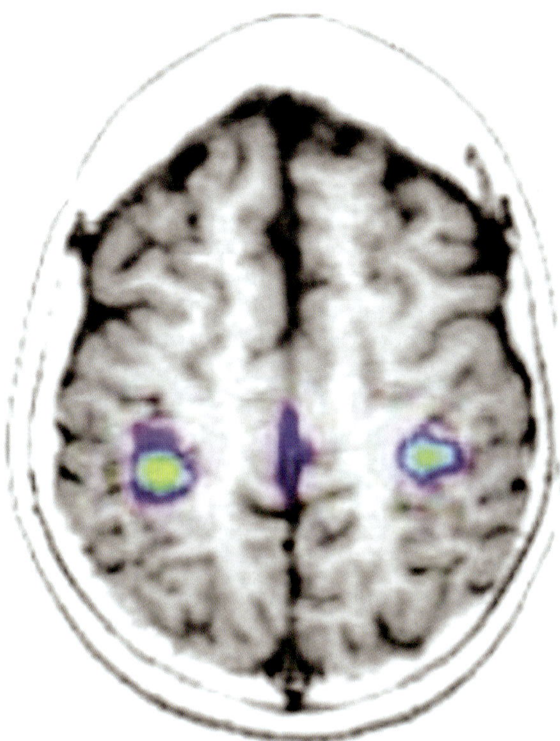

**Figure 15.10.** Finger tapping task activation map of the left hand in a right-handed patient. There is bilateral motor cortex activation with slight right-sided dominance.

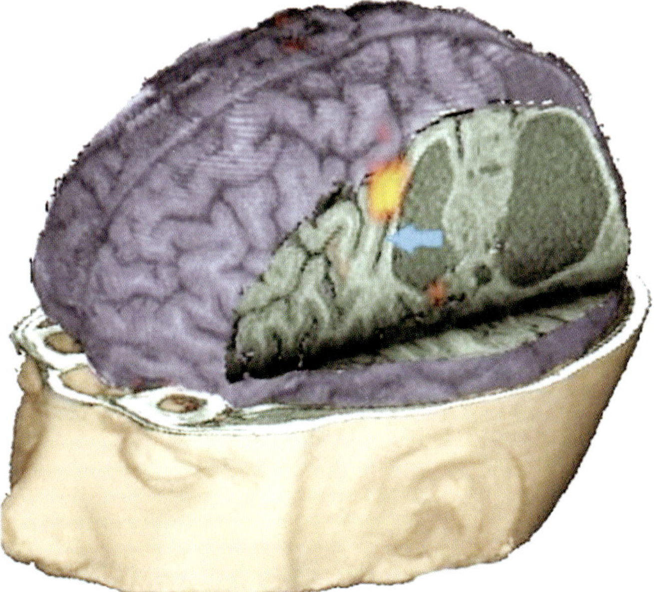

**Figure 15.11.** Right finger-tapping task in patient with large tumor. Three-dimensional fMRI that demonstrates a large left parietal ganglioglioma. The left motor cortex is located by the central sulcus (blue arrow). This is displaced rostrally by the tumor. Small activation is also seen of the right motor cortex.

version of the non-nutritive high amplitude sucking procedure. This procedure is originally performed by presenting a verbal stimulus (e.g., the syllable /pa/) to an infant with a pacifier in its mouth. This results in a high frequency of strong sucking. Repeated presentation of the stimulus results in a gradual decrease in the intensity of sucking. When such habituation occurs, a new speech stimulus is presented to reinitiate the sucking. The paradigm has shown that newborns and infants are able to perform phonemic discrimination and extract differences between allophonic words such as nitrate and night rate.[80] The task with fMRI consists of placing the child in the magnet with a pacifier and delivering the mother's voice through headphones during ON epochs to elicit the sucking response. During the OFF epoch, her voice is halted. Motor activation can be obtained using this paradigm in a sedated infant (Figure 15.12). The areas activated are bilateral, located on the homunculus caudal to the hand area representing the mouth and tongue region.

Cortical activation has been described on fMRI exams by brief innocuous electrical stimuli applied to the fingers in adults.[81] Other stimuli include automated quantitative heat and cold. These techniques may be potentially used as a passive technique in children who are sedated or comatose; however, to date, no studies in children have been reported using these methods. Swallowing studies in children have demonstrated activation in pre- and postcentral gyrus, superior motor cortex, insula, inferior frontal cortex, Heschl's gyrus, lenticular nucleus, and nucleus ambiguous.[82] The significance of these findings may aid in the development of novel rehabilitative strategies in compromized patients.

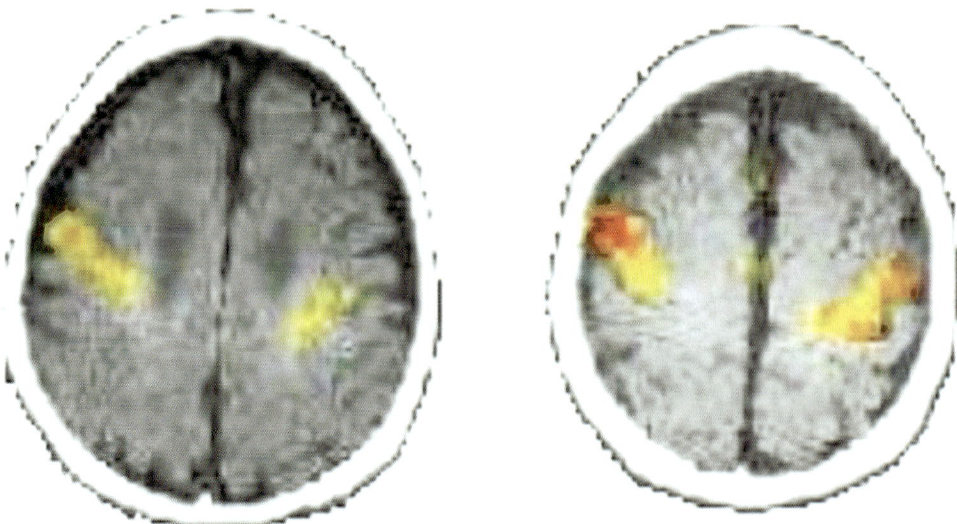

**Figure 15.12.** Motor activation of the oral facial cortex associated with sucking reflex in sedated two-month-old. There is bilateral activation of the precentral gyri in the oral facial region. This is related with the habituation–dishabituation of high-amplitude sucking in response to linguistic stimuli.

The concordance of motor fMRI and intraoperative electrophysiology utilizing somatosensory-evoked potential and direct cortical stimulation is excellent.[83,84]

Sensory activation in children has been obtained using tactile stimulation of the hand by rubbing the patient's palm and fingers with a mildly abrasive surface.[76]

### Cognitive Function Mapping

#### *Auditory*

Primary auditory function is crucial to the normal development of the language system.[35,85,86]

Evaluation of learning and other higher cognitive functions are now starting to be evaluated with fMRI. Numerous studies have been performed comparing dyslexic to normal children, looking at patterns of activation of reading paradigms. Dyslexic children have less activation in left temporal–parietal cortex.[87] They show significant hyperactivation in the left inferior frontal gyrus.[69] In auditory tasks, dyslexic children had more inferior temporal activation than normal children when judging phonological differences. They show less middle frontal gyrus and more left orbito-frontal gyrus activation than normal children in lexical judgment.[88]

## ADHD

Attention deficit hyperactivity disorder (ADHD) lacks clear anatomical markers.[89] These children have a characteristic of impairment of inhibition. They demonstrate different areas of activation related to inhibition tasks when compared to normal children. Difficulty with compliance in ADHD patients is expected. However, with the use of the proper paradigms, fMRI has been proven to be feasible in ADHD patients. These tasks include sustained visual vigilance,[90] inhibition of motor response also known as go-no-go paradigm,[90] delayed and stop motor response,[91] and Stroop and Stroop-like tasks (Figure 15.13).[92] These tasks are starting to be used to compare ADHD and normal children. Normal activation to inhibition tasks show activation in bilateral inferior frontal gyri, anterior cingulate gyrus, the superior parietal lobules (predominantly on the left), and the inferior parietal lobules for the sustained visual paradigm. Adolescents show a lower response in the right mesial prefrontal cortex, right inferior prefrontal cortex, and left caudate nucleus during the go-no-go-task. Attention deficit hyperactivity disorder patients show less activation of the anterior cingulate gyrus on Stroop paradigms than normal patients.[92,93] Attention deficit hyperactivity disorder patients increase their striatal activation as compared to normal patients.[91] Functional MRI based on T2 relaxometry, which measures the steady-state blood flow and tests for enduring medication effects in specific regions of the brain, has been utilized to assess the function of the basal ganglia of normal children and patients with ADHD.[94] There appears to be a strong correlation of T2 relaxation

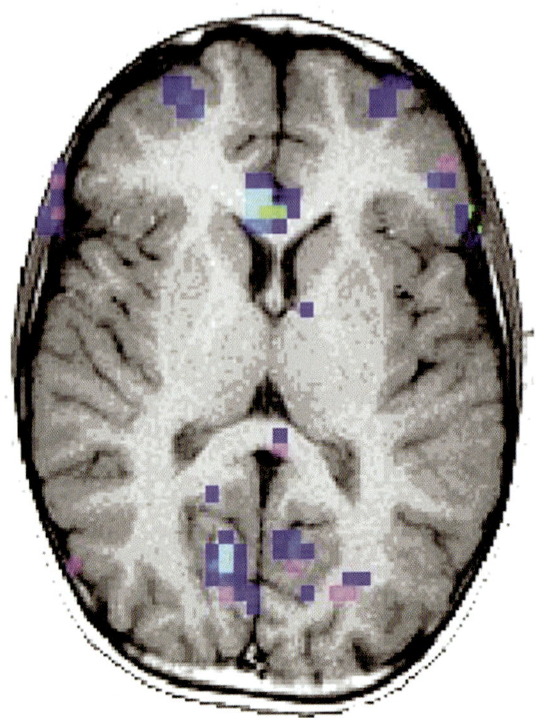

**Figure 15.13.** Functional MRI image of normal child performing STROOP. Activation in the anterior cingulate gyrus and bilateral middle frontal gyrus is associated with inhibition tasks. The bilateral calcarine cortex is related to the visual demands of the task.

times of the caudate and putamen with the child's capacity to sit still and accomplish a computerized attention task. Treatment with methylphenidate significantly decreased the T2 relaxation times in the ADHD group.[94]

## Memory

The neural substrate of memory is poorly understood despite the immense effort from different neuroscience fields. The complexity of memory is manifest in the difficulties and challenges observed in trying to design reliable paradigms involving memory encoding. To date, no replicable and accurate paradigms have been presented for the assessment of the mechanisms underlying memory. Some results have been obtained in both adults and children performing working memory tasks. It has been shown that spatial working memory tasks applied in children between 8 to 11 years elicit fMRI activation in several cortical areas, including the dorsal aspects of the prefrontal cortex and in the posterior parietal and anterior cingulate gyrus.[95] Utilizing a non-spatial

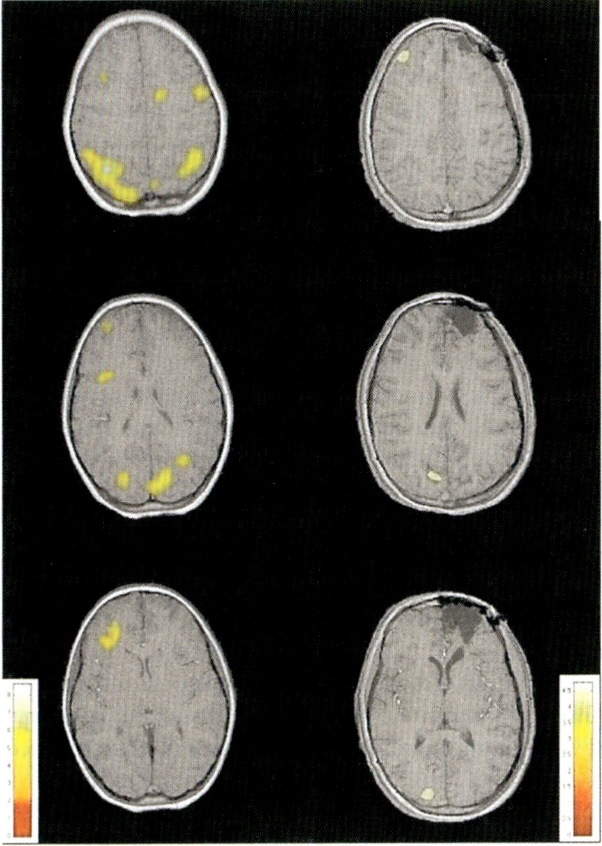

**Figure 15.14.** In a working memory *N*-back task, two children with TBI show diminished performance and display more focal activation than their age, gender, handedness, and performance-matched controls. Shown here: Normal female control 10 year old (left) versus severe female 9 year old traumatic brain injury [TBI], (right). Right hemisphere is depicted on left. Scales depict *T*-values. From Newsome, Hunter, and Levin, Baylor College of Medicine, with permission.

task an increase of signal intensity in children ages 9 to 11 has been demonstrated in the bilateral inferior and middle frontal gyri with dominance on the left.[16] Others describe right hemisphere lateralization for spatial working memory (Figure 15.14).[96]

Functional MRI evaluation of memory has potential clinical applications in the work-up of temporal lobe epilepsy (TLE). Differences of activation in the mesial aspect of the temporal lobes, elicited by mental navigation and recall tasks, lateralized the side of seizure onset in 90% of patients with symptomatic TLE.[97]

## Other fMRI Studies on Cognition

Fragile X syndrome is one of the most common genetic causes of developmental and learning problems.[98] Magnetic resonance imaging is

showed a shift of activation for both receptive and expressive language tasks to the right hemisphere, mirroring those previously found in the left hemisphere.[114]

Disinhibition and enlargement of the motor cortex associated with the removed limb in patients amputated during childhood have been demonstrated with transcranial magnetic stimulation and confirmed by fMRI.[114] These patients also show ipsilateral functional reorganization. Another example of brain plasticity is seen in three adolescents with brachial plexus injury who underwent nerve transfer surgery. The expected activation of the intercostal nerve along the hemoncal was found transferred to the ellow region in these patients.

## Epilepsy

Functional MRI techniques and applications have been utilized in seizure localization in patients with frequent reliable epileptic discharges. Cortical activation triggered by seizures provokes a BOLD effect (Figure 15.16). This may be localized with fMRI if the seizure is captured in the MR scanner and does not produce head movement. An ictal fMRI in a four-year-old boy with frequent partial motor seizures

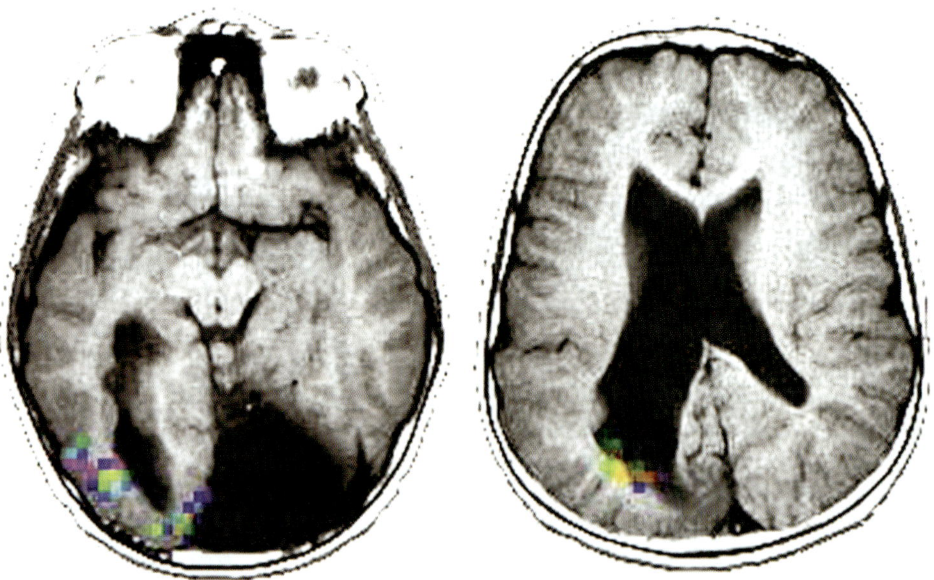

**Figure 15.16.** Seizure localization with fMRI. Ten-year-old epileptic boy with frequent visual auras lasting 20 to 60 seconds, often accompanied by left facial twitching. Electroencephalogram is localized to the right posterior quadrant. During the fMRI for visual assessment, the patient reported one aura of unknown duration. A pedestal design paradigm was applied retrospectively using the pre-aural period as the OFF epoch. Different durations of the ON epoch were tried between 20 and 60 seconds to correspond to the known aural length. The ON epoch that resulted in the best activation was used. The remaining timepoints were used as the second OFF epoch. Activation was obtained in cortical and subcortical areas of the right occipital lobe. This was confimed intraoperatively by electrocorticography.

has demonstrated the epileptic focus.[117] The paradigm consisted of contrasting periods of clinical seizures to baseline images acquired during a ten-minute sequence. Another incidental ictal activity was mapped with fMRI in a 16-year-old boy performing different tasks for presurgical mapping of a dysplastic lesion.[118] Subclinical ictal activity has also been detected with fMRI, and confirmed with invasive monitoring in adolescent patients with frequent partial motor seizures.[119]

Electroencephalogram recording during fMRI data acquisition has been performed.[120] This technique allows interictal spikes captured by the scalp electrodes to trigger fMRI acquisitions.[120–122] The epilepsy focus may be demonstrated in up to 60% of cases. Epileptogenic areas of the frontal, occipital, and parietal lobes were reliably detected. Areas close to the sinuses that create a profound paramagnetic effect on the images are not well served with this technique. This unfortunately occurs in the mesial temporal region, which is the most frequent epileptogenic region. A different approach, based on the degree of the activation, may allow MRI to localize the seizure origin in cases of occipital lobe epilepsy using a visual paradigm.[123]

## Conclusions

Functional MRI has begun to show considerable clinical benefits in the understanding of crucial aspects of cognitive development in both normal and impaired children. Presurgical mapping of eloquent brain regions with MRI will increase in utility as alternative procedures are more invasive and costly. Functional MRI will challenge today's gold standards and create new gold standards in understanding the complex cognitive functions in the child's brain. Functional MRI shows promise in the field of seizure focus localization and may become one of the principals tools for the work-up of epilepsy. Conditions such as ADHD, autism , dyslexia, and psychiatric disorders will be better diagnosed and understood. Treatment will be better tailored and monitored with MRI. The clinical contribution of fMRI in the understanding of physiologic processes of the brain will be as significant as MRI in the understanding of anatomic abnormalities.

## References


1. Pauling L, Coryell CD. The magnetic properties and structure of hemoglobin, oxyhemoglobin and carbonmonoxyhemoglobin. *Proc Natl Acad Sci U S A*. 1936;22:210–216.
2. Kwong KK, Belliveau JW, Chesler DA, et al. Dynamic magnetic resonance imaging of human brain activity during primary sensory stimulation. *Proc Natl Acad Sci U S A*. 1992;89:5675–5679.
3. Castellanos FX, Giedd JN, Marsh WL, et al. Quantitative brain magnetic resonance imaging in attention-deficit hyperactivity disorder. *Arch Gen Psychiatry*. 1996;53:607–616.
4. Filipek PA. Quantitative magnetic resonance imaging in autism: the cerebellar vermis. *Curr Opin Neurol*. 1995;8:134–138.

5. Leonard CM, Voeller KK, Lombardino LJ, et al. Anomalous cerebral structure in dyslexia revealed with magnetic resonance imaging. *Arch Neurol.* 1993;50:461–469.
6. Pfefferbaum A, Mathalon DH, Sullivan EV, et al. A quantitative magnetic resonance study of changes in brain morphology from infancy to late adulthood. *Arch Neurol.* 1994;51:874–887.
7. Reiss AL, Abrams MT, Singer HS, et al. Brain development, gender and IQ in children. A volumetric imaging study. *Brain.* 1996;119:1763–1774.
8. Barkovich AJ, Kjos BO, Jackson D Jr., et al. Normal maturation of the neonatal and infant brain: MR imaging at 1.5 T. *Radiology.* 1988;166:173–180.
9. Staudt M, Krageloh-Mann I, Grodd W. [Normal myelination in childhood brains using MRI—a meta analysis]. *Rofo Fortschr Geb Rontgenstr Neuen Bildgeb Verfahr.* 2000;172:802–811.
10. Huttenlocher PR. Synaptic density in human frontal cortex—developmental changes and effects of aging. *Brain Res.* 1979;163:195–205.
11. Huttenlocher PR. Morphometric study of human cerebral cortex development. *Neuropsychologia.* 1990;28:517–527.
12. Chugani HT, Phelps ME, Mazziotta JC. Positron emission tomography study of human brain functional development. *Ann Neurol.* 1987;22:487–497.
13. D'Esposito M, Zarahn E, Aguirre GK, et al. The effect of normal aging on the coupling of neural activity to the bold hemodynamic resopnse. *Neuroimage.* 1999;10:6–14.
14. Huettel SA, Singerman JD, McCarthy G. The effects of aging upon the hemodynamic response measuredby functional MRI. *Neuroimage.* 2001;13:161–175.
15. Uftring SJ, Wachtel SR, Chu D, et al. An fMRI study of the effect of amphetamine on brain activity. *Neuropsychopharmacology.* 2001;25:925–935.
16. Casey B, Cohen JD, Jezzard P, et al. Activation of prefrontal cortex in children during a nonspatial working memory task with functional MRI. *Neuroimage.* 1995;2:221–229.
17. Galliard WD, Hertz-Pannier L, Mott SH, et al. Functional anatomy of cognitive development: fMRI of verbal fluency in children and adults. *Neurology.* 2000;54:180–185.
18. Volpe JJ. Neurology of the Newborn. Philadelphia, PA: WB Saunders; 1995:53–58.
19. Rubia K, Overmeyer S, Taylor E, et al. Functional frontalisation with age: mapping neurodevelopmental trajectories with fMRI. *Neurosci Biobehav Rev.* 2000;24:13–19.
20. Klingberg T, Vaidya CJ, Gabrieli JD, et al. Myelination and organization of the frontal white matter in children: a diffusion tensor MRI study. *Neuroreport.* 1999;10:2817–2821.
21. Huttenlocher PR, Dabholkar AS. Regional differences in synaptogenesis in human cerebral cortex. *J Comp Neurol.* 1997;387:167–178.
22. Bookheimer SY, Dapretto M, Cohen MS, et al. Functional MRI of the hippocampus during short-term memory tasks: parametric responses to task difficulty and stimulus novelty. *Neuroimage.* 1996;3:S531.
23. Raichle ME, Fiez JA, Videen TO, et al. Practice-related changes in human brain functional anatomy during non-motor learning. *Cereb Cortex.* 1994;4:8–26.
24. Price C, Wise R, Ramsay S, et al. Regional response differences within the human auditory cortex when listening to words. *Neurosci Lett.* 1992;146:179–182.

25. Poldrack RA, Pare-Blagoev EJ, Grant PE. Pediatric functional magnetic resonance imaging: progress and challenges. *Top Magn Reson Imaging*. 2002;13:61–70.
26. Slifer KJ, Cataldo MF, Cataldo MD, et al. Behavior analysis of motion control for pediatric neuroimaging. *J Appl Behav Anal*. 1993;26:469–470.
27. Rosenberg DR, Sweeney JA, Gillen JS, et al. Magnetic resonance imaging of children without sedation: preparation with stimulation. *J Am Acad Child Adolesc Psychiatry*. 1997;36:853–859.
28. Yamada H, Sadato N, Konishi Y, et al. A milestone for normal development of the infantile brain detected by functional MRI. *Neurology*. 2000; 55:218–223.
29. Born AP, Miranda MJ, Rostrup E, et al. Functional magnetic resonance imaging of the normal and abnormal visual system in early life. *Neuropediatrics*. 2000;31:24–32.
30. Altman NR, Bernal B. Brain activation in sedated children: auditory and visual functional MR imaging. *Radiology*. 2001;221:56–63.
31. Morita T, Kochiyama T, Yamada H, et al. Difference in the metabolic response to photic stimulation of the latral geniculate nucleus and the primary visual cortex of infants: a fMRI study. *Neurosci Res*. 2000;38:63–70.
32. Souweidane MM, Kim KH, McDowall R, et al. Brain mapping in sedated infants and young children with passive-functional magnetic resonance imaging. *Pediatr Neurosurg*. 1999;30:86–92.
33. Meek JH, Firbank M, Elwell CE, et al. Regional hemodynamic responses to visual stimulation in awake infants. *Pediatr Res*. 1998;43:840–843.
34. Born AP, Law I, Lund TE, et al. Is the negative BOLD response in sedated children caused by age or state of alertness? Paper presented at: Annual Meeting of the American Society of Neuroradiology; May 13–17, 2002; Vancouver B.C., Canada.
35. Anderson AW, Marois R, Colson ER, et al. Neonatal auditory activation detected by functional magnetic resonance imaging. *Magn Reson Imaging*. 2001;19:1–5.
36. Martin E, Joeri P, Loenneker T, et al. Visual processing in infants and children studied using functional MRI. *Pediatr Res*. 1999;46:135–140.
37. Talairach J, Tournoux P. A co-planar stereotactic atlas of the human brain. Stuttgart, Germany: Thieme.
38. Fischl B, Sereno MI, Tootell RB, et al. High-resolution intersubject averaging and a coordinate system for the cortical surface. *Hum Brain Mapp*. 1999;8:272–284.
39. Kastrup A, Kruger G, Neumann-Haefelin T, et al. Changes of cerebral blood flow, oxygenation, and oxidative metabolism during graded motor activation. *Neuroimage*. 2002;15:74–82.
40. Just MA, Carpenter PA, Keller TA, et al. Brain activation modulated by sentence comprehension. *Science*. 1996;274:114–116.
41. Cohen JD, Forman SD, Braver TS, et al. Activation of the prefrontal cortex in a nonspatial working memory task with functional MRI. *Hum Brain Mapp*. 1994;1:293–304.
42. Cohen MS, DuBois RM. Stability, repeatability and the expression of signal magnitude in functional magnetic resonance imaging. *J Magn Reson Imaging*. 1999;10:33–40.
43. Hertz-Pannier L, Gaillard WD, Mott SH, et al. Noninvasive assessment of language dominance in children and adolescents with functional MRI: a preliminary study. *Neurology*. 1997;48:1003–1012.

44. Gaillard WD, Grandin CB, Xu B. Developmental aspects of pediatric MRI: considerations for image acquisition, analysis and interpretation. *Neuroimage*. 2001;13:239–249.
45. Binder JR, Swanson SJ, Hammeke TA, et al. Determination of langugage dominance using functional MRI: a comparison with the Wada test. *Neurology*. 1996;46:978–984.
46. Stapleton SR, Kiriakopoulos E, Mikulis D, et al. Combined utility of functional MRI, cortical mapping, and frameless stereotaxy in the resection of lesions in eloquent areas of brain in children. *Pediatr Neurosurg*. 1997;26: 68–82.
47. Miki A, Liu GT, Fletcher DW, et al. Ocular dominance in anterior fisual cortex in a child demonstrated by the use of fMRI. *Pediatr Neurosurg*. 2001;24:232–234.
48. Sie LTL, Rombouts SARB, Scheltens P, et al. Functional MRI of the visual cortex in sedated children with periventricular echodensities. *Dev Med Child Neurol*. 2001;43:486–490.
49. Choi MY, Lee K-M, Hwang J-M, et al. Comparison between anisometropic and strabismic amblyopia using functional magnetic resonance imaging. *Br J Opthalmol*. 2001;85:1052–1056.
50. Spreen O, Risser AH, Edgell D. Cognitive development in relation to the development of the nervous system. In: Developmental Neuropsychology. Oxford: Oxford University Press; 1999:57–77.
51. Johansson B, Wedenberg E, Westin B. Measurement of tone response by human fetus. *Acta Otolaryngol (Stockh)*. 1964;57:188.
52. Hykin J, Moore R, Duncan K, et al. Fetal brain activity demonstrated by functional magnetic resonance imaging. *Lancet*. 1999;354:645–646.
53. Boakye M, Huckins SC, Szeverenyi NM, et al. Functional magnetic resonance imaging of somatosensory cortex activity produced by electrical stimulation of the median nerve or tactile stimulation of the index finger. *J Neurosurg*. 2000;93:774–783.
54. Benson DF, Ardila A. Aphasia: A Clinical Perspective. New York: Oxford University Press; 1996:34.
55. Ojemann G. Cortical organization of language. *J Neurosci*. 1991;11:2281–2287.
56. Chapman SB, McKinnon L. Discussion of developmental plasticity: factors affecting cognitive outcome after pediatric traumatic brain injury. *J Commun Disord*. 2000;33:333–344.
57. Jacobs KM, Graber KD, Kharazia VN, et al. Postlesional epilepsy: the ultimate brain plasticity. *Epilepsia*. 2000;41 (Suppl6):S153–161.
58. Schwartzkroin PA. Mechanisms of brain plasticity: from normal brain function to pathology. *Int Rev Neurobiol*. 2001;45:1–15.
59. Benbadis SR, Binder JR, Swanson SJ, et al. Is speech arrest during wada testing a valid method for determining hemispheric representation of language. *Brain Lang*. 1998;65:441–446.
60. Spreer J, Arnold S, Quiske A, et al. Determination of hemisphere dominance for language: comparison of frontal and temporal fMRI activation with intracarotid amytal testing. *Neuroradiology*. 2002;44:467–474.
61. Yetkin FZ, Swanson S, Fischer M, et al. Functional MR of frontal lobe activation: comparison with Wada language results. *AJNR Am J Neuroradiol*. 1998;19:1095–1098.
62. Lehericy S, Cohen L, Bazin B, et al. Functional MR evaluation of temporal and frontal langugage dominance compared with the Wada test. *Neurology*. 2000;54:1625–1633.

63. Ruge MI, Victor J, Hosain S, et al. Concordance between functional magnetic resonance imaging and intraoperative language mapping. *Stereotact Funct Neurosurg*. 1999;72:95–102.
64. Schlosser MJ, Luby M, Spencer DD, et al. Comparative localization of auditory comprehension by using functional magnetic resonance imaging and cortical stimulation. *J Neurosurg*. 1999;91:626–635.
65. Jayakar P, Bernal B, Medina LS, et al. False lateralization of language cortex on functional MRI after a cluster of focal seizures. *Neurology*. 2002;58:490–492.
66. Krings T, Topper R, Willmes K, et al. Activation in primary and secondary motor areas in patients with CNS neoplasms and weakness. *Neurology*. 2002;58:381–390.
67. Helmstaedter C, Kurthen M, Linke DB, et al. Patterns of language dominance in focal left and right hemisphere epilepsies: relation to MRI findings, EEG, sex, and age at onset of epilepsy. *Brain Cogn*. 1997;33:135–150.
68. Saltzman J, Smith ML, Scott K. The impact of age at seizure onset on the likelihood of atypical language representation in children with intractable epilepsy. *Brain Cogn*. 2002;48:517–520.
69. Georgiewa P, Rzanny R, Hopf JM, et al. fMRI during word processing in dyslexic and normal reading children. *Neuroreport*. 1999;10:3459–3465.
70. Lee BC, Kuppusamy K, Grueneich R, et al. Hemispheric language dominance in children demonstrated by functional magnetic resonance imaging. *J Child Neurol*. 1999;14:78–82.
71. Holland SK, Plante E, Weber Byars A, et al. Normal fMRI brain activation patterns in children performing a verb generation task. *Neuroimage*. 2001; 14:837–843.
72. Rutten GJ, van Rijen PC, van Veelen CW, et al. Language area localization with three-dimensional functional magnetic resonance imaging matches intrasulcal electrostimulation in Broca's area. *Ann Neurol*. 1999;46:405–408.
73. Ulualp SO, Biswal BB, Yetkin FZ, et al. Functional magnetic resonance imaging of auditory cortex in children. *Laryngoscope*. 1998;108:1782–1786.
74. Kansaku K, Yamaura A, Kitazawa S. Sex differences in lateralization revealed in the posterior language areas. *Cereb Cortex*. 2000;10:866–872.
75. Gaillard WD, Pugliese M, Grandin CB, et al. Cortical localization of reading in normal children, an fMRI language study. *Neurology*. 2001;57: 47–54.
76. Hirsch J, Ruge MI, Kim KHS, et al. An integrated functional magnetic resonance imaging procedure for preoperative mapping of cortical areas associated with tactile, motor, language, and visual functions. *Neurosurgery*. 2000;47:711–721.
77. Lee CC, Jack C Jr., Riederer SJ. Mapping of the central sulcus with functional MR: active versus passive activation tasks. *AJNR Am J Neuroradiol*. 1998;19:847–852.
78. Roux F-E, Ibarrola D, Tremoulet M, et al. Methodological and technical issues for integrating functional magnetic resonance imaging data in a neuronavigational system. *Neurosurgery*. 2001;49:1145–1156.
79. Staudt M, Pieper T, Grodd W, et al. Functional MRI in a 6-year-old boy with unilateral cortical malformation: concordant representation of both hands in the unaffected hemisphere. *Neuropediatrics*. 2001;32:159–161.
80. Hohne EA, Jusczyk PW. Two-month-old infants' sensitivity to allophonic differences. *Percept Psychophys*. 1994;56:613–623.

81. Deuchert M, Ruben J, Schwiemann J, et al. Event-related fMRI of the somatosensory system using electrical finger stimulation. *Neuroreport.* 2002;13:365–369.
82. Hartnick CJ, Rudolph C, Willging JP, et al. Functional magnetic resonance imaging of the pediatric swallow: imaging the cortex and the brainstem. *Laryngoscope.* 2001;111:1183–1191.
83. Puce A, Constable RT, Luby ML, et al. Functional magnetic resonance imaging of sensory and motor cortex: comparison with electrophysiological localization. *J Neurosurg.* 1995;83:262–270.
84. Yousry TA, Schmidt UD, Jassoy AG, et al. Topography of the cortical motor hand area: prospective study with functional MR imaging and direct motor mapping at surgery. *Radiology.* 1995;195:23–29.
85. Paradise JL, Dollaghan CA, Campbell TF, et al. Language, speech sound production, and cognition in three-year-old children in relation to otitis media in their first three year of life. *Pediatrics.* 2000;105:1119–1130.
86. Sininger YS, Doyle KJ, Moore JK. The case for early identification of hearing loss in children. Auditory system development, experimental auditory deprivation, and development of speech perception and hearing. *Pediatr Clin North Am.* 1999;46:1–14.
87. Temple E, Poldrack RA, Salidis J, et al. Disrupted neural responses to phonological and orthographic processing in dyslexic children: an fMRI study. *Neuroreport.* 2001;12:299–307.
88. Corina DP, Richards TL, Serafini S, et al. fMRI auditory language differences between dyslexic and able reading chldren. *Neuroreport.* 2001;12: 1195–1201.
89. Baumeister AA, Hawkins MF. Incoherence of neuroimaging studies of attention deficit/hyperactivity disorder. *Clin Neuropharmacol.* 2001;24:2–10.
90. Sunshine JL, Lewin JS, Wu DH, et al. Functional MR to localize sustained visual attention activation in patients with attention deficit hyperactivity disorder: a pilot study. *AJNR Am J Neuroradiol.* 1997;18.
91. Vaidya CJ, Austin G, Kirkorian G, et al. Selective effects of methylphenidate in attention deficit hyperactivity disorder: a functional magnetic resonance study. *Proc Natl Acad Sci U S A.* 1998;95:14494–14499.
92. Bush G, Frazier JA, Rauch SL, et al. Anterior cingulate cortex dysfunction in attention-deficit/hyperactivity disorder revealed by fMRI and the counting Stroop. *Biol Psychiatry.* 1999;45:1542–1552.
93. Peterson BS, Skudlarski P, Gatenby JC, et al. An fMRI study of Stroop word-color interference: evidence for cingulate subregions subserving multiple distributed attentional systems. *Biol Psychiatry.* 1999;45:1237–1258.
94. Teicher MH, Anderson CM, Polcari A, et al. Functional deficits in basal ganglia of children with attention-deficit/hyperactivity disorder shown with functional magnetic resonance imaging relaxometry. *Nat Med.* 2000;6: 470–473.
95. Nelson CA, Monk CS, Lin J, et al. Functional neuroanatomy of spatial working memory in children. *Dev Psychol.* 2000;36:109–116.
96. Thomas KM, Casey BJ. Functional MRI in pediatrics. In: Moonen CTW, ed. Functional MRI. Berlin, Germany: Springer; 1999:513–523.
97. Jokeit H, Okujava M, Woermann FG. Memory fMRI lateralizes temporal lobe epilepsy. *Neurology.* 2001;57:1786–1793.
98. Crawford DC, Acuna JM, Sherman SL. fMRI and the fragile X syndrome: human genome epidemiology review. *Genet Med.* 2001;3:359–371.
99. Guerreiro MM, Camargo EE, Kato M, et al. Fragile X syndrome. Clinical, electroencephalographic and neuroimaging characteristics. *Arq Neuropsiquiatr.* 1998;56:18–23.

100. Eliez S, Blasey CM, Freund LS, et al. Brain anatomy, gender and IQ in children and adolescents with fragile X syndrome. *Brain*. 2001;124:1610–1618.
101. Tamm L, Menon V, Johnston CK, et al. fMRI study of cognitive interference processing in females with fragile X syndrome. *J Cogn Neurosci*. 2002;14:160–171.
102. Swerdlow NR, Karban B, Ploum Y, et al. Tactile prepuff inhibition of startle in children with Tourette's syndrome: in search of an "fMRI-friendly" startle paradigm. *Biol Psychiatry*. 2001;50:578–585.
103. Biswal BB, Ulmer JL, Krippendorf RL, et al. Abnormal cerebral activation associated with a motor task in Tourette syndrome. *AJNR Am J Neuroradiol*. 1998;19:1509–1512.
104. Oktem F, Diren B, Karaagaoglu E, et al. Functional magnetic resonance imaging in children with Asperger's syndrome. *J Child Neurol*. 2001;16: 253–256.
105. Muller RA, Pierce K, Ambrose JB, et al. Atypical patterns of cerebral motor activation in autism: a functional magnetic resonance study. *Biol Psychiatry*. 2001;49:665–676.
106. Schneider G. Early lesions and abnormal neuronal connections. *Trends Neurosci*. 1981;4:187–192.
107. Hebb D. The effect of early and late brain injury upon test scores, and the nature of normal adult intelligence. *Proc Am Phil Soc*. 1942;85:275–292.
108. Maegaki Y, Yamamoto T, Takeshita K. Plasticity of central motor and sensory pathways in a case of unilateral extensive cortical dysplasia: investigation of magnetic resonance imaging, transcranial magnetic stimulation and short-latency somatosensory evoked potentials. *Neurology*. 1995;45:2255–2261.
109. Purdy SC, Kelly AS, Thorne PR. Auditory evoked potentials as measures of plasticity in humans. *Audiol Neurootol*. 2001;6:211–215.
110. Papanicolaou AC, Simos PG, Breier JI, et al. Brain plasticity for sensory and linguistic functions: a functional imaging study using magnetoencephalography with children and young adults. *J Child Neurol*. 2001;16: 241–252.
111. Benecke R, Meyer BU. Magnetic stimulationof corticonuclear systems and of cranial nerves in man: physiological basis and clinical application. *Electroencephalogr Clin Neurophysiol*. 1991;43 (Suppl):333–343.
112. Muller RA, Rothermel RD, Behen ME, et al. Language organization in patients with early and late left-hemispheric lesion: a PET study. *Neuropsychologia*. 1999;37:545–557.
113. Hertz-Pannier L, Chiron C, Van de Morteele P, et al. Non-invasive assessment of language dominance in children and adolescents with functional MRI: a preliminary study. *Neurology*. 1997;205:534.
114. Hertz-Pannier L, Chiron C, Jambaque I, et al. Late plasticity for language in a child's non-dominant hemisphere: a pre-and post-surgery fMRI study. *Brain*. 2002;125:361–372.
115. Hamzei F, Liepert J, Dettmers C, et al. Structural and functional cortical abnormalities after upper limb amputation during childhood. *Neuroreport*. 2000;12:957–962.
116. Iwase Y, Mashiko T, Ochiai N, et al. Postoperative changes on functional mapping of the motor cortex in patients with brachial plexus injury: comparative study of magnetoencephalography and functional magnetic resonance imaging. *J Orthop Sci*. 2001;6:397–402.
117. Jackson GD, Connelly A, Cross JH, et al. Functional magnetic resonance imaging of focal seizures. *Neurology*. 1994;44:850–856.

118. Schwartz TH, Resor SR Jr., De La Paz R. Functional magnetic resonance imaging localization of ictal onset to a dysplastic cleft with simultaneous sensorimotor mapping: intraoperative electrophysiological confirmation and postoperative follow-up: technical note. *Neurosurgery*. 1998;43:639–644.
119. Detre JA, Sirven JI, Alsop DC, et al. Localization of subclinical ictal activity by functional magnetic resonance imaging: correlation with invasive monitoring. *Ann Neurol*. 1995;38:618–624.
120. Krakow K, Lemieux L, Messina D, et al. Spatio-temporal imaging of focal interictal epileptiform activity using EEG-triggered functional MRI. *Epileptic Disord*. 2001;3:67–74.
121. Krakow K, Woermann FG, Symms MR, et al. EEG-triggered functional MRI of interictal epileptiform activity in patients with partial seizures. *Brain*. 1999;122:1679–1688.
122. Lazeyras F, Blanke O, Perrig S, et al. EEG-triggered functional MRI in patients with pharmacoresistant epilepsy. *J Magn Reson Imaging*. 2000;12:177–185.
123. Matsuoka LK, Anderson AW, Gore JC, et al. Functional magnetic resonance imaging identifies abnormal visual cortical function in patients with occipital lobe epilepsy. *Epilepsia*. 1999;40:1248–1253.

# 16

# fMRI of Clinical Pain

Karen D. Davis

## Introduction

### The Pain Experience

Pain is a subjective experience. Although we can objectively measure the functionality of aspects of the nervous system that likely contribute to pain—such as peripheral nerve conduction, neuronal responses to noxious stimuli, etc.—the actual pain experience can only be assessed from subjective reports. The lack of objective measures of pain can lead to misunderstandings and under-appreciation of the totality of the pain experience. However, the maturation of functional brain imaging technologies now provides an opportunity to develop an objective correlate of the subjective pain experience.

It is important to recognize that pain encompasses more than one dimension. In 1968, Melzack and Casey[1] described a multistage framework for the pain experience: First, a sensation of pain due to activation of a central pain center; second, an evaluation and perception of the pain, leading to the third stage of pain affect and motivation. The second and third stages contribute to various pain reactions. Central modulation is also an important factor on the overall pain experience.[2] More recently, additional factors such as salience, past experience, gender, culture, and attention have been shown to impact the pain experience.[3–6]

A modern view of pain is that it is experienced along several dimensions so that its location can be detected, its intensity can be sensed, its texture based on sensory qualities can be appreciated, its meaning and value can be interpreted and assessed based on context, past experience, and future needs to react emotionally to construct motor reactions and coping strategies.

## Suitability of fMRI for the Study of Pain

Functional magnetic resonance imaging (fMRI) can demonstrate identifiable MRI signals within specific brain regions during application of a sensory stimulus (e.g., touch) or during performance of a motor task (e.g., digit movement). This new technique has been used for the study of pain. There are, however, certain restrictions on the use of fMRI to study pain. An fMRI activation map is achieved when the MRI signals recorded during a task are compared to a reference signal—typically obtained during a control state or rest. The absolute numerical values of the MRI signals at any one timepoint are not meaningful unless compared to other timepoints within that scanning session, unlike other imaging techniques that can record signal values that actually represent a physiological measure (e.g., blood flow, receptor occupation, etc.). It is not possible to evaluate the meaning of the fMRI numerical values if there is only one state throughout the scan. Simply stated, fMRI tells us how the brain responds to a stimulus. Therefore, fMRI studies often are referred to as activation studies. Functional fMRI studies of pain require subjects to be in both a pain state and a control state. The end result of this technical caveat is that fMRI is best suited to study acute, experimental pain rather than chronic pain. Thus, the field of imaging pain was initially directed towards understanding the brain mechanisms underlying acute experimental pain. However, the findings from these acute pain studies are crucial to the understanding of normal brain mechanisms underlying both acute and clinical pain. More recently, creative solutions have emerged to provide opportunities to study some clinical and chronic pain states.

An important issue that must be considered in all pain imaging studies is the multiple systems that are affected when a pain stimulus is expected and then actually delivered, or when pain is experienced. As noted above, pain is a multidimensional experience; therefore, the pain can invoke attention, anticipation (possibly of more pain), cardiovascular changes, memories, stress, and motor responses. Each of these outcomes may be associated with increased, decreased, or modulation of activity, particularly in the forebrain region. Furthermore, if the pain is being assessed during the scan, there may also be brain activations due to this assessment (e.g., motor responses, evaluative responses, attentional responses). Such confounds need to be controlled for and carefully considered in the fMRI data interpretation.

One technical obstacle that is inherent to pain fMRI studies is the ability to deliver the stimulus modality of choice. All devices used for fMRI must be MR-compatible. This is not a problem for simple nonmetallic mechanical devices such as von Frey probes or brushes. However, other devices (TENS, thermal stimulators, lasers, etc.) may require special shielding or modification to avoid interference (noise) during imaging. Magnetic resonance-compatible response devices (e.g., button press boxes, trackball) are readily available.

## fMRI of Acute, Nonclinical Pain

Studies of acute, nonclinical pain have examined the forebrain responses to various types of noxious stimuli. For technical reasons, the earliest studies were restricted to single-subject designs and imaging within a limited number of brain slices.[5,7–17] Despite these limitations (including statistical power problems), this approach was quite useful to ask very specific questions about particular brain regions, as well as to investigate individual variations in pain responses. Technical improvements in the late 1990s made it possible to acquire whole brain coverage during a single imaging session, and also to average/combine data across subjects. One of the major advantages of this approach is improved statistical power. Additionally, group studies allow inferences about common pain mechanisms. However, it should be noted that group-average maps have reduced spatial resolution and represent only those areas of activation that generally are common to the subject population. Figure 16.1 shows an example of group-averaged pain-related activity in the primary somatosensory cortex (S1) and single-subject pain-related activity in secondary somatosensory

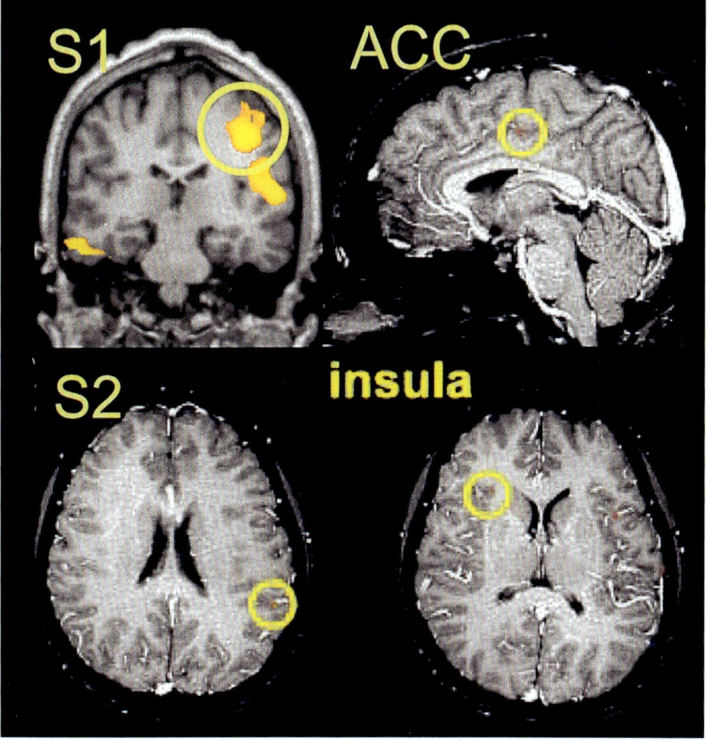


**Figure 16.1.** Acute cutaneous pain-related activity in the primary somatosensory cortex (S1), secondary somatosensory cortex (S2), anterior cingulate cortex (ACC), and the anterior insula (see encircled areas). The S1 activation is taken from group-averaged data, whereas the other examples are taken from a single subject analysis. From the lab of Karen D. Davis, with permission.

cortex (S2), the anterior cingulate cortex (ACC), and the anterior insula. Of note are the small discrete activations in the single subjects. Because these activations are likely to show some anatomic variability from subject to subject, successful group averaging of relatively commonly located activations require spatial smoothing, which tends then to result in the somewhat blurred group images such as the S1 example.

Acute pain group studies have examined the responses to mechanical, thermal (hot/cold), electrical, or chemical stimuli applied to the skin, muscle, and viscera. Most studies have used a block-design approach whereby the repeated painful and control stimuli (or rest) are interleaved with relatively long stimulus durations (15 to 60 seconds). A few studies have found that an event-related approach using shorter stimuli (e.g., thermal, laser) can also be effective.[10,18,19] The general consensus of most acute pain imaging studies is that there are multiple cortical areas that respond during painful stimulation, including S1, S2, insula, ACC, prefrontal cortex and various motor nuclei (e.g., SMA, M1, cerebellum, basal ganglia). However, there is considerable variability across studies and across subjects. Much of this variability can be attributed to the level and type of stimulus used to evoke pain. Such variability in stimulation methods led to varying amounts and quality of pain experiences and related responses.[5,20,21] More recently, fMRI studies of pain have been designed to address specific aspects of the pain experience. There is some evidence for the involvement of S1, S2, insula, ACC, and even some motor areas in the intensity aspect of pain.[5,13] With the ACC, several studies have shown a segregation of pain intensity-, motor-, and attention-related responses.[8,18,22] However, a recent study emphasized the difficulty in identifying brain areas related to a specific aspect of the pain experience due to the overlap of intensity information within the affect, feature extraction, motor control, and attention components of pain.[23] Anticipation of pain has also been shown to be a powerful modulator of activity in pain-related areas such as S1, insula, and the ACC,[19,24] although there may be some segregation of pain-related and anticipation-related activations within the insula, ACC, and cerebellum.[16]

## fMRI of Clinical Pain

Despite the growing number of fMRI studies of acute, nonclinical pain, imaging clinical pain with fMRI is in its infancy. However, a few strategies have been devised to study patients with different types of clinical pain using fMRI.

### Allodynia

Allodynia refers to the pain that is evoked by stimuli that are not normally painful (e.g., light touch or cool temperatures). Allodynia is commonly experienced in normal individuals after a cut, burn, or insect bite. However, allodynia is also a common component of some types of chronic pain, particularly neuropathic pain.[25] The most popular experimental model of allodynia is the capsaicin model. Topical or subcutaneous capsaicin readily produces a pronounced burning pain that is followed by a state of mechanical allodynia (pain to the touch) within a large region surrounding the capsaicin site. An fMRI study of capsaicin-induced allodynia found that touching allodynic skin evoked a greater response than touching non-allodynic skin, particularly in the prefrontal cortex.[26] In a single case report of central pain and allodynia following stroke, a cool stimulus applied to the allodynic skin (but not the normal skin) evoked responses in the S2/insula area (Figure 16.2).[27] These studies corroborate the concept that the cortex can reflect the perceptual response to a stimulus rather than the physical properties of the stimulus. A related clinical disorder is fibromyalgia that is characterized by diffuse pain and tenderness. fMRI studies have been performed that show evidence of augmentation of pain processing in this disorder (Figure 16.3).[28,29]

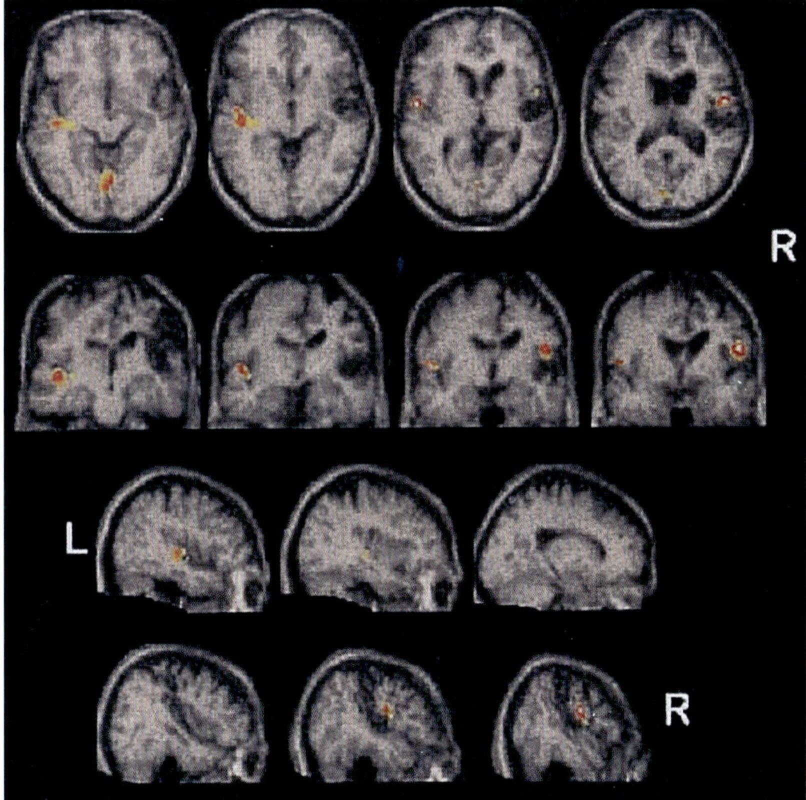


**Figure 16.2.** Left-sided allodynia-related activity (due to a non-noxious cool stimulus moved across the skin) in the S2/insula area of a patient with central pain following a stroke involving the right S1, S2, and ACC. See Peyron and colleagues[20] for details. Reprinted with permission from Peyron R, Garcia-Larrea L, Gregoire MC, Convers P, Richard A, Lavenne F, et al. Parietal and cingulated processes in central pain. A combined positron emission tomography (PET) and functional magnetic resonance imaging (fMRI) study of an unusual case. *Pain* 2000;84(1):77–87.

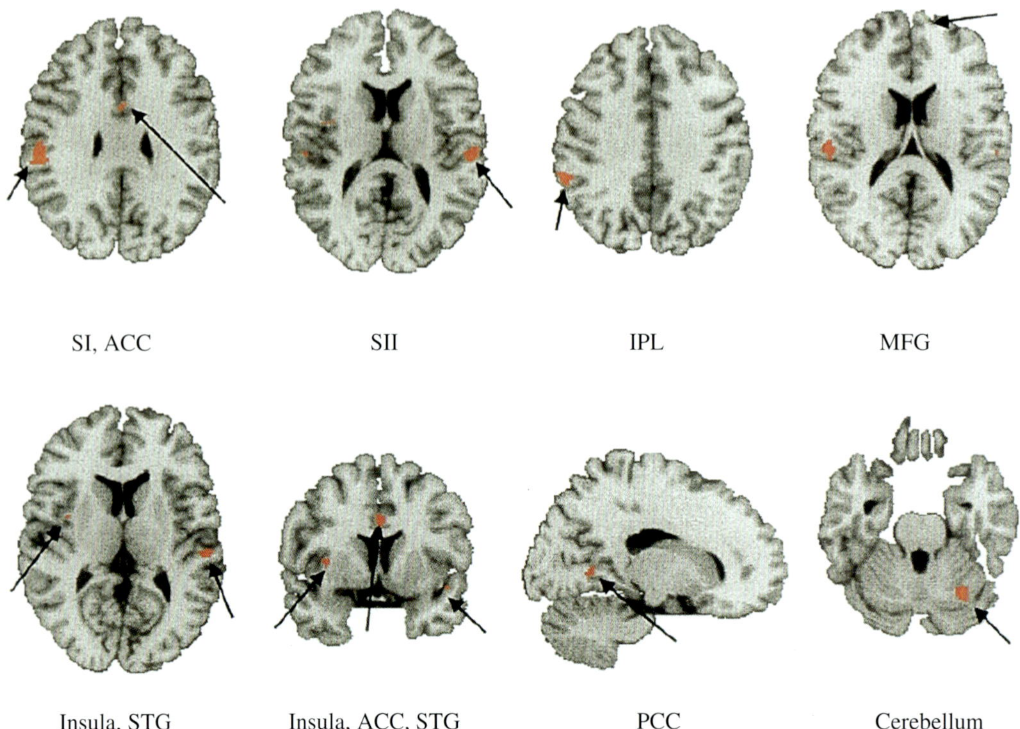


**Figure 16.3.** Comparison of the effects of similar stimulus pressures in patients and controls. Results of unpaired *t*-tests of the mean difference in signal (**arrows**) between painful pressure and innocuous touch for each group are shown in standard space superimposed on an anatomic image of a standard brain. Image are shown in radiologic view, with the right brain shown on the left. Regions in which the response in patients was significantly greater than the response in controls are shown in red; regions in which the response in controls was significantly greater than that in patients are shown in green. The level of significance was adjusted for multiple comparisons at $P < 0.05$. Patients showed significant activations that were significantly different from the activation in the healthy controls in the SI, IPL, insula, posterior cingulate cortex (PCC), SII, ATG, and cerebellum. The peak of the significant difference in anterior cingulate cortex (ACC) is in the right hemisphere, although the activation is near the midline and spreads into both hemispheres. Significant increases in the contralateral STG and in a scond region of ipsilateral cerebellum are not shown. In contrast to these regions of significantly greater signal differences in patients, the similar stimulus pressures resulted in 1 region of significantly increased stimulus intensity in control subjects, located in the medial frontal gyrus (MFG). (See Gracely RH et al.,[28] with permission.) *Source*: Gracely RH, Petzke F, Wolf JM, Clauw DJ. Functional magnetic resonance imaging evidence of augmented pain processing in fibromyalgia. *Arthritis Rheum* 2002;46:1333–1343.

## Visceral Pain

To date, there have been only a few preliminary fMRI studies of visceral pain (e.g., esophageal, rectal), and many have been restricted to normal subject populations.[30,31] These studies generally found that that cortical areas associated with somatic pains were activated during acute visceral pain. Figure 16.4 shows an example of the cortical activations found during painful distention of the esophagus in normal subjects. The development of methods to study visceral pain in control subjects is extremely important to provide a framework from which to study patients with visceral pain. Recent fMRI reports of rectal-evoked

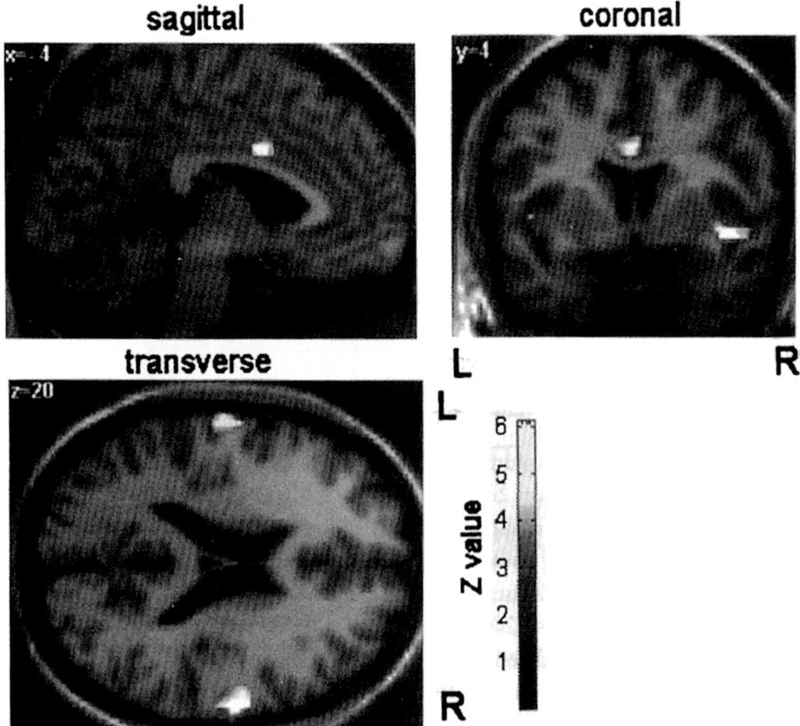


**Figure 16.4.** Cortical activations associated with painful distention of the esophagus in a normal volunteer. Note the activations in the anterior cingulate cortex (sagittal view), right insula (coronal view), and parietal opercula (axial view). Reprinted with permission from Binkofski F, Schnitzler A, Enck P, Frieling T, Posse S, Seitz RJ, et al. Somatic and limbic cortex activation in esophageal distention: A functional magnetic resonance imaging study. *Ann Neurol* 1998;44:811–815. Reprinted with permission of John Wiley and Sons. Inc. (Neurologic coordinates)

activations in patients with irritable bowel syndrome and inflammatory bowel disease suggest abnormal cortical processing in these patient groups.[32,33] Because many patients with visceral pain display visceral hyperalgesia (e.g., irritable bowel syndrome), it is important to monitor the pain evoked by test stimuli during fMRI so that the brain activations can be related to the patient's pain.[34]

### Headache

Migraine headaches often are preceded by particular prodrome symptoms such as visual, somatosensory, or motor disturbances. The phenomena known as cortical spreading depression is thought to be related to these auras.[35] An fMRI study of migraine visual aura found a period of reduced visual responsiveness that spread across the occipital cortex during the aura (Figure 16.5).[36,37] These studies support the concept of cortical spreading depression in the etiology of aura. In-depth fMRI studies of the subsequent pain phase of migraine have not yet been published.

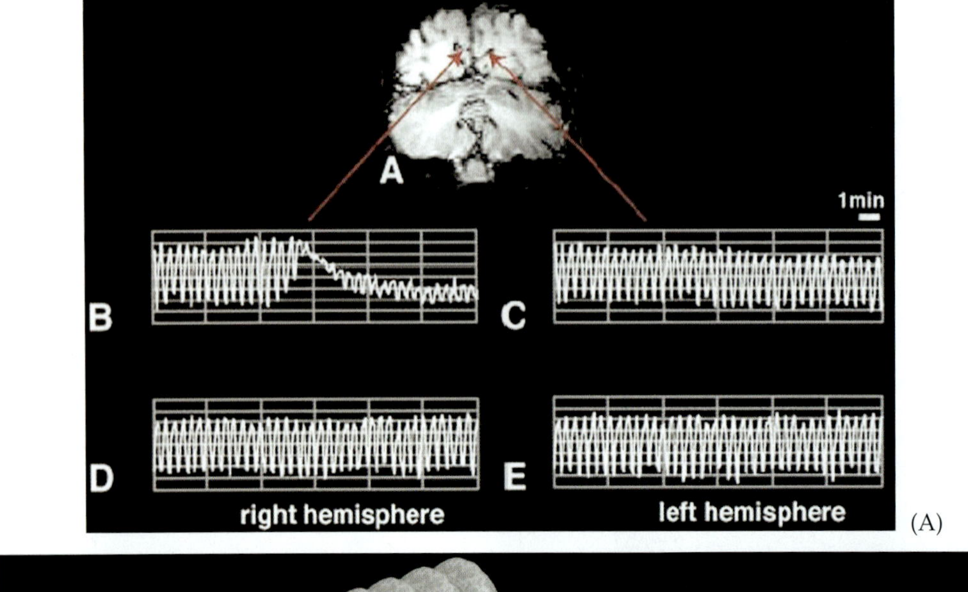


(A)

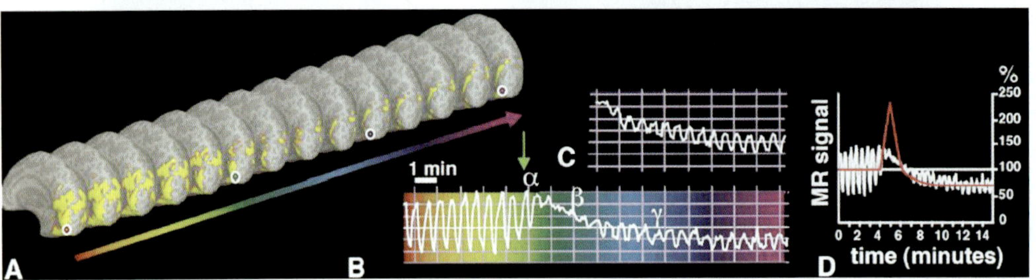


(B)

**Figure 16.5.** (A) Ictal and interictal BOLD responses in human visual cortex. A representative functional MRI slice is shown *(A)*. The slice plane was oriented near-perpendicular to the calcarine fissure, so that cerebellum occupies the lower portion of the figure, and occipital lobe occupies the upper portion. *(B–E)* Representative BOLD responses over time, taken from single voxels within homologous areas of the occipital lobe (*B and D, Right* vs. *C* and *E, Left*), as designated by green arrows. Time is shown on the $x$ axis, and levels of MR modulation are shown on the $y$ axis. The stimulus-driven signal oscillation in *B–E* is the BOLD responses to 16-s presentations of the checkerboard visual stimulus (on response), relative to the intervening 16-s presentations of a black screen with a fixation point (off response). (*D* and *E*) Normal BOLD modulation during an interictal period for each hemisphere. (*B* and *C*) The BOLD responses during a migraine aura affecting only the right hemisphere (*B*) Perturbations did not appear in the left hemisphere during the ictal (*C*), or interictal scans (*D* and *E*). (B) Time-dependent BOLD activity changes from a single region of interest in VI, acquired before and during episodes of either spontaneous (*C*) or induced (*B*) visual aura. (*A*) A series of anatomical images, including BOLD activity on "inflated" cortical hemispheres showing the medial bank (similar to a conventional mid-sagittal view). Images were sampled at 32-s intervals, showing the same region of interest (circles) in V1. (*B*) The MR signal perturbation over time from the circled region of interest; the perturbation is similar to that in Fig. 16.5A. Variations in time are color-coded (deep red to magenta), and the four colored circles match corresponding times within the V1 region of interest. The slice prescription failed to include a few mm in the most posterior part of the occipital pole in that induced attack, so activation is not revealed in any of these images. *B* shows that before the onset of the aura, the BOLD response to visual stimulation shows a normal, oscillating activation pattern. After the onset of aura (green arrow), the BOLD response showed a marked increase in mean level (α), a marked suppression to light modulation (β), followed by a partial recovery of the response to light modulation at decreased mean level (γ; –3% to –6%). (*C*) Data from a spontaneous attack (subject M.C.), captured ≈18 min after the onset of the visual symptoms affecting the right hemifield. The data represent the time course in left visual area V1, at an eccentricity of ≈20° of visual angle. (*D*) A superimposition of CBF changes seen in the rat during CSD (as described by Lauritzen et al.) with the MR signal data shown in *A*. Note that the timing of the hyperemia (3–4.5 min in CSD vs. 3.3 ± 1.9 min in migraine aura) is remarkably similar in these two quite different data sets. The amplitude of the hyperemia is different in the two conditions, presumably because of differences in the blood flow measurement techniques used (laser doppler versus BOLD) and the nonlinear relationship between blood flow and BOLD signal. *Source*: Hadjikhani N, Sanchez DR, Wu O, Schwartz D, Bakker D, Fischl B, et al. Mechanisms of migraine aura revealed by functional MRI in human visual cortex. *Proc Natl Acad Sci USA*. 2001;98(8):4687–4692.

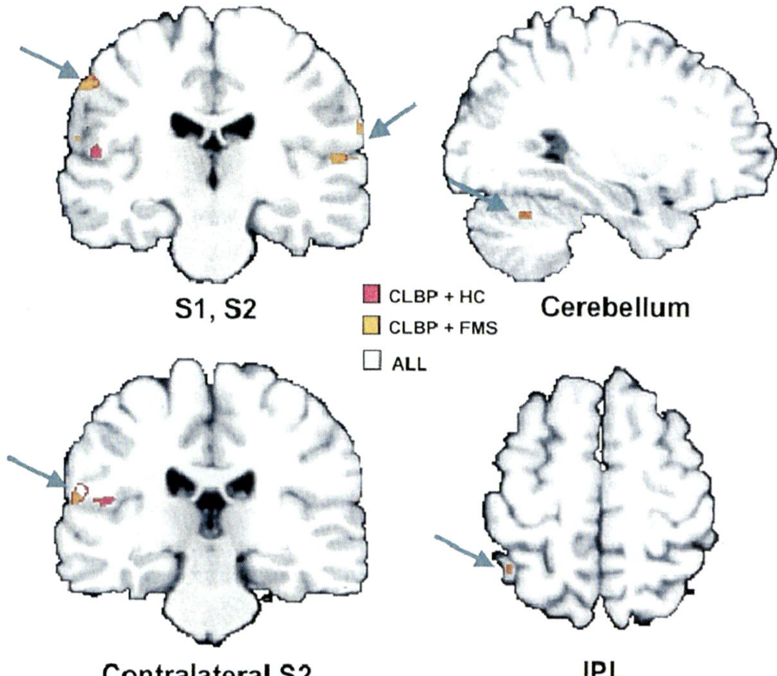


**Figure 16.6.** Overlapping neuronal activations under the equal stimulus condition. In the chronic low back pain (CLBP), fibromyalgia syndrome (FMS), and healthy control (HC) groups under the equal pressure condition, significant increases in pain-related neuronal activations (**arrows**) are demonstrate in standard space superimposed on a structural T1-weighted magnetic resonance image. Images are shown in radiologic view, with the right brain shown on the left. Overlapping activations appear in the indicated colors. Equal pressure intensities result in 5 overlapping areas of neuronal activation in the CLBP and FMS groups (in the contralateral S1, S2, and inferior parietal lobule [IPL], and in ipsilateral S2 and cerebellum), but in only 1 overlapping area of neuronal activation among the HC, CLBP, and FMS groups (in the contralateral S2). *Source*: Giesecke T, Gracely RH, Grant MAB, et al. Evidence of augmented central pain processing in idiopathic chronic lower back pain. *Arthritis Rheum* 2004;50:613–623.

## Low Back Pain

There is a limited number of studies of back pain using fMRI. In a recent case report, a patient was scanned during alternating periods of rest and straight leg raises.[38] Psychophysical monitoring prior to the scan confirmed that the patient's back pain was exacerbated during the leg raises. This preliminary study did not provide detailed results, but was nonetheless instructive in demonstrating the feasibility of modulating chronic pain for future studies.

Another study examined a group of patients with idiopathic chronic low back pain (LBP), fibromyalgia and normals.[39] It showed that patients with CLBP and fibromyalgia have increased pressure-pain sensitivity at a site distant from their region of clinical pain. These findings are consistent with the presence of central augmentation of pain processing (Figure 16.6).

## Phantom Pain

Following amputation, a majority of patients experience phantom pain—pain that is experienced as arising in the missing limb. Phantom pains can take many forms, including feelings of burning pain, shooting pain, cramping pain, or that something is penetrating the limb. Most theories of phantom pain include abnormal processing and plasticity in the central nervous system (CNS).[40–42] These theories are based mostly on animal studies because there is limited opportunity to obtain data in humans. However, thalamic electrophysiological recordings[43] and imaging studies (with electric source imaging, MEG, PET, or EEG[44–48] in amputees support the concept that central plasticity impacts on phantom phenomena. The precise effect is still unknown, but recent fMRI studies have provided some insight into the functionality of the sensorimotor cortex in patients with phantom pain. One group[49] found a shift in center of the primary sensorimotor representation of the lip into the region normally representing the absent limb in amputees with phantom pain. Furthermore, when these amputees imagined moving their missing limb, there was activation of the face area of sensorimotor cortex. Interestingly, these signs of plasticity were not observed in amputees who had no pain after using a myoelectric prosthesis. Another group[50] reported similar regions of motor cortex activation during actual finger movements compared to imagining moving the missing fingers, but they noted an increased area of S1 when an amputee imagined their phantom pain versus nonpainful phantom limb manipulation. A slightly different aspect of plasticity was investigated by another group,[51] who obtained fMRI data in upper-extremity amputees during movements of their intact stump and shoulder. This study found that movements of the stump or shoulder on the amputated side produced more widespread primary and supplemental motor cortex activation than on the intact side. The presence of phantom pain also enhanced this effect. The abnormal findings on the amputated side were attributed to an increased excitability. A single case report of increased S1 during painful and nonpainful stimulation of the stump versus contralateral intact skin[52] corroborates this concept. The aforementioned studies demonstrate the applicability of fMRI in studies of the mechanisms of phantom pain.

## Spinal and Brain Stimulation

Preliminary studies have demonstrated the utility of fMRI in a small number of chronic pain patients with implanted spinal[53] and brain[54] stimulators. In both studies, trial stimulation prior to fMRI was effective in reducing the patient's chronic intractable pain. During the imaging sessions, stimulators were turned on for short periods of time to evoke tingling sensations. The stimulation evoked activation of S1, S2, insula, and ACC. Larger-scale studies are needed to provide detailed information about the mechanism of brain and spinal stimulation effects on pain. However, these types of studies require extreme caution to protect against potentially harmful effects of using implanted stimulation devices in an MR environment.

## Challenges in Imaging Chronic and Clinical Pains

The fMRI technique basically relies on an activation strategy whereby a statistical analysis is performed on brain images obtained in two states (e.g., pain and nonpain) (see above); therefore, the fundamental challenge in chronic/clinical pain studies is to manipulate the pain state during a single imaging session—either to increase or decrease the pain. If the patient experiences ongoing spontaneous pain, then the manipulation must decrease the pain (e.g., short-acting analgesics, distraction). Conversely, if the patient does not have spontaneous pain, but does have evoked pain (e.g., allodynia, back pain), then an appropriate stimulus is used to invoke the pain; therefore, this approach can provide information about the cortical areas active when the patient is experiencing their clinical pain. However, a related type of study can be done to investigate how a patient with one type of pain responds to other types of pain. This type of study may provide insight into more general abnormalities in cortical pain responsiveness.

Because clinical pain can often change on a daily basis, another challenge is to have insight into what the patient is feeling during the imaging session. Some labs developed methods for monitoring pain levels during imaging of acute pain.[10,13,55,56,57] These methods should be used to differentiate cortical responses related to the pain experience rather than merely to the presence of a stimulus because the two types of responses may differ under normal and pathological conditions; for instance, a light brush stimulus is perceived as a nonpainful touch under normal conditions, but in an allodynic state, this same stimulus evokes pain.

## Future Applications

Despite technical difficulties, the fMRI technique has great potential for the study of clinical pain. One area for future development is in the study of analgesic drug effects. Several PET studies have already been conducted that demonstrate the forebrain action of opiate agonists such as (remi)fentanyl in suppressing regional cerebral blood flow and responses to noxious stimuli in regions[58,59] associated with pain perception. Another area for further development is in patients with neuropathic pain conditions, especially in cases with associated allodynia or hyperalgesia. These patients are well suited for fMRI study because their pain can be evoked by mechanical or thermal stimuli. Other conditions that are characterized by evokable pain, such as joint and muscle disorders, would also be suited for study using fMRI.

## References

1. Melzack R, Casey KL. Sensory, motivational, and central control determinants of pain: a new conceptual model. In: Kenshalo D, ed. The Skin Senses. Springfield: C.C. Thomas; 1968:423–439.

2. Melzack R, Wall PD. Pain mechanisms: A new theory. *Science.* 1965;150: 971–979.
3. Rainville P. Brain mechanisms of pain affect and pain modulation. *Curr Opin Neurobiol.* 2002;12(2):195–204.
4. Casey KL, Lorenz J. The determinants of pain revisited: coordinates in sensory space. *Pain Res Manag.* 2000;5:197–204.
5. Bushnell MC, Duncan GH, Hofbauer RK, Ha B, Chen JI, Carrier B. Pain perception: is there a role for primary somatosensory cortex? *Proc Natl Acad Sci U S A.* 1999;96(14):7705–7709.
6. Berkley KJ. Sex differences in pain. *Behav Brain Sci.* 1997;20:371–380.
7. Davis KD, Wood ML, Crawley AP, Mikulis DJ. fMRI of human somatosensory and cingulate cortex during painful electrical nerve stimulation. *Neuroreport.* 1995;7:321–325.
8. Davis KD, Taylor SJ, Crawley AP, Wood ML, Mikulis DJ. Functional MRI of pain- and attention-related activations in the human cingulate cortex. *J Neurophysiol.* 1997;77:3370–3380.
9. Bucher SF, Dieterich M, Wiesmann M, Weiss A, Zink R, Yousry TA, et al. Cerebral functional magnetic resonance imaging of vestibular, auditory, and nociceptive areas during galvanic stimulation. *Ann Neurol.* 1998;44: 120–125.
10. Davis KD, Kwan CL, Crawley AP, Mikulis DJ. Event-related fMRI of pain: entering a new era in imaging pain. *Neuroreport.* 1998;9:3019–3023.
11. Davis KD, Kwan CL, Crawley AP, Mikulis DJ. Functional MRI study of thalamic and cortical activations evoked by cutaneous heat, cold and tactile stimuli. *J Neurophysiol.* 1998;80:1533–1546.
12. Disbrow E, Buonocore M, Antognini J, Carstens E, Rowley HA. Somatosensory cortex: a comparison of the response to noxious thermal, mechanical, and electrical stimuli using functional magnetic resonance imaging. *Hum Brain Mapp.* 1998;6:150–159.
13. Porro CA, Cettolo V, Francescato MP, Baraldi P. Temporal and intensity coding of pain in human cortex. *J Neurophysiol.* 1998;80:3312–3320.
14. Becerra LR, Breiter HC, Stojanovic M, Fishman S, Edwards A, Comite AR, et al. Human brain activation under controlled thermal stimulation and habituation to noxious heat: an fMRI study. *Magn Reson Med.* 1999;41(5): 1044–1057.
15. Gelnar PA, Krauss BR, Sheehe PR, Szeverenyi NM, Apkarian AV. A comparative fMRI study of cortical representations for thermal painful, vibrotactile, and motor performance tasks. *Neuroimage.* 1999;10(4):460–482.
16. Ploghaus A, Tracey I, Gati JS, Clare S, Menon RS, Matthews PM, et al. Dissociating pain from its anticipation in the human brain. *Science.* 1999; 284(5422):1979–1981.
17. Davis KD, Kwan CL, Crawley AP, Mikulis DJ. fMRI of cortical and thalamic activations correlated to the magnitude of pain. In: Devor M, Rowbotham MC, Wiesenfeld-Hallin Z, eds. Progress in Pain Research and Management, Proceedings of the 9th World Congress on Pain. Seattle, WA: IASP Press; 2000:497–505.
18. Buchel C, Bornhovd K, Quante M, Glauche V, Bromm B, Weiller C. Dissociable neural responses related to pain intensity, stimulus intensity, and stimulus awareness within the anterior cingulate cortex: A parametric single-trial laser functional magnetic resonance imaging study. *J Neurosci.* 2002;22(3):970–976.
19. Sawamoto N, Honda M, Okada T, Hanakawa T, Kanda M, Fukuyama H, et al. Expectation of pain enhances responses to nonpainful somatosensory

stimulation in the anterior cingulate cortex and parietal Operculum/Posterior insula: an event-related functional magnetic resonance imaging study. *J Neurosci.* 2000;20(19):7438–7445.
20. Peyron R, Laurent B, Garcia-Larrea L. Functional imaging of brain responses to pain. A review and meta-analysis (2000). *Neurophysiol Clin.* 2000;30(5):263–288.
21. Davis KD. Studies of pain using fMRI. In: Bushnell MC, Casey KL, eds. Pain Imaging. Seattle, WA: IASP Press; 2000:195–210.
22. Kwan CL, Crawley AP, Mikulis DJ, Davis KD. An fMRI study of the anterior cingulate cortex and surrounding medial wall activations evoked by noxious cutaneous heat and cold stimuli. *Pain.* 2000;85:359–374.
23. Coghill RC, Sang CN, Maisog JM, Iadarola MJ. Pain intensity processing within the human brain: A bilateral, distributed mechanism. *J Neurophysiol.* 1999;82(4):1934–1943.
24. Porro CA, Baraldi P, Pagnoni G, Serafini M, Facchin P, Maieron M, et al. Does anticipation of pain affect cortical nociceptive systems? *J Neurosci.* 2002;22(8):3206–3214.
25. IASP Task Force on Taxonomy. Classification of chronic pain. Descriptions of chronic pain syndromes and definitions of pain terms. 2nd ed. Seattle, WA: IASP Press; 1994.
26. Baron R, Baron Y, Disbrow E, Roberts TP. Brain processing of capsaicin-induced secondary hyperalgesia: a functional MRI study. *Neurology.* 1999; 53(3):548–557.
27. Peyron R, Garcia-Larrea L, Gregoire MC, Convers P, Richard A, Lavenne F, et al. Parietal and cingulate processes in central pain. A combined positron emission tomography (PET) and functional magnetic resonance imaging (fMRI) study of an unusual case. *Pain.* 2000;84(1):77–87.
28. Gracely RH, Petzke F, Wolf JM, Clauw DJ. Functional magnetic resonance imaging evidence of augmented pain processing in fibromyalgia. Arthritis Rheum 2002;46:1333–1343.
29. Gracely RH, Gerssei ME, Giesecke T. et al. Pain catastrophizing and neural responses to pain among persons with fibromyalgia. Brain 2004; Feb. 11.
30. Binkofski F, Schnitzler A, Enck P, Frieling T, Posse S, Seitz RJ, et al. Somatic and limbic cortex activation in esophageal distention: A functional magnetic resonance imaging study. *Ann Neurol.* 1998;44:811–815.
31. Baciu MV, Bonaz BL, Papillon E, Bost RA, Le Bas JF, Fournet J, et al. Central processing of rectal pain: a functional MR imaging study. *AJNR Am J Neuroradiol.* 1999;20(10):1920–1924.
32. Mertz H, Morgan V, Tanner G, Pickens D, Price R, Shyr Y, et al. Regional cerebral activation in irritable bowel syndrome and control subjects with painful and nonpainful rectal distention. *Gastroenterology.* 2000;118(5):842–848.
33. Bernstein CN, Frankenstein UN, Rawsthorne P, Pitz M, Summers R, McIntyre MC. Cortical mapping of visceral pain in patients with GI disorders using functional magnetic resonance imaging. *Am J Gastroenterol.* 2002; 97(2):319–327.
34. Kwan CL, Diamant NE, Mikulis DJ, Davis KD. Percept-related fMRI of rectal-evoked sensations in irritable bowel syndrome. [abstract] *Soc Neurosci.* 2002.
35. James MF, Smith JM, Boniface SJ, Huang CLH, Leslie RA. Cortical spreading depression and migraine: new insights from imaging? *Trends Neurosci.* 2001;24(5):266–271.

36. Cao Y, Welch KM, Aurora S, Vikingstad EM. Functional MRI-BOLD of visually triggered headache in patients with migraine. *Arch Neurol.* 1999;56(5): 548–554.
37. Hadjikhani N, Sanchez DR, Wu O, Schwartz D, Bakker D, Fischl B, et al. Mechanisms of migraine aura revealed by functional MRI in human visual cortex. *Proc Natl Acad Sci U S A.* 2001;98(8):4687–4692.
38. Apkarian AV, Krauss BR, Fredrickson BE, Szeverenyi NM. Imaging the pain of low back pain: functional magnetic resonance imaging in combination with monitoring subjective pain perception allows the study of clinical pain states. *Neurosci Lett.* 2001;299(1–2):57–60.
39. Giesecke T, Gracely RH, Grant MAB, et al. Evidence of augmented central pain processing in idiopathic chronic lower back pain. Arthritis Rheum 2004;50:613–623.
40. Sherman RA, Sherman CJ, Parker L. Chronic phantom and stump pain among American veterans: results of a survey. *Pain.* 1984;18:83–95.
41. Katz J, Melzack R. Pain 'memories' in phantom limbs: review and clinical observations. *Pain.* 1990;43:319–336.
42. Ramachandran VS, Hirstein W. The perception of phantom limbs—The D.O. Hebb lecture. *Brain.* 1998;121:1603–1630.
43. Davis KD, Kiss ZHT, Luo L, Tasker RR, Lozano AM, Dostrovsky JO. Phantom sensations generated by thalamic microstimulation. *Nature.* 1998;391:385–387.
44. Elbert T, Flor H, Birbaumer N, Knecht S, Hampson S, Larbig W, et al. Extensive reorganization of the somatosensory cortex in adult humans after nervous system injury. *Neuroreport.* 1994;5:2593–2597.
45. Kew JJM, Halligan PW, Marshall JC, Passingham RE, Rothwell JC, Ridding MC, et al. Abnormal access of axial vibrotactile input to deafferented somatosensory cortex in human upper limb amputees. *J Neurophysiol.* 1997;77:2753–2764.
46. Yang TT, Gallen CC, Ramachandran VS, Cobb S, Schwartz BJ, Bloom FE. Noninvasive detection of cerebral plasticity in adult human somatosensory cortex. *Neuroreport.* 1994;5:701–704.
47. Birbaumer N, Lutzenberger W, Montoya P, Larbig W, Unertl K, Töpfner S, et al. Effects of regional anesthesia on phantom limb pain are mirrored in changes in cortical reorganization. *J Neurosci.* 1997;17:5503–5508.
48. Willoch F, Rosen G, Tölle TR, Oye I, Wester HJ, Berner N, et al. Phantom limb pain in the human brain: Unraveling neural circuitries of phantom limb sensations using positron emission tomography. *Ann Neurol.* 2000; 48(6):842–849.
49. Lotze M, Flor H, Grodd W, Larbig W, Birbaumer N. Phantom movements and pain. An fMRI study in upper limb amputees. *Brain.* 2001;124(Pt 11): 2268–2277.
50. Hugdahl K, Rosen G, Ersland L, Lundervold A, Smievoll AI, Barndon R, et al. Common pathways in mental imagery and pain perception: an fMRI study of a subject with an amputated arm. *Scand J Psychol.* 2001;42(3): 269–275.
51. Dettmers C, Adler T, Rzanny R, Van Schayck R, Gaser C, Weiss T, et al. Increased excitability in the primary motor cortex and supplementary motor area in patients with phantom limb pain after upper limb amputation. *Neurosci Lett.* 2001;307(2):109–112.
52. Condes-Lara M, Barrios FA, Romo JR, Rojas R, Salgado P, Sanchez-Cortazar J. Brain somatic representation of phantom and intact limb: a fMRI study case report. *Eur J Pain.* 2000;4(3):239–245.

53. Kiriakopoulos ET, Tasker RR, Nicosia S, Wood ML, Mikulis DJ. Functional magnetic resonance imaging: A potential tool for the evaluation of spinal cord stimulation: Technical case report. *Neurosurgery.* 1997;41:501–504.
54. Rezai AR, Lozano AM, Crawley AP, Joy ML, Davis KD, Kwan CL, et al. Thalamic stimulation and functional magnetic resonance imaging: localization of cortical and subcortical activation with implanted electrodes. Technical note. *J Neurosurg.* 1999;90(3):583–590.
55. Apkarian AV, Darbar A, Krauss BR, Gelnar PA, Szeverenyi NM. Differentiating cortical areas related to pain perception from stimulus identification: temporal analysis of fMRI activity. *J Neurophysiol.* 1999;81(6): 2956–2963.
56. Davis KD, Pope GE, Crawley AP, Mikulis DJ. Neural correlates of prickle sensation: a percept-related fMRI study. *Nat Neurosci.* 2002;5:1121–1122.
57. Davis KD, Pope GE, Crawley AP, Mikulis DJ. Perceptual illusion of "paradoxical heat" engages the insular cortex. *J Neurophysiol.* 2004;92(2): 1248–1251.
58. Casey KL, Svensson P, Morrow TJ, Raz J, Jone C, Minoshima S. Selective opiate modulation of nociceptive processing in the human brain. *J Neurophysiol.* 2000;84(1):525–533.
59. Wagner KJ, Willoch F, Kochs EF, Siessmeier T, Tolle TR, Schwaiger M, et al. Dose-dependent regional cerebral blood flow changes during remifentanil infusion in humans: a positron emission tomography study. *Anesthesiology.* 2001;94(5):732–739.

# 17

# Pharmacological Applications of fMRI

Betty Jo Salmeron and Elliot A. Stein

## Introduction

Over the last few years, functional magnetic resonance imaging (fMRI) has developed rapidly into a powerful means of investigating both the pharmacological effects of drugs on neuronal activity and, with the ability to make real-time measurements of specific behaviors and physiological processes, the correlation of those neuronal changes with changes in behavior and various markers of the internal milieu. This prospect of combining powerful, noninvasive brain imaging with careful behavioral, cognitive, and physiological monitoring holds tremendous opportunity for advancing not only our understanding of fundamental brain mechanisms, but also clinical applications such as diagnostic procedures, medications development, treatment matching, and outcomes prediction.

Historically, invasive techniques such as single-cell electrophysiology have been utilized to monitor specific neurons or groups of neurons in awake, behaving subjects. However, invasive monitoring is, for the most part, only feasible in animals and is limited in the number of brain areas and cells that can be simultaneously examined. Given such limitations, indirect methods have been developed to study changes in neuronal activity related to brain function. Electroencephalography (EEG) methods appeared initially in the early part of the twentieth century,[1] offering temporal resolution in the tens to hundreds of milliseconds range,[2] almost as rapid as single-cell recording. Such techniques allow recording from multiple brain regions while simultaneously measuring central nervous system (CNS) output (behavior and changes in internal milieu). These methods, while continually improving in both hardware and software, still offer relatively poor and uncertain spatial resolution. Subsequently, various semiinvasive ways of indirectly measuring changes in neuronal activity have been developed that measure changes in regional cerebral blood flow (rCBF) and glucose utilization (CMRglu).[3] These rely on the tight coupling of neuronal activity to metabolism (see below) and require the administration of a radiotracer. Still more recently, radiotracers have been and are continuing to be developed to measure changes in receptor density and occupancy that may reflect acute, as well as chronic, effects of drug administration on specific neurotransmitter systems.

Using such radiolabeled methods, observations can be made regarding brain areas that are activated by a drug, the correlation of neuronal activity with subjective and objective state of being, and changes in task-related neuronal activity and brain chemistry following acute and/or chronic drug administration. Positron emission tomography (PET), with its ability to visualize radiolabeled molecules in the brain, is ideally suited to studying changes in receptor/transporter density or occupancy and can be used to elucidate the brain distribution of a radiolabeled drug. Positron emission tomagraphy can also be used to study drug- or task-related changes in neuronal activity by directly measuring rCBF ([$H_2{}^{15}O$]) or CMRglu ($^{18}F$ deoxy-glucose utilization). Unfortunately, the limited temporal resolution of these methods (on the order of tens of seconds to tens of minutes[4]) and their limited within-subjects repeatability due to dosimetry limits and/or isotope half-life make them ill-suited to studying dynamic changes after drug administration, especially for short-acting drugs whose effects may have dissipated before the radiotracer uptake period is complete. In addition, many small limbic structures (e.g., nucleus accumbens, amygdala) thought to be intimately involved in the actions of drugs of abuse and therapeutic psychotropic medications are difficult to visualize with PET given the limited spatial resolution of the technique.

In contrast, functional magnetic resonance imaging (fMRI) provides temporal and spatial resolution that make it ideal for studying the acute effects of rapidly acting drugs and the neuronal circuits underlying the effects of drugs on subjective state- and task-related activation. Further, fMRIs virtually infinite repeatability makes it attractive for studying the chronic effects of drugs. Like the above [$H_2{}^{15}O$] PET method, fMRI shares the property of being an indirect measure of neuronal activity based on changes in blood flow and metabolism that are tightly coupled to neuronal activity. Unlike [$H_2{}^{15}O$] PET, however, blood oxygen level-dependent (BOLD) fMRI (currently the most commonly used fMRI method) derives its signal not only from changes in rCBF and regional cerebral blood volume (rCBV), but also from changes in the amount of deoxygenated hemoglobin, related to changes in oxygen metabolism in activated neural tissue. In fact, change in the amount of deoxygenated hemoglobin accounts for the bulk of the change in the BOLD signal.[5] The MR signal is, therefore, one step further removed from the actual neuronal activity, adding another layer of uncertainty about the relationship of the signal to the underlying neuronal activity. Nevertheless, in the approximately 10 years since the first fMRI studies on humans were published,[6,7] several lines of research have demonstrated excellent agreement between BOLD measures of neuronal activity and more-established electrophysiological measures.[8–12] As such, BOLD fMRI promises to provide the most powerful means yet for noninvasively monitoring human brain activity with temporal resolution approaching real time.

To elucidate the potential difficulties in combining BOLD fMRI with drug administration, this chapter begins by briefly reviewing the basics of BOLD fMRI and discusses potential ways to experimentally address these issues. Design and analysis issues specific to combining BOLD with pharmacological inquiries (phMRI) also are discussed. Selected research is presented to illustrate both the potential and the pitfalls in using phMRI to study the acute effects of rapidly acting drugs and the effects of drugs on various cognitive tasks and other activation paradigms, both in healthy and diseased populations. The final section discusses potential future directions for phMRI applications in research and clinical medicine.

## BOLD fMRI Basics Pertinent to Pharmacological Applications

Although all of the intricacies of neuronal vascular coupling have not as yet been fully elucidated, regional BOLD signal increases, under normal physiological conditions, have been hypothesized to result from increases in rCBF, rCBV, and local oxygen concentration that are tightly coupled with neuronal activation.[5] As currently understood, the increased blood flow following neuronal activity is much larger than the activity-induced increase in oxygen extraction, thus decreasing the local concentration of deoxy-hemoglobin. Oxyhemoglobin and deoxyhemoglobin differ in magnetic susceptibility (the propensity of a substance to generate an extraneous magnetic field when placed in an external field). Because oxyhemoglobin is diamagnetic whereas deoxyhemoglobin is paramagnetic, the decrease in deoxyhemoglobin results in greater local field homogeneity and, therefore, increased MR signal.

The dependence of the BOLD signal on blood flow changes raises two issues for phMRI. First, the administration of a pharmacological agent may potentially alter the relationship between rCBF and neuronal activity. While it is clear that rCBF is tightly coupled to neuronal activation,[13,14] the coupling transduction mechanism is still not clear. Proposed mechanisms include direct innervation of blood vessels by neurons or glial cells (the so-called neurogenic hypotheses[14,15]) and/or the release of diffusible coupling factors by activated neurons or neighboring glia (the metabolic hypothesis).[16–18] For the latter, proposed diffusible coupling factors include metabolic byproducts and/or small molecules directly or indirectly involved in cell–cell signaling such as $H^+$, $Ca^{2+}$, $K^+$, NO, endotholin, trigeminal peptides, and such neurotransmitters as dopamine, norepinephrine, adenosine and acetylcholine.[16,18] Because many drugs, either acutely or chronically, are capable of altering levels of any number of these proposed coupling factors, drug administration could alter the BOLD signal independent of neuronal activity by either altering neuronal activation–rCBF coupling factors and/or by acting directly on cerebral blood vessels to induce changes in rCBF and/or rCBV.

A second issue that must be considered when combining BOLD fMRI with drug administration is the possibility that the drug may cause global changes in cardiovascular tone that could alter global CBF and CBV independent of neuronal activity, thus altering the BOLD signal independent of neuronal activity changes (see Table 17.1 on pp. 461–463). Indeed, global cerebral vasodilatation induced by five-percent $CO_2$ inhalation has been shown to reduce the BOLD response to finger tapping,[19] presumably due to reaching the vasodilatory limit of the vascular bed, the consequence of which would be the false-negative interpretation of an absence of task-induced neuronal activity. In contrast, Corfield and colleagues[20] reported that breathing four-percent $CO_2$ produced not only an increase in baseline BOLD signal, but also preserved the BOLD response (% signal change above the tonic vasodilatation) to visual stimulation, suggesting that if one stays within the vasodilatory dynamic range, an additive effect on rCBF is measurable. Thus, manipulations of CBF and CBV independent of neuronal activity can, but do not necessarily, interfere with BOLD signal from an activation paradigm.

These studies point to one potential way to address the question of whether a pharmacological manipulation has affected the ability to detect a true, neuronally coupled BOLD signal. If a well-characterized task whose performance should not be altered by the drug in question can be shown to elicit a similar BOLD response in the presence and absence of the drug, one may infer that coupling mechanisms remain intact such that any induced changes in global cardiovascular or cerebrovascular tone have not affected the BOLD signal transduction mechanisms. Such an approach was employed by Rao and colleagues[21] to demonstrate the feasibility of using BOLD to investigate cognitive changes after methylphenidate administration. Using the well-characterized task of finger tapping to a metronome set at different rates,[22] they demonstrated no change in task performance or BOLD response after methylphenidate administration, although modest changes in cardiovascular tone (increased heart rate) were evident, suggesting that coupling mechanisms and vascular responsivity remained intact after methylphenidate administration. As such, changes in BOLD activation during cognitive task performance in the presence of methylphenidate administration may therefore be assumed to result from changes in neuronal activation. A similar strategy was employed by Gollub and colleagues,[23] who demonstrated no change in the % BOLD signal change to visual stimulation after acute cocaine administration in the face of a modest decrease in global CBF.

Given that the BOLD signal is several steps removed from neuronal activation, and that several of these steps may be susceptible to drug effects independent of neuronal activation (see Figure 17.1), it is essential that all phMRI studies include an appropriate control procedure in an attempt to demonstrate that the mechanisms resulting in the BOLD signal have not been directly altered by the drug. Finger tapping to an auditory or visual metronome is appealing for several reasons. First, it

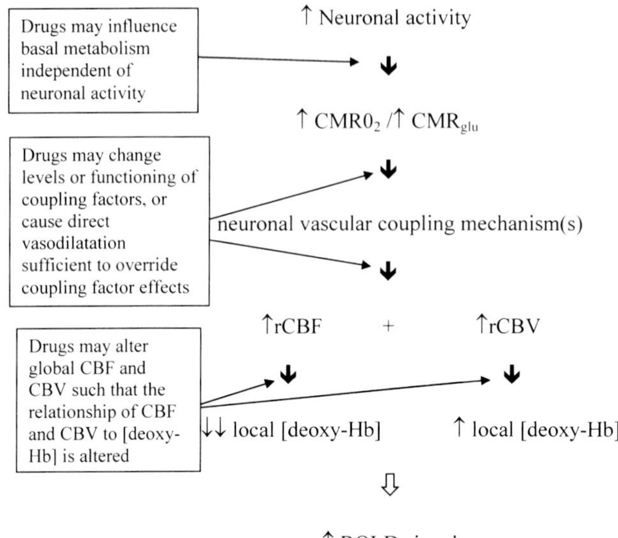


**Figure 17.1.** Pharmacologic agents might alter the relationship of BOLD signal to neuronal activity independent of direct changes in neural activity at any point indicated by a closed arrow.

is a simple task, easily taught, and whose performance is both very good at baseline and, after limited practice, not likely to improve in the presence of acute drug. A motor task also allows for a measurable behavioral output to ensure that subjects have not been affected by excessive sedation or other gross disruptions of attention. In contrast, if a purely sensory task is used (e.g., flashing visual checkerboard or auditory tone presentations), there may be questions about the equivalency of the attention paid to the stimulus before and after drug administration that could independently alter the signal.[24–26] Because sensory-paced finger tapping includes both a sensory and motor component, sensory brain regions also may be examined with the knowledge that similar attention has been exerted to the sensory stimulus in the presence and absence of the drug. The presentation of stimuli at varying rates, known to produce linearly varying changes in BOLD signal,[22] provides an examination of the integrity of the signal across a range of task demands, thus providing a more complete examination of the neuronal vascular coupling dynamic range under the drug challenge.

Unfortunately, some drugs may not be amenable to such a validation procedure because their sites of action are mediated more globally than locally, thus precluding the possibility of finding a task unaffected by the drug administration. In such cases, data from complementary techniques, as well as differential analyses of the BOLD signal, may help interpret otherwise ambiguous results; for example, in addition to its psychogenic properties, alcohol is known to alter cerebral metabolism and oxygen consumption and to directly cause cerebral vasodilatation.[27] Electroencephalgraphy studies, reflecting summated neuronal synaptic activity, have shown decreased amplitude in several somatosensory and visual evoked potential components and a decrease in the normal right dominant hemispheric asymmetry of visual evoked potentials.[28–30] Therefore, it is likely that BOLD signal under the influence of alcohol will be altered by mechanisms both related and unrelated to neuronal activity, making interpretation problematic, even without considering potential effects of alcohol on neuronal vascular coupling.

Levin and colleagues[31] used BOLD fMRI to examine the effect of alcohol on the primary visual cortex response to photic stimulation. Subjects underwent BOLD imaging sessions of 30-second blocks of darkness alternating with a diffuse red flash pattern before and 50 minutes after consuming an alcohol- or placebo-containing drink. They reported that the amplitude of the BOLD response to photic stimulation was diminished by about 33% after alcohol consumption, and the normal right predominant asymmetry in BOLD response was likewise diminished. Taken by themselves, such decreases in the BOLD response could be attributed to reaching the limit on the dynamic range of the cerebral vasculature as a consequence of the direct vasodilatory effects of alcohol. Indeed, similar results with acetazolamide were interpreted in this fashion[32] before this diuretic was demonstrated to have a direct suppressive effect on brain function that could also contribute to the results.[33] Instead, Levin and colleagues argued that their results reflected, at least in part, a true suppression of neural function by alcohol. They supported this claim by citing data gathered from other modalities, including a PET study,[34] demonstrating consistent fractional rCBF changes to photic stimulation across a range of baseline CBF values manipulated by inducing hypo- and hypercapnea. Second, they noted the similarity between their results and those obtained with evoked potentials,[28–30] a measure that has been used in other settings[8–10] to support the assertion that BOLD changes reflect changes in neuronal activity.

Seifritz and colleagues[35] illustrated a further refinement of this approach, taking into account what is known about alcohol's effect on rCBF. Recognizing that ethanol produces vasodilatation, they modeled the relationship between rCBF and BOLD signal changes. Assuming that ethanol caused a ten percent increase in baseline flow, they used the resulting Flow–BOLD-Dependence curve to assert that the ethanol reduction in BOLD signal to acoustic stimulation after alcohol was seven to twelve percent greater than could be explained by direct vasodilatation alone. They attributed this excess BOLD reduction to ethanol's suppression of neuronal activity.

## Acute Drug Challenges

After first establishing that an interpretable BOLD signal can be obtained following acute administration of a specified drug-dose range, it is then possible to consider using phMRI to investigate the drug's direct CNS actions. At this point, another feature of BOLD becomes important in design issues. Unlike some fMRI methods, such as arterial spin labeling (ASL) and dynamic contrast gadolinium-enhanced flow and volume measures, BOLD produces a signal that is measured in arbitrary units; thus, resting data between scan sessions or runs within a session are not directly comparable. Therefore, in order to use BOLD to study such direct acute drug effects, the onset of drug action must be rapid enough to complete a study in one session in the scanner, generally limited to about two hours, beyond which most participants have great difficulty remaining stationary. Ideally, then, the drug must have a rapid onset of action and be administered in such a way that its effect peaks early, making it simpler to determine when looking for the drug response in the brain. Most often such pharmacokinetic considerations lead to choosing intravenous drug delivery because this route provides rapid, relatively uniform, and unambiguous drug uptake.

After appropriate choice of the pharmacological agent to study and control procedures, the next major issue is how to identify a significant BOLD drug response. Of the several methods recently proposed, perhaps the most straightforward approach is to compare the post-drug mean BOLD signal with the pre-drug signal. For example, Breiter and colleagues[36] used the Kolmogorov–Smirnov test, a nonparametric *t*-test, to determine the regional localization of BOLD changes after intravenous cocaine administration. While certainly valid, such an analysis does not take full advantage of the magnitude, polarity, and temporal information available in the BOLD time series.

An alternative approach put forward is based on the hypothesis that the drug-induced BOLD effect follows a single-dose, one-compartment pharmacokinetic model and applies analytical methods that take advantage of the temporal richness of the BOLD signal. This pattern-recognition approach uses appropriate onset and offset times and significant peak signal changes based upon known pharmacokinetics and/or concomitant serum drug levels. When coupled with a similar analysis after a placebo (saline) injection, which would presumably reflect experimental noise, a false-positive rate associated with a given set of criteria for activated voxels can be established.[37,38] This approach has been used to identify the sites of action of intravenous nicotine.[39] This study included multiple drug doses in order to determine dose-related brain responses, further increasing confidence that identified regions were directly affected by the drug. After a placebo injection of saline, three consecutive one-minute injections were given approximately 30 minutes apart in increasing dose order (0.75, 1.5 and 2.25 mg/70 kg). Using the pharmacokinetic modeling described above (Figure 17.2), dose-dependent activation was seen in numerous brain regions, including the nucleus accumbens, amygdala, anterior cingulate, and frontal lobes (Figure 17.3). Animal studies have repeatedly associated these areas with the reinforcing properties of drugs of abuse,[40,41] suggesting that nicotine is working through common mechanisms in the human brain. A similar approach has recently been applied to study the acute effects of cocaine.[42]

A promising approach that has been underutilized in phMRI is a class of analysis techniques termed non-hypothesis driven or data

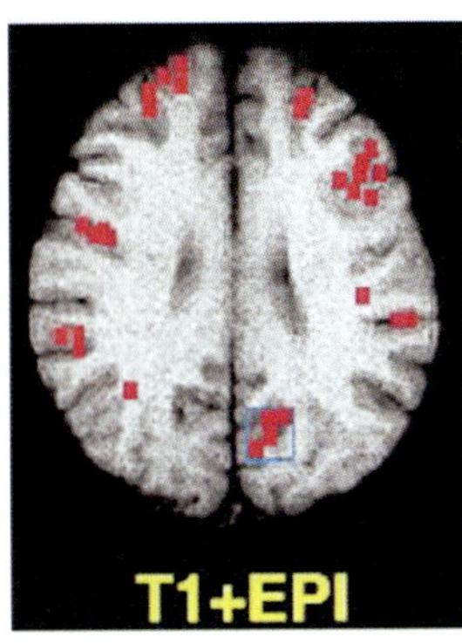


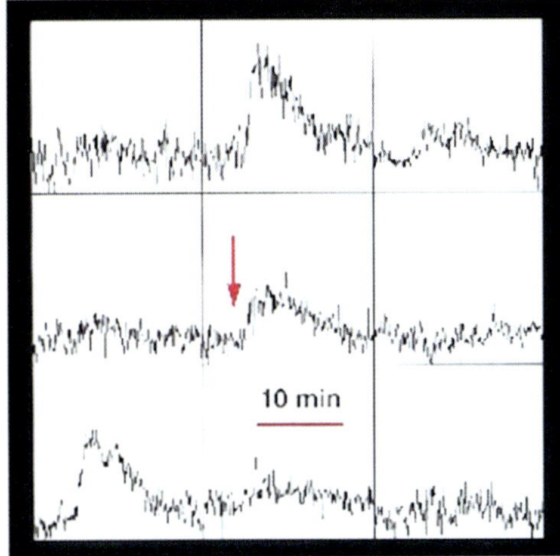


**Figure 17.2.** Fast spin-echo planar image of nicotine-activated voxels (red boxes) superimposed on T1-weighted anatomical image. Time series data for the nine voxels outlined in blue on the left are shown on the right. Red arrow indicates start of one-minute injection.[39] Reprinted from Stein EA, Pankiewicz J, Harsch HH, et al. Nicotine-induced limbic cortical activation in the human brain: a functional MRI study. *Am J Psychiatry*. 1998;155:1009–1015. Copyright © 1998, the American Psychiatric Association. http://ajp.psychiatryonline.org. Reprinted by permission.

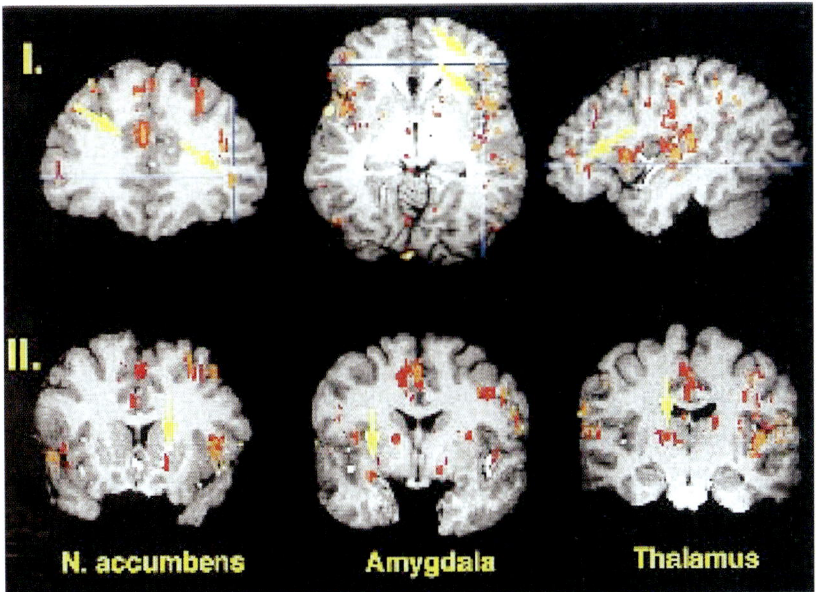


**Figure 17.3.** Areas significantly activated by nicotine injection compared to saline injection. Top row shows three views through the same point (indicated by blue cross-hairs). Arrows indicate anterior cingulate, lateral orbital gyrus, insula, nucleus accumbens, amygdala, and thalamus.[39] Reprinted from Stein EA, Pankiewicz J, Harsch HH, et al. Nicotine-induced limbic cortical activation in the human brain: a functional MRI study. *Am J Psychiatry*. 1998;155:1009–1015. Copyright © 1998, the American Psychiatric Association. http://ajp.psychiatryonline.org. Reprinted by permission.

driven. These methods seek out underlying structure in the data without the use of any a priori model. Of these, the most promising approach is independent components analysis.[43] Independent components analysis decomposes the fMRI data into a set of component time series, each of which is associated with a spatially independent map. An advantage to independent components analysis is that the component time series can be correlated, which could allow separating signal from drug-induced neuronal activity from possibly similar low-frequency signal drifts often seen in BOLD imaging. Difficulties include identifying the drug-related component(s) and the lack of standard group-inference methods. Other data-driven methods that could be utilized in phMRI include temporal clustering[44] and fuzzy clustering (see, for example, Fadili and colleagues[45]). None of these methods have yet been applied to phMRI studies and await validation and application.

The temporal resolution of BOLD fMRI and the ability to simultaneously gather behavioral responses during experiments has been exploited by a number of investigators to assess brain areas of activation that specifically correlate with the induced subjective drug effects. For example, Breiter and colleagues[36] collected self-ratings of high, rush, craving, and low once per minute before and after intravenous cocaine administration, and subsequently used these ratings as input functions in a cross-correlation analysis to determine those brain areas whose signal change accompanied the reported feeling state. Using this analysis, rush was found to be related to BOLD signal in the ventral tegmentum, caudate nucleus, and lateral prefrontal cortex, whereas correlations with craving were seen in the nucleus accumbens and some lateral prefrontal regions, among others (Figure 17.4). Other concurrently gathered data, including such physiological measures as skin temperature or galvanic skin response, also can be used as analysis input vectors (e.g., Patterson and colleagues[46]).

## Drug Challenges and Activation Paradigms

In contrast to the above discussion of acute drug effects, many of the more interesting actions of pharmacologic agents may only be apparent when an appropriate neural system is activated. Such task activation could occur:

1. simultaneously with drug administration (e.g., comparing passive to self-administration of drugs of abuse),
2. in advance of drug (e.g., administering a drug of abuse after a craving stimulus compared with after a neutral stimulus), or
3. after a stable drug effect has been achieved (e.g., elucidating methylphenidate's effects on sustained attention by activating the system with a continuous performance task).

For drugs whose onset of action requires more time than that observable during a single scanner session, an activation paradigm as in Example 3 above is required because, as noted, resting BOLD data between sessions is not directly comparable. For medications such as

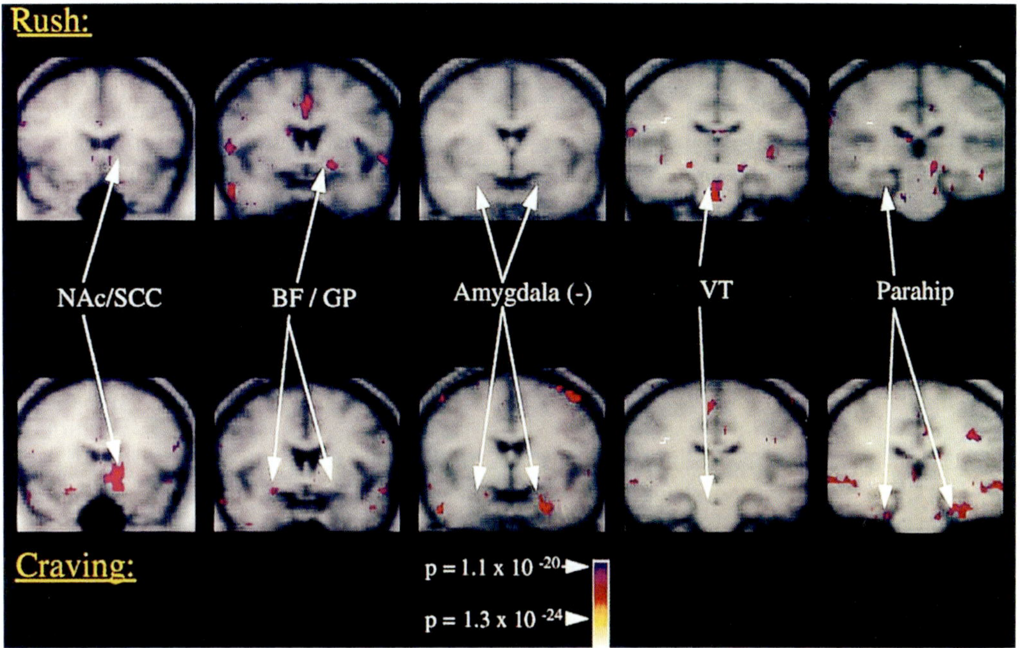


**Figure 17.4.** Correlations of self-reported rush and craving with BOLD data after cocaine injection. Reprinted from *Neuron*, Vol. 19, Breiter HC, Gollub RL, Weisskoff RM et al, Acute effects of cocaine on human brain activity and emotion, 591–611. Copyright © 1997, with permission from Elsevier.

antidepressants and antipsychotics, whose onset of action is measured in weeks, one must carefully choose an appropriate activation paradigm in order to study these drug's brain effects. For example, if an antipsychotic is hypothesized to improve cognitive functioning in patients with schizophrenia, one must first clarify exactly what functions are thought to be improved and develop or apply tasks that measure that specific cognitive construct before and after medication treatment. Such task comparisons, however, raise yet another complication, namely, the interpretation of activation to a cognitive task when the behavioral performance may or may not be altered as a consequence of the drug treatment.

When task performance differs following drug administration, it may be difficult to determine if neural changes seen are responsible for the difference in performance or simply reflect the fact that the task was not being performed to the same degree of accuracy under the two conditions; for example, the direct effect of a drug may be sedation, mediated by brain stem mechanisms. Cognitive task performance and neural activation may be altered secondary to the sedative effect. This secondary effect could not be distinguished from a direct effect on cognitive brain areas without further control procedures built into the experiment. Conversely, differences in neural activation when performance is unchanged may reflect changes in the efficiency of the neural circuits involved or may reflect changes in background activity that may have nothing to do with the cognitive function of interest. Interpretation of such results becomes quite problematic.

There are several ways one might consider addressing these issues; each may be appropriate in different circumstances and care must be taken to examine the implications of such choices to ensure the study question can be addressed. As a general rule, including as much parametric variation as possible, both in doses of drug and in level of task difficulty coupled with Latin square order controls, makes results easier to interpret. Additionally, matched nontreatment (and in some cases, nondiseased) control populations are strongly recommended to control for the repeated effects of time and learning. A discussion of several designs and their particular strengths and weaknesses follows, with illustrative studies presented where available.

### *Event Related Design*

Using an event-related design allows for the analysis to include only those trials in which the task was completed successfully.[47] Event-related design is appropriate for tasks in which each trial is a self-contained event and not dependent on overall task behavior. Using an event-related design for comparisons across drug conditions requires that there be enough correct trials in each condition to make statistically reliable comparisons. The study by Thiel and colleagues[48] illustrates such an approach. That study examined the effect of scopolamine and lorazepam on face repetition priming. The task required categorizing faces, some of which were presented during an earlier phase of the experiment, as famous or nonfamous. Performance in the various task conditions ranged from about 70 to 90%. Thiel and colleagues only compared activation on trials that were categorized correctly, thus eliminating the extraneous variability that might be introduced by including trials in which the task was not correctly accomplished (note: while it has been argued that the metabolic consequences of task performance are independent of outcome, but rather reflect effort of processing, thus making parsing data by performance superfluous, it is not possible to test this hypothesis without also knowing that equal effort is being exerted across conditions. This is very difficult to demonstrate. As such, parsing data by outcome may serve a useful role in equalizing treatment effects.)

Another example currently underway in our lab is the use of a go-no go task to examine the effect of medication treatment on children with attention deficit hyperactivity disorder (ADHD). The task, a version of which has been used successfully in an event-related design,[49] requires responding to Xs and Ys in a stream of letters, but only if they alternate in their presentation. By examining neural responses to successful inhibitions, one can determine if the drug has had an effect on the neural circuits underlying this cognitive construct. By comparing successful inhibitions in healthy children with successful inhibitions in children with ADHD in the presence and absence of drug, one might be able to determine if the drug has normalized neural activity or changed it in some other way. By looking separately at failures of inhibition, one might be able to determine what goes awry in the circuit when children with ADHD fail to inhibit appropriately.

### *Block Design with Parametric Variation of Level of Difficulty*

For tasks best suited to a block design, it may be possible to get roughly equivalent performance across drug conditions using different levels of task difficulty. However, care must be taken to ensure that changing task difficulty does not change the underlying cognitive process in question. An example of a situation in which this may be appropriate is when studying working memory with an *n*-back task. The constant updating of information in working memory is the process of interest, not the individual responses to targets. The task is therefore well-suited to a block design. Task difficulty can be manipulated by varying the *n* or by changing the rate or duration of stimulus presentation. Varying the level of difficulty within the task (e.g., random alternating blocks of each of the *n* backs) such that performance can be matched in the presence and absence of drug at some difficulty levels, but remains different at other difficulty levels provides more information to interpret the meaning of any activation differences found. Using a block design (with fixed task difficulty but in contrast to a low-level control task), Lawrence and colleagues[50] found that transdermal nicotine replacement improved task performance in cigarette smokers and increased brain activation to a rapid visual information-processing task in the parietal cortex, thalamus, and caudate, whereas nicotine induced a generalized increase in occipital cortex activity. Based on these findings, it was suggested that nicotine improves attention in smokers by enhancing activation in areas traditionally associated with visual attention, arousal, and motor (Figure 17.5).

### *Use of Tasks Whose Performance Is Measured by Changes in Reaction Time*

Some tasks measure performance solely in terms of reaction time. Such tasks have an advantage for scanning because the same task is clearly being performed both in the presence and absence of drug, but with varying efficiency. An example of such an approach is seen in Furey and colleagues.[51] This study examined the effects of physostigmine on working memory performance using a delayed face match to sample paradigm that allowed for separate examination of the encoding phase, memory delay phase, and recognition phase. This simple task, with nearly perfect performance by most normal subjects, shows reaction-time improvements under physostigmine. In addition, BOLD activity was enhanced in extrastriate pathways and decreased in some prefrontal regions following physostigmine administration, especially during the encoding phase. This effect was interpreted as being due to a reduced demand on prefrontal function secondary to enhanced efficiency of the encoding, maintenance, and recall systems.

### *Use of Activation Paradigms in Which BOLD Signal in Particular Brain Structures Is the Outcome of Interest*

Certain drug effects may alter neural responses to particular stimuli in structures inherently interesting for the drug being studied; for example, depression is thought to relate, at least in part, to aberrant processing of emotional stimuli by particular brain structures. Probing the response of particular structures to affectively charged stimuli

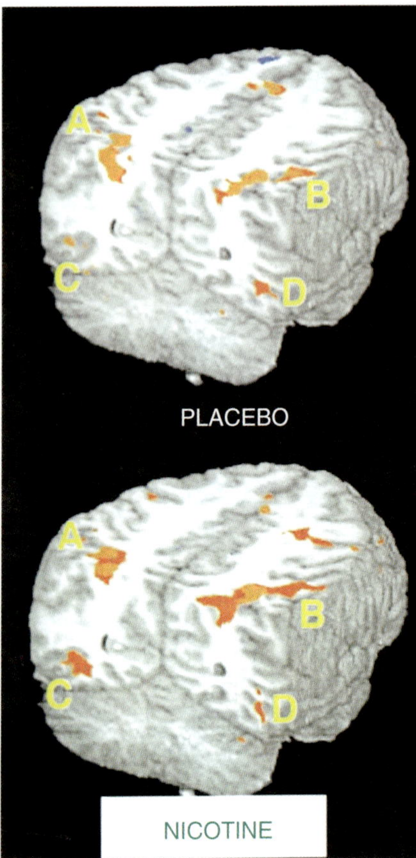


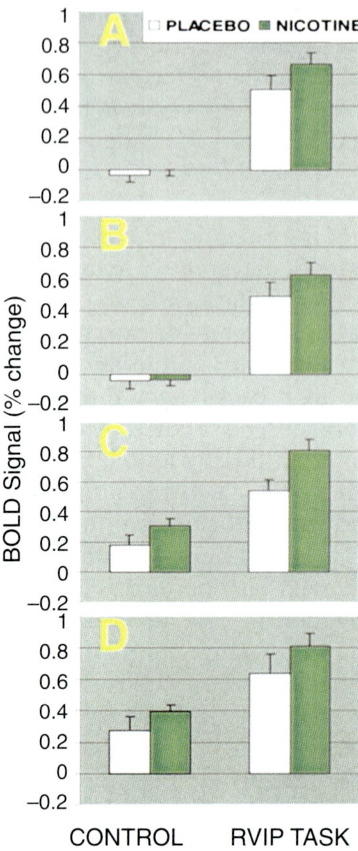


**Figure 17.5.** Enhancement of activation to RVIP task in smokers treated with nicotine patch in bilateral parietal (A and B) and occipital (C and D) regions. Reprinted from *Neuron*, Vol. 36, Lawrence NS, Ross TJ, Stein EA, Cognitive mechanisms of nicotine on visual attention, 539–538. Copyright © 2002, with permission from Elsevier.

during a depressive episode and after successful treatment with an antidepressant may help to elucidate the action of these drugs in the brain. Using such an approach, Sheline and colleagues[52] investigated the amygdala response to masked fearful faces in depressed subjects before and after treatment with the selective serotonin reuptake inhibitor, sertraline. Depressed subjects showed increased responses in the left amygdala to all faces, especially fearful faces. Amygdala response decreased bilaterally after treatment.

Use of a more complex neural response is illustrated in Stephan and colleagues.[53] Noting that the cognitive dysmetria model of schizophrenia hypothesizes that altered connectivity in brain circuits may underlie many of the deficits seen in the disorder, as well as the improvements seen with neuroleptic treatment, they examined the functional connectivity (the intercorrelation of time series between two areas) between the cerebellum and other areas activated by a finger-tapping task before and after treatment with olanzapine. They found that olanzapine caused widespread changes in cerebellar functional connectivity, especially in the prefrontal cortex and medial dorsal thalamus. Functional connectivity also has been used to demonstrate disruptions in visual cortex and motor cortex functional connectivity after cocaine injection (Figure 17.6).

## Future Directions

Using the BOLD technique with phMRI offers excellent spatial and temporal resolution and virtually unlimited repeatability. With careful attention to appropriate validation procedures for each drug as outlined above, BOLD phMRI investigations should provide consider-

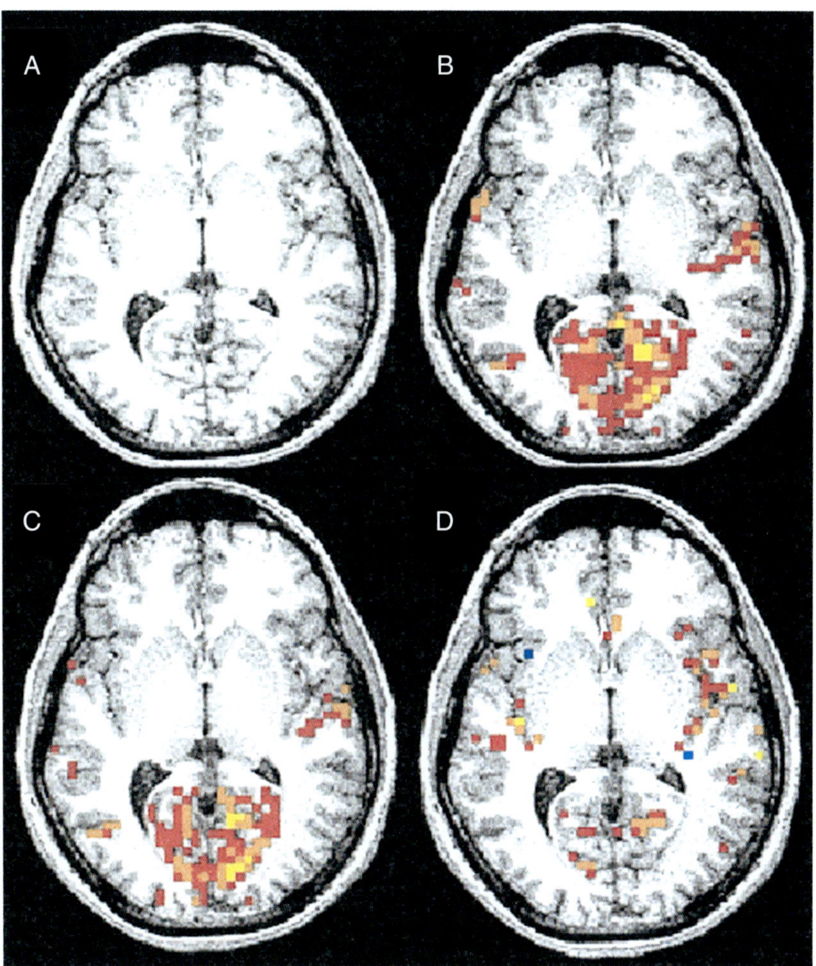


**Figure 17.6.** (A) High-resolution anatomical image through visual cortex. (B) Functional connectivity map generated at rest for a reference voxel in visual cortex. (C) Functional connectivity map for same reference voxel after saline injection. (D) Functional connectivity map for same reference voxel after cocaine injection. Reprinted from Li SJ, Biswal B, Li Z, et al. Cocaine administration decreases functional connectivity in human primary visual and motor cortex as detected by functional MRI. *Mag Reson Med*. 2000;43:45–51. Copyright © 2000. Reprinted with permission of Wiley-Liss, Inc., a subsidiary of John Wiley & Sons, Inc.

able new information on how drugs affect resting neural activity and neural activity underlying specific cognitive and affective processes that may be modulated by drugs. However, BOLD phMRI only indirectly measures neural activity as reflected by changes in rCBF/rCBV and oxygenation and is measured in arbitrary units not directly comparable between sessions. By combining BOLD phMRI investigations with other MR techniques such as ASL, dynamic susceptibility contrast (DSC) MRI, and magnetic resonance spectroscopy (MRS), as well as with other imaging modalities, such as PET, broader investigations of the influence of drugs on neural functioning may be conducted.

Arterial spin labeling is an MRI technique that measures blood flow by applying an inversion radio frequency (RF) pulse to arterial blood as it enters a brain section of interest. This pulse alters the spins of water molecules that can be measured as this labeled blood travels into the tissue of interest. Arterial spin labeling is thought to provide better neuronal spatial fidelity than BOLD because the majority of the signal comes from the arterial side of the capillary bed rather than the venous side, where veins may also drain tissue some distance from the primary site of neuronal activity. Importantly, ASL can provide a quantitative measure of blood flow (reported in mL/100g/min), thus allowing for between-session comparisons. However, ASL is currently limited to a few brain slices, and the contrast-to-noise ratio is considerably lower than that obtained with BOLD. With sufficient technical improvements, ASL may eventually replace BOLD as the technique of choice in some applications, offering the significant advantages of producing a quantifiable signal that is more directly related to neural activity while retaining the noninvasive characteristic of BOLD fMRI. To date, ASL has been used in combination with BOLD phMRI in order to provide quantifiable blood flow measures that can be compared in the presence and absence of drug, regardless of the amount of time between baseline and drug condition measures.[21,23]

Dynamic susceptibility contrast MRI relies on the administration of a paramagnetic contrast agent to enhance the sensitivity of fMRI signals and was, in fact, utilized before echo planar BOLD imaging became the standard.[55] This method can detect both global and regional CBF and CBV changes. Global measures can be useful for detecting changes in hemodynamics due to drug-induced alterations in systemic cardiovascular status. Such changes may alter BOLD signal independent of changes in neural activity, as discussed earlier. Gadolinium (Gd) is the only contrast agent currently available for human use. Its short half-life limits CBV measures to those gathered on the first pass of a bolus through the brain. Monocrystalline iron oxide nanocolloid (MION) is a contrast agent currently available only for animal use. Its long intravascular half-life (four hours in rats) allows for tracking of local changes in CBV (a signal closer to changes in neural activity than BOLD) on a time frame similar to that attainable with BOLD and has been successfully used to map the actions of cocaine in rats.[56–58] As longer half-life agents become available for human use, DSC MRI may prove useful for experiments currently conducted using BOLD, providing similar advantages as ASL, with the drawback, however, of being a more invasive procedure. To date, DSC MRI has been used to document decreases in CBV after administration of cocaine[59] and to investigate CBV changes following administration of lorazepam to subjects with and without a family history of alcoholism.[60]

Magnetic resonance spectroscopy is a technique that exploits small differences in how magnetic nuclei ($^{1}$H, $^{13}$C, $^{19}$F, $^{23}$Na, $^{7}$Li, and $^{31}$P) behave. When placed in a strong magnetic field, these nuclei spin at a unique frequency that is altered slightly by chemical bonding. By detecting these frequencies, it is possible to measure these elements incorporated into certain compounds in the brain; for example, the three $^{31}$P atoms present in adenosine 5′-triphosphate can be distinguished from one another.[61] To allow direct evaluation of glucose utilization, $^{1}$H MRS can be used to detect metabolites produced during glycolysis. It also can determine concentrations of *n*-acetyl aspartate (NAA), a presumptive marker of neuronal viability, myoinositol (MI), a presumed marker of glial activity, $\gamma$ amino butyric acid (GABA), and glutamate/glutamine pools in the brain. However, the MR signal contains both metabolic and neurotransmitter pools of the chemicals, making interpretation of the findings difficult.

In addition, because $^{7}$Li and $^{19}$F are essentially not present in the brain under normal circumstances, levels of drugs containing these elements, such as $LiCO_3$ and fluoxetine, can be measured with MRS with the potential of using such an approach to follow changes in brain levels over the course of treatment. The signal measured with MRS is small, currently requiring measurement over relatively large areas of brain averaged over many minutes. However, because the signal magnitude scales with field strength, further advancements in functional MRS are expected as machines with higher static magnetic field strengths become available.

Magnetic resonance spectroscopy has already proved useful in understanding several aspects of the complex effect of pharmacologic agents on brain metabolism. Progress has been made in understanding the relationship between drug dose and plasma and brain levels of several medications.[62–66] Magnetic resonance spectroscopy has also been used to examine the effects of chronic drug administration on various MRS-visible metabolic substrates and products; for example, increases in GABA has been demonstrated following topiramate treatment,[67] and lower-than-normal basal ganglia choline:creatinine ratios have been shown to increase in depressed subjects successfully treated with fluoxetine.[68] Alterations in NAA and MI have been observed in chronic cocaine and methamphetamine abusers[69–71] that might relate to the neuronal consequences of chronic abuse of these substances. Magnetic resonance spectroscopy has also demonstrated a similar effect of tamoxefin and estrogen on brain metabolism in elderly women.[72] By combining MRS with BOLD phMRI studies, it may be possible to integrate metabolic and functional consequences of drug administration, thereby enhancing the global understanding of how pharmacological agents affect brain functioning.

While less than optimal as a measure of the direct actions of a drug on neuronal activity, PET is the only method currently capable of evaluating neurotransmitter systems by determining levels of specific receptors, transmitters, and transporters. An exciting possibility for the future is to combine phMRI studies with PET studies characterizing specific neurotransmitter systems, and then to correlate these characterizations with the function of particular structures and/or circuits, both at baseline and under the influence of a drug. This may aid not only in understanding the actions of drugs, but also in elucidating the pathophysiology of various disease states; for example, dopamine transporter levels have been shown to be elevated in ADHD and to be lower following methylphenidate (a DAT blocker) treatment.[73] However, while the group difference was significant, several subjects fell clearly within the normal range prior to treatment, and several subjects demonstrated decreased DAT levels well below the normal range after treatment. Combining phMRI studies manipulating selected cognitive functions under methylphenidate with PET or SPECT studies of transporter levels could add considerably to our understanding of the pathophysiology of ADHD, in particular the role of the dopamine transporter. It also may help elucidate issues of multiple endophenotypes in this disorder. Eventually, studies of this kind may be useful in therapeutic drug-choice selections and in maximizing medication responses. A summary of studies using phMRI is shown in Table 17.1.

In sum, phMRI promises to provide considerable information about acute drug effects on neural activity in the human brain and how and where a drug interacts with specific cognitive and affective task-related activity. The ability to measure these changes in virtual real time and within repeated-measure design greatly adds to the utility of this noninvasive technique. When used in combination with other imaging methods that allow for evaluation of metabolic and neurotransmitter system consequences of drug administration, phMRI should provide a means to more completely characterize neural systems than ever before possible. Such characterization should have significant implications for medications development, individualized treatment matching, outcomes prediction, and possibly novel, more accurate differential diagnostic procedures.

## Acknowledgment

The authors gratefully acknowledge the contributions of Dr. Thomas Ross to discussions related to data analysis methods.

Table 17.1. Summary of Studies Using phMRI

| Acute drug effects | | | |
|---|---|---|---|
| Authors | Subjects | FMRI paradigm | Results |
| Bloom et al., 2001[19] | Frequent marijuana users | Two doses i.v. THC on different occasions | Multiple areas of ↓ signal including NAcc, orbitofrontal cortex, and cerebellum. Some ↑ signal seen in visual cortex |
| Breiter et al., 1997[17] | 17 cocaine-dependent subjects | Double-blind placebo-controlled cocaine injection (single dose, two sessions) | ↑ signal in multiple areas including VTA, NAcc, cingulate, frontal areas, hippocampus, and insula |
| Mu et al., 2001[9] | 26 regular cocaine users | 3 sessions: single-blinded saline and 1 of 3 cocaine doses in each session | Dose related signal ↓: NAcc, Ant. Cing, hippocampus, L amygdala, and others<br>Dose related signal ↑: L-sided Post. Cing., amygdala, caudate/putamen<br>R-sided insula, Ant. Cing. |
| Stein et al., 1998[4] | 16 healthy smokers | Saline and 3 doses of nicotine given 20 minutes apart in ascending order in cumulative dosing paradigm | Dose-related activation in NAcc, cingulate, amygdala, and frontal lobes |

| Drug on task effects | | | |
|---|---|---|---|
| Authors | Subjects | FMRI paradigm | Results |
| Furey et al., 2000[16] | 7 healthy adults | Delayed face match-to-sample paradigm on 2 occasions: i.v. bolus + drip physostigmine or saline prior to and during experiment | Physostigmine ↑ selectivity of extrastriate response, esp. during encoding; ↑ ventral extrastriate, ↓ prefrontal cortex during maintenance |
| Kimberg et al., 2001[12] | 11 healthy adults | Verbal 2-back WM, WCST, motor response task on and off bromocriptine | Bromocriptine generally reduced task related activity in all 3 tasks. |
| Levin et al., 1998[11] | 15 healthy adults | Photic stimulation before and after oral ETOH ($n = 10$) or placebo ($n = 5$) | 33% ↓ in visual cortex activation after ETOH |
| Mattay et al., 2000[10] | 10 healthy adults | no-back, 2-back & 3-back WM task 2° after D-amph. or placebo | D-amph. ↓ activation in no-back, ↑ activation in 3-back, esp. in those whose performance worsened |
| Seifritz et al., 2000[7] | 11 healthy adults | 2 sessions: tone presented 3 times before and after oral ETOH or placebo | ETOH ↓ response to acoustic stimulation |

*Continued*

Table 17.1. *Continued*

| Drug on task effects | | | |
|---|---|---|---|
| Authors | Subjects | FMRI paradigm | Results |
| Thiel et al., 2002[3] | 47 healthy adults | Scopolamine, lorazepam, or placebo given prior to showing faces to subjects; Scanning in a face recognition paradigm followed | Scopolamine impaired priming and showed none of the repetition effects seen after placebo and lorazepam. |
| Wise et al., 2002[2] | 9 healthy male adults | Noxious thermal stimulation of back of hand before, during, and after remifentanil infusion | Remifentanil ↓ pain-related BOLD response in insula and anterior cingulate |
| Loubinoux et al., 1999[15] | 12 healthy right-handed adults (6 male) | Auditorily paced sequential opposition of thumb and fingers before and after fenozolone or fluoxetine | Both drugs produced more focused activation in sensorimotor areas, greater involvement of posterior supplemental motor area, and ↓ cerebellar activation |
| Sperling et al., 2002[8] | 10 right-handed healthy male adults | Face–name associative encoding paradigm after scopolamine, lorazepam or placebo (×2) (4 sessions, total) | ↓ extent and magnitude of activation in hippocampal, fusiform, and prefrontal regions after scopolamine or lorazepam |

| Drug on task in disease state | | | |
|---|---|---|---|
| Authors | Subjects | FMRI paradigm | Results |
| Honey et al., 1999[13] | 20 medicated schizophrenic patients; 10 healthy controls | Verbal WM task at baseline (all subjects) and 6 weeks later (schizophrenics subjects only); 1/2 switched to risperidone after baseline | Risperidone ↑ activation in right prefrontal cortex, suppl. motor area, and posterior parietal cortex |
| Howard et al., 1996[14] | 2 narcoleptic subjects; 3 healthy controls | Periodic visual and auditory stimuli before and after amphetamine | Narcoleptics- ↑ activation in 1° & assoc. cortices Controls-small ↓ activation on amphetamine |
| Sheline et al., 2001[6] | 11 major depression patients; 11 matched controls | Masked faces paradigm before and after 8 weeks of sertraline treatment (patients only) | ↑ L amygdala response in depressed subjects, esp. to fearful faces at baseline ↓ bilat. amygdala response to all faces after successful sertraline treatment |
| Stephan et al., 2001[5] | 6 subjects w/schizophrenia 6 healthy controls | Seed–voxel correlation analysis using ant. cerebellum seed voxel during finger tapping in two conditions: drug-free and olanzapine treated | Olanzapine normalized connectivity patterns for right, but not left cerebellum |
| Vaidya et al., 1998[1] | 10 8–13 y.o. ADHD males, 6 healthy matched controls | Go-no go task on and off methylphenidate | Methylphenidate ↑ striatal activation in ADHD, ↓ striatal activation in controls; no change or small ↑ in frontal activation in both groups |

| | | | |
|---|---|---|---|
| **Braus et al., 1999[18]** | **40 schizophrenic subjects (14 first- episode unmedicated, 13 stable on typical meds, 13 stable on atypical meds), 15 normal controls** | **Self-paced sequential finger opposition of left hand** | **First-episode schizophrenics and controls activated similarly; typical neuroleptics ↓ activation in bilateral sensorimotor areas. Typical and atypical neuroleptics ↓ activation in supplementary motor area** |

i.v. (intravenous), THC (tetrahydrocannabinol), NAcc (nucleus accumbens), VTA (ventral tegmental area), Ant. Cing. (anterior cingulate), L (left), R (right), Post. Cing. (posterior cingulate), WCST (Wisconsin card sorting task), ETOH (ethanol), WM (working memory), D-amph. (dextro-amphetamine), ADHD (attention-deficit/hyperactivity disorder)

1. Vaidya CJ, Gabrieli JD. Searching for a neurobiological signature of attention deficit hyperactivity disorder. *Mol Psychiatry.* 1999;4:206–208.
2. Wise RG, Rogers R, Painter D, et al. Combining fMRI with a pharmacokinetic model to determine which brain areas activated by painful stimulation are specifically modulated by remifentanil. *Neuroimage.* 2002;16:999–1014.
3. Thiel CM, Henson RN, Dolan RJ. Scopolamine but not lorazepam modulates face repetition priming: a psychopharmacological fMRI study. *Neuropsychopharmacology.* 2002;27:282–292.
4. Stein EA, Pankiewicz J, Harsch HH, et al. Nicotine-induced limbic cortical activation in the human brain: a functional MRI study. *Am J Psychiatry.* 1998;155:1009–1015.
5. Stephan KE, Magnotta VA, White T, et al. Effects of olanzapine on cerebellar functional connectivity in schizophrenia measured by fMRI during a simple motor task. *Psychol Med.* 2001;31:1065–1078.
6. Sheline YI, Barch DM, Donnelly JM, Ollinger JM, Snyder AZ, Mintun MA. Increased amygdala response to masked emotional faces in depressed subjects resolves with antidepressant treatment: an fMRI study. *Biol Psychiatry.* 2001;50:651–658.
7. Seifritz E, Bilecen D, Hanggi D, et al. Effect of ethanol on BOLD response to acoustic stimulation: implications for neuropharmacological fMRI. *Psych Res.* 2000;99:1–13.
8. Sperling R, Greve D, Dale A, et al. Functional MRI detection of pharmacologically induced memory impairment. *Proc Natl Acad Sci U S A.* 2002;99:455–460.
9. Mu Q, Ross T, Risinger RC, et al. Dose-dependent responses of acute cocaine administration in humans using fMRI. *Neurosci Abs.* 2001.
10. Mattay VS, Callicott JH, Bertolino A, et al. Effects of dextroamphetamine on cognitive performance and cortical activation. *Neuroimage.* 2000;12:268–275.
11. Levin JM, Ross MH, Mendelson JH, et al. Reduction in BOLD fMRI response to primary visual stimulation following alcohol ingestion. *Psychiatry Res.* 1998;82:135–146.
12. Kimberg DY, Aguirre GK, Lease J, D'Esposito M. Cortical effects of bromocriptine, a D-2 dopamine receptor agonist, in human subjects, revealed by fMRI. *Hum Brain Mapp.* 2001;12:246–257.
13. Honey GD, Bullmore ET, Soni W, Varatheesan M, Williams SC, Sharma T. Differences in frontal cortical activation by a working memory task after substitution of risperidone for typical antipsychotic drugs in patients with schizophrenia. *PNAS.* 1999;96:13432–13437.
14. Howard RJ, Ellis C, Bullmore ET, et al. Functional echoplanar brain imaging correlates of amphetamine administration to normal subjects and subjects with the narcoleptic syndrome. *Magn Reson Imaging.* 1996;14:1013–1016.
15. Loubinoux I, Boulanouar K, Ranjeva JP, et al. Cerebral functional magnetic resonance imaging activation modulated by a single dose of fluoxetine and fenozolone during hand sensorimotor tasks. *J Cereb Blood Flow Metab.* 1999;19:1365–1375.
16. Furey ML, Pietrini P, Haxby JV. Cholinergic enhancement and increased selectivity of perceptual processing during working memory. *Science.* 2000;290:2315–2319.
17. Breiter HC, Gollub RL, Weisskoff RM, et al. Acute effects of cocaine on human brain activity and emotion. *Neuron.* 1997;19:591–611.
18. Braus DF, Ende G, Weber-Fahr W, et al. Antipsychotic drug effects on motor activation measured by functional magnetic resonance imaging in schizophrenic patients. *Schizophr Res.* 1999;39:19–29.
19. Bloom AS, Risinger RC, Ross TJ, Sanders J, Stein EA. Dose-dependent effects of tetrahydrocannabinol (THC) on brain activity and perfusion in humans: a functional magnetic resonance imaging study. *Soc Neurosci Abstr.* 2001;27:668.9.

## References

1. Berger H. Uber das elektrenkephalogramm des menschen. *Archiv fur Psychiatrie und Nervenkrankheiten.* 1929;87:527–570.
2. Knight RT. Electrophysiology in behavioral neurology. In: Mesulam M-M, ed. *Principles of Behavioral Neurology.* Philadelphia: FA Davis; 1985:327–346.
3. Sokoloff L. *Metabolic Probes of Central Nervous System Activity in Experimental Animals and Man. Magnes Lecture Series.* Vol. 1. Sunderland, MA: Sinauer Associates Inc.; 1984.
4. Kotrla KJ. Functional Neuroimaging in Psychiatry. In: Yudofsky SC, Hales RE, eds. *The American Psychiatric Press Textbook of Neuropsychiatry.* Washington DC: American Psychiatric Press; 1997:239–270.
5. Ogawa S, Lee TM, Kay AR, Tank DW. Brain magnetic resonance imaging with contrast dependent on blood oxygenation. *Proc Natl Acad Sci USA.* 1990;87:9868–9872.
6. Kwong KK, Belliveau JW, Chesler DA, et al. Dynamic magnetic resonance imaging of human brain activity during primary sensory stimulation. *Proc Natl Acad Sci USA.* 1992;89:5675–5679.
7. Bandettini PA, Wong EC, Hinks RS, Tikofsky RS, Hyde JS. Time course EPI of human brain function during task activation. *Magn Reson Med.* 1992;25:390–397.
8. Bonmassar G, Anami K, Ives J, Belliveau JW. Visual evoked potential (VEP) measured by simultaneous 64-channel EEG and 3T fMRI. *Neuroreport.* 1999;10:1893–1897.
9. Arthurs OJ, Williams EJ, Carpenter TA, Pickard JD, Boniface SJ. Linear coupling between functional magnetic resonance imaging and evoked potential amplitude in human somatosensory cortex. *Neuroscience.* 2000;101: 803–806.
10. Menon V, Ford JM, Lim KO, Glover GH, Pfefferbaum A. Combined event-related fMRI and EEG evidence for temporal-parietal cortex activation during target detection. *Neuroreport.* 1997;8:3029–3037.
11. Heeger DJ, Huk AC, Geisler WS, Albrecht DG. Spikes versus BOLD: what does neuroimaging tell us about neuronal activity? *Nat Neurosci.* 2000;3: 631–633.
12. Logothetis NK, Pauls J, Augath M, Trinath T, Oeltermann A. Neurophysiological investigation of the basis of the fMRI signal. *Nature.* 2001;412: 150–157.
13. Roy CS, Sherrington CS. On the regulation of the blood supply of the brain. *J Physiol.* 1890;11:85–108.
14. Kuschinsky W, Wahl M. Local chemical and neurogenic regulation of cerebral vascular resistance. *Physiol Rev.* 1978;58:656–689.
15. Iadecola C. Neurogenic control of the cerebral microcirculation: is dopamine minding the store? *Nat Neurosci.* 1998;1:263–265.
16. Mraovitch S, Sercombe R. *Neurophysiological Basis of Cerebral Blood Flow Control: An Introduction.* London, England: John Libbey & Company, Ltd; 1996.
17. Villringer A, Dirnagl U. Coupling of brain activity and cerebral blood flow: basis of functional neuroimaging. *Cerebrovasc Brain Metab Rev.* 1995;7: 240–276.
18. Brian JE, Jr, Faraci FM, Heistad DD. Recent insights into the regulation of cerebral circulation. *Clin Exper Pharmacol Physiol.* 1996;23:449–457.
19. Bandettini PA, Wong EC. A hypercapnia-based normalization method for improved spatial localization of human brain activation with fMRI. *NMR Biomed.* 1997;10:197–203.

20. Corfield DR, Murphy K, Josephs O, Adams L, Turner R. Does hypercapnia-induced cerebral vasodilation modulate the hemodynamic response to neural activation? *Neuroimage.* 2001;13:1207–1211.
21. Rao SM, Salmeron BJ, Durgerian S, et al. Effects of methylphenidate on functional MRI blood-oxygen-level-dependent contrast. *Am J Psychiatry.* 2000;157:1697–1699.
22. Rao SM, Bandettini PA, Binder JR, et al. Relationship between finger movement rate and functional magnetic resonance signal change in human primary motor cortex. *J Cereb Blood Flow Metab.* 1996;16:1250–1254.
23. Gollub RL, Breiter HC, Kantor H, et al. Cocaine decreases cortical cerebral blood flow but does not obscure regional activation in functional magnetic resonance imaging in human subjects. *J Cereb Blood Flow Metab.* 1998; 18:724–734.
24. Hall DA, Haggard MP, Akeroyd MA, et al. Modulation and task effects in auditory processing measured using fMRI. *Hum Brain Mapp.* 2000;10: 107–119.
25. Martin E, Thiel T, Joeri P, et al. Effect of pentobarbital on visual processing in man. *Hum Brain Mapp.* 2000;10:132–139.
26. Born AP, Rostrup E, Miranda MJ, Larsson HB, Lou HC. Visual cortex reactivity in sedated children examined with perfusion MRI (FAIR). *Magn Reson Imaging.* 2002;20:199–205.
27. Mathew R, Wilson W. Substance abuse and cerebral blood flow. *Am J Psychiatry.* 1991;148:292–305.
28. Rhodes LE, Obitz FW, Creel D. Effect of alcohol and task on hemispheric asymmetry of visually evoked potentials in man. *Electroencephalogr Clin Neurophysiol.* 1975;38:561–568.
29. Porjesz B, Begleiter H. Alcohol and bilateral evoked brain potentials. *Adv Exper Med Biol.* 1975;59:553–567.
30. Lewis EG, Dustman RE, Beck EC. The effects of alcohol on visual and somato-sensory evoked responses. *Electroencephalogr Clin Neurophysiol.* 1970;28:202–205.
31. Levin JM, Ross MH, Mendelson JH, et al. Reduction in BOLD fMRI response to primary visual stimulation following alcohol ingestion. *Psychiatry Res.* 1998;82:135–146.
32. Bruhn H, Kleinschmidt A, Boecker H, Merboldt KD, Hanicke WJF. The effect of acetazolamide on regional cerebral blood oxygenation at rest and under stimulation as assessed by MRI. *J Cereb Blood Flow Metab.* 1994;14: 742–748.
33. Oishi M, Mochizuki Y, Hara M, Takasu T. P300 and xenon computed tomography before and after intravenous injection of acetazolamide. *Arch Neurol.* 1995;52:850–851.
34. Shimosegawa E, Kanno I, Hatazawa J, et al. Photic stimulation study of changing the arterial partial pressure level of carbon dioxide. *J Cereb Blood Flow Metab.* 1995;15:111–114.
35. Seifritz E, Bilecen D, Hanggi D, et al. Effect of ethanol on BOLD response to acoustic stimulation: implications for neuropharmacological fMRI. *Psychiatry Res.* 2000;99:1–13.
36. Breiter HC, Gollub RL, Weisskoff RM, et al. Acute effects of cocaine on human brain activity and emotion. *Neuron.* 1997;19:591–611.
37. Ward BD, Garavan H, Ross TJ, Bloom AS, Cox RW, Stein EA. Nonlinear regression for fMRI time series analysis. *Neuroimage.* 1998;7:S767.
38. Bloom AS, Hoffmann RG, Fuller SA, Pankiewicz J, Harsch HH, Stein EA. Determination of drug-induced changes in functional MRI signal using a pharmacokinetic model. *Hum Brain Mapp.* 1999;8:235–244.

39. Stein EA, Pankiewicz J, Harsch HH, et al. Nicotine-induced limbic cortical activation in the human brain: a functional MRI study. *Am J Psychiatry.* 1998;155:1009–1015.
40. Wise RA, Hoffman DC. Localization of drug reward mechanisms by intracranial injections. *Synapse.* 1992;10:247–263.
41. Self DW. Neural substrates of drug craving and relapse in drug addiction. *Ann Med.* 1998;30:379–389.
42. Mu Q, Ross T, Risinger RC, et al. Dose-dependent responses of acute cocaine administration in humans using fMRI. *Neurosci Abs.* 2001.
43. McKeown MJ, Makeig S, Brown GG, et al. Analysis of fMRI data by blind separation into independent spatial components. *Hum Brain Mapp.* 1998;6: 160–188.
44. Liu Y, Gao JH, Liu HL, Fox PT. The temporal response of the brain after eating revealed by functional MRI. *Nature.* 2000;405:1058–1062.
45. Fadili MJ, Ruan S, Bloyet D, Mazoyer B. A multistep unsupervised fuzzy clustering analysis of fMRI time series. *Hum Brain Mapp.* 2000;10: 160–178.
46. Patterson JCN, Ungerleider LG, Bandettini PA. Task-independent functional brain activity correlation with skin conductance changes: an fMRI study. *Neuroimage.* 2002;17:1797–1806.
47. Donaldson DI, Buckner RL. Trying versus succeeding: event-related designs dissociate memory processes. *Neuron.* 1999;22:412–414.
48. Thiel CM, Henson RN, Dolan RJ. Scopolamine but not lorazepam modulates face repetition priming: a psychopharmacological fMRI study. *Neuropsychopharmacology.* 2002;27:282–292.
49. Garavan H, Ross TJ, Stein EA. Right hemispheric dominance of inhibitory control: an event-related functional MRI study. *Proc Natl Acad Sci USA.* 1999;96:8301–8306.
50. Lawrence NS, Ross TJ, Stein EA. Cognitive mechanisms of nicotine on visual attention. *Neuron.* 2002;36:539–548.
51. Furey ML, Pietrini P, Haxby JV. Cholinergic enhancement and increased selectivity of perceptual processing during working memory. *Science.* 2000;290:2315–2319.
52. Sheline YI, Barch DM, Donnelly JM, Ollinger JM, Snyder AZ, Mintun MA. Increased amygdala response to masked emotional faces in depressed subjects resolves with antidepressant treatment: an fMRI study. *Biol Psychiatry.* 2001;50:651–658.
53. Stephan KE, Magnotta VA, White T, et al. Effects of olanzapine on cerebellar functional connectivity in schizophrenia measured by fMRI during a simple motor task. *Psychol Med.* 2001;31:1065–1078.
54. Li SJ, Biswal B, Li Z, et al. Cocaine administration decreases functional connectivity in human primary visual and motor cortex as detected by functional MRI. *Magn Reson Med.* 2000;43:45–51.
55. Belliveau JW, Rosen BR, Kantor HL, et al. Functional cerebral imaging by susceptibility-contrast NMR. *Magn Reson Med.* 1990;14:538–546.
56. Chen YCI, Galpern WR, Brownell AL, et al. Detection of dopaminergic neurotransmitter activity using pharmacologic MRI: correlation with PET, microdialysis, and behavioral data. *Magn Reson Med.* 1997;38: 389–398.
57. Mandeville JB MJ, Ayata C, Moskowitz MA, Weisskoff RM, Rosen BR. MRI measurement of the temporal evolution of relative CMRO(2) during rat forepaw stimulation. *Magn Reson Med.* 1999;42:944–951.
58. Marota JJA, Mandeville JB, Weisskoff RM, Moskowitz MA, Rosen BR, Kosofsky BE. Cocaine activation discriminates projections by temporal response: an fMRI study in rat. *Neuroimage.* 2000;11:13–23.

59. Kaufman MJ, Levin JM, Maas LC, et al. Cocaine decreases relative cerebral blood volume in humans: a dynamic susceptibility contrast magnetic resonance imaging study. *Psychopharmacology.* 1998;138:76–81.
60. Streeter CC, Ciraulo DA, Harris GJ, et al. Functional magnetic resonance imaging of alprazolam-induced changes in humans with familial alcoholism. *Psychiatry Res.* 1998;82:69–82.
61. Aellig WH. Nuclear magnetic resonance in clinical pharmacology and measurement of therapeutic response. *Br J Clin Pharmacol.* 1990;29:157–167.
62. Gonzalez RG, Guimaraes AR, Sachs GS, Rosenbaum JF, Garwood M, Renshaw PF. Measurement of human brain lithium in vivo by MR spectroscopy. *AJNR Am J Neuroradiol.* 1993;14:1027–1037.
63. Henry ME, Moore CM, Kaufman MJ, et al. Brain kinetics of paroxetine and fluoxetine on the third day of placebo substitution: a fluorine MRS study. *Am J Psychiatry.* 2000;157:1506–1508.
64. Kato T, Takahashi S, Inubushi T. Brain lithium concentration by 7Li- and 1H-magnetic resonance spectroscopy in bipolar disorder. *Psychiatry Res.* 1992;45:53–63.
65. Komoroski RA, Newton JE, Sprigg JR, Cardwell D, Mohanakrishnan P, Karson CN. In vivo 7Li nuclear magnetic resonance study of lithium pharmacokinetics and chemical shift imaging in psychiatric patients. *Psychiatry Res.* 1993;50:67–76.
66. Renshaw PF, Guimaraes AR, Fava M, et al. Accumulation of fluoxetine and norfluoxetine in human brain during therapeutic administration. *Am J Psychiatry.* 1992;149:1592–1594.
67. Petroff OA, Hyder F, Mattson RH, Rothman DL. Topiramate increases brain GABA, homocarnosine, and pyrrolidinone in patients with epilepsy. *Neurology.* 1999;52:473–478.
68. Sonawalla SB, Renshaw PF, Moore CM, et al. Compounds containing cytosolic choline in the basal ganglia: a potential biological marker of true drug response to fluoxetine. *Am J Psychiatry.* 1999;156:1638–1640.
69. Li S-J, Wang Y, Pankiewicz J, Stein EA. Neurochemical adaptation to cocaine abuse: reduction of N-acetyl aspartate in thalamus of human cocaine abusers. *Biol Psychiatry.* 1999;45:1481–1487.
70. Ernst T, Chang L, Leonido-Yee M, Speck O. Evidence for long-term neurotoxicity associated with methamphetamine abuse: A 1H MRS study. *Neurology.* 2000;54:1344–1349.
71. Chang L, Mehringer CM, Ernst T, et al. Neurochemical alterations in asymptomatic abstinent cocaine users: a proton magnetic resonance spectroscopy study. *Biol Psychiatry.* 1997;42:1105–1114.
72. Ernst T, Chang L, Cooray D, et al. The effects of tamoxifen and estrogen on brain metabolism in elderly women. [comment]. *J Natl Cancer Inst.* 2002; 94:592–597.
73. Krause KH, Dresel SH, Krause J, Kung HF, Tatsch K. Increased striatal dopamine transporter in adult patients with attention deficit hyperactivity disorder: effects of methylphenidate as measured by single photon emission computed tomography. *Neurosci Lett.* 2000;285:107–110.

# 18

# Cognitive Neuroscience Applications

Mark D'Esposito

## Introduction

Cognitive neuroscience is a discipline that attempts to determine the neural mechanisms underlying cognitive processes. Specifically, cognitive neuroscientists test hypotheses about brain–behavior relationships organized along two conceptual domains: *functional specialization*—the idea that functional modules exist within the brain, that is, areas of the cerebral cortex that are specialized for a specific cognitive process, and *functional integration*—the idea that a cognitive process can be an emergent property of interactions among a network of brain regions that suggests that a brain region can play a different role across many functions.

Early studies of brain–behavior relationships consisted of careful observation of individuals with neurological injury resulting in focal brain damage. The idea of functional specialization evolved from hypotheses that damage to a particular brain region was responsible for a given behavioral syndrome that was characterized by a precise neurological examination; for instance, the association of nonfluent aphasia with right-sided limb weakness implicated the left hemisphere as the site of language abilities. Moreover, upon the death of a patient with a neurological disorder, clinicopathological correlations provided confirmatory information about the site of damage causing a specific neurobehavioral syndrome such as aphasia; for example, in 1861, Paul Broca's observations of nonfluent aphasia in the setting of a damaged left inferior frontal gyrus cemented the belief that this brain region was critical for speech output.[1] The introduction of structural brain imaging more than 100 years after Broca's observations, first with computerized tomography and later with magnetic resonance imaging (MRI), paved the way for more precise anatomical localization in the living patient of the cognitive deficits that develop after brain injury. The superb spatial resolution of structural neuroimaging has reduced the reliance on the infrequently obtained autopsy for making brain–behavior correlations.

Functional neuroimaging, broadly defined as techniques that measure brain activity, has expanded our ability to study the neural basis of cognitive processes. One such method, functional MRI (fMRI) has emerged as an extremely powerful technique that affords excellent spatial and temporal resolution. Measuring regional brain activity in healthy subjects while they perform behavioral tasks links localized brain activity with specific behaviors; for example, functional neuroimaging studies have demonstrated that the left inferior frontal gyrus is consistently activated during the performance of speech-production tasks in healthy individuals.[2] Such findings from functional neuroimaging are complementary to findings derived from observations of patients with focal brain damage. This chapter focuses on the principles underlying fMRI as a cognitive neuroscience tool for exploring brain–behavior relationships.

## Inference in Functional Neuroimaging Studies of Cognitive Processes

Insight regarding the link between brain and behavior can be gained through a variety of approaches. It is unlikely that any single neuroscience method is sufficient to investigate fully any particular question regarding the mechanism underlying cognitive function. From a methodological point of view, every method will offer different temporal and spatial resolution. From a conceptual point of view, every method will provide data that will support different types of inferences that can be drawn from it. Thus, data obtained addressing a single question but derived from multiple methods can provide more comprehensive and inferentially sound conclusions.

Functional neuroimaging studies support inferences about the association of a particular brain system with a cognitive process. However, it is difficult to prove in such a study that the observed activity is necessary for an isolated cognitive process because perfect control over a subject's cognitive processes during a functional neuroimaging experiment is never possible. Even if the task a subject performs is well designed, it is difficult to demonstrate conclusively that he/she is differentially engaging a single identified cognitive process. The subject may engage in unwanted cognitive processes that either have no overt measurable effects, or are perfectly confounded with the process of interest. Consequently, the neural activity measured by the functional neuroimaging technique may result from some confounding neural computation that is itself not necessary for executing the cognitive process seemingly under study. In other words, functional neuroimaging is an observational, correlative method.[3] It is important to note that the inferences that can be drawn from functional neuroimaging studies such as fMRI apply to all methods of physiological measurement [e.g., electroencephalogram (EEG) or magnetoencephalogram.]

The inference of necessity cannot be made without showing that inactivating a brain region disrupts the cognitive process in question. However, unlike precise surgical or neurotoxic lesions in animal models, lesions in patients are often extensive, damaging local neurons and fibers of passage; for example, damage to prominent white matter tracts can cause cognitive deficits similar to those produced by cortical lesions, such as the amnesia resulting from lesions of the fornix, the main white matter pathway projecting from the hippocampus.[4] In addition, connections from region A may support the continued metabolic function of region B, but region A may not be computationally involved in certain processes undertaken by region B. Thus, damage to region A could impair the function of region B via two possible mechanisms: (1) diaschisis[5] and (2) retrograde transsynaptic degeneration. Consequently, studies of patients with focal lesions cannot conclusively demonstrate that the neurons within a specific region are themselves critical to the computational support of an impaired cognitive process.

Empirical studies using lesion and electrophysiologic methods demonstrate these issues regarding the types of inferences that can logically be drawn from them. In monkeys, single-unit recording reveals neurons in the lateral prefrontal cortex that increase their firing during the delay between the presentation of information to be remembered and a few seconds later when that information must be recalled.[6,7] These studies are taken as evidence that persistent neural activity in the prefrontal cortex is involved in temporary storage of information, a cognitive process known as working memory. The necessity of prefrontal cortex for working memory was demonstrated in other monkey studies showing that prefrontal lesions impair performance on working memory tasks, but not on tasks that do not require temporarily holding information in memory.[8] Persistent neural activity during working memory tasks are also found in the hippocampus.[9,10] Hippocampal lesions, however, do not impair performance on most working memory tasks,[11] which suggests that the hippocampus is involved in maintaining information over short periods of time, but is not necessary for this cognitive operation. Observations in humans support this notion. For example, the well-studied patient H.M., with complete bilateral hippocampal damage and the severe inability to learn new information, could nevertheless perform normally on working memory tasks such as digit span.[12] The hippocampus is implicated in long-term memory, especially when relations between multiple items or multiple features of a complex novel item must be retained. Thus, the hippocampus may only be engaged during working memory tasks that requires someone to subsequently remember novel information.[13]

When the results from lesion and functional neuroimaging studies are combined, a stronger level of inference emerges. As in the examples of Broca's aphasia or working memory, a lesion of a specific brain region causes impairment of a given cognitive process, and when engaged by an intact individual, that cognitive process evokes neural activity in the same brain region. In this type of finding, the inference that this brain region is computationally necessary for the cognitive process is stronger than data derived from each study performed in isolation. Thus, lesion and functional neuroimaging studies are complementary, each providing inferential support that the other lacks.

Other types of inferential failure can occur in the interpretation of functional neuroimaging studies when other common assumptions do not hold true. First, it is assumed that if a cognitive process activates a particular brain region (evoked by a particular task), the neural activity in that brain region must depend on engaging that particular cognitive process; for example, a brain region showing greater activation during the presentation of faces than to other types of stimuli, such as photographs of cars or buildings, is considered to engage face perception processes. However, this region also may support other higher-level cognitive processes such as memory processes, in addition to lower-level perceptual processes.[14] Second, it is assumed that if a particular brain region is activated during the performance of a cognitive task, the subject must have engaged the cognitive process supported by that region during the task; for example, observing activation of the frontal lobes during a mental rotation task, it was proposed that subjects engaged working memory processes to recall the identity of the rotated target.[15] (They derived this assumption from other imaging studies showing activation of the frontal lobes during working memory tasks.) However, in this example, because some other cognitive process supported by the frontal lobes could have activated this region,[16] one cannot be sure that working memory was engaged leading to the activation of the frontal lobes.

In summary, interpretation of the results of functional neuroimaging studies attempting to link brain and behavior rests on numerous assumptions. Familiarity with the types of inferences that can and cannot be drawn from these studies should be helpful for assessing the validity of the findings reported by such studies.

## Functional MRI as a Cognitive Neuroscience Tool

Functional MRI has become the predominant functional neuroimaging method for studying the neural basis of cognitive processes in humans. Compared to its predecessor, positron emission tomography (PET) scanning, fMRI offers many advantages; for example, MRI scanners are much more widely available, and imaging costs are less expensive because MRI does not require a cyclotron to produce radioisotopes. Magnetic resonance imaging is also a noninvasive procedure because there is no requirement for injection of a radioisotope into the bloodstream. In addition, given the half-life of available radioisotopes, PET scanning is unable to provide comparable temporal resolution to that of fMRI, which can provide images of behavioral events occurring on the order of seconds rather than the summation of many behavioral events over tens of seconds.

In selected circumstances, however, PET can provide an advantage over fMRI for studying certain questions concerning the neural basis of cognition; for example, at present, fMRI does not adeguately image the regions within the orbitofrontal cortex and the anterior or inferior temporal lobe because of the susceptibility artifact near the interface of the brain and sinuses. These artifacts worsen at higher magnetic fields (i.e., 3 or 4 Tesla), and such scanners are becoming commonly available and increasingly utilized by cognitive neuroscientists. Improvements in pulse sequences for acquiring fMRI data and development of algorithms for distortion correction of images should eventually eliminate or reduce these artifacts.[17–19] Currently, however, such sequences and methods are not widely available and implemented. Position emission tomography scanning may remain desirable or necessary when studying certain populations of individuals; for example, amnesic patients resulting from cerebral anoxia often have implanted cardiac pacemakers precluding them from having an MRI scan due to the magnetic field. However, PET scanning is unacceptable for studies of children due to the radiation exposure.

The MRI scanner, compared to a behavioral testing room, is less than ideal for performing most cognitive neuroscience experiments. Experiments are performed in the awkward position of lying on one's back, often requiring subjects to visualize the presentation of stimuli through a mirror in an acoustically noisy environment. Moreover, most individuals develop some degree of claustrophobia due to the small bore of the MRI scanner and find it difficult to remain completely motionless for a long duration of time that is required for most experiments (e.g., usually 60 to 90 minutes). These constraints of the MRI scanner make it especially difficult to scan children, which has resulted in many fewer fMRI studies involving children than adults.[20,21] In addition, it has been a technical challenge to develop equipment within the MRI environment that successfully presents different types of stimuli to the individual (e.g., olfactory, tactile), as well as to collect ancillary response or physiological data necessary for a particular experiment.

All sensory systems have been investigated with fMRI, including the visual, auditory, somatosensory, olfactory, and gustatory systems. Each system requires different technologies for successful presentation of relevant stimuli within an MRI environment. At the time of this writing, very few off-the-shelf commercial products exist that are MRI compatible, and most in use today have been engineered locally by individual laboratories. Most published fMRI studies have utilized visual stimuli, although great strides have been made to allow the presentation of other types of stimuli. Details regarding the issues related to presenting visual and auditory stimuli in the MRI environment can be reviewed furthered in a comprehensive chapter on the topic by Savoy and colleagues.[22] In brief, the most common means of presenting visual stimuli is via a LCD projector system, with the sophistication of the system depending on the quality of image resolution required for the experiment. Several options exist for auditory stimuli, such as piezoelectric or electrostatic headphones. However, the biggest challenge is the acoustically noisy scanner environment. The pulsing of the fMRI gradient coils is the source of such noise, making the study of auditory processes challenging;[23,24] for example, during echoplanar imaging within a 4 Tesla magnet using a high-performance head gradient set, sound levels can reach 130 decibels. As a reference point, Food and Drug Administration (FDA) safety regulations require no greater than an average of 105 decibels for one hour. With placement of absorbing materials within the scanner and on the walls of the room, as well as a fiberglass bore liner surrounding the gradient set, we have been able to reduce sound levels by about 25 decibels. For further discussion concerning sound reduction techniques, refer to the chapter on Auditing MRI. One of the biggest technical challenges within an MRI scanner has been the ability to present olfactory stimuli. However, sophisticated MR-compatible olfactometers have been designed and utilized successfully. Such methods use a nasal-mask in which the change from odorant to no-odorant conditions occurs within a few milliseconds.[25,26]

Acquiring ancillary electrophysiological data such as electromyographic recordings to measure muscle contraction or electrodermal responses to measure autonomic activity enhances many cognitive neuroscience experiments. Devices have been developed that are MR compatible for these types of measurements, as well other physiological measures such as heart rate, electrocardiography, oxygen saturation, and respiratory rate. The recording of eye movements is becoming commonplace in MRI scanners, predominantly with the use of an infrared video camera equipped with long-range optics.[27,28] Video images of the pupil–corneal reflection can be sampled at 60/120/240 hertz, allowing for the accurate (less than one degree) localization of gaze within 50 horizontal and 40 vertical degrees of visual angle. Although most behavioral tasks used in cognitive neuroscience experiments rely on collecting manual responses, the ability to reliably collect verbal responses without significant artifact being introduced into the data has been demonstrated by several laboratories.[29–31]

Electroencephalogram recordings also have been performed successfully during MRI scanning.[32,33] However, the recording of event-related potentials, a signal that is much smaller in amplitude than the signal in EEG, can be more difficult in a magnetic field due to artifacts induced by gradient pulsing and head movement from cardiac pulsation. New monitoring devices and algorithms to remove artifact are being developed, allowing for reliable measurements of event-related potentials during MRI scanning.[34,35]

In summary, most initial challenges facing performing cognitive and behavioral experiments within the MRI environment have been overcome, creating an environment that is comparable to standard psychophysical testing labs outside of a scanner. Although individual laboratories have achieved most of these advancements, MRI scanners originally designed for clinical use by manufacturers are now being designed with consideration of many of these research-related issues.

### *Temporal Resolution*

Two types of temporal resolution need to be considered for cognitive neuroscience experiments. First, what is the briefest neural event that can be detected as an fMRI signal? Second, how close together can two neural events occur and be resolved as separable fMRI signals?

The time scale on which neural changes occur are quite rapid; for example, neural activity in the lateral intraparietal area of monkeys increases within 100 milliseconds of the visual presentation of a saccade target.[36] In contrast, the fMRI signal gradually increases to its peak magnitude within four to six seconds after an experimentally induced brief (less than one second) change in neural activity, and then decays back to baseline after several more seconds.[37–39] This slow time course of fMRI signal change in response to such a brief increase in neural activity is informally referred to as the BOLD fMRI hemodynamic response, or simply, the hemodynamic response (see Figure 18.1). Thus, neural dynamics and neurally evoked hemodynamics, as measured with fMRI, are on quite different time scales.

The sluggishness of the hemodynamic response limits the temporal resolution of the fMRI signal to hundreds of milliseconds to seconds as opposed to the millisecond temporal resolution of electrophysiological recordings of neural activity, such as from single-unit recording in monkeys and EEG or magnetoencephalogram in humans. However, it has been clearly demonstrated that brief changes in neural activity can be detected with reasonable statistical power using fMRI; for example, appreciable fMRI signal can be observed in sensorimotor cortex in association with single finger movements[40] and in visual cortex during very briefly presented (34 milliseconds) visual stimuli.[41] In contrast, the temporal resolution of fMRI limits the detection of sequential changes in neural activity that occurs rapidly with respect to the hemodynamic response. That is, the ability to resolve the changes in the fMRI signal associated with two neural events, often requires the separation of those events by a relatively long period of time compared with the width of the hemodynamic response. This is because two neural events closely spaced in time will produce a hemodynamic response that reflects the accumulation from both neural events, making it difficult to estimate the contribution of each individual neural event. In general, evoked fMRI responses to discrete neural events separated by at least four seconds appear to be within the range of resolution.[42] However, provided that the stimuli are presented randomly, studies have shown significant differential functional responses between two events (e.g., flashing visual stimuli) spaced as closely as 500 milliseconds apart.[43–45] The effect at fixed and randomized intertrial intervals on the BOLD signal is illustrated in Figure 18.2.

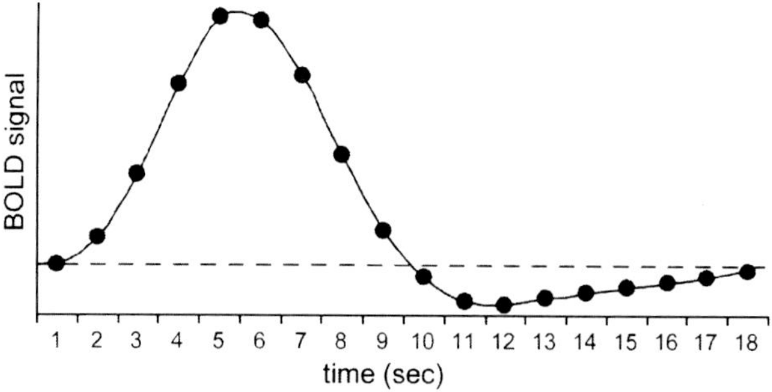


**Figure 18.1.** A typical hemodynamic response (i.e., fMRI signal change in response to a brief increase of neural activity) from the primary sensorimotor cortex. The fMRI signal peaked approximately five seconds after the onset of the motor response (at time zero).

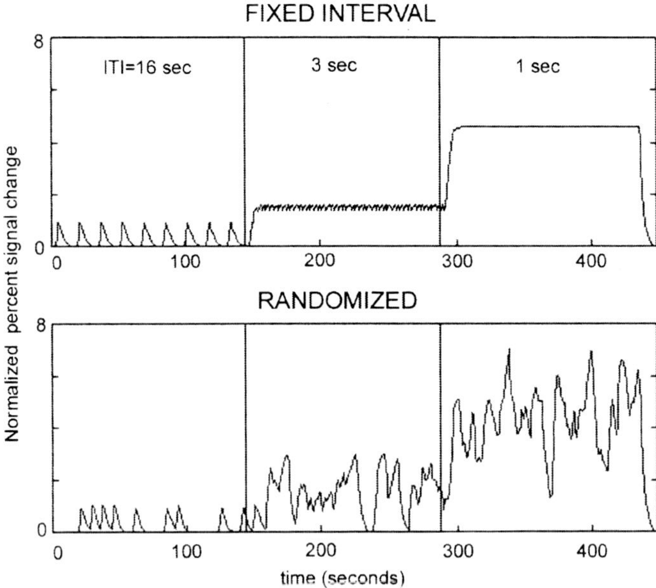


**Figure 18.2.** Effect of fixed versus randomized intertrial intervals on the BOLD fMRI signal. Adapted from Burock MA, Buckner RL, Woldorff MG, Rosen BR, Dale AM. Randomized event related experimental designs allow for extremely rapid presentation rates using functional MRI. *Neuroreport*. 1998;9:3735–3739.

In some tasks, the order of individual trial events cannot be randomized; for example, in certain types of working memory tasks, the presentation of the information to be remembered during the delay period, and the period when the subject must recall the information, are individual trial events whose order cannot be randomized. In these types of tasks, short time scales (less than four seconds) cannot be temporally resolved. These temporal resolution issues in fMRI have been extensively considered regarding their impact on experimental design.[46,47]

### *Spatial Resolution*

It has yet to be determined how precisely the measured BOLD fMRI signal, which arises from the vasculature, reflects adjacent neural activity. Thus, the ultimate spatial resolution of BOLD fMRI is unknown. Functional MRI studies in both monkey and man at high field (4 to 4.7 Tesla) have demonstrated that BOLD signal can be obtained with high spatial resolution—approximately $0.75 \times 0.75\,\text{mm}^2$ in-plane resolution.[48,49] In monkeys, with novel approaches such as using a small, tissue-compatible, intraosteally implanted radiofrequency coil, ultra high spatial resolution of $125 \times 125\,\mu\text{m}^2$ has been obtained.[50] Using this method, Logothetis and colleagues[50] demonstrated cortical lamina-specific activation in a task that compared responses to moving stimuli with those elicited by flickering stimuli. This contrast elicited BOLD signal mostly in the granular layers of the striate cortex of the monkey, which are known to have a high concentration of directionally selective cells. Advances in such methods would allow for imaging of hundreds of neurons per voxel as opposed to hundreds of thousands of neurons per voxel, which is more typical for a human cognitive neuroscience fMRI experiment.

Virtually all fMRI studies model the large BOLD signal increase, which is due to a local low-deoxyhemoglobin state (see Figure 18.1), in order to detect changes correlating with a behavioral task. However, optical imaging studies have demonstrated that preceding this large positive response is an initial negative response reflecting a localized increase in oxygen consumption, causing a high-deoxyhemoglobin state.[51] This early hemodynamic response is called the initial dip and is thought to be more tightly coupled to the actual site of neural activity evoking the BOLD signal as compared to the later positive portion of the BOLD response; for example, Kim and colleagues,[52] scanning cats in a high field scanner, demonstrated that the early negative BOLD response (e.g., initial dip) produced activation maps that were consistent with orientation columns within visual cortex. This finding is quite remarkable given that the average spacing between two adjacent orientation columns in cortex is approximately one millimeter. In contrast, the activation maps produced by the delayed positive BOLD response appeared more diffuse, and cortical columnar organization could not be identified.[52] Thus, empirical evidence suggests that deriving activation maps by correlating behavioral responses with the initial dip may markedly improve spatial resolution. However, it is important to note that observation of the initial dip of the BOLD signal has been inconsistently observed in humans across laboratories for reasons that are still unclear. Several groups, however, were able to detect columnar architecture (in this case, ocular dominance columns) by modeling the positive BOLD response in humans scanning at 4 Tesla.[49,53] These investigators attributed their success to optimized radiofrequency coils, limiting head motion, optimizing slice orientation, and the enhanced signal-to-noise ratio (SNR) provided by a high magnetic field.

Another unique method for improving spatial resolution has been called functional magnetic resonance–adaptation (fMR-A), which could provide a means for identifying and assessing the functional attributes of sharply defined neuronal populations within a given region of the brain.[54] Even if the spatial resolution of fMRI evolves to the point of being able to resolve a population of a few hundred neurons within a voxel, it is still likely that this small population will contain neurons with very different functional properties that will be averaged together. The adaptation method is based on several basic principles. First, repeated presentation of the same type of stimuli (i.e., a picture of the one object) causes neurons to adapt to those stimuli (i.e., neuronal firing is reduced). Second, if these neurons are then exposed to a different type of stimulus (i.e., a picture of another object) or a change in some property of the stimulus (i.e., the same object in a different orientation), recovery from adaptation can be assessed (i.e., whether or not the BOLD signal returns to its original state). If the signal remains adapted, it implies that the neurons are invariant to the attribute that was changed. If the signal recovers from the adapted

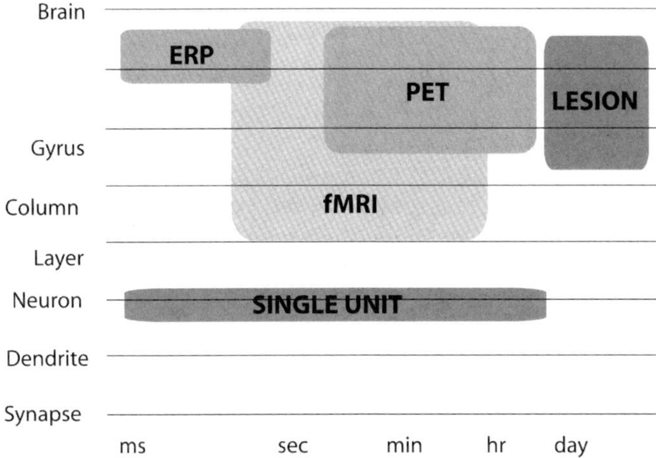


**Figure 18.3.** Temporal and spatial resolution of different neuroscience methods. Adapted from Churchland PS, Sejnowski TJ. Perspectives on cognitive neuroscience. *Science*. 1988;242:741–745. Copyright © 1988 AAAS.

state, it would imply that the neurons are sensitive to that attribute; for example, Grill-Spector and colleagues demonstrated that an area of lateral occipital cortex thought to be important for object recognition was less sensitive to changes in object size and position as compared to changes in illumination and viewpoint.[55] Thus, with this method, it is possible to investigate the functional properties of neuronal populations with a level of spatial resolution that is beyond that obtained from conventional fMRI data analysis methods.

Considering all the neuroscientific methods available today for studying human brain–behavior relationships, fMRI provides an excellent balance of temporal and spatial resolution (see Figure 18.3). Improvements on both fronts will clearly add to the increasing popularity of this method.

## Issues in Functional MRI Experimental Design

Numerous options exist for designing experiments using fMRI (see Chapter 3 by Aguirre for more in-depth discussion of experimental design). The prototypical fMRI experimental design consists of two behavioral tasks presented in blocks of trials alternating over the course of a scanning session, and the fMRI signal between the two tasks is compared. This is known as a blocked design; for example, a given block might present a series of faces to be viewed passively, which evokes a particular cognitive process, such as face perception. The experimental block alternates with a control block, which is designed to evoke all of the cognitive processes present in the experimental block except for the cognitive process of interest. In this experiment, the control block may comprise a series of objects. In this way, the stimuli used in experimental and control tasks have similar visual attributes, but differ in the attribute of interest (i.e., faces). The inferential framework of cognitive subtraction[56] attributes differences in neural activity between the two tasks to the specific cognitive process (i.e., face perception). Cognitive subtraction was originally conceived by Donders[57] in the late 1800s for studying the chronometric substrates of cognitive processes (see Sternberg[58]) and was a major innovation in imaging.[56,59]

The assumptions required for cognitive subtraction may not always hold and could produce erroneous interpretation of functional neuroimaging data.[42] Cognitive subtraction relies on two assumptions: pure insertion and linearity. Pure insertion implies that a cognitive process can be added to a preexisting set of cognitive processes without affecting them. This assumption is difficult to prove because one needs an independent measure of the preexisting processes in the absence and presence of the new process.[58] If pure insertion fails as an assumption, a difference in the neuroimaging signal between the two tasks might be observed, not because a specific cognitive process was engaged in one task and not the other, but because the added cognitive process and the preexisting cognitive processes interact.

An example of this point is illustrated in working memory studies using delayed-response tasks.[60] These tasks (for an example, see Jonides and colleagues[61]) typically present information that the subject must remember (engaging an encoding process), followed by a delay period during which the subject must hold the information in memory over a short period of time (engaging a memory process), followed by a probe that requires the subject to make a decision based on the stored information (engaging a retrieval process). The brain regions engaged by evoking the memory process theoretically are revealed by subtracting the BOLD signal measured by fMRI during a block of trials that the subject performs that do not have a delay period (only engaging the encoding and retrieval processes) from a block of trials with a delay period (engaging the encoding, memory, and retrieval processes). In this example, if the addition or insertion of a delay period between the encoding and retrieval processes affects these other behavioral processes in the task, the result is failure to meet the assumptions of cognitive subtraction. That is, these non-memory processes may differ in delay trials and no-delay trials, resulting in a failure to cancel each other out in the two types of trials that are being compared.

Empirical evidence of such failure exists.[62] For example, Figure 18.4 demonstrates BOLD signal derived from the prefrontal cortex from a subject performing a delayed response task similar to the tasks described above. The left side of the figure illustrates BOLD signal consistent with delay period activity, whereas the right side of the figure illustrates BOLD signal from another region of prefrontal cortex that did not display sustained activity during the delay, yet showed greater activity in the delay trials as compared to the trials without a delay. In any blocked functional neuroimaging study that compares delay versus no-delay trials with subtraction, such a region would be detected and likely assumed to be a memory region. Thus, this result provides empirical grounds for adopting a healthy doubt regarding the inferences drawn from imaging studies that rely exclusively on cognitive subtraction.

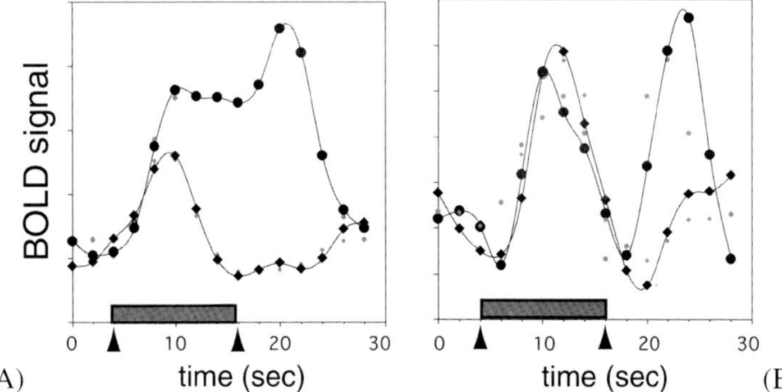


**Figure 18.4.** Data derived from the performance of a normal subject on a spatial delayed-response task. This task comprised both delay trials (circles), as well as trials without a delay period (no-delay trials; diamonds). (A) Trial-averaged fMRI signal from prefrontal cortex that displayed delay-correlated activity. The gray bar along the $x$-axis denotes the 12-second delay period during delay trials. The delay trials display a level of fMRI signal greater than baseline throughout the period of time corresponding to the retention delay (taking into account the delay and dispersion of the fMRI signal). The peaks seen in the signal correspond to the encoding and retrieval periods. (B) Trial-averaged fMRI signal from a region in prefrontal cortex that did not display the characteristics of delay-correlated activity. This region displays a significant functional change associated with the no-delay trials, and a significant functional change associated with the encoding and retrieval periods of the delay trials, but not one associated with the retention delay of delay trials. Adapted from Zarahn E, Aguirre GK, D'Esposito M. Temporal isolation of the neural correlates of spatial mnemonic processing with fMRI. *Cogn Brain Res.* 1999;7:255–268.

In functional neuroimaging, the transform between the neural signal and the hemodynamic response (measured by fMRI) must also be linear for the cognitive subtractive method to yield valid results. In other words, it is assumed that the BOLD signal being measured is approximately proportional to the local neural activity that evokes it. Surprisingly, although thousands of empirical studies using fMRI to study brain–behavior relationships have been published, only a handful exist that have explored the neurophysiological basis of the BOLD signal (for reviews, see Attwell and Iadecola[63] and Heeger and Ress[64]). In several studies, linearity did not strictly hold for the BOLD fMRI system, but the linear transform model was reasonably consistent with the data; for example, Boynton and colleagues tested whether BOLD signal in response to long duration stimuli can be predicted by summing the responses to shorter duration stimuli.[39] Using pulses of flickering checkerboard patterns and measuring within human primary visual cortex, these investigators found that the BOLD signal response to various durations of stimulus presentation (6, 12, or 24 seconds) could be predicted from the responses they obtained from shorter stimulus presentations; for example, the BOLD signal response to a six-second pulse could be predicted from the summation of the BOLD signal response to the three-second pulse with a copy of the same response delayed by three seconds. However, temporal summation did not always hold, and there are clearly nonlinear effects in the transform of neural activity to a hemodynamic response that must be considered.[65–68] If these nonlinearities lead to saturation of the BOLD effect at a certain stimulus intensity, erroneous interpretation of particular results of fMRI experiments may occur.

Another class of experimental designs, called event-related fMRI, attempt to detect changes associated with individual trials, as opposed to the larger unit of time comprising a block of trials.[69,70] Each individual trial may be composed of one behavioral event, such as the presentation of a single stimulus (e.g., a face or object to be perceived), or several behavioral events, such as in the delayed-response task described above, (e.g., an item to be remembered, a delay period, and a motor response in a delayed-response task); for example, with an event-related design, activity within the prefrontal cortex has consistently been shown to correlate with the delay period,[62] supporting the role of the PFC in temporarily maintaining information. This finding is consistent with single-neuron recording studies in the PFC of monkeys.[7] Event-related designs offer numerous advantages; for example, it allows for stimulus or trial randomization, avoiding the behavioral confounds of blocked trials. It also permits the separate analysis of functional responses, which are identified only in retrospect (i.e., trials on which the subject made a correct or incorrect response). Of course, an experiment does not have to be limited to either a block or event-related designs—a mixed-type (both event-related and blocked) design, where particular trial types are randomized within a block, is perfectly feasible. In this type of design, both item-related processes (e.g., transient responses to stimuli), as well as state-related processes (processes sustained throughout a block of trials or a task)[71,72] are perfectly feasible. Overall, much flexibility exists in the type of experimental design that can be utilized in an fMRI experiment, and continued innovation in this area will greatly expand the types of neuroscientific questions that can be addressed.

## Issues in Interpretation of fMRI Data

### *Statistics*

Many statistical techniques are used for analyzing fMRI data, but no single method has emerged as the ideal or gold standard (see Chapter 3 by Aguirre for more in-depth discussion of statistical analysis of fMRI data). The analysis of any fMRI experiment designed to contradict the null hypothesis (i.e., there is no difference between experimental conditions) requires inferential statistics. If the difference between two experimental conditions is too large to reasonably be due to chance, then the null hypothesis is rejected in favor of the alternative hypothesis, which typically is the experimenter's hypothesis (e.g., the fusiform gyrus is activated to a greater extent by viewing faces than objects). Unfortunately, because errors can occur in any statistical test, experimenters will never know when an error is committed, and they can only try to minimize them.[73] Knowledge of several basic statistical issues provides a solid foundation for the correct interpretation of the data derived from functional neuroimaging studies.

Two types of statistical errors can occur. A Type I error is committed when the null hypothesis is falsely rejected when it is true, that is, a difference between experimental conditions is found but a difference does not truly exist. This type of error is also called a false-positive error. In a functional neuroimaging study, a false-positive error would be finding a brain region activated during a cognitive task, when actually it is not. A Type II error is committed when the null hypothesis is accepted when it is false, that is, no difference between experimental conditions exists when a difference does exist. This type of error is called a false-negative error. A false-negative error in a functional neuroimaging study would be failing to find a brain region activated during the performance of a cognitive task when actually it is.

In fMRI experiments, like all experiments, a tolerable probability for Type I error, typically less than five percent, is chosen for adequate control of specificity, that is, control of false-positive rates. Two features of imaging data can cause unacceptable false-positive rates, even with traditional parametric statistical tests. First, there is the problem of multiple comparisons. For the typical resolution of images acquired during fMRI scans, the full extent of single slice (matrix-$128^2$, slice-5 mm) of the human brain could comprise 15000 voxels. Thus, with any given statistical comparison of two experimental conditions, there are actually 15000 statistical comparisons being performed. With such a large number of statistical tests, the probability of finding a false-positive activation, that is, committing a Type I error, somewhere in the brain increases. Several methods exist to deal with this problem. One method, a Bonferroni correction, assumes that each statistical test is independent and calculates the probability of Type I error by dividing the chosen probability ($p = 0.05$) by the number of statistical tests performed. Another method is based on Gaussian field theory,[74] and calculates the probability of Type I error when imaging data are spatially smoothed. Many other methods for determining thresholds of statistical maps are proposed and utilized,[75,76] but unfortunately, no single method has been universally accepted. Nevertheless, all fMRI studies must apply some type of correction for multiple comparisons to control the false-positive rate.

The second feature that might increase the false-positive rate is the noise in fMRI data. Data from BOLD fMRI are temporally autocorrelated, with more noise at some frequencies than at others. The shape of this noise distribution is characterized by a 1/frequency function, with increasing noise at lower frequencies.[77] Traditional parametric and nonparametric statistical tests assume that the noise is not temporally autocorrelated, that is, each observation is independent. Therefore, any statistical test used in fMRI studies must account for the noise structure of fMRI data. If not, the false-positive rates will inflate.[77,78]

Type II error is rarely considered in functional neuroimaging studies. When a brain map from an fMRI experiment is presented, several areas of activation are typically attributed to some experimental manipulation. The focus of most imaging studies is on brain activation, whereas it is often implicitly assumed that all of the other areas (typically, most of the brain) were not activated during the experiment. Power as a statistical concept refers to the probability of correctly rejecting the null hypothesis.[73] As the power of a fMRI study to detect changes in brain activity increases, the false-negative rate decreases. Unfortunately, power calculations for particular fMRI experiments are rarely performed, although this methodology is evolving.[79–81] Reports that specific brain areas were not active during an experimental manipulation should provide an estimate of the power required for detection of a change in the region. All experiments should be designed to maximize power. Relatively simple strategies can increase power in an fMRI experiment in certain circumstances, such as increasing the amount of imaging data collected or increasing the number of subjects studied. It is also important to note that task designs can affect sensitivity;[82] for example, because BOLD fMRI data are temporally autocorrelated, experiments with fundamental frequencies in the lower range (e.g., a boxcar design with 60-second epochs) will have reduced sensitivity due to the presence of greater noise at these lower frequencies. Finally, in a study that simultaneously measured neural signal via intracortical recording and BOLD signal in a monkey, it was observed that the SNR of the neural signal was, on average, at least one order of magnitude higher than that of the BOLD signal. The investigators of this study concluded that "the statistical and thresholding methods applied to the hemodynamic responses probably underestimate a great deal of actual neural activity related to a stimulus or task."[83] Thus, the magnitude of Type II error in BOLD fMRI may currently be underestimated and warrants further consideration in the interpretation of almost any cognitive neuroscience experiment.

### *Altered Hemodynamic Response*

When comparing changes in BOLD signal levels within the brain of an individual subject across different cognitive tasks and making conclusions regarding changes in neural activity and the pattern of activity, numerous assumptions are made regarding the steps comprising neurovascular coupling (stimulus → neural activity → hemodynamic response → BOLD signal) and the regional variability of the metabolic and vascular parameters influencing the BOLD signal. It should be obvious that fMRI studies of cognition and behavior of individuals with local vascular compromise or diffuse vascular disease (e.g., patients with strokes or normal elderly) are potentially problematic; for example, many fMRI studies have sought to identify age-related changes in the neural substrates of cognitive processes. These studies that directly compare changes in BOLD signal intensity across age groups rely upon the assumption of age-equivalent coupling of neural activity to BOLD signal. However, there is empirical evidence that suggests that this general assumption may not hold true. Extensive research on the aging neurovascular system has revealed that it undergoes significant changes in multiple domains in a continuum throughout the human lifespan, probably as early as the fourth decade (for a review, see Farkas and Luiten[84]). These changes affect the vascular ultrastructure,[85] the resting cerebral blood flow (CBF),[86,87] the vascular responsiveness of the vessels,[88] and the cerebral metabolic rate of oxygen consumption.[89,90] Aging is also frequently associated with comorbidities such as diabetes, hypertension, and hyperlipidemia, all of which may affect the BOLD signal by affecting CBF and neurovascular coupling.[91] Any one of these age-related differences in the vascular system could conceivably produce age-related differences in BOLD fMRI signal responsiveness, greatly affecting the interpretation of results from such studies.

Our laboratory compared the hemodynamic response function (HRF) characteristics in the sensorimotor cortex of young and older subjects in response to a simple motor reaction-time task.[92] The provisional assumption was made that there was identical neural activity between the two populations based on physiological findings of equivalent movement-related electrical potentials in subjects under similar conditions.[93] Thus, it was presumed that any changes that were observed in BOLD fMRI signal between young and older individuals in motor cortex would be due to vascular, and not neural, activity changes in normal aging. Several important similarities and differences were observed between age groups. Although there was no significant difference in the shape of the hemodynamic response curve or peak amplitude of the signal, a significantly decreased SNR in the BOLD signal was found in older individuals as compared to young individuals. This was attributed to a greater level of noise in the older individuals. A decrease in the spatial extent of the BOLD signal was also observed in older individuals compared to younger individuals in sensorimotor cortex (i.e., the median number of suprathreshold voxels). Similar results have been replicated by two other laboratories.[94,95] These findings suggest that there is some property of the coupling between neural activity and BOLD signal that changes with age.

The notion that vascular differences among individuals may affect BOLD signal is especially a concern when considering studies of patient populations with known vascular changes such as stroke. A recent fMRI study addressed the issue of the influence of vascular factors on the BOLD signal in a symptomatic stroke population.[96] They analyzed the time course of the BOLD HRF in the sensorimotor cortex of patients with an isolated subcortical lacunar stroke compared to a group of age-matched controls. They found a decrease in the rate of rise and the maximal BOLD HRF to a finger- or hand-tapping task in both the sensorimotor cortex of the hemisphere affected by the stroke and the unaffected hemisphere. These investigators proposed that, given the widespread changes of these BOLD signal differences, the change was unlikely a direct consequence of the subcortical lacunar stroke, but rather a manifestation of preexisting diffuse vascular pathology.

In summary, comparing BOLD signal in two different groups of individuals that may differ in their vascular system should be done with caution; for example, in one scenario, a comparison of activation of young and elderly individuals during a cognitive task may show less activation by elderly (as compared to young subjects) in some brain regions, but greater activation in other regions (e.g., see Rypma and colleagues[97]). In this scenario, it is unlikely that regional variations in the hemodynamic coupling of neural activity to imaging signal would account for such age-related differences in patterns of activation. In another scenario, a comparison of young and elderly subjects may show less activation by elderly (as compared to young subjects) in some brain regions, but no evidence of greater activation in any other region. In this case, it is possible that the observed age-related differences are not due to differences in intensity of neural activity, but rather to other non-neuronal contributions to the imaging signal, that is, neurovascular coupling. Several statistical approaches towards the imaging data are being developed that will attempt to address these potential confounds.[72,98,99]

## Types of Hypotheses Tested Using fMRI

Functional neuroimaging experiments test hypotheses regarding the anatomical specificity for cognitive processes (functional specialization), basic mechanisms of cognition (cognitive theory), and direct or indirect interactions among brain regions (functional integration). The experimental design and statistical analyses chosen will determine the types of questions that can be addressed. Ultimately, the most powerful approach for the testing of theories on brain–behavior relationships is the analysis of converging data from multiple methods.

### Functional Specialization

The major focus of fMRI studies of cognition is testing theories on functional specialization. The concept of functional specialization is based on the premise that functional modules exist within the brain, that is, areas of the cerebral cortex are specialized for a specific cognitive process; for example, facial recognition is a critical primary function likely served by a functional module. Prosopagnosia is the selective inability to recognize faces. Patients with prosopagnosia, however, can recognize familiar faces, such as those of relatives, by other means, such as the voice, dress, or body shape. Other types of visual recognition, such as identifying common objects, are normal. Prosopagnosia arises from lesions of the inferomedial temporo-occipital lobe, which usually are due to a stroke within the posterior cerebral artery circulation. No lesion studies have precisely localized the area crucial for facial perception. However, they provide strong evidence that a brain area is specialized for processing faces. Functional imaging studies have provided anatomical specificity for such a module; for example, Kanwisher and colleagues[100] used fMRI to test a group of healthy individuals and found that the fusiform gyrus was significantly more active when the subjects viewed faces than when they viewed assorted common objects. The specificity of a fusiform face area was further demonstrated by the finding that this area also responded significantly more strongly to passive viewing of faces than to scrambled two-tone faces, front-view photographs of houses, and photographs of human hands. These elegant experiments allowed the investigators to reject alternative functions of the face area, such as visual attention, subordinate-level classification, or general processing of any animate or human forms, demonstrating that this region selectively perceives faces.

## Cognitive Theory

An exciting new direction for studies using functional neuroimaging are those that test theories of the underlying mechanisms of cognition; for example, an fMRI study[101] attempted to answer the question, "To what extent does perception depend on attention?" One hypothesis is that unattended stimuli in the environment receive very little processing,[102] but another hypothesis is that the processing load in a relevant task determines the extent to which irrelevant stimuli are processed.[103] These alternative hypotheses were tested by asking normal individuals to perform linguistic tasks of low or high load while ignoring irrelevant visual motion in the periphery of a display. Visual motion was used as the distracting stimulus because it activates a distinct region of the brain (cortical area MT or V5, another functional module in the visual system). Activation of area MT would indicate that irrelevant visual motion was processed. Although task and irrelevant stimuli were unrelated, fMRI of motion-related activity in MT showed a reduction in motion processing during the high-processing load condition in the linguistic task. These findings support the hypothesis that perception of irrelevant environmental information depends on the information processing load that is currently relevant and being attended to. Thus, by the finding that perception depends on attention, this fMRI experiment provides insight regarding underlying cognitive mechanism.

## Functional Integration

Functional neuroimaging experiments can also test hypotheses about interactions between brain regions by focusing on covariances of activation levels between regions.[104,105] These covariances reflect functional connectivity, a concept that was originally developed in reference to temporal interactions among individual neurons.[106] Newer approaches, often using a statistical test called structural equation modeling, attempt to determine whether covariances among brain regions result from direct or indirect interactions, a concept called effective connectivity. Using this method, McIntosh and colleagues[105] found shifting prefrontal and limbic interactions in a working memory task for faces as the retention delay increased (see Figure 18.5). The different interactions between brain regions at short and long delays were interpreted as a functional change; for example, strong corticolimbic interactions were found at short delays, but at longer delays, when the image of the face was more difficult to maintain, strong fronto-cingulate-occipital interactions were found. The investigators postulated that the former finding was due to maintaining an iconic facial representation, and that the latter finding was due to an expanded encoding strategy, resulting

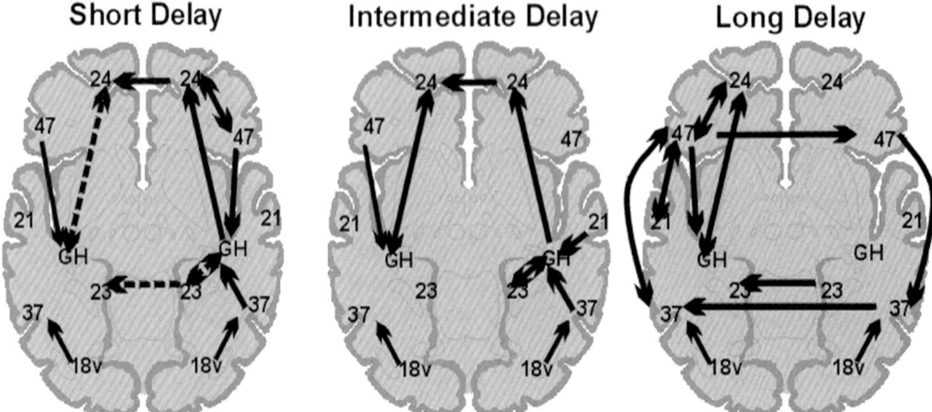


**Figure 18.5.** Network analysis of fMRI data during performance of a working memory task cross three different delay periods.[105] Areas of correlated increases in activation (*solid lines*) and areas of correlated decreases in activation (*dotted lines*) are shown. Note the different pattern of interactions among brain regions at short and long delays. Adapted from McIntosh AR, Grady CL, Haxby JV, Ungerleider LG, Horwitz B. Changes in limbic and prefrontal functional interactions in working memory task for faces. *Cereb Cortex*. 1996;6:571–584.

in more resilient memory. By characterizing changes in regional activity and the interactions between regions over time, the network analysis in this study added to the original analysis, that of only assessed regional changes in mean activity.

## Integration of Multiple Methods

The most powerful approach toward understanding brain–behavior relationships comes from analyzing converging data from multiple methods. There are several ways in which different methods can provide complementary data; for example, one method can provide superior spatial resolution (e.g., fMRI), whereas the other can provide superior temporal resolution (e.g., event-related potetials). In addition, the data from one method may allow for different conclusions to be drawn from it, such as whether a particular brain region is necessary to implement a cognitive process (i.e., lesion methods) or whether it is only involved during its implementation (i.e., physiological methods). The following sections describe examples of such approaches.

### Combined fMRI/Lesion Studies

The combined use of functional neuroimaging and lesions studies can be illustrated with studies of the neural basis of semantic memory, the cognitive system that represents our knowledge of the world. Early studies of patients with focal lesions supported the notion that the temporal lobes mediate the retrieval of semantic knowledge[107]; for example, patients with temporal lobe lesions may show a disproportionate impairment in the knowledge of living things (e.g., animals) compared with nonliving things. Other patients have a disproportionate deficit in knowledge of nonliving things.[108] These observations led to the notion that the semantic memory system is subdivided into different sensorimotor modalities, that is, living things, compared with nonliving things, are represented by their visual and other sensory attributes (e.g., a banana is yellow), whereas nonliving things are represented by their function (e.g., a hammer is a tool but comes in many different visual forms). The small number of patients with these deficits, and often large lesions, limits precise anatomical–behavioral relationships. However, functional neuroimaging studies in normal subjects can provide spatial resolution that the lesion method lacks.[109]

These original observations regarding the neural basis of semantic memory conflicted with functional neuroimaging studies consistently showing activation of the left inferior frontal gyrus (IFG) during the retrieval of semantic knowledge; for example, an early cognitive activation PET study revealed IFG activation during a verb-generation task compared with a simple word-repetition task.[59] A subsequent fMRI study[110] offered a fundamentally different interpretation of the apparent conflict between lesion and functional neuroimaging studies of semantic knowledge: left IFG activity is associated with the need to select some relevant feature of semantic knowledge from competing alternatives, not retrieval of semantic knowledge per se. This interpretation was supported by an fMRI experiment in normal individuals in which selection, but not retrieval, demands were varied across three semantic tasks. In a verb-generation task, in a high-selection condition, subjects generated verbs to nouns with many appropriate associated responses without any clearly dominant response (e.g., wheel), but in a low-selection condition, nouns with few associated responses or with a clear dominant response (e.g., scissors) were used. In this way, all tasks required semantic retrieval, and differed only in the amount of selection required. The fMRI signal within the left IFG increased as the selection demands increased (see Figure 18.6). When the degree of semantic processing varied independently of selection demands, there was no difference in left IFG activity, suggesting that selection, not retrieval, of semantic knowledge drives activity in the left IFG.

To determine if left IFG activity was correlated with, but not necessary for, selecting information from semantic memory, the same task used during the fMRI study was used to examine the ability of patients with focal frontal lesions to generate verbs.[111] Supporting the earlier claim regarding left IFG function derived from an fMRI study,[110] the overlap of the lesions in patients with deficits on this task corresponded to the site of maximum fMRI activation in healthy young subjects during the verb-generation task (see Figure 18.6). In this example, the approach of using converging evidence from lesion and fMRI studies differs in a subtle but important way from the study described earlier that isolated the face-processing module. Patients with left IFG lesions do not present with an identifiable neurobehavioral syndrome reflecting the nature of the processing in this region. Guided by the fMRI results from healthy young subjects, the investigators studied patients with left IFG lesions to test a hypothesis regarding the necessity of

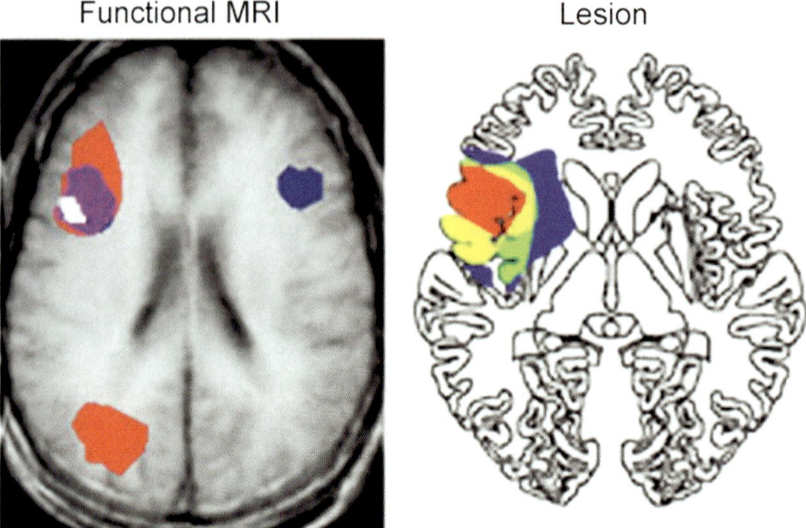


**Figure 18.6.** Regions of overlap of fMRI activity in healthy human subjects (left side of figure) during the performance of three semantic memory tasks, with the convergence of activity within the left inferior frontal gyrus (white region). Adapted from Thompson-Schill SL, D'Esposito M, Aguirre GK, Farah MJ. Role of left inferior prefrontal cortex in retrieval of semantic knowledge: a reevaluation. *Proc Natl Acad Sci USA*. 1997;94:14792–14797. Copyright © 1997 National Academy of Sciences, U.S.A. Regions of overlap of lesion location in patients with selection-related deficits on a verb-generation task (right side of figure) with maximal overlap within the left inferior frontal gyrus (red region). Adapted from Thompson-Schill SL, Swick D, Farah MJ, D'Esposito M, Kan IP, Knight RT. Verb generation in patients with focal frontal lesions: a neurophysiological test of neuroimaging findings. *Proc Natl Acad Sci USA*. 1998;95: 15855–15960. Copyright © 1998 National Academy of Sciences, U.S.A. (Neurologic coordinates)

this region in a specific cognitive process. Coupled with the well-established finding that lesions of the left temporal lobe impair semantic knowledge, these studies further our understanding of the neural network mediating semantic memory.

### Combined fMRI/Transcranial Magnetic Stimulation Studies

Transcranial magnetic stimulation (TMS) is a noninvasive method that can induce a reversible virtual lesion of the cerebral cortex in a normal human subject.[112] Using both fMRI and TMS provides another means of combining brain activation data with data derived from the lesion method. There are several advantages for using TMS as a lesion method. First, brain injury likely results in brain reorganization after the injury, and studies of patients with lesions assume that the non-lesioned brain areas have not been affected, whereas, in TMS, it is performed on the normal brain. Another advantage for using TMS is that it has excellent spatial resolution and can target specific locations in the brain, whereas lesions in patients with brain injury are markedly variable in location and size across individuals. Such an approach can be illustrated in a recent investigation of the role of the medial frontal cortex in task-switching.[113] In this study, subjects first performed an fMRI study that identified the regions that were active when they stayed on the current task versus when they switched to a new task. It was found that medial frontal cortex is activated when switching between tasks. In order to determine if the medial frontal cortex was necessary for the processes involved in task-switching, the same paradigm was utilized during inactivation of the medial frontal cortex with TMS. Guided by the locations of activation observed in the fMRI study, and using a MRI-guided frameless stereotaxic procedure, it was found that applying a TMS pulse over the medial frontal cortex disrupted performance only during trials during which the subject was required to switch between tasks. Transcranial magnetic stimulation over adjacent brain regions did not show this effect. Additionally, the excellent temporal resolution of TMS allowed the investigators to stimulate during precise periods of the task, determining that the observed effect was during the time when the subjects were presented a cue, indicating they must switch tasks prior to the actual performance of the new task. Thus, combining the results from both fMRI and TMS, it was concluded that medial prefrontal cortex was essential for allowing individuals to intentionally switch to a new task.

### Combined fMRI/Event-Related Potential Studies

The strength of combining these two methods is coupling the superb spatial resolution of fMRI with the superb temporal resolution of event-related potential recording. An example of such a study was reported by Dehaene and colleagues, who asked the question "Does the human capacity for mathematical intuition depend on linguistic competence or on visuospatial representations?" In this study, subjects performed two addition tasks—one in which they were instructed to select the correct sum from two numerically close numbers (exact condition) and one in which there were instructed to estimate the result and select the closest number (approximate condition). During fMRI scanning, greater bilateral parietal lobe activation was observed in the approximation condition as compared to the exact condition. Because this activation was outside the perisylvian language zone, it was taken as support that visuospatial processes were engaged during the cognitive operations involved in approximate calculation. Greater left lateralized frontal lobe activation was observed to be greater in the exact condition as compared to the approximate condition, which was taken as evidence for language-dependent coding of exact addition facts. In order to consider an alternative explanation of the fMRI findings, the investigators also performed an ERP study. The alternative explanation was that in both the exact and approximate tasks, subjects would compute the exact result using the same representation for numbers, but later processing, when they had to make a decision as to the correct choice, was what led to the differences in brain activation. Because fMRI does not offer adequate temporal resolution to resolve these two behavioral events that occur on brief time scale, event-related potential was the appropriate method to test this hypothesis. In the event-related potential study, it was demonstrated that the evoked neural response during exact and approximate trials already differed significantly during the first 400 milliseconds of a trial before subjects had to make a decision.

## Summary

Functional MRI is an extremely valuable tool for studying brain–behavior relationships, as it is widely available, noninvasive, and has superb temporal and spatial resolution. New approaches in fMRI experimental design and data analysis are appearing in the literature at an almost exponential rate, leading to numerous options for testing hypotheses on brain–behavior relationships. Combined with information from other complimentary methods, such as the study of patients with focal lesions, healthy individuals with transcranial magnetic stimulation, or event-related potentials, data from fMRI studies provide new insights regarding the organization of the cerebral cortex, as well as the neural mechanisms underlying cognition.

## References

1. Broca P. Remarques sur le siege de la faculte du langage articule suivies d'une observation d'amphemie (perte de al parole). *Bull Mem Soc Anat Paris*. 1861;36.
2. Buckner RL, Raichle ME, Petersen SE. Dissociation of human prefrontal cortical areas across different speech production tasks and gender groups. *J Neurophysiol*. 1995;74:2163–2173.
3. Sarter M, Bernston G, Cacioppo J. Brain imaging and cognitive neuroscience: toward strong inference in attributing function to structure. *Am Psychol*. 1996;51:13–21.
4. Gaffan D, Gaffan EA. Amnesia in man following transection of the fornix: a review. *Brain*. 1991;114:2611–2618.
5. Feeney DM, Baron JC. Diaschisis. *Stroke*. 1986;17:817–830.
6. Fuster JM, Alexander GE. Neuron activity related to short-term memory. *Science*. 1971;173:652–654.
7. Funahashi S, Bruce CJ, Goldman-Rakic PS. Mnemonic coding of visual space in the monkey's dorsolateral prefrontal cortex. *J Neurophysiol*. 1989; 61:331–349.
8. Funahashi S, Bruce CJ, Goldman-Rakic PS. Dorsolateral prefrontal lesions and oculomotor delayed-response performance: Evidence for mnemonic "scotomas". *J Neurosci*. 1993;13:1479–1497.
9. Watanabe T, Niki H. Hippocampal unit activity and delayed response in the monkey. *Brain Res*. 1985;325:241–254.
10. Cahusac PM, Miyashita Y, Rolls ET. Responses of hippocampal formation neurons in the monkey related to delayed spatial response and object-place memory tasks. *Behav Brain Res*. 1989;33:229–240.
11. Alvarez P, Zola-Morgan S, Squire LR. The animal model of human amnesia: long-term memory impaired and short-term memory intact. *Proc Natl Acad Sci U S A*. 1994;91:5637–5641.
12. Corkin S. Lasting consequences of bilateral medial temporal lobectomy: clinical course and experimental findings in H.M. *Sem Neurol*. 1984;4: 249–259.
13. Ranganath C, D'Esposito M. Medial temporal lobe activity associated with active maintenance of novel information. *Neuron*. 2001;31:865–873.
14. Druzgal TJ, D'Esposito M. Activity in fusiform face area modulated as a function of working memory load. *Brain Res Cogn Brain Res*. 2001;10: 355–364.

15. Cohen MS, Kosslyn SM, Breiter HC, et al. Changes in cortical activity during mental rotation: a mapping study using functional MRI. *Brain.* 1996;119:89–100.
16. D'Esposito M, Ballard D, Aguirre GK, Zarahn E. Human prefrontal cortex is not specific for working memory: a functional MRI study. *Neuroimage.* 1998;8:274–282.
17. Abduljalil AM, Robitaille PM. Macroscopic susceptibility in ultra high field MRI. *J Comput Assist Tomogr.* 1999;23:832–841.
18. Abduljalil AM, Kangarlu A, Yu Y, Robitaille PM. Macroscopic susceptibility in ultra high field MRI. II: acquisition of spin echo images from the human head. *J Comput Assist Tomogr.* 1999;23:842–844.
19. Zeng H, Constable RT. Image distortion correction in EPI: comparison of field mapping with point spread function mapping. *Magn Reson Med.* 2002;48:137–146.
20. Casey BJ, Thomas KM, Davidson MC, Kunz K, Franzen PL. Dissociating striatal and hippocampal function developmentally with a stimulus-response compatibility task. *J Neurosci.* 2002;22:8647–8652.
21. Schlaggar BL, Brown TT, Lugar HM, Visscher KM, Miezin FM, Petersen SE. Functional neuroanatomical differences between adults and school-age children in the processing of single words. *Science.* 2002;296:1476–1479.
22. Savoy RL, Ravicz ME, Gollub R. The psychophysiological laboratory in the magnet: stimulus delivery, response recording, and safety. In: Moonen CTW, Bandettini PA, eds. *Functional MRI.* Berlin: Springer; 1999:347–365.
23. Edminster WB, Talavage TM, Ledden PJ, Weisskoff RM. Improved auditory cortex imaging using clustered volume acquisitions. *Hum Brain Mapp.* 1999;7:88–97.
24. Belin P, Zatorre RJ, Hoge R, Evans AC, Pike B. Event-related fMRI of the auditory cortex. *Neuroimage.* 1999;10:417–429.
25. Sobel N, Prabhakaran V, Hartley CA, et al. Blind smell: brain activation induced by an undetected air-borne chemical. *Brain.* 1999;122(Pt 2): 209–217.
26. Sobel N, Prabhakaran V, Desmond JE, Glover GH, Sullivan EV, Gabrieli JD. A method for functional magnetic resonance imaging of olfaction. *J Neurosci Methods.* 1997;78:115–123.
27. Gitelman DR, Parrish TB, LaBar KS, Mesulam MM. Real-time monitoring of eye movements using infrared video-oculography during functional magnetic resonance imaging of the frontal eye fields. *Neuroimage.* 2000;11:58–65.
28. Kimmig H, Greenlee MW, Gondan M, Schira M, Kassubek J, Mergner T. Relationship between saccadic eye movements and cortical activity as measured by fMRI: quantitative and qualitative aspects. *Exp Brain Res.* 2001;141:184–194.
29. Palmer ED, Rosen HJ, Ojemann JG, Buckner RL, Kelley WM, Petersen SE. An event-related fMRI study of overt and covert word stem completion. *Neuroimage.* 2001;14:182–193.
30. Fu CH, Morgan K, Suckling J, et al. A functional magnetic resonance imaging study of overt letter verbal fluency using a clustered acquisition sequence: greater anterior cingulate activation with increased task demand. *Neuroimage.* 2002;17:871–879.
31. Barch DM, Sabb FW, Carter CS, Braver TS, Noll DC, Cohen JD. Overt verbal responding during fMRI scanning: empirical investigations of problems and potential solutions. *Neuroimage.* 1999;10:642–657.
32. Goldman RI, Stern JM, Engel J Jr., Cohen MS. Acquiring simultaneous EEG and functional MRI. *Clin Neurophysiol.* 2000;111:1974–1980.

33. Lazeyras F, Zimine I, Blanke O, Perrig SH, Seeck M. Functional MRI with simultaneous EEG recording: feasibility and application to motor and visual activation. *J Magn Reson Imaging*. 2001;13:943–948.
34. Kruggel F, Herrmann CS, Wiggins CJ, von Cramon DY. Hemodynamic and electroencephalographic responses to illusory figures: recording of the evoked potentials during functional MRI. *Neuroimage*. 2001;14:1327–1336.
35. Kruggel F, Wiggins CJ, Herrmann CS, von Cramon DY. Recording of the event-related potentials during functional MRI at 3.0 Tesla field strength. *Magn Reson Med*. 2000;44:277–282.
36. Gnadt JW, Andersen RA. Memory related motor planning activity in posterior parietal cortex of macaque. *Exp Brain Res*. 1988;70:216–220.
37. Aguirre GK, Zarahn E, D'Esposito M. The variability of human, BOLD hemodynamic responses. *Neuroimage*. 1998;8:360–369.
38. Bandettini PA, Wong EC, Hinks RS, Tikofsky RS, Hyde JS. Time course of EPI of human brain function during task activation. *Magn Reson Med*. 1992;25:390–397.
39. Boynton GM, Engel SA, Glover GH, Heeger DJ. Linear systems analysis of functional magnetic resonance imaging in human V1. *J Neurosci*. 1996;16:4207–4221.
40. Kim SG, Richter W, Ugurbil K. Limitations of temporal resolution in fMRI. *Magn Reson Med*. 1997;37:631–636.
41. Savoy RL, Bandettini PA, O'Craven KM, et al. Pushing the temporal resolution of fMRI: studies of very brief stimuli, onset of variability and asynchrony, and stimulu-correlated changes in noise. *Proc Soc Magn Reson Med*. 1995;3:450.
42. Zarahn E, Aguirre GK, D'Esposito M. A trial-based experimental design for functional MRI. *Neuroimage*. 1997;6:122–138.
43. Burock MA, Buckner RL, Woldorff MG, Rosen BR, Dale AM. Randomized event-related experimental designs allow for extremely rapid presentation rates using functional MRI. *Neuroreport*. 1998;9:3735–3739.
44. Clark VP, Maisog JM, Haxby JV. fMRI studies of visual perception and recognition using a random stimulus design. *Soc Neurosci Abstr*. 1997;23:301.
45. Dale AM, Buckner RL. Selective averaging of rapidly presented individual trials using fMRI. *Hum Brain Mapp*. 1997;5:1–12.
46. Miezin FM, Maccotta L, Ollinger JM, Petersen SE, Buckner RL. Characterizing the hemodynamic response: effects of presentation rate, sampling procedure, and the possibility of ordering brain activity based on relative timing. *Neuroimage*. 2000;11:735–759.
47. D'Esposito M, Zarahn E, Aguirre GK. Event-related functional MRI: implications for cognitive psychology. *Psychol Bull*. 1999;125:155–164.
48. Logothetis NK, Guggenberger H, Peled S, Pauls J. Functional imaging of the monkey brain. *Nat Neurosci*. 1999;2:555–562.
49. Cheng K, Waggoner RA, Tanaka K. Human ocular dominance columns as revealed by high-field functional magnetic resonance imaging. *Neuron*. 2001;32:359–374.
50. Logothetis N, Merkle H, Augath M, Trinath T, Ugurbil K. Ultra high-resolution fMRI in monkeys with implanted RF coils. *Neuron*. 2002;35:227–242.
51. Malonek D, Grinvald A. Interactions between electrical activity and cortical microcirculation revealed by imaging spectroscopy: implications for functional brain mapping. *Science*. 1996;272:551–554.
52. Kim SG, Duong TQ. Mapping cortical columnar structures using fMRI. *Physiol Behav*. 2002;77:641–644.

53. Menon RS, Ogawa S, Strupp JP, Ugurbil K. Ocular dominance in human V1 demonstrated by functional magnetic resonance imaging. *J Neurophysiol*. 1997;77:2780–2787.
54. Grill-Spector K, Malach R. fMR-adaptation: a tool for studying the functional properties of human cortical neurons. *Acta Psychol (Amst)*. 2001;107:293–321.
55. Grill-Spector K, Kushnir T, Edelman S, Avidan G, Itzchak Y, Malach R. Differential processing of objects under various viewing conditions in the human lateral occipital complex. *Neuron*. 1999;24:187–203.
56. Posner MI, Petersen SE, Fox PT, Raichle ME. Localization of cognitive operations in the human brain. *Science*. 1988;240:1627–1631.
57. Donders FC. Over de snelheid van psychische processen. Onderzoekingen gedaan in het Physiologisch Laboratorium der Utrechtsche Hoogeschool. *Tweede Reeks*. 1868;II:92–120.
58. Sternberg S. The discovery of processing stages: extensions of Donders' method. *Acta Psychol*. 1969;30:276–315.
59. Petersen SE, Fox PT, Posner MI, Mintun M, Raichle ME. Positron emission tomographic studies of the cortical anatomy of single word processing. *Nature*. 1988;331:585–589.
60. Fuster J. *The Prefrontal Cortex: Anatomy, Physiology, and Neuropsychology of the Frontal Lobes*. Raven Press: New York; 1997.
61. Jonides J, Smith EE, Koeppe RA, Awh E, Minoshima S, Mintun MA. Spatial working memory in humans as revealed by PET. *Nature*. 1993;363:623–625.
62. Zarahn E, Aguirre GK, D'Esposito M. Temporal isolation of the neural correlates of spatial mnemonic processing with fMRI. *Cogn Brain Res*. 1999;7:255–268.
63. Attwell D, Iadecola C. The neural basis of functional brain imaging signals. *Trends Neurosci*. 2002;25:621–625.
64. Heeger DJ, Ress D. What does fMRI tell us about neuronal activity? *Nat Rev Neurosci*. 2002;3:142–151.
65. Friston KJ, Josephs O, Rees G, Turner R. Nonlinear event-related responses in fMRI. *Magn Reson Med*. 1998;39:41–52.
66. Glover GH. Deconvolution of impulse response in event-related BOLD fMRI. *Neuroimage*. 1999;9:416–429.
67. Miller KL, Luh WM, Liu TT, et al. Nonlinear temporal dynamics of the cerebral blood flow response. *Hum Brain Mapp*. 2001;13:1–12.
68. Vazquez AL, Noll DC. Nonlinear aspects of the BOLD response in functional MRI. *Neuroimage*. 1998;7:108–118.
69. D'Esposito M, Zarahn E, Aguirre GK. Event-related fMRI: implications for cognitive psychology. *Psychol Bull*. 1999;125:155–164.
70. Rosen BR, Buckner RL, Dale AM. Event-related functional MRI: past, present, and future. *Proc Natl Acad Sci U S A*. 1998;95:773–780.
71. Donaldson DI, Petersen SE, Ollinger JM, Buckner RL. Dissociating state and item components of recognition memory using fMRI. *Neuroimage*. 2001;13:129–142.
72. Mitchell KJ, Johnson MK, Raye CL, D'Esposito M. fMRI evidence of age-related hippocampal dysfunction in feature binding in working memory. *Brain Res Cogn Brain Res*. 2000;10:197–206.
73. Keppel G, Zedeck S. *Data Analysis for Research Design*. New York: W.H. Freeman & Company; 1989.
74. Worsley KJ, Friston KJ. Analysis of fMRI time-series revisited—again. *Neuroimage*. 1995;2:173–182.
75. Forman SD, Cohen JD, Fitzgerald M, Eddy WF, Mintun MA, Noll DC. Improved assessment of significant activation in functional magnetic

resonance imaging (fMRI): use of a cluster-size threshold. *Magn Reson Med*. 1995;33:636–647.
76. Everitt BS, Bullmore ET. Mixture model mapping of the brain activation in functional magnetic resonance images. *Hum Brain Mapp*. 1999;7:1–14.
77. Zarahn E, Aguirre GK, D'Esposito M. Empirical analyses of BOLD fMRI statistics. I. Spatially unsmoothed data collected under null-hypothesis conditions. *Neuroimage*. 1997;5:179–197.
78. Aguirre GK, Zarahn E, D'Esposito M. Empirical analyses of BOLD fMRI statistics. II. Spatially smoothed data collected under null-hypothesis and experimental conditions. *Neuroimage*. 1997;5:199–212.
79. D'Esposito M, Ballard D, Zarahn E, Aguirre GK. The role of prefrontal cortex in sensory memory and motor preparation: an event-related fMRI study [see comments]. *Neuroimage*. 2000;11:400–408.
80. Zarahn E, Slifstein M. A reference effect approach for power analysis in fMRI. *Neuroimage*. 2001;14:768–779.
81. Van Horn JD, Ellmore TM, Esposito G, Berman KF. Mapping voxel-based statistical power on parametric images. *Neuroimage*. 1998;7:97–107.
82. Aguirre GK, D'Esposito M. Experimental design for brain fMRI. In: Moonen CTW, Bandettini PA, eds. *Functional MRI*. Berlin: Springer Verlag; 1999:369–380.
83. Logothetis NK, Pauls J, Augath M, Trinath T, Oeltermann A. Neurophysiological investigation of the basis of the fMRI signal. *Nature*. 2001; 412:150–157.
84. Farkas E, Luiten PG. Cerebral microvascular pathology in aging and Alzheimer's disease. *Prog Neurobiol*. 2001;64:575–611.
85. Fang HCH. Observations on aging characteristics of cerebral blood vessels, macroscopic and microscopic features. In: Gerson S, Terry RD, eds. *Neurobiology of Aging*. New York: Raven Press; 1976.
86. Bentourkia M, Bol A, Ivanoiu A, et al. Comparison of regional cerebral blood flow and glucose metabolism in the normal brain: effect of aging. *J Neurol Sci*. 2000;181:19–28.
87. Schultz SK, O'Leary DS, Boles Ponto LL, Watkins GL, Hichwa RD, Andreasen NC. Age-related changes in regional cerebral blood flow among young to mid-life adults. *Neuroreport*. 1999;10:2493–2496.
88. Yamamoto M, Meyer JS, Sakai F, Yamaguchi F. Aging and cerebral vasodilator responses to hypercarbia: responses in normal aging and in persons with risk factors for stroke. *Arch Neurol*. 1980;37:489–496.
89. Yamaguchi T, Kanno I, Uemura K, et al. Reduction in regional cerebral rate of oxygen during human aging. *Stroke*. 1986;17:1220–1228.
90. Takada H, Nagata K, Hirata Y, et al. Age-related decline of cerebral oxygen metabolism in normal population detected with positron emission tomography. *Neurol Res*. 1992;14:128–131.
91. Claus JJ, Breteler MM, Hasan D, et al. Regional cerebral blood flow and cerebrovascular risk factors in the elderly population. *Neurobiol Aging*. 1998;19:57–64.
92. D'Esposito M, Zarahn E, Aguirre GK, Rypma B. The effect of normal aging on the coupling of neural activity to the bold hemodynamic response. *Neuroimage*. 1999;10:6–14.
93. Cunnington R, Iansek R, Bradshaw JL, Phillips JG. Movement-related potentials in Parkinson's disease. Presence and predictability of temporal and spatial cues. *Brain*. 1995;118:935–950.
94. Buckner RL, Snyder AZ, Sanders AL, Raichle ME, Morris JC. Functional brain imaging of young, nondemented, and demented older adults. *J Cogn Neurosci*. 2000;12(Suppl 2):24–34.

95. Huettel SA, Singerman JD, McCarthy G. The Effects of Aging upon the Hemodynamic Response Measured by Functional MRI. *Neuroimage.* 2001;13:161–175.
96. Pineiro R, Pendlebury S, Johansen-Berg H, Matthews PM. Altered hemodynamic responses in patients after subcortical stroke measured by functional MRI. *Stroke.* 2002;33:103–109.
97. Rypma B, Prabhakaran V, Desmond JE, Gabrieli JD. Age differences in prefrontal cortical activity in working memory. *Psychol Aging.* 2001;16: 371–384.
98. Jonides J, Marshuetz C, Smith EE, Reuter-Lorenz PA, Koeppe RA, Hartley A. Age differences in behavior and PET activation reveal differences in interference resolution in verbal working memory. *J Cogn Neurosci.* 2000;12:188–196.
99. Rypma B, D'Esposito M. Isolating the neural mechanisms of age-related changes in human working memory. *Nat Neurosci.* 2000;3:509–515.
100. Kanwisher N, McDermott J, Chun MM. The fusiform face area: a module in huma extrastriate cortex specialized for face perception. *J Neurosci.* 1997;17:4302–4311.
101. Rees G, Frith CD, Lavie N. Modulating irrelevant motion perception by varying attentional load in an unrelated task. *Science.* 1997;278:1616–1619.
102. Treisman AM. Strategies and models of selective attention. *Psychol Rev.* 1969;76:282–299.
103. Lavie N, Tsal Y. Perceptual load as a major determinant of the locus of selection in visual attention. *Percept Psychophys.* 1994;56:183–197.
104. Buchel C, Coull JT, Friston KJ. The predictive value of changes in effective connectivity for human learning. *Science.* 1999;283:1538–1541.
105. McIntosh AR, Grady CL, Haxby JV, Ungerleider LG, Horwitz B. Changes in limbic and prefrontal functional interactions in a working memory task for faces. *Cereb Cortex.* 1996;6:571–584.
106. Gerstein GL, Perkel DH, Subramanian KN. Identification of functionally related neural assemblies. *Brain Res.* 1978;140:43–62.
107. McCarthy RA, Warrington EK. Disorders of semantic memory. *Philos Trans R Soc Lond B Biol Sci.* 1994;346:89–96.
108. Warrington EST. Category specific semantic impairments. *Brain.* 1984;107: 829–854.
109. Thompson-Schill SL. Neuroimaging studies of semantic memory: inferring "how" from "where". *Neuropsychologia.* 2003;41:280–292.
110. Thompson-Schill SL, D'Esposito M, Aguirre GK, Farah MJ. Role of left inferior prefrontal cortex in retrieval of semantic knowledge: a reevaluation. *Proc Natl Acad Sci U S A.* 1997;94:14792–14797.
111. Thompson-Schill SL, Swick D, Farah MJ, D'Esposito M, Kan IP, Knight RT. Verb generation in patients with focal frontal lesions: a neuropsychological test of neuroimaging findings. *Proc Natl Acad Sci U S A.* 1998;95: 15855–15860.
112. Pascual-Leone A, Tarazona F, Keenan J, Tormos JM, Hamilton R, Catala MD. Transcranial magnetic stimulation and neuroplasticity. *Neuropsychologia.* 1999;37:207–217.
113. Rushworth MF, Hadland KA, Paus T, Sipila PK. Role of the human medial frontal cortex in task switching: a combined fMRI and TMS study. *J Neurophysiol.* 2002;87:2577–2592.
114. Churchland PS, Sejnowski TJ. Perspectives on cognitive neuroscience. *Science.* 1988;242:741–745.

# 19

# Clinical Overview and Future fMRI Applications

Scott H. Faro and Feroze B. Mohamed

The past ten years (1990–2000) had been designated the decade of the brain, as this has been the one of the subjects of major research focus worldwide in medical sciences. During this period there has been tremendous research in brain sciences leading to numerous technological developments and establishment of fundamental clinical protocols to understand brain functions. The next decade beginning the twenty-first century will continue the momentum of brain research; this is evident from the numerous publications in scientific journals. This is currently one of the most exciting and progressive times in scientific advancement in the field of brain function, and functional magnetic resonance imaging (fMRI) represents one of the most advanced and potentially enlightening techniques that have ever been developed. According to published reports, the number of published research papers using fMRI has increased exponentially from two in 1990 to over 3877 currently (May 2005).

The field of fMRI has two major areas of research interest. The first is within the field of cognitive neuroscience, which focuses on understanding all aspects of cognition. The second is the use of fMRI to localize eloquent regions in the brain for a variety of clinical applications. This book has focused primarily on the new and emerging clinical applications of fMRI as applied to humans, as well as an introduction of the basic physics and physiological principles of fMRI.

The current clinical applications include all aspects of pediatric and adult cognitive brain imaging. There has never previously been a non-invasive technique with high spatial and temporal resolution to define brain activation. One of the main indications for clinical fMRI is evaluation of eloquent areas of the brain, such as the cortical spinal tract, in relation to a focal parenchymal brain region, such as a neoplasm or arterial venous malformation. The uses of fMRI to localize language and memory centers in relation to a frontal lobe or temporal lobe lesion are becoming a commonplace procedure for presurgical evaluation.

Currently, there is a large volume of research that has investigated the language and memory centers, and there is ongoing research to evaluate the comparison between the intracarotid amobarbital procedure commonly known as WADA and fMRI. For a full review of this topic, see the chapters on fMRI of Memory, fMRI of Language, and fMRI WADA evaluation. The current gold standard for language localization is the WADA test and interoperative cortical stimulation mapping. These tests have the obvious limitations related to the invasive nature of both procedures and the relative lack of spatial resolution for both techniques. Functional MRI has been shown to predict postoperative language defects, as well as, and perhaps better than, the WADA test. An argument can be made that it is not necessary to compare fMRI directly to WADA in reference to language localization. It is anticipated that, in the near future, fMRI will become the gold standard for language localization. This promising technique currently has limitations in that there are no current language activation paradigms that have been described in the literature that are associated with a prominent anterior temporal lobe activation. It is known that the dominant anterior temporal lobe does contribute to cognitive language function and anterior temporal lobectomy may be associated with postoperative deficits involving language function. In general, there is great acceptance of language fMRI to localize the receptive (Wernicke) and expressive (Broca) regions of the language function. The majority of these studies have evaluated a single cognitive test for functional evaluation of Wernicke's and Broca's Areas. There is a promising new fMRI method that uses multiple tasks and a composite analysis to increase sensitivity of these language centers.

Functional MRI of memory continues to be an active area of cognitive and clinical research. The WADA test has been considered the gold standard for clinical memory testing; however, there are recognized problems with this test. Intrinsically, the WADA test is invasive and uses a limited number of cognitive tests. Additionally, there are concerns of validity of the patient response that is being obtained in a potentially compromised cognitive state during the intra-arterial–induced anesthesia of the dominant and nondominant hemispheres. In general, the memory component is a challenge with both the WADA testing and fMRI. Functional MRI has great potential due to its noninvasive nature and the ability to test a large number of cognitive tasks in a more natural cognitive state. Current research is actively being performed to develop evidence-based proof for the memory component for fMRI. It is clear that currently both fMRI and traditional WADA testing are complimentary, and within a few years, standards will be developed for fMRI as the primary preoperative evaluation for language and memory function.

Functional MRI of memory has also been extended to patients with dementia and normal age-related memory changes. These are three functionally anatomical memory systems that include episodic memory, semantic memory, and working memory. Episodic memory has been the most studied, and changes include a reduction in prefrontal symmetric activation, greater prefrontal connectivity, and an alteration in the frontal temporal activation. The current primary clinical application and research focus has been Alzheimer's disease. When testing for episodic and coding, there is decreased activation within the hippocampus, and when testing for the retrieval component of episodic memory, there is a reduction in activation within the prefrontal cortex region. These observations exemplify the power of fMRI to evaluate a unique activation pattern in certain disease states. Alzheimer's disease represents a very important clinical disease that is increasing in frequency and these new techniques have a great potential for early detection and subsequent early treatment for this disease. Additionally, there is potential for fMRI to aid in treatment planning, management, and optimization of drug therapy for these patients.

One of the largest areas of fMRI clinical research includes the psychiatric and mental illnesses. There has been a large body of research that investigated the functional patterns related to a variety of disorders, which includes the autism spectrum disorders; substance abuse and dependence: schizophrenia; depression and bipolar disorder; obsessive/compulsive disorder; and a variety of affective behavioral disorders. In relation to the autism spectrum disorders, it is the hope that fMRI can help characterize more accurately subsets of autism that can help in strategic treatment planning; for example, it has been demonstrated that patients with an autistic disorder demonstrate an alternate method of facial processing when compared to normal controlled subjects. This has been shown to cause a decreased activation within the amygdala and fusiform face region.

Investigations of patients with schizophrenia also demonstrate a promising use of fMRI that has defined cortical dysfunction, which showed a decrease in activation in both the sensory and motor cortex and supplementary motor area. Areas of fMRI research such as this may allow for investigation of the effects of medication on patients with schizophrenia and related disorders. There has been initial fMRI research that has investigated major depression and bipolar disorder. In depression, patients have shown an increased area of activation within the medial and prefrontal cortex and in the right cingulate gyrus during viewing of a video presentation that induced the motion of sadness compared to normal controls. These studies are limited, but suggest future potential for use of fMRI as a clinical tool, perhaps in relation to therapeutic modulation of these disorders. Patient's with obsessive/compulsive disorder that are on medication have demonstrated an increased activation in the medial orbital frontal, lateral frontal, anterior temporal, anterior cingulate, as well as within the basal and ganglia. The group of affective disorders also represents a large population of patients and fMRI has demonstrated increased activity within the amygdala, which is involved in the perception of emotion with special emphasis on fear. It has been well-understood that the limbic structures such as the amygdala play a crucial role in emotional processing, and they also interact with the prefrontal cortex that may influence affected responses. The understanding of these focused areas of brain activation may help in further understanding these disease processes and potential changing activation patterns with therapeutic drugs that may develop into a major clinical tool in patient care.

Another area of active investigation is substance abuse and dependence, which has begun to elucidate unique patterns in patients with a drug addiction; for example, individuals addicted to cocaine demonstrate increased activation in the anterior cingulate and decreased frontal lobe activation during a stimulus that elicits a desire for cocaine use. Additionally, cocaine-related reduction in cortical activation in the primary visual cortex and primary motor cortex has been shown in long-term cocaine users. There has also been work with chronic marijuana use that has demonstrated increase activation within a cingulate cortex that has not been demonstrated in the normal controls. This is consistent with a specific pattern of cortical activation in this drug-abuse population.

Another important field of the clinical fMRI involves pediatric applications. There are unique challenges in relation to pediatric imaging that includes patient motion, pediatric sedation-related issues and challenges with stimulus activation in developing young patients. As with adults, the fMRI has been used for presurgical mapping of eloquent areas of the brain in relation to a neoplasm or arterial venous malformation. Language mapping within the first few years of infancy is a challenge, although it has been assessed using passive paradigms. An example is localizing language development to the left dominant hemisphere with the activation task of listening to the mother's voice. Language and memory mapping in older cooperative children are similar to language mapping in adults.

One of the most exciting areas of fMRI applications relates to pharmacology. Functional MRI has the ability to explore the pharmacology effects of drugs in relation to a variety of clinical disorders that include drug addiction, for example alcohol and cocaine; affective disorders, which include schizophrenia and depression; and tension and anxiety and related disorders such as ADHD. The field of pharmacological fMRI (pfMRI) holds great promise to improve our understanding of acute and chronic drug affects on neuronal activation. The power of this new field of pfMRI lies in the noninvasive technique to measure drug effects within the brain with real-time imaging and with the ability to repeat experiments within the same sitting. Pharmacological fMRI will not only improve our knowledge of the fundamental brain mechanisms related to these disorders, but will also aid in medication development, treatment planning, and clinical outcome predictions.

Visual cortex fMRI has added a great body of knowledge to the field of visual neuroscience. Currently, the clinical use of fMRI in relation to the optic pathway is limited. Future applications include studying the functional reorganization of the optic pathway in patients with damage to the visual centers within the brain. Additionally, in young patients with amblyopia and anisometropia, fMRI may contribute to early diagnosis and characterization of improving the visual acuity, therefore assisting in treatment planning. Optic neuritis is a common demyelinating process that affects the optic nerve and may present an isolated unilateral disease; however, this may represent an early presentation for multiple sclerosis. Studies demonstrating fMRI-related changes of a contralateral demyelinating process may one day lead to an early diagnosis and treatment for multiple sclerosis.

The field of fMRI as it relates to clinical pain is in its infancy. Studies have begun to investigate aspects of acute and chronic pain. The study of pain has traditionally been related to subjective changes in the patient. The fMRI allows for an objective evaluation of the specific areas of brain activation related to pain. The initial investigations of fMRI of pain include allodynia, visceral pain (e.g., irritable bowel syndrome), headaches, low back pain, and phantom pain. Functional MRI may aid in the study of analgesic drug effects, which will aid in drug modification and objective characterization of the pain process.

An upcoming area of important clinical research is the use of fMRI for the auditory system. One of the primary technical challenges in auditory studies is scanner noise, and this is now being controlled with active noise-cancellation systems that can present a nondistorted auditory stimulus. An important future potential use of fMRI is for the presurgical evaluation of patients who are candidates for cochlear implants. In patients with a hearing deficit, fMRI can aid in choosing the optimal middle ear for cochlear implantation surgery. Additionally, fMRI can evaluate for any functional brain reorganization of the auditory cortex in patients with congenital deafness. Functional MRI also has potential use in the evaluation of patients with tinnitus, as it provides a quantitative measure of perceived auditory stimulation and may potentially be useful to evaluate the effects of various treatments. The fMRI auditory pattern also may help characterize subtypes of patients with tinnitus, which will help guide patient therapy.

A very important clinical application of fMRI relates to epilepsy. This is particularly important with patients with intractable seizures that are being considered for epilepsy surgery. As previously described, the eloquent regions of the brain that relate to language, memory, or the sensory motor strip can be defined in relation to a seizure focus. Functional MRI may also define the functional asymmetries in brain activation, which will help in the lateralization and localization of an epileptogenic focus. Current research is also focused on the use of ictal and interictal BOLD signal changes to help define an epileptogenic region.

The current trend, which uses neuro-image guidance during a surgical procedure, will also involve the use of functional fMRI data superimposed on high-resolution MRI data to aid in the neurosurgical treatments of pathologic brain lesions. Future advancements will include real-time fMRI, perhaps in the neurosurgical suite, with advancements in interoperative MRI. In addition to these clinical research investigations, there are ongoing technical advances in the field of fMRI that include the use of high field strength MRI scanners (3 Tesla or greater), as well as advancements in gradient strengths, imaging coil design, advancement of computer speed, and software.

Most of the current applications of fMRI involve a qualitative analysis of focal anatomic regions of activation in relation to a specific task. Future applications of fMRI may involve quantitative analysis of a region of activation using a novel activation task such as a graded stimulus task as a component of their analysis. This field of research will begin to investigate the concepts of neuronal recruitment, which represents the number of activated neurons and neuronal enhancement that defines the magnitude of the degree of neuronal activation.

Current technological limitations such as magnet field strength imposes constraints on such studies in terms of signal-to-noise ratios (SNR) and in-plane resolution; however, several studies using the existing MRI methods have shown promising results and trends in that direction. Our group has investigated quantitative fMRI of the visual cortex using a graded luminous-intensity contrast stimuli in normal patients and patients with multiple sclerosis using a 1.5 Tesla MRI system. This study demonstrated an increasing number of activated voxels within the primary visual cortex, with increasing luminous intensity stimuli that is consistent with neuronal recruitment (Figure 19.1). We have investigated the quantitative analysis of common voxels within the primary visual cortex in a normal population with increasing luminous contrast and demonstrated a trend in increasing a bold signal with no definitive increase, suggesting that no significant neuronal enhancement was present. These fMRI patterns may represent additional physiologic data in relation to neuronal activation. This activation pattern may yield another set of criteria to define a pathologic process and be useful to define unique patterns of different disease states that will characterize clinical subdivisions within a given pathologic process. Functional MRI will enhance our knowledge of pathologic processes that affect the brain. In the future, these activation patterns may possibly be used as a marker of a disease and the spectrum of abnormality within the disease.

One of the primary goals of any new scientific investigation is to improve our knowledge of the basic pathophysiology of a disease. Functional MRI has shown a tremendous potential in a variety of applications in both the cognitive and clinical neural sciences. Besides the main-stream studies, several other fMRI applications are being studied

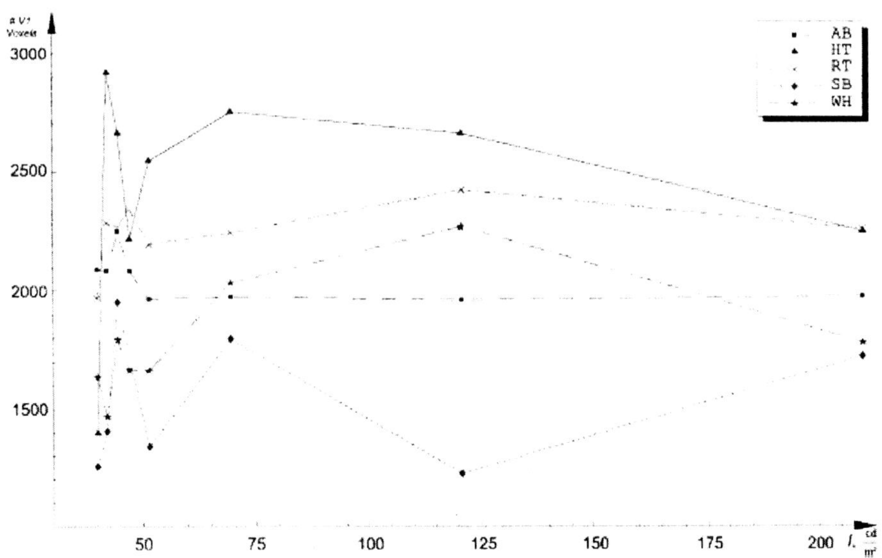


**Figure 19.1.** The number of significant voxels within the primary visual cortex as a function of luminance intensity.

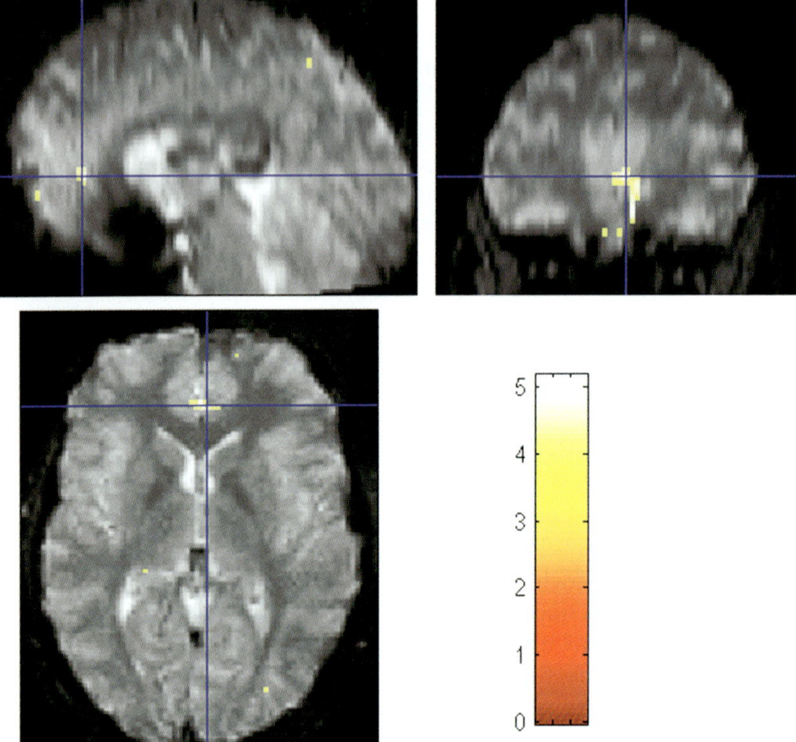


**Figure 19.2.** Functional MRI of a normal subject during deception showing focal activation in the anterior cingulate.

and developed. They range from in utero fMRI to fMRI of yawing, truth, and deception. Our group has investigated fMRI of cognitive truth, as well as the possible use of fMRI to define the potential patterns of activation in relation to a deceptive process (Figure 19.2). These are some examples of powerful uses of fMRI and demonstrate that this new technique is truly boundless in its potential applications.

The field of fMRI is in its infancy, and although the field is relatively new, there has already been a tremendous body of knowledge created. Functional MRI has grown into a vital new area of clinical research and applications. Recently, it was reported in the *Journal of Neuroscience* that there are now 58 research-oriented MRI centers worldwide, and the number is growing rapidly. Functional MRI has its origin in the academic centers throughout the world and is now ready to enter the clinical realm of medicine and surgery.

# Appendix

## Independent Component Analysis and fMRI Imaging

Christopher G. Green, Victor Haughton, and Dietmar Cordes

### Introduction

Independent component analysis (ICA)[1–9] is a statistical method for estimating a collection of unobservable signals from observations of their mixtures. This scenario falls into the more general class of blind source separation (BSS) problems, in which we wish to recover the original source signals and the method of mixing solely from measurements of their mixtures and certain assumptions about the sources. Independent component analysis, which assumes that the sources are statistically independent, has emerged as a powerful tool for solving (BSS) problems. It has also shown great promise in the fields of exploratory data analysis[3] and feature extraction.[10]

The classical example of a blind source separation problem is the cocktail party problem, in which there are $N$ distinct conversations being held at a party and $M$ microphones placed throughout the room recording the conversations. The recorded sounds are linear mixtures of the actual conversations, and the task is to recover the individual conversations from the mixtures. Separating and selectively tuning to the individual conversations has proven to be quite difficult computationally. Independent component analysis is one of many methods that attempt to perform this separation, and, in the special case of instantaneous mixing (no time delays and no echoes), arguably one of the more successful.

Independent component analysis is also an example of unsupervised learning. In *unsupervised learning*, a representation of the data is constructed from the data alone, that is, without outside assistance from a "teacher." (Contrast this with *supervised learning*, where feedback from an external omniscient observer is used to modify the representation iteratively.) Learning a representation of the data is equivalent to estimating the hidden factors responsible for the data. It can be proven that linear ICA provides a linear representation of the data that is as structured as possible from an information-theoretic standpoint.[7]

Independent component analysis was pioneered in the early 1980s by Herault, Jutten, and Ans,[1] and later advanced by Common,[3] Bell and

Sejnowski,[4] and Hyvärinen and Oja,[5] among others. The field is growing in popularity and applicability, as is evidenced by the recent appearance of texts devoted to the subject.[7–9]

## Review of Relevant Mathematical Concepts

### Introduction

In the present work, it will be assumed that the reader is familiar with elementary mathematical concepts such as random variables, expectation, and variance. A thorough review of these concepts can be found in any standard textbook on probability.

For brevity, the following notational conventions will be adopted. Random variables will usually be denoted by $X$, while $\mathbf{X}$ will usually stand for a random vector of dimension $M$. Probability density functions (pdfs) will be denoted by $p(X)$ or $p(\mathbf{X})$, as appropriate. The expectation operator will be denoted by $E\langle\rangle$. We will use $\mu$ to denote the population mean $E\langle X\rangle$ of the distribution and to denote the population variance $E\langle(X-\mu)^2\rangle$.

### Kurtosis

*Kurtosis* is a mathematical quantity that roughly describes the peakedness of a distribution. Kurtosis usually is normalized so that a Gaussian distribution has a kurtosis of zero. Random variables having a positive kurtosis are called *supergaussian*, whereas those with a negative kurtosis are called *subgaussian*. Supergaussian random variables are characterized by pdfs that are relatively large near their mean $\mu$ and have heavier tails than a Gaussian. A typical example is a random variable with a Laplace distribution (Figure A.1). Subgaussian random variables, on the other hand, typically have flat or bimodal distributions. The uniform distribution (shown in Figure A.1 for the interval [−6,6]) is an example of a subgaussian distribution.

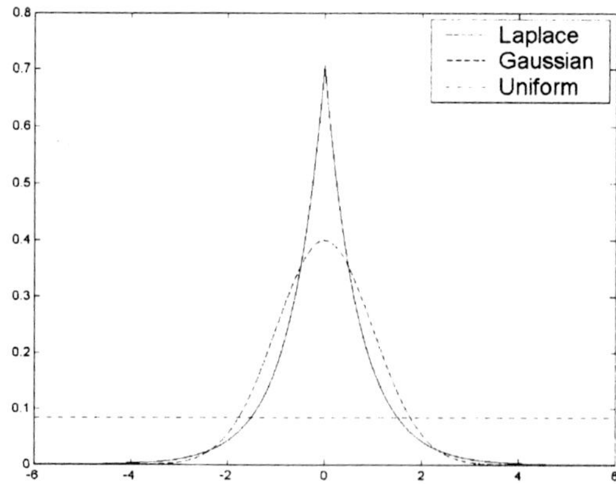


**Figure A.1.** Examples of supergaussian, Gaussian, and subgaussian distributions.

### Entropy and Mutual Information

In information theory, *entropy* measures the average amount of information that an observation of $\mathbf{X}$ yields. The entropy of $\mathbf{X}$ is given by the equation

$$H[\mathbf{X}] \equiv -E\langle \log p(\mathbf{X}) \rangle. \tag{A.1}$$

Entropy is small for distributions whose mass is concentrated on certain values (for example, the Laplace distribution shown in Figure A.1): because the values of a random variable coming from such a distribution are known a priori to be localized to small regions with high probability, observation of these variables does not convey much information.

On the other hand, it can be demonstrated that of all distributions with zero mean and a fixed covariance matrix $\mathbf{\Sigma}$ the zero-mean multivariate Gaussian distribution with covariance matrix $\mathbf{\Sigma}$ has the largest entropy.[12] Hence, from an information-theoretic viewpoint, the Gaussian distribution is the most random of all distribution.[17]

A closely related concept is that of *mutual information*, which measures the amount of information about one random variable that is contained in another. Equivalently, mutual information is the amount of uncertainty in one random variable that is cleared up by observation of another random variable. It can be shown that the mutual information $I[\mathbf{X}; \mathbf{Y}]$ between two random vectors $\mathbf{X}$ and $\mathbf{Y}$ is always nonnegative, and equals zero precisely when $\mathbf{X}$ and $\mathbf{Y}$ are independent. This agrees with our intuition about independent random variables—observation of either of a pair of independent random variables conveys no information about the other, so their mutual information should be zero.

### Principal Component Analysis

*Principal component analysis* (PCA) computes a linear transformation of the observed data such that the resulting observations are uncorrelated. The covariance matrix $\mathbf{\Sigma}$ of the data has a factorization of the form $\mathbf{\Sigma} = \mathbf{P\Lambda P}^T$, where $\mathbf{\Lambda}$ is a diagonal matrix and $\mathbf{P}$ is matrix such that $\mathbf{P}^{-1} = \mathbf{P}^T$[13]. The transformation $\mathbf{Y} = \mathbf{P}^T(\mathbf{X} - \overline{\mathbf{X}})$ then yields a coordinate system in which the components of $\mathbf{Y}$ have mean zero and are uncorrelated.

## Independent Component Analysis

Recall that the aim of ICA is to estimate a collection of unobservable source signals $\mathbf{S} = [s_1 \ldots s_N]^T$ solely from measurements of their (possibly noisy) mixtures $\mathbf{X} = [x_1 \ldots x_M]^T$ and certain assumptions about the sources. In the simplest formulation of ICA, linear mixing can be assumed, that is, that there exists an $M \times N$ mixing matrix $\mathbf{A}$ such that $\mathbf{X} = \mathbf{AS}$. For the linear ICA problem, $M \geq N$ is usually assumed, so that $\mathbf{A}$ has rank $N$. (The need for this condition arises from standard results in matrix algebra on the solvability of linear equations.[13]) When $M < N$

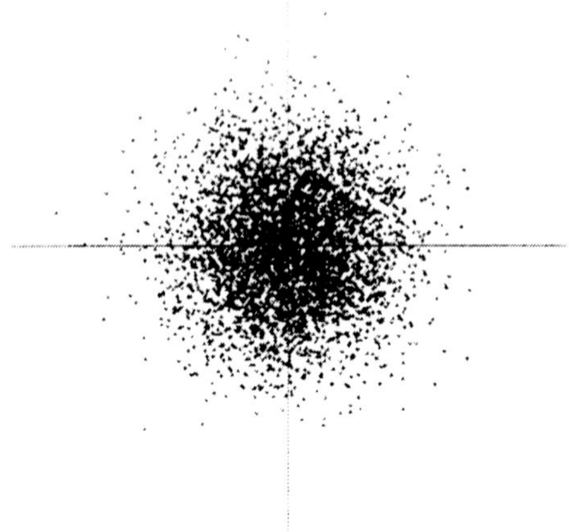

**Figure A.2.** Scatterplot of a mixture of Gaussian signals. The cloud is rotationally symmetric, so no amount of rotation will yield any new information.

(the so-called underdetermined case), modifications must be made to standard linear ICA methods.[14] To simplify this presentation, attention will be restricted to the case of a square ($N \times N$) mixing matrix for the remainder of this article.

Obviously, given only **X**, it is impossible to determine the pair (**A**, **S**) uniquely; certain structural assumptions must be made about **A** and **S** to be able to solve this problem. In ICA, it is assumed that the source signals **S** are mutually statistically independent, that is, that the joint probability density function $p(\mathbf{S})$ of **S** equals the product of the marginal probability density functions $p_i(s_i)$ of the individual sources. Roughly speaking, this assumption means that information about any one signal $s_i$ conveys no information about any other signal $s_j$, $i \neq j$.

Some caveats regarding ICA are to be noted:

(1) We can only recover the sources up to a scale change, for we may multiply any source by any non-zero number so long as we divide the corresponding column of **A** by the same number. Moreover, the order of the sources is ambiguous, since permuting the rows or columns of **A** does not affect our ability to solve **X** = **AS**.

(2) Independent component analysis cannot separate a mixture of Gaussian signals. This follows from the observations that (a) a sum of Gaussian random variables is another Gaussian random variable; and (b) the Gaussian distribution is rotationally symmetric (see Figure A.2). Therefore, the directions of the original signals cannot be inferred from rotations of the mixture alone. The upshot of this is that ICA can extract one Gaussian source from a data set; multiple Gaussian sources, if present, will be agglomerated in this one source.

(3) Independent component analysis assumes that statistical properties of the source signals are unchanging over time. In practice, this is not always true, and it is currently unknown exactly how the breakdown of this assumption affects ICA.

It is sufficient to estimate only the mixing matrix **A**, for then the estimate of the sources is simply $\mathbf{S} = \mathbf{A}^{-1}\mathbf{X}$. It turns out that it is easier (from a numerical standpoint) to estimate $\mathbf{W} \equiv \mathbf{A}^{-1}$, so that the source estimate is given by $\mathbf{S} = \mathbf{WX}$.

The general idea underlying ICA algorithms is to find the unmixing matrix **W** that makes the estimate sources **WX** as independent as possible. This is achieved by constructing a contrast function (a function to be optimized) involving the unmixing matrix **W** that quantifies the independence of the estimated sources. This function, when optimized with respect to **W**, gives not only the best estimate of **W**, but also the most statistically independent sources.

There are several different flavors of ICA. Their differences arise from their measure of independence and/or their contrast functions. The one that will be discussed here is called the Information Maximization method.

## Information Maximization

The Information Maximization (or Infomax, for short) principle is based upon a study by Nadal and Parga[15] demonstrating that a nonlinear network transmits the most information when its weights and transfer function are chosen to produce outputs that are as statistically independent as possible. Intuitively, this statement makes sense: the closer the outputs are to independent, the less redundancy between them and the more information they can carry. The (Bell and Sejnowski) Infomax algorithm[4,8] is a learning rule for a neural network that performs this maximization.

To use the Infomax algorithm, the unmixing process is viewed as a neural network whose inputs are the observations **X** and whose outputs are the sources **S**. The observations are multiplied by **W**, a matrix containing the weights of the neural network, and fed-forward to a nonlinear function $\mathbf{g} = (g_1, \ldots, g_N)$ (see Figure A.3). The nonlinear function **g**, through its Taylor series expansion, allows the network to utilize information contained in the higher-order statistics of $\mathbf{U} = \mathbf{WX}$.[8]

In view of Nadal and Parga's result, we seek to maximize the joint entropy of the output sources over all possible weight matrices **W**. Upon carrying out the requisite manipulations, we arrive at the Infomax learning rule of Bell and Sejnokswi[4,8,16]

$$\begin{aligned} \mathbf{W}_{\text{new}} &= \mathbf{W}_{\text{old}} + \Delta\mathbf{W}, \\ \Delta\mathbf{W} &= \alpha[\mathbf{I} - \varphi(\mathbf{u})\mathbf{u}^{\mathrm{T}}]\mathbf{W}_{\text{old}}, \end{aligned} \tag{A.2}$$

where $\alpha$ is an adjustable scalar (the learning rate) and the score function $\varphi(\mathbf{u})$ is defined as

$$\varphi(\mathbf{u}) = -\frac{1}{p(\mathbf{u})}\frac{\partial p(\mathbf{u})}{\partial \mathbf{u}}. \tag{A.3}$$

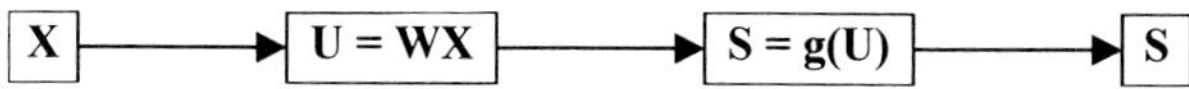


**Figure A.3.** Neural network depiction of ICA.

The score function is implicitly a function of the source densities, and therefore plays a crucial role in determining what kinds of sources ICA will detect. In the original study by Bell and Sejnowski,[4] the nonlinearity was fixed to be a logistic function. This choice is generally good for detecting supergaussian distributions, but cannot be used to detect subgaussian or skewed distributions. Shortly thereafter, Girolami and Fyfe[17] and Lee and colleagues[18] derived an extended Infomax algorithm that overcame this limitation. The extended Infomax algorithm is more robust than the original Infomax algorithm in the sense that it is capable of separating mixtures of supergaussian and subgaussian sources.

Finally, it is noted that the Infomax learning rule can be derived by many other approaches, such as Maximum Likelihood Estimation.[8]

## ICA and fMRI

### Introduction

In this section, a description of how ICA may be used to analyze functional magnetic resonance imaging (fMRI) data will be provided. Functional MRI data consist of a series of three-dimensional (3D) matrices collected over time. At each time point, the MR-induced signals from the brain are sampled over a discrete grid of volume elements (voxels). In the most common setup, the entries in the data matrix for a given time point are the magnitudes of the measured signals at the corresponding voxels. The signals obtained from the scanner are assumed to be a linear mixture of signals arising from various biological processes, some of which are presumed to be a associated with the administered functional task. We desire to recover spatial activation maps and time courses of activity related to the functional task in question. Independent component analysis provides one manner of accomplishing this goal.[20]

Because the fMRI data set contains both spatial and temporal information, it is theoretically possible to look for signals independent over space (spatial ICA) or over time (temporal ICA). In practice, however, it is very difficult to obtain accurate and meaningful results from a temporal ICA of fMRI data due to severe dimensionality issues (more will be said about this later). Therefore, spatial ICA is the method of choice for fMRI.

A spatial ICA, performed on the full fMRI dataset, will yield statistically independent spatial maps (areas of brain activation) and their corresponding time courses. The consequences of this decomposition are twofold: (1) the voxels of a given map effectively function as a mathematical unit; and (2) the activity produced by each such unit is independent of the activity produced by any other unit.

The interpretation of these abstract units requires researcher intervention. Spatial ICA assumes only that the source signals underlying the observed signals have independent distributions over space (an assumption justified from fMRI, positron emission tomography (PET), and electroencephalogram (EEG) studies demonstrating that brain activity is sparse and highly localized[8]); it does not make any assumptions about underlying functional organization of the brain. It is up to the researcher to identify physiologically relevant components. Typically, some knowledge of the task design is needed to make this identification (see below).

As stated in earlier, ICA is ideal for exploratory data analysis. Independent component analysis, in contrast to traditional confirmatory (hypothesis-based) methods, can be used to examine data in the absence of a priori knowledge of the hemodynamic response or of the paradigm. Furthermore, whereas simple correlation with a reference function can only detect consistently task-related (CTR) activity, ICA is capable of detecting CTR, transiently task-related (TTR), slowly varying, quasiperiodic, and movement-related activity.[20]

Another important difference between ICA and confirmatory methods is the lack of an associated level of significance.[20] This is not a significant drawback, however, as one can determine the statistical significance of a spatial map using advanced statistical techniques such as the jackknife or the bootstrap.[20] One can also use receiver operating characteristic (ROC) methods to evaluate the accuracy of independent components.[21]

Independent component analysis should be considered complementary to available hypothesis-based methods. It can be used to gain valuable insight into the data and can provide a researcher with many new ideas for further exploration.

## Implementation

The data from a scan are placed into a matrix **X** indexed by time and voxel: the columns of **X** correspond to time courses of individual voxels while its rows correspond to the voxel intensities in a given volume (see Figure A.4). Due to its simplicity and the size of the data, the linear ICA model is usually employed for fMRI: we seek an unmixing matrix **W** such that the source estimates **S** are maximally statistically independent.

To simplify the calculations, the mean of each input signal is removed. To improve the convergence of ICA methods further, the input data are then *whitened*: the input signals are decorrelated and normalized to unit variance.

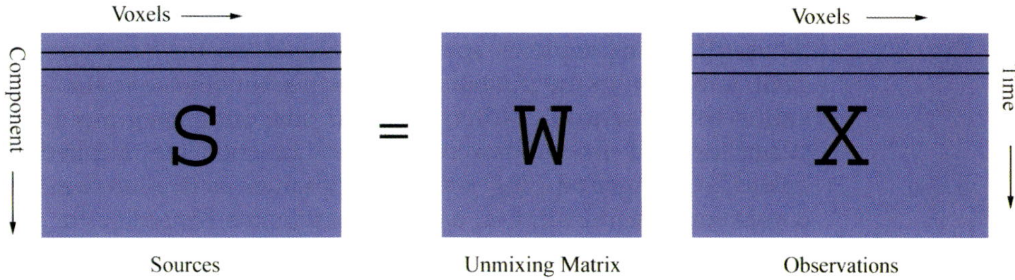


**Figure A.4.** Graphical depiction of ICA setup.

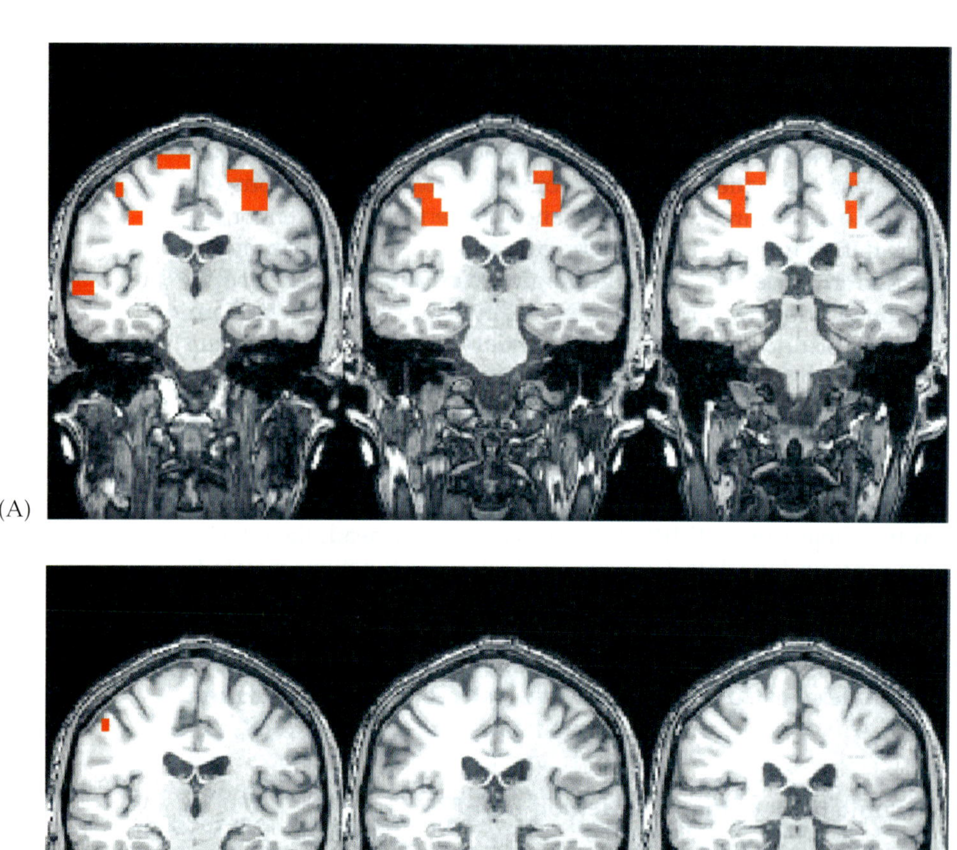


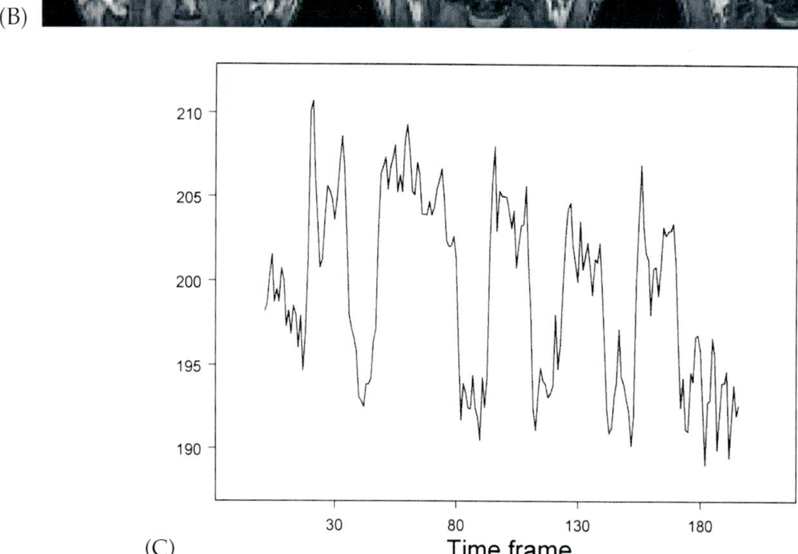


**Figure A.5.** Comparison of maps prepared with ICA (A) and with the conventional reference function (B) in a patient who performed the finger-tapping task incorrectly. In the ICA map, activation is evident in the sensorimotor cortex and SMA, whereas in the map prepared with the reference function, less activation is evident in either area. The error in the performance is demonstrated by the time course of the independent component (C) in which the second epoch of finger tapping was not terminated on time and each subsequent performance of the task was displaced in time.

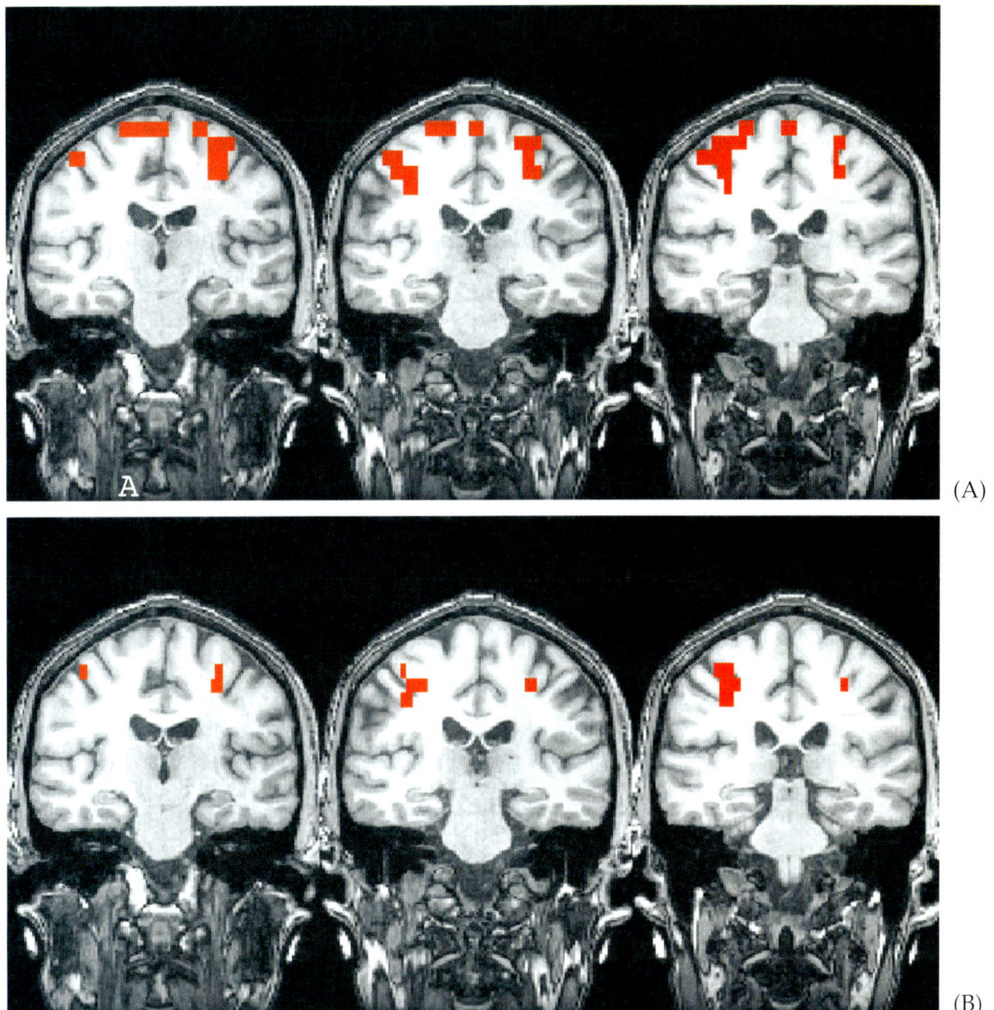


**Figure A.6.** Comparison of activation maps prepared with ICA (A) and with the conventional reference function (B) in a patient who moved during the performance of the finger-tapping task. The ICA map shows robust activation in the sensorimotor cortices bilaterally and in the supplementary motor area (SMA). With the reference function, activation in the sensorimotor cortex is less apparent, and is unapparent in the SMA. Motion analysis was carried out in AFNI (Robert Cox, NIH). The amount of movement during the acquisition is shown in (C) in which yaw (top line), pitch, roll, A-P, R-L, and I-S motion (bottom row) are graphed. The effect of motion on the time course of activation is shown in (D).

17. Girolami M, Fyfe C. Extraction of independent signal sources using a deflationary exploratory projection pursuit network with lateral inhibition. *IEE Proc Vision Image Signal Processing J.* 1997;144(5):299–306.
18. Lee T-W, Girolami M, Sejnowski TJ. Independent component analysis using an extended infomax algorithm for mixed sub-gaussian and super-gaussian sources. *Neural Comput.* 1999;11:417–441.
19. Huber PJ. Projection pursuit. *Ann Stat.* 1985;13(2):435–475.
20. McKeown MJ, Makeig S, Brown GG, Jung T-P, Kindermann SS, Bell AJ, Sejnowski TJ. Analysis of fMRI data by blind separation into independent spatial components. *Hum Brain Mapp.* 1998;6:160–188.
21. Esposito F, Formisano E, Seifritz E, Goebel R, Morrone R, Tedeschi G, Di Salle F. Spatial independent component analysis of functional MRI time-series: To what extend do results depend on the aligorithm used? *Hum Brain Mapp.* 2002;16:146–157.
22. Calhoun VD, Adali T, Pearlson GD, Pekar JJ. A method for group inferences from functional MRI data independent component analysis. *Hum Brain Mapp.* 2001;14:140–151.
23. Green CG, Nandy RR, Cordes D. PCA Preprocessing of fMRI Data Adversely Affects the Results of ICA. Paper presented at: ISMRM 10th Scientific Meeting and Exhibition; May 18–24, 2002; Honolulu, Hawaii.
24. Brockwell PJ, Davis RJ. *Time Series: Theory and Methods.* New York: Springer-Verlag; 1993.
25. Beckmann CF, Noble JA, Smith SM. Investigating the intrinsic dimensionality of FMRI data for ICA. Paper presented at: Seventh International. Conference on Functional Mapping of the Human Brain; 2001.

# Index